World Health Organization Classification of Tumours

WHO 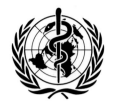 OMS

International Agency for Research on Cancer (IARC)

Pathology and Genetics of Head and Neck Tumours

Edited by

Leon Barnes

John W. Eveson

Peter Reichart

David Sidransky

IARCPress

Lyon, 2005

World Health Organization Classification of Tumours

Series Editors   Paul Kleihues, M.D.
                  Leslie H. Sobin, M.D.

Pathology and Genetics of Head and Neck Tumours

Editors   Leon Barnes, M.D.
           John W. Eveson, M.D.
           Peter Reichart, M.D.
           David Sidransky, M.D.

Coordinating Editor   Wojciech Biernat, M.D.

Layout   Vanessa Meister
          Marlen Grassinger
          Stephan Rappo
          Sibylle Söring

Illustrations   Nobert Wey
                 Thomas Odin

Printed by   Team Rush
              69603 Villeurbanne, France

Publisher   IARC*Press*
             International Agency for
             Research on Cancer (IARC)
             69008 Lyon, France

This volume was produced in collaboration with the

International Academy of Pathology (IAP)

and the

Department of Pathology, University Hospital, Zurich, Switzerland

The WHO Classification of Head and Neck Tumours
presented in this book reflects the views of a Working Group that convened for an
Editorial and Consensus Conference in Lyon, France,
July 16-19, 2003.

Members of the Working Group are indicated
in the List of Contributors on page 371.

Published by IARC Press, International Agency for Research on Cancer,
150 cours Albert Thomas, F-69008 Lyon, France

Format for bibliographic citations:
Barnes L., Eveson J.W., Reichart P., Sidransky D. (Eds.): World Health Organization
Classification of Tumours. Pathology and Genetics of Head and Neck Tumours.
IARC Press: Lyon 2005

IARC Library Cataloguing in Publication Data

Pathology and genetics of head and neck tumours / edited by Leon Barnes ... [et al.].

(World Health Organization classification of tumours ;)

1. Head and Neck Neoplasms – genetics   2. Head and Neck Neoplasms – pathology
3. Odontogenic Tumors – genetics   4. Odontogenic Tumors – pathology
I. Barnes, Leon II. Series

ISBN   92 832 2417 5   (NLM Classification WE 707)

Contents

CHAPTER 1

Tumours of the Nasal Cavity and Paranasal Sinuses

Although the nasal cavity and paranasal sinuses occupy a relatively small anatomical space, they are the site of origin of some of the more complex, histologically diverse group of tumours in the entire human body. These include neoplasms derived from mucosal epithelium, seromucinous glands, soft tissues, bone, cartilage, neural/neuroectodermal tissue, haematolymphoid cells and the odontogenic apparatus. Many of the tumours are similar to those found elsewhere in the body but a few, such as the olfactory neuroblastoma, are unique to this site.

WHO histological classification of tumours of the nasal cavity and paranasal sinuses

Malignant epithelial tumours

Squamous cell carcinoma	8070/3
Verrucous carcinoma	8051/3
Papillary squamous cell carcinoma	8052/3
Basaloid squamous cell carcinoma	8083/3
Spindle cell carcinoma	8074/3
Adenosquamous carcinoma	8560/3
Acantholytic squamous cell carcinoma	8075/3
Lymphoepithelial carcinoma	8082/3
Sinonasal undifferentiated carcinoma	8020/3
Adenocarcinoma	
Intestinal-type adenocarcinoma	8144/3
Non-intestinal-type adenocarcinoma	8140/3
Salivary gland-type carcinomas	
Adenoid cystic carcinoma	8200/3
Acinic cell carcinoma	8550/3
Mucoepidermoid carcinoma	8430/3
Epithelial-myoepithelial carcinoma	8562/3
Clear cell carcinoma N.O.S.	8310/3
Myoepithelial carcinoma	8982/3
Carcinoma ex pleomorphic adenoma	8941/3
Polymorphous low-grade adenocarcinoma	8525/3
Neuroendocrine tumours	
Typical carcinoid	8240/3
Atypical carcinoid	8249/3
Small cell carcinoma, neuroendocrine type	8041/3

Benign epithelial tumours

Sinonasal papillomas	
Inverted papilloma	
(Schneiderian papilloma, inverted type)	8121/1
Oncocytic papilloma	
(Schneiderian papilloma, oncocytic type)	8121/1
Exophytic papilloma	
(Schneiderian papilloma, exophytic type)	8121/0
Salivary gland-type adenomas	
Pleomorphic adenoma	8940/0
Myoepithelioma	8982/0
Oncocytoma	8290/0

Soft tissue tumours

Malignant tumours	
Fibrosarcoma	8810/3
Malignant fibrous histiocytoma	8830/3
Leiomyosarcoma	8890/3
Rhabdomyosarcoma	8900/3
Angiosarcoma	9120/3
Malignant peripheral nerve sheath tumour	9540/3
Borderline and low malignant potential tumours	
Desmoid-type fibromatosis	8821/1
Inflammatory myofibroblastic tumour	8825/1
Glomangiopericytoma	
(Sinonasal-type haemangiopericytoma)	9150/1
Extrapleural solitary fibrous tumour	8815/1

Benign tumours

Myxoma	8840/0
Leiomyoma	8890/0
Haemangioma	9120/0
Schwannoma	9560/0
Neurofibroma	9540/0
Meningioma	9530/0

Tumours of bone and cartilage

Malignant tumours	
Chondrosarcoma	9220/3
Mesenchymal chondrosarcoma	9240/3
Osteosarcoma	9180/3
Chordoma	9370/3
Benign tumours	
Giant cell lesion	
Giant cell tumour	9250/1
Chondroma	9220/0
Osteoma	9180/0
Chondroblastoma	9230/0
Chondromyxoid fibroma	9241/0
Osteochondroma (exostosis)	9210/0
Osteoid osteoma	9191/0
Osteoblastoma	9200/0
Ameloblastoma	9310/0
Nasal chondromesenchymal hamartoma	

Haematolymphoid tumours

Extranodal NK/T cell lymphoma	9719/3
Diffuse large B-cell lymphoma	9680/3
Extramedullary plasmacytoma	9734/3
Extramedullary myeloid sarcoma	9930/3
Histiocytic sarcoma	9755/3
Langerhans cell histiocytosis	9751/1

Neuroectodermal

Ewing sarcoma	9260/3
Primitive neuroectodermal tumour	9364/3
Olfactory neuroblastoma	9522/3
Melanotic neuroectodermal tumour of infancy	9363/0
Mucosal malignant melanoma	8720/3

Germ cell tumours

Immature teratoma	9080/3
Teratoma with malignant transformation	9084/3
Sinonasal yolk sac tumour (endodermal sinus tumour)	9071/3
Sinonasal teratocarcinosarcoma	
Mature teratoma	9080/0
Dermoid cyst	9084/0

Secondary tumours

---

[1] Morphology code of the International Classification of Diseases for Oncology (ICD-O) {821} and the Systematized Nomenclature of Medicine (http://snomed.org). Behaviour is coded /0 for benign tumours, /3 for malignant tumours, and /1 for borderline or uncertain behaviour.

TNM classification of carcinomas of the nasal cavity and paranasal sinuses

TNM classification [1,2]

TNM classification of carcinomas of the nasal cavity and sinuses

T – Primary tumour

TX   Primary tumour cannot be assessed
T0   No evidence of primary tumour
Tis   Carcinoma in situ

Maxillary sinus

T1   Tumour limited to the antral mucosa with no erosion or destruction of bone
T2   Tumour causing bone erosion or destruction, including extension into hard palate and/or middle nasal meatus, except extension to posterior antral wall of maxillary sinus and pterygoid plates
T3   Tumour invades any of the following: bone of posterior wall of maxillary sinus, subcutaneous tissues, floor or medial wall of orbit, pterygoid fossa, ethmoid sinuses
T4a   Tumour invades any of the following: anterior orbital contents, skin of cheek, pterygoid plates, infratemporal fossa, cribriform plate, sphenoid or frontal sinuses
T4b   Tumour invades any of the following: orbital apex, dura, brain, middle cranial fossa, cranial nerves other than maxillary division of trigeminal nerve V2, nasopharynx, clivus

Nasal cavity and ethmoid sinus

T1   Tumour restricted to one subsite of nasal cavity or ethmoid sinus, with or without bony invasion
T2   Tumour involves two subsites in a single site or extends to involve an adjacent site within the nasoethmoidal complex, with or without bony invasion
T3   Tumour extends to invade the medial wall or floor of the orbit, maxillary sinus, palate, or cribriform plate
T4a   Tumour invades any of the following: anterior orbital contents, skin of nose or cheek, minimal extension to anterior cranial fossa, pterygoid plates, sphenoid or frontal sinuses
T4b   Tumour invades any of the following: orbital apex, dura, brain, middle cranial fossa, cranial nerves other than V2, nasopharynx, clivus

N – Regional lymph nodes [3]

NX   Regional lymph nodes cannot be assessed
N0   No regional lymph node metastasis
N1   Metastasis in a single ipsilateral lymph node, 3 cm or less in greatest dimension
N2   Metastasis as specified in N2a, 2b, 2c below
N2a   Metastasis in a single ipsilateral lymph node, more than 3 cm but not more than 6 cm in greatest dimension
N2b   Metastasis in multiple ipsilateral lymph nodes, none more than 6 cm in greatest dimension
N2c   Metastasis in bilateral or contralateral lymph nodes, none more than 6 cm in greatest dimension
N3   Metastasis in a lymph node more than 6 cm in greatest dimension
Note: Midline nodes are considered ipsilateral nodes.

M – Distant metastasis

MX   Distant metastasis cannot be assessed
M0   No distant metastasis
M1   Distant metastasis

Stage grouping

Stage 0	Tis	N0	M0
Stage I	T1	N0	M0
Stage II	T2	N0	M0
Stage III	T1, T2	N1	M0
	T3	N0, N1	M0
Stage IVA	T1, T2, T3	N2	M0
	T4a	N0, N1, N2	M0
Stage IVB	T4b	Any N	M0
	Any T	N3	M0
Stage IVC	Any T	Any N	M1

---

[1] {947,2418}.
[2] A help desk for specific questions about the TNM classification is available at www.uicc.org/index.php?id=508 .
[3] The regional lymph nodes are the cervical nodes

Tumours of the nasal cavity and paranasal sinuses: Introduction

L. Barnes
L.L.Y. Tse
J.L. Hunt

M. Brandwein-Gensler
H.D. Curtin
P. Boffetta

Anatomy

The nasal cavities are separated in the midline by the nasal septum. Each cavity is wide caudally, and narrow cranially. The roof of the nasal cavity is formed by the thin (0.5 mm) cribriform plate. The floor is the hard palate, formed by the palatine processes of the maxillae and the horizontal portions of the palatine bones. The lateral nasal wall contains the maxillary and ethmoid ostia, plus three or four turbinates. These turbinates are delicate scroll-like projections of bone and vascular soft tissue that become smaller as they ascend in the nasal cavity. They attach to the lateral nasal wall anteriorly, and have a free edge posteriorly. The turbinates are covered with a thick mucous membrane and contain a dense, thick-walled venous plexus. The upper margins of the nasal fossa are bound laterally by the superior nasal turbinate and adjacent lateral nasal wall, and medially by the nasal septum. This region is the olfactory recess and it has a yellowish epithelium, the olfactory mucosa (OM). This mucosa contains bipolar olfactory nerve fibers that cross through the cribriform plate. The terminal axons of the olfactory nerves extend to the free surface of the epithelium, where they expand into knob-like protrusions bearing cilia (olfactory cilia). Bowman's glands, or olfactory glands, within the lamina propria appear similar to serous minor salivary glands.

The nasal cavity and paranasal sinuses are lined by Schneiderian mucosa, consisting of pseudostratified columnar ciliated epithelium with interspersed goblet cells. The lamina propria within the paranasal sinuses, especially the maxillary antrum, is loose and well vascularized, with seromucinous glands, and can easily become polypoid as a result of edema. The goblet cell component of the mucosal surface and seromucinous glands is variable. In chronic sinusitis, goblet cell hyperplasia can result in a papillary mucosal lesion.

The major portion of the nasal septum is formed by the perpendicular plate of the ethmoid bone posteriorly and the septal cartilage anteriorly. The vomer completes the posteroinferior portion of the septum. The septum is lined by relatively thin, ciliated respiratory mucosa, which may regularly undergo squamous metaplasia. The underlying thin lamina propria, although containing seromucinous glands, is tethered to the septal cartilage, restricting reactive polyp formation.

The frontal sinus

These paired sinuses reside between the internal and external cranial tables and drain either via a nasofrontal duct into the frontal recess or more directly into the anterior infundibulum, or less often, into the anterior ethmoid cells, which in turn will open into the infundibulum of the bulla ethmoidalis.

Ethmoid complex

This paired complex of sinuses contains 3-18 cells that are grouped as anterior, middle, or posterior, according to the location of their ostia. There is an inverse relationship between the number and size of the cells. Generally, the posterior cells are both larger and fewer than the anterior cells. Each ethmoid labyrinth lies between the orbit and the upper nasal fossa. The left and right groups of ethmoid cells are connected in the midline by the cribriform plate (nasal roof) of the ethmoid bone. The cribriform plate is an important landmark in evaluation of

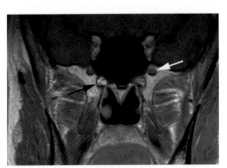

Fig. 1.1 Normal coronal T1 WI shows foramen rotundum (white arrow) and entrance to the Vidian canal (black arrow).

sinonasal tumour stage - violation of the cribriform plate signifies direct extension of the tumour into the anterior cranial fossa. The crista galli is a distinctive pointed bony landmark that extends from the midline of the cribriform plate upward into the floor of the anterior cranial fossa. The perpendicular plate of the ethmoid bone extends downward from the cribriform plate to contribute to the nasal septum. The medial wall of each ethmoid labyrinth is formed by a thin lamella of bone from which arise the middle, superior, and supreme turbinates. The lateral ethmoid wall is formed by the thin lamina papyracea, which separates the ethmoid cells from the orbit. This is yet another important landmark for tumour staging. Tumour violation of the lamina papyracea may necessitate including the orbit and globe with the surgical resection. This area should be sampled in a maxillectomy specimen a) if the globe has not been removed (as the lamina papyracea represents the lateral orbital margin), or b) if orbital exenteration has been performed. The roof of the ethmoid complex is formed by a medial extension of the orbital plate of the frontal bone, which projects to articulate with the cribriform plate. This is often referred to as the fovea ethmoidalis.

Sphenoid sinus

The average adult sphenoid sinus measures 20 mm high, 23 mm long, and 17 mm wide. The relationship of the posterior extension of the sphenoid in relation to the sella turcica is variable. The sphenoid sinus septum is usually in the midline, and anteriorly aligned with the nasal septum. However, it can also deviate far to one side creating two unequal sinus cavities. With the exception of the sinus roof, the other sinus walls are of variable thickness depending on the degree of pneumatization. The sphenoid roof is thin, often measuring only 1 mm. (planum sphenoidale), and is vulnerable to perforation during surgery. The sinus roof relates to the floor of the anterior cranial fossa, anteriorly; the optic chiasm and the sella turcica, posteriorly. The lateral sphenoid wall is related to the orbital apex, the optic canal, the optic nerve, and the cavernous sinus, containing the internal carotid artery. The sinus floor is the roof of the nasopharynx, and the anterior sinus wall is the back of the nasal fossa.

Maxillary sinus
The maxillary sinus lies within the body of the maxillary bone. Behind the orbital rims, each sinus roof/orbital floor slants obliquely upward so that the highest point of the sinus is in the posteromedial portion, lying directly beneath the orbital apex. The medial antral wall is the inferior lateral wall of the nasal cavity ("party wall"). The curved posterolateral wall separates the sinus from the infratemporal fossa. The anterior sinus wall is the facial surface of the maxilla that is perforated by the infraorbital foramen below the orbital rim. The floor of the sinus is lowest near the second premolar and first molar teeth and usually lies 3-5 mm below the nasal floor. The lower expansion of the antrum is intimately related to dentition. The location of the maxillary sinus ostia, is high on the medial wall. They drain through the ethmoidal infundibulum and then the nasal fossa. This pattern of drainage in the erect position is accomplished by intact ciliary action. The maxillary hiatus is a bony window leading to the interior of the maxillary sinus. The hiatus is normally partially covered by portions of four bones: the perpendicular plate of the palatine bone, posteriorly; the lacrimal bone, anterosuperiorly; the inferior turbinate, inferiorly; and above the turbinate attachment, the uncinate process of the ethmoid bone.

Epidemiology

Carcinomas of the nasal cavity and paranasal sinuses account for 0.2-0.8% of all malignant neoplasms and 3% of those occurring in the head and neck {169,2378}. Sixty percent of sinonasal tumours originate in the maxillary sinus, 20-30% in the nasal cavity, 10-15% in the ethmoid sinus, and 1% in the sphenoid and frontal sinuses {1493,2186}. When considering the paranasal sinuses alone, 77% of malignant tumours arise in the maxillary sinus, 22% in the ethmoid sinus and 1% in the sphenoid and frontal

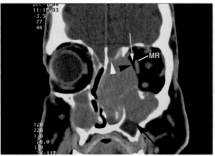

Fig. 1.2 Malignancy of ethmoid and nasal cavity. Coronal CT with contrast. The tumour erodes the cribriform plate and fovea ethmoidalis (white arrowhead). The lamina papyracea is eroded (black arrowhead) but the fat (white arrow) medial to the medial rectus (MR) is normal. The orbital fat is not invaded. The margin (black arrow) of the tumour in the maxillary sinus is separable from the obstructed secretions because of different densities.

sinuses {2378}. Malignant neoplasms of this region may lead to significant morbidity and disfigurement.

The incidence of cancer of the nasal cavity and paranasal sinuses (sinonasal cancer) is low in most populations (<1.5/100,000 in men and <1.0/100,000 in women). Higher rates are recorded in Japan and certain parts of China and India. Squamous cell carcinomas are the commonest. Time trends have shown in most populations a stable incidence or a small decline in recent decades.

Etiology

Occupational exposure to wood dust, in particular to dust of hard woods such as beech and oak, is the main known risk factor for sinonasal cancer. The increase in risk (in the order of 5-50 fold) is strongest for adenocarcinomas and for cancers originating from the sinuses. The effect is present after 40 or more years since first exposure and persists after cessation of exposure. An increased risk of sinonasal cancer has been shown among workers in nickel refining and chromate pigment manufacture, but not among workers exposed to these metals in other processes, such as plating and welding. Among other suspected occupational carcinogens are formaldehyde, diisopropyl sulfate and dichloroethyl sulfide.

A relatively weak (relative risks in the range 2-5) but consistent association has been shown between tobacco smoking

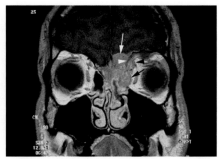

Fig. 1.3 Malignancy of upper nasal cavity invading orbital fat and extending intracranially. The tumour (white arrow) extends through the roof of the ethmoid and along the roof of the orbit (white arrowhead). The tumour bulges (black arrow) the periorbita near the medial rectus but breaks through into the orbital fat more superiorly (black arrowhead). Note that the tumour enhances intermediately and less intensely than the mucosa.

and sinonasal cancer, in particular squamous cell carcinoma. Exposure to Thorotrast, a radioactive contrast agent, represents an additional risk factor.

Imaging

Modern imaging plays a key role in the evaluation of sinonasal tumours {2423}. The anatomy of the lesion can be defined with the exact margins clearly delineated in almost every case. Imaging is a dominant factor in determining surgical approach and is an integral part of radiation therapy planning. Computed tomography (CT) and magnetic resonance imaging (MRI) provide significant information about the texture, the margins, the effect on bone and even the vascularity. In addition, some findings are typical for a particular diagnosis, and although biopsy is still required for ascertaining the nature of the lesion, the imaging appearance may help limit the list of differential diagnoses.

Staging and surgical planning
The spread of a sinonasal tumour intracranially or into the orbit and the relationship of tumour to the optic nerve and carotid artery are important features that can be delineated with imaging.

Tumour can invade the orbit through the lamina papyracea or the roof of the maxillary sinus. Even if the bony wall is apparently destroyed, orbital fat may not be invaded {515}. A smooth bowing of the soft tissue interface with the orbital fat

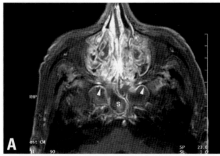 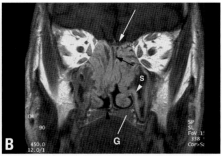 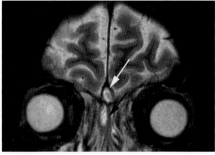

Fig. 1.4 Sinonasal polyps with multiple obstructed sinuses. **A** Axial T1 WI after intravenous gadolinium. The enhancing mucosa (arrowheads) lines the obstructed sphenoid sinus (S). The sinus was also dark on T2WI indicating high protein and long standing obstruction. **B** Coronal T1WI shows cascading polyps filling the nasal cavity. The secretions in the maxillary sinus (S) are dark and the lining mucosa (white arrowhead) is visible. The nasal septum (black arrow) is intact. Hard palate - (black arrowhead), minor salivary glands at roof of mouth (G), olfactory bulb (white arrow).

Fig. 1.5 Sinonasal polyps. Coronal T2WI. The secretions in the sinus (S) are dark indicating high protein desiccated secretions. Compare to high signal of the edematous mucosa. Intact nasal septum (black arrow), crista galli (white arrow).

suggests that the lesion is contained by periorbital fascia. Infiltration or irregularity of this margin suggests extension into the fat or true orbital invasion. The thin line of fat between the medial rectus muscle and the lamina papyracea is a key landmark in the evaluation of orbital extension of ethmoid neoplasms.

The key landmarks for the assessment of intracranial extension of tumour are the roof of the ethmoid, the cribriform plate and the crista galli. Elevation or frank invasion of the dura may be evaluated using MRI.

A tumour in the maxillary sinus region may extend posteriorly and laterally through the bony wall into the pterygopalatine fossa and the infratemporal fossa. Tumour can invade the pterygopalatine fossa area either by direct extension or by following the nerves. From there, perineural extension of tumour in the foramen rotundum and Vidian canal may result in intracranial spread {516}.

Tumour may spread from the sphenoid sinus region, laterally into the cavernous sinus through the very thin layer of bone separating these two structures. If the bone is intact, the tumour is likely contained within the sinus.

Radiographic signs

Bone changes can give an indication of the aggressiveness of a tumour {2038}. In general, slowly growing lesions, such as Schneiderian papillomas, appear to push bone as they slowly remodel the osseous structure. More aggressive lesions, such as squamous cell carcinoma, can aggressively destroy bony walls leaving only a few remaining fragments {2425}. Occasionally, however, malignant lesions can cause bowing rather than infiltrating destruction of bone {2424}.

The integrity of the thin plates of bone in the ethmoid sinus as well as the bony walls of the sphenoid sinus and the bony nasal septum also suggests that malignancy is unlikely.

Mineralization can be seen in several tumours, such as ring-like calcifications in cartilage lesions as well as calcifications in olfactory neuroblastomas {2130}. Meningioma can cause hyperostosis and can also calcify.

Tumour location plays a significant role in differential diagnosis. Tumours in the region of the cribriform plate and upper nasal cavity suggest diagnoses such as olfactory neuroblastoma or meningioma. Inverted Schneiderian papilloma occurs predominantly along the lateral wall of

the nasal cavity or the medial maxillary sinus {534}. In the lower maxilla, odontogenic lesions should be considered. Such lesions arise in the bone of the alveolar process and as they grow elevate the floor of the maxillary sinus. Fibroosseous lesions enter the differential diagnosis when a radiodense lesion arises from or follows the contour of bone. Correlation of imaging studies with histologic appearance is crucial in the evaluation of bony lesions.

Squamous cell carcinoma

B.Z. Pilch
J. Bouquot
L.D.R. Thompson

Definition
A malignant epithelial neoplasm originating from the mucosal epithelium of the nasal cavities or paranasal sinuses that includes a keratinizing and a non-keratinizing type.

ICD-O codes
Squamous cell carcinoma 8070/3
Verrucous carcinoma   8051/3
Papillary squamous cell carcinoma
                          8052/3
Basaloid squamous cell carcinoma
                          8083/3
Spindle cell carcinoma   8074/3
Adenosquamous carcinoma
                          8560/3
Acantholytic squamous cell
carcinoma   8075/3

Synonyms
Keratinizing squamous cell carcinoma: squamous cell carcinoma.
Nonkeratinizing carcinoma: Schneiderian carcinoma, cylindrical cell carcinoma, transitional (cell) carcinoma, Ringertz carcinoma, respiratory epithelial carcinoma.

Epidemiology
Sinonasal squamous cell carcinoma is rare, accounting for <1% of malignant tumours and only about 3% of malignancies of the head and neck {169,2758}. The disease appears to be more common in Japan than in the West {2205}. It is extremely rare in children, and men are more commonly affected (about 1.5 times) than women. Patients are generally about 55-65 years of age {502,2758}.

Etiology
Reported risk factors have included exposure to nickel, chlorophenols, and textile dust, prior Thorotrast instillation, smoking, and a history or concurrence of sinonasal (Schneiderian) papilloma.
Human papillomavirus (HPV) has been found in some cases, especially those associated with inverted Schneiderian papilloma {303}, but a definite etiologic role has not been clearly established. Formaldehyde, despite the results of animal experiments, has not been found to be a definite risk factor in humans {502,1443,1571,2205,2904}.

Localization
Sinonasal squamous cell carcinomas occur most frequently in the maxillary sinus (about 60-70%), followed by the nasal cavity (about 12-25%), ethmoid sinus (about 10-15%) and the sphenoid and frontal sinuses (about 1%) {131,502}. Squamous cell carcinoma of the nasal vestibule should be considered a carcinoma of the skin rather than sinonasal mucosal epithelium {2566}.

Clinical features
Symptoms include nasal fullness, stuffiness, or obstruction; epistaxis; rhinorrhea; pain; paraesthesia; fullness or swelling of the nose or cheek or a palatal bulge; a persistent or non-healing nasal sore or ulcer; nasal mass; or, in advanced cases, proptosis, diplopia, or lacrimation {131,502,2758}. Radiologic studies such as CT scan or MRI may delineate the extent of the lesion, the presence of bony invasion, and extension to neighbouring structures such as the orbit, pterygopalatine or infratemporal spaces.

Macroscopy
Sinonasal squamous cell carcinomas may be exophytic, fungating, or papillary; friable, haemorrhagic, partially necrotic, or indurated; demarcated or infiltrative.

Tumour spread and staging
Nasal cavity carcinomas can spread to adjacent sites in the nasal cavity or to the ethmoid sinus, or can extend to involve

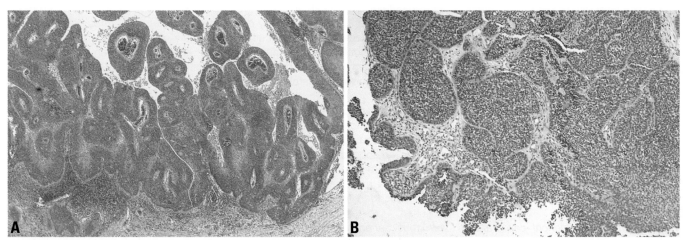

Fig. 1.6 A Non-keratinizing papillary squamous cell carcinoma. Multiple complex papillary projections lined by thickened epithelium. Lymphocytic response is present at the pushing border of infiltration. **B** Squamous cell carcinoma, non-keratinizing. Islands of cohesive tumour cells invading into the underlying stroma. Surface carcinoma in-situ is seen.

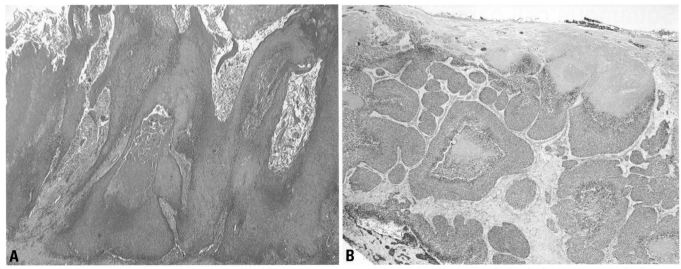

Fig. 1.7 A Nasal verrucous carcinoma "Church-spire" type hyperkeratosis, parakeratosis and a broad pushing border of infiltration in a non-atypical epithelium support the diagnosis. **B** Basaloid squamous cell carcinoma. A characteristic feature is the presence of comedonecrosis in the center of the neoplastic lobules. Surface is ulcerated.

the contralateral nasal cavity, bone, maxillary sinus, palate, skin and soft tissues of the nose, lip, or cheek, cribriform plate, or cranial cavity. Maxillary sinus carcinomas may spread to the nasal cavities, palate, other paranasal sinuses, skin or soft tissues of the nose or cheek, orbit, cranial contents, or the pterygopalatine and infratemporal spaces {131,2418}. Lymph node metastases are less common than in squamous cell carcinomas of other sites in the head and neck.

Histopathology

Keratinizing squamous cell carcinoma

This tumour is histologically identical to squamous cell carcinomas of other mucosal sites in the head and neck. There is histologic evidence of squamous differentiation, in the form of extracellular keratin or intracellular keratin (pink cytoplasm, dyskeratotic cells) and/or intercellular bridges. Tumour cells are generally apposed to one another in a "mosaic tile" arrangement. The tumour may be arranged in nests, masses, or as small groups of cells or individual cells. Invasion occurs as blunt projections or ragged, irregular strands. There is often a desmoplastic stromal reaction. The carcinomas may be well, moderately, or poorly differentiated.

Non-keratinizing (cylindrical cell, transitional) carcinoma

This is a distinctive tumour of the sinonasal tract characterized by a plexi-

form or ribbon-like growth pattern. It invades into the underlying tissue with a smooth, generally well-delineated border. Therefore, definite evidence of stromal invasion may be difficult to appreciate, although a degree of invasion by irregular small nests or strands may be present. There is typically a lack of maturation in the epithelial nests or ribbons, as in transitional cell carcinoma of the urinary tract, which this tumour subtype resembles. Cytologic atypia is present to a significant degree. As its name implies, this tumour does not generally evince histologic evidence of keratinization, although some degree may be seen. When keratinization is significant, there is morphologic overlap with keratinizing squamous cell carcinoma. Occasional mucus-containing cells can be seen. The tumour may be moderately or poorly differentiated; the latter type is difficult to recognize as squamous, and must be differentiated from olfactory neuroblastomas or neuroendocrine carcinomas.

Variants of squamous cell carcinoma

Variants of squamous cell carcinoma are rare in the sinonasal tract. They are similar to the analogous tumours occurring with greater frequency in other sites in the head and neck and are more completely described in the corresponding sections.

Verrucous carcinoma of the nasal and paranasal sinuses is very rare. It is a low-grade variant of squamous cell carcinoma characterized by a papillary or warty

exophytic mass of very well-differentiated, keratinized epithelium {899,1955, 2118,2278}. The maxillary sinus is the most common site, followed by the nasal fossa. Rare nasopharyngeal lesions have encroached on the nasal sinus {1199,1872}.

Papillary squamous cell carcinoma {2488} is an exophytic squamous cell carcinoma with a papillary configuration composed of thin fingers of tumour surrounding fibrovascular cores.

Basaloid squamous cell carcinoma is uncommon in the sinonasal tract {2786}. It is an aggressive variant of squamous cell carcinoma that is characterized by rounded nests of cytologically highly atypical and mitotically-active basaloid epithelial cells, with high nuclear/cytoplasmic ratios and hyperchromatic nuclei. There is often comedo-type necrosis. A pseudoglandular or strand-like arrangement, reminiscent of the architecture of an adenoid cystic carcinoma, is often present, as is the production of basement membrane-like material. Squamous differentiation is invariably present, either in basaloid nests, as separate foci of tumour, or as surface epithelial carcinoma or carcinoma in-situ.

Spindle cell carcinoma is characterized by a biphasic pattern of squamous cell carcinoma as well as a generally much larger component of malignant spindled cells, reminiscent of a sarcoma. The squamous component may be scant or even inapparent on light microscopy. In the latter circumstance, immunohistochemical or ultrastructural evidence of epithelial differentiation is required for the diagnosis. The spindle cell component is characteristically immunohistochemically vimentin-positive, and keratin positivity may be scant, difficult to demonstrate, or even absent.

Adenosquamous carcinoma is uncommon in the sinonasal tract, and is more completely described in the sections on oral and laryngeal tumours. Briefly, it is generally considered as a variant of squamous cell carcinoma in which a surface mucosal component of squamous cell carcinoma is present. There is also a component of carcinoma with definite glandular differentiation in the form of ductules or tubules, often intimately admixed with the squamous cell carcinoma. The mere presence of intracellular mucin is not sufficient for the diagnosis.

Acantholytic squamous cell carcinoma is exceedingly rare in the sinonasal tract.

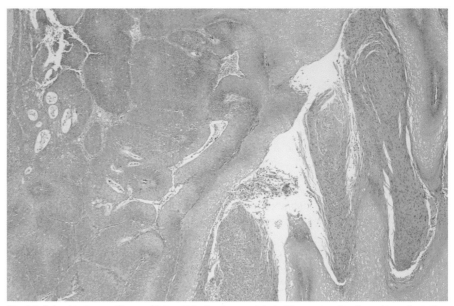

Fig. 1.8 Schneiderian papilloma with keratinization is associated with an area of malignant transformation into a squamous cell carcinoma with severe cytologic atypia.

Precursor lesions

Precursor lesions for sinonasal squamous cell carcinomas are considerably less well defined than for oral or laryngeal carcinomas. The sinonasal Schneiderian (inverted) papilloma appears to be a precursor lesion; the frequency of association has been estimated at about 10% {173}. Although squamous metaplasia may precede the development of sinonasal squamous carcinoma, a predisposing role for such metaplasia in the development of carcinoma has not been clearly established.

Prognosis and predictive factors

Patients with nasal squamous cell carcinomas generally present earlier than patients with maxillary cancers and, not surprisingly, fare better than the latter group. Nasal squamous cell carcinomas rarely metastasize to lymph nodes, and recurrences, when they occur, do so quickly {131}. Advanced local disease worsens the prognosis. The overall 5-year survival for nasal squamous cell carcinomas is about 60%. Squamous carcinomas of the maxillary sinus have a more ominous prognosis. They are likely to be large and extensive when diagnosed. Prognosis correlates with stage. Patients with the non-keratinizing type of carcinoma tend to do better than those with the keratinizing type {502}. The overall 5-year survival of patients with maxillary sinus squamous carcinoma is about 42% {131}.

Lymphoepithelial carcinoma

W.Y.W. Tsang
J.K.C. Chan

Definition
Lymphoepithelial carcinoma is a poorly differentiated squamous cell carcinoma or histologically undifferentiated carcinoma accompanied by a prominent reactive lymphoplasmacytic infiltrate, morphologically similar to nasopharyngeal carcinoma.

ICD-O code   8082/3

Synonyms
Undifferentiated carcinoma; undifferentiated carcinoma with lymphocytic stroma; undifferentiated carcinoma of nasopharyngeal type; lymphoepithelioma-like carcinoma

Epidemiology
Sinonasal lymphoepithelial carcinoma is rare, and most reported cases have originated from Southeast Asia, where nasopharyngeal carcinoma is also prevalent {1216,1480,1558,2910}. It affects adults in the fifth to seventh decades, and there is a male predominance of approximately 3:1.

Etiology
Nearly all sinonasal lymphoepithelial carcinomas show a strong association with Epstein-Barr virus (EBV) {801,1216,1480,1558,2910}.

Localization
Sinonasal lymphoepithelial carcinomas are more common in the nasal cavity than in the paranasal sinuses, although both sites may be involved simultaneously. The tumours may show local invasion of the palate, orbit, and base of skull.

Clinical features
Patients present with nasal obstruction, bloody nasal discharge or epistasis. Intracranial extension of tumour may cause proptosis and cranial nerve palsy {1216,1480}. There may be cervical lymph node and/or distant metastasis at presentation. Examination and biopsy of the nasopharynx is required to exclude loco-regional spread from a primary nasopharyngeal carcinoma.

Histopathology
The tumour infiltrates the mucosa in the form of irregular islands and sheets, usually without a desmoplastic stroma. The tumour cells possess relatively monotonous vesicular nuclei with prominent nucleoli. The cytoplasm is lightly eosinophilic, with indistinct cell borders, resulting in a syncytial appearance. The tumour cells may also appear plump spindly, with streaming of nuclei. Intraepithelial spread of tumour may sometimes be seen in the overlying epithelial lining. Necrosis and keratinization are usually not evident. The tumour is infiltrated by variable numbers of lymphocytes and plasma cells. In general, the inflammatory infiltrate is less prominent than that seen in nasopharyngeal carcinoma. In some cases, the inflammatory cells may even be sparse {1216,1480}. The epithelial nature of the tumour can be confirmed by immunostaining for pan-cytokeratin and epithelial membrane antigen. EBV encoded RNA (EBER) is strongly expressed by the tumour cells in most cases {801,1216,1480,1558,2910}.

Differential diagnosis
Sinonasal lymphoepithelial carcinoma must be distinguished from the vastly more aggressive sinonasal undifferentiated carcinoma (SNUC). The presence of lymphoplasmacytic infiltrates, although helpful, cannot be relied on solely in making the distinction. SNUC is characterized by tumour cells with nuclear pleomorphism, high mitotic rate and frequent necrosis. EBV status is also helpful since SNUC, except for rare cases from Asians, are EBV-negative {1216,1480, 1558}. Other important differential diagnoses are malignant melanoma and non-Hodgkin lymphoma.

Prognosis and predictive factors
The tumour responds favourably to local-regional radiotherapy even in the presence of cervical lymph node metastasis {623,1216,1480}. Distant metastasis (most often to bone), however, is associated with a poor prognosis.

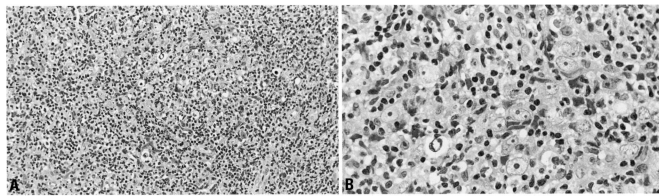

Fig. 1.9 Primary lymphoepithelial carcinoma of the nasal cavity. **A** The intimate intermingling of the carcinoma cells with lymphoid cells imparts a lymphoma-like appearance. **B** Large carcinoma cells with indistinct cell borders, vesicular nuclei and prominent nucleoli are admixed with numerous small lymphocytes..

Sinonasal undifferentiated carcinoma

H.F. Frierson, Jr.

Definition
A highly aggressive and clinicopathologically distinctive carcinoma of uncertain histogenesis that typically presents with locally extensive disease. It is composed of pleomorphic tumour cells with frequent necrosis, and should be differentiated from lymphoepithelial carcinoma and olfactory neuroblastoma.

ICD-O code   8020/3

Synonym
Anaplastic carcinoma

Epidemiology
The tumour is rare, with fewer than 100 reported cases. The age range is broad (third to ninth decade), and the median age is in the sixth decade {350,1216}. There is a male predominance (2-3:1).

Etiology
The neoplasm is typically negative for Epstein-Barr virus {350,1216}. Some cases have occurred after prior radiation therapy for nasopharyngeal carcinoma {1216}.

Localization
The nasal cavity, maxillary antrum, and ethmoid sinus are typically involved alone or in combination. The neoplasm also commonly extends to other contiguous sites.

Clinical features
Patients have multiple nasal/paranasal sinus symptoms, usually of relatively short duration, including nasal obstruction, epistaxis, proptosis, periorbital swelling, diplopia, facial pain, and symptoms of cranial nerve involvement.

Macroscopy
The tumour is usually larger than 4 cm. It is fungating, with poorly defined margins, bone destruction, and invasion of adjacent structures {2038}.

Tumour spread and staging
In addition to involvement of multiple sinuses, the neoplasm destroys sinus walls and orbital bones. Penetration into the cranial cavity is frequent. Less often, there is extension into the nasopharynx or oral cavity. The tumour can metastasize to cervical lymph nodes and distant sites (such as liver, lung, bone) {1216}.

Histopathology
Sinonasal undifferentiated carcinoma forms nests, lobules, trabeculae and sheets, in the absence of squamous or glandular differentiation. Severe dysplasia of the overlying surface epithelium has been noted in a few instances.
The nuclei are medium to large-sized, surrounded by small amounts of eosinophilic cytoplasm that lacks a syncytial quality. The nucleoli are variable in size, but most often, they are single and prominent. The mitotic rate is very high and there is often prominent tumour necrosis and apoptosis. Lymphovascular invasion is often prominent.

Immunohistochemistry
The carcinoma is immunoreactive for pan-cytokeratins and simple keratins (CK7, CK8 and CK19), but not CK4, CK5/CK6 and CK14 {801}. Less than half of the cases have been reported to be positive for epithelial membrane antigen, neuron specific enolase, or p53 {350}. The tumour is negative for CEA, while positivity for synaptophysin, chromogranin, or S100 protein is only rarely observed {350,1216}.

Electron microscopy
Ultrastructurally, cells with occasional small desmosomes and rare dense core granules have been noted {819}.

Histogenesis
This is a tumour of uncertain histogenesis, but with unique clinicopathologic characteristics. It should be differentiated from other specific types of carcinoma and non-epithelial tumours with round cells.

Prognosis and predictive factors
Despite aggressive management, the prognosis is poor, with median survival of less than 18 months {350,1216}, and 5-year survival of less than 20% {856}. Recent results suggest that more promising outcome may be achieved by combining chemoradiation and radical resection {1802}.

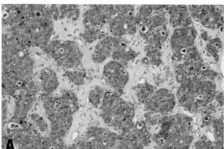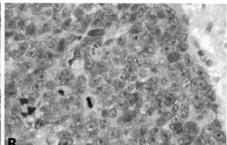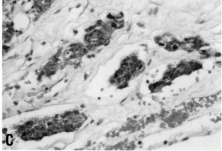

Fig. 1.10 Sinonasal undifferentiated carcinoma. **A** Small nests of tumour cells with or without interconnections are frequently observed. **B** The cells usually have prominent nucleoli. The mitotic rate is high. **C** Conspicuous invasion of vascular spaces.

Adenocarcinoma

A. Franchi
M. Santucci
B.M. Wenig

These are glandular malignancies of the sinonasal tract, excluding defined types of salivary gland carcinoma. Two main categories are recognized: (1) intestinal-type adenocarcinoma, and (2) non-intestinal-type adenocarcinoma, which can be further divided into low-grade and high-grade subtypes. Overall, adenocarcinomas and salivary-type carcinomas comprise 10-20% of all sinonasal primary malignant tumours.

Intestinal-type adenocarcinomas

Definition
A primary malignant glandular tumour of the nasal cavity and paranasal sinuses histologically resembling adenocarcinoma or adenoma of the intestines, or exceptionally normal small intestinal mucosa.

ICD-O code
8144/3

Synonyms
Colonic-type adenocarcinoma, enteric-type adenocarcinoma.

Epidemiology
The frequency of intestinal type adenocarcinomas (ITACs) among primary sinonasal malignancies is difficult to ascertain. Most series report a pronounced male predominance, possibly because of occupational exposure. Patients have ranged in age from 12 to 86 years at the time of diagnosis (mean 58 years) {124}.

Etiology
The causal relationship of wood dust and leather dust with the development of sinonasal ITACs has been established by several epidemiological studies from different countries {1594}. In this setting, dust particle size is important because those smaller than 5 μm reach the lower respiratory tract, while larger particles are accumulated in the nasal mucosa. However, the carcinogens involved in the onset of ITACs in wood workers and leather workers have not yet been clearly identified. Biologically active substances which can be present in wood and leather dusts include alkaloids, saponins, stilbenes, aldehydes, quinones, flavonoids, resins, oil, steroids, terpenes, fungal proteins, and tannins {1341}.

Association has also been reported for agricultural workers, food manufacturers, and motor-vehicle drivers among men, and for textile occupations among women {1443}.

Localization
ITACs involve the ethmoid sinus, nasal cavities and maxillary sinus in approximately 40%, 27% and 20% of cases, respectively. In the nasal cavities, the inferior and middle turbinates are the sites of predilection. For larger destructive lesions it may be impossible to ascertain the exact site of origin. Advanced tumours tend to invade the orbit, the pterygopalatine and infratemporal fossae, and the cranial cavity. About 10% of cases show lymph node involvement at presentation {124,1341, 2234}.

Clinical features
Most patients present with unilateral nasal obstruction, rhinorrhea and epistaxis. Advanced tumours may cause pain, neurologic disturbances, exophthalmos and visual disturbances.

Imaging
Computed tomography (CT) and magnetic resonance imaging (MRI) are used for diagnosis of early lesions, defining the extent of disease and detection of early recurrence. CT best shows sites of bone destruction, while MRI best delineates soft tissue extension {1537}.

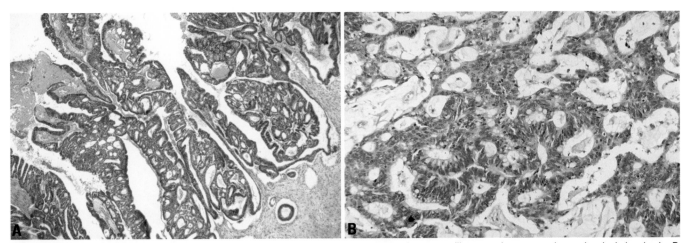

Fig. 1.11 Intestinal-type adenocarcinoma **A** Well differentiated intestinal type adenocarcinoma shows a papillary growth pattern and occasional tubular glands. **B** Higher power view of a moderately differentiated intestinal type adenocarcinoma, showing glandular structures formed by cylindrical and goblet cells.

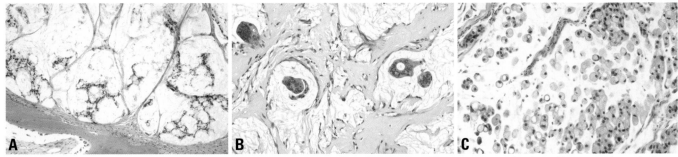

Fig. 1.12 Intestinal-type adenocarcinoma **A** Mucinous intestinal-type adenocarcinoma invading bone. The tumour has an alveolar architecture and strands of neoplastic cells with clear mucus-containing cytoplasm are present within mucus pools. **B** Mucinous intestinal-type adenocarcinoma showing small glands and solid islands floating in abundant mucous substance. **C** Mucinous intestinal-type adenocarcinoma formed by signet ring cells.

Macroscopy

ITACs present as an irregular exophytic pink or white mass bulging in the nasal cavity or paranasal sinus, often with a necrotic friable appearance. Some lesions are gelatinous.

Histopathology

Two classifications of ITACs have been proposed. Barnes divided these tumours into 5 categories: papillary, colonic, solid, mucinous and mixed. Kleinsasser and Schroeder divided ITACs into four categories: papillary tubular cylinder cell (PTCC) types I-III (I = well-differentiated, II = moderately-differentiated, III = poorly-differentiated) {799,804,1333}, alveolar goblet type, signet-ring type and transitional type. Either classification is acceptable, but for simplicity the Barnes classification is preferred and will be the one utilized in this description. The most common histologic types seen in association with wood workers as well as in sporadic cases are the papillary and colonic types {124,1333}.

The papillary type (papillary tubular cylinder cell I or well-differentiated adenocarcinoma), which accounts for approximately 18% of cases, shows a predominance of papillary architecture with occasional tubular glands, minimal cytologic atypia, and rare mitotic figures. The colonic type (papillary tubular cylinder II or moderately-differentiated adenocarcinoma), representing approximately 40% of cases, shows a predominance of tubulo-glandular architecture, rare papillae, increased nuclear pleomorphism and mitotic activity.

The solid type (papillary tubular cylinder III or poorly-differentiated adenocarcinoma), representing approximately 20% of cases, shows a loss of differentiation, characterized by solid and trabecular growth with isolated tubule formation, marked increase in number of smaller cuboidal cells with nuclear pleomorphism, round vesicular nuclei, prominent nucleoli and increased mitotic figures.

Analogous to colonic adenocarcinoma, some ITACs are predominantly comprised of abundant mucus and are classified as the mucinous type. The mucinous type (alveolar goblet cell and signet ring) includes two growth patterns. In one pattern, there are solid clusters of cells, individual glands, signet ring cells, short papillary fronds with or without fibrovascular cores; mucin is predominantly intracellular and a mucomyxoid matrix may be present. The other pattern shows the presence of large, well-formed glands distended by mucus and extracellular mucin pools {799,804,1333}. In the latter type, pools of extracellular mucin are separated by thin connective tissue septa creating an alveolar type pattern. Predominantly cuboidal or goblet tumour cells are present in single layers at the periphery of mucus lakes.

Mucus extravasation may elicit an inflammatory response that can include multinucleated giant cells. {799}.

The mixed type (transitional) is composed of an admixture of two or more of the previously defined patterns.

Irrespective of the histologic type, ITACs histologically simulate normal intestinal mucosa and may include villi, Paneth cells, enterochromaffin cells and muscularis mucosae {1739}. In rare instances, the tumour is so well differentiated that it is composed of well-formed villi lined by columnar cells resembling normal resorptive cells; in some cases, bundles of smooth muscle cells resembling muscularis mucosae may also be identified under the villi.

Immunohistochemistry

ITACs are diffusely positive for epithelial markers including pancytokeratin, epithelial membrane antigen, B72.3, Ber-EP4, BRST-1, Leu-M1, and human milk fat globule (HMFG-2) {1687}. They show CK20 positivity (73%) and variable CK7

Table 1.1 Classification and survival of intestinal-type adenocarcinoma

Barnes {124}	Klesinsasser and Schroeder {1333}	3-year cumulative survival[b]
Papillary-type	PTCC-I[a]	82%
Colonic-type	PTCC-II	54%
Solid-type	PTCC-III	36%
Mucinous type	Alveolar goblet	48%
	Signet-ring	0%
Mixed	Transitional	71%

[a]PTCC, papillary tubular cylinder cell
[b]Survival data derived from Kleinsasser and Schroeder {1333}

reactivity (43% to 93% of cases) {800}. CDX-2, a nuclear transcription factor involved in the differentiation of intestinal epithelial cells and diffusely expressed in intestinal adenocarcinomas, is commonly expressed in ITACs {800}. Information on CEA staining in ITACs is conflicting {1687,2660}. Scattered or groups of chromogranin-positive cells are frequently identified {1687}; these neuroendocrine cells may express a variety of hormone peptides, including serotonin, cholecystokinin, gastrin, somatostatin and leu-enkephalin {163}.

Electron microscopy
ITAC demonstrates features of the intestinal epithelium {163}. Columnar cells present regular microvilli with cores of microfilaments that combine to form a band that inserts into the zonula adherens of the junctional complexes. Glycocalyceal bodies as characteristic of intestinal-type epithelium may be identified between the microvilli. Endocrine cells with neurosecretory granules, Paneth cells with large exocrine granules, and goblet cells containing several mucin droplets in the apical cytoplasm are present in variable numbers.

Precursor lesions
The frequent presence of squamous metaplasia and/or dysplasia of the sinonasal epithelium in the vicinity of the tumour impairs mucociliary clearance, resulting in prolonged contact of carcinogenic substances with the mucosa {2789}.

Histogenesis
It has been hypothesized that ITAC derives from a stem cell capable of undergoing differentiation into various type of epithelial cells (resorptive cells, goblet cells, neuroendocrine cells, Paneth cells) {1739}.

Genetics
Genetic data are limited {2012,2013, 2218,2829}. K-RAS or H-RAS mutation has been detected in only about 15% of cases {2012,2218}. TP53 mutations are reported in 18-44% of cases {2013,2829}; mutations consist more frequently of C:G to A:T transitions and involve the CpG dinucleotides. Other gene alterations include loss of heterozygosity (LOH) at 17p13 and 9q21, and promoter methylation of p14(ARF) and

p16(INK4a). A close association between TP53, p14(ARF) and p16(INK4a) gene deregulation has been found in tumours from individuals occupationally exposed to dusts {2013}.

Prognosis and predictive factors
Sinonasal ITACs are generally locally aggressive tumours with frequent local failure (about 50% of cases), whereas metastasis to cervical lymph nodes and spread to distant sites are infrequent (about 10% and 20%, respectively) {124,799,804,1333}. The 5-year cumulative survival rate is around 40%, with most deaths occurring within 3 years. Since most patients present with advanced local disease, clinical staging generally has no relevant prognostic significance.
The histologic subtype has been identified as indicative of clinical behaviour in different series {124,799,804,1333}. The papillary type (papillary tubular cylinder cell adenocarcinoma I = well-differentiated adenocarcinoma) has a more indolent course, with little tendency to distant spread (5-year survival rate of about 80%). Conversely, the solid type (papillary tubular cylinder cell adenocarcinoma III = poorly differentiated adenocarcinoma) and mucinous type adenocarcinoma have a very poor survival. Other factors that have been associated with a more aggressive behaviour are: H-RAS mutation, chromogranin expression and c-erbB-2 expression {855,1687,2012}.
Although it has been suggested that ITACs occurring in occupational exposed individuals have a better prognosis than sporadic ITACs {124}, this has not been confirmed in other reports {799}.

Sinonasal non-intestinal-type adenocarcinoma

ICD-O code   8140/3

Synonyms
Sinonasal low-grade adenocarcinoma, terminal tubulus adenocarcinoma, sinonasal tubulopapillary low-grade adenocarcinoma.

Definition
Adenocarcinomas arising in the sinonasal tract that are not of minor salivary gland origin and do not demonstrate histopathologic features of the sinonasal intestinal-type adenocarcinoma. These adenocarcinomas are divided into low- and high-grade subtypes.

Epidemiology
Sinonasal non-intestinal-type adenocarcinomas predominantly occur in adults but have been identified over a wide age range from 9-80 years {1044}. The average patient age at presentation of low-grade adenocarcinomas is 53 years while that of high-grade ones is 59 years {1044}. There is a slight male predominance for the low-grade adenocarcinomas but a more marked male predilection in the high-grade ones {1044}.

Etiology
There are no known occupational or environmental etiological factors.

Localization
The low-grade non-intestinal-type adenocarcinomas predilect to the ethmoid sinus (to a lesser extent as compared with the intestinal-type), and the high-grade non-intestinal-type adenocarcinomas predilect to the maxillary sinus

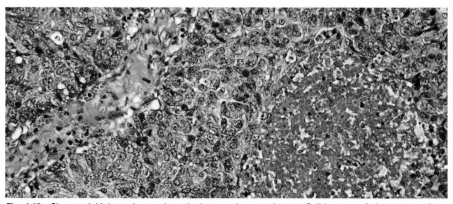
Fig. 1.13 Sinonasal high-grade non-intestinal-type adenocarcinoma. Solid areas of the tumour show marked nuclear pleomorphism as well as an area of comedo-type necrosis.

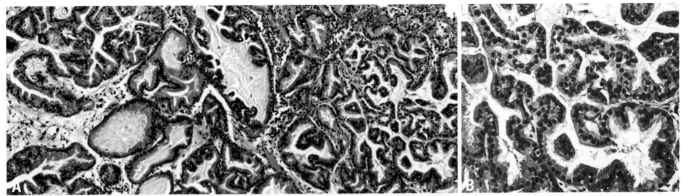

Fig. 1.14 Sinonasal (mucosal) non-intestinal-type adenocarcinoma. **A** Complex glandular growth and focal papillary architecture. **B** The glands are lined by a single layer of cuboidal to columnar appearing cells with uniform, round nuclei, single small identifiable nucleoli and eosinophilic appearing cytoplasm.

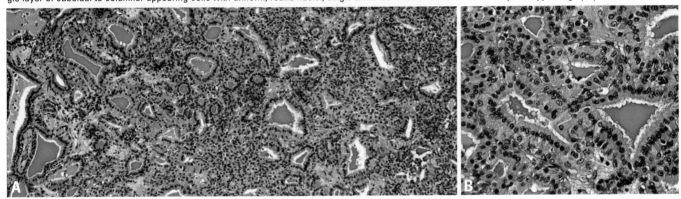

Fig. 1.15 Sinonasal low-grade non-intestinal-type adenocarcinoma. **A** Complex glandular growth including back-to-back glands lacking an intervening fibrovascular stroma is characteristically seen. **B** The glands are comprised of a single layer of nonciliated columnar cells with uniform, round nuclei, granular eosinophilic cytoplasm. The cells vary from orderly linear arrangement to stratification with loss of nuclear polarity.

{1044}. Either tumour type may also originate in the nasal cavity, other paranasal sinuses, or in multiple sinonasal sites in various combinations {1044}.

Clinical features

For low-grade adenocarcinomas, patients primarily present with nasal obstruction and epistaxis. Pain is an infrequent feature {1044}. The duration of symptoms ranges from 2 months to five years, with a median of 5.5 months.

For high-grade adenocarcinomas, the presenting symptoms include nasal obstruction, epistaxis, pain and facial deformity (e.g., proptosis). The duration of symptoms ranges from two weeks to five years with a median of 2.5 months {1044}.

Macroscopy

The appearance varies, including well demarcated to poorly-defined and invasive, flat to exophytic or papillary growths with a tan/white to pink colour and a friable to firm consistency.

Histopathology

The low-grade non-intestinal-type adenocarcinomas are circumscribed or invasive, and have a glandular or papillary growth. Numerous uniform small glands or acini are arranged in a back-to-back or coalescent pattern with little or no intervening stroma. Occasionally, large, irregular cystic spaces can be seen. The glands are lined by a single layer of nonciliated, cuboidal to columnar cells with uniform, round nuclei which may be limited to the basal aspect of the cells or may demonstrate pseudostratification with loss of nuclear polarity. The cytoplasm is eosinophilic. Cellular pleomorphism is mild to moderate. While occasional mitotic figures may be seen, atypical mitoses and necrosis are absent. Variants include papillary, clear cell and oncocytic adenocarcinomas. Multiple morphologic patterns may be present in a single neoplasm. Despite the relatively bland histology, the complexity of growth, absence of myoepithelial/basal cell component, absence of encapsulation and invasion into the submucosa permit a diagnosis of

malignancy to be made.

The high-grade non-intestinal-type adenocarcinomas are invasive tumours with a predominantly solid growth pattern, but glandular and papillary patterns can also be present. These tumours are characterized by moderate to marked cellular pleomorphism, high mitotic activity, including atypical forms, and necrosis.

Prognosis and predictive factors

The treatment for sinonasal non-intestinal-type adenocarcinomas is complete surgical excision generally via a lateral rhinotomy; depending on the extent and histology of the neoplasm, the surgery varies from local excision to more radical procedures (maxillectomy, ethmoidectomy and additional exenterations). Radiotherapy may be utilized for extensive disease or for higher-grade neoplasms. The low-grade neoplasms have an excellent prognosis, while high-grade neoplasms have a dismal prognosis with a 3-year survival rate of only approximately 20% {1044}.

Salivary gland-type carcinomas

J.W. Eveson

Salivary gland neoplasms of the sinonasal tract are uncommon, and the majority are malignant {1039}. For details see Chapter 5 on tumours of salivary glands.

ICD-O codes

Adenoid cystic carcinoma 8200/3
Acinic cell carcinoma   8550/3
Mucoepidermoid carcinoma
                                      8430/3
Epithelial-myoepithelial carcinoma
                                      8562/3
Clear cell carcinoma   8310/3

Adenoid cystic carcinoma

Adenoid cystic carcinoma is the most frequent malignant salivary gland-type tumour of the sinonasal tract. The age range is from 11-92 years {1039}. The majority develop in the maxillary sinus (about 60%) and nasal cavity (about 25%) {130}. The disease is often insidious, and symptoms include nasal obstruction, epistaxis, and pain, paraesthesia or anaesthesia. Swelling of the palate or face, and loosening of the teeth may be the presenting symptom. Many tumours are large and extensively infiltrative at the time of diagnosis. These tumours can be difficult to detect on plain film radiographs and often extend widely through bone before there is radiographical evidence of osseous destruction. In addition, the true extent of tumour spread is often underestimated by imaging techniques. The long-term prognosis is poor and the 10-year survival rate is only 7% {2444}. Most patients die as a result of local spread rather than metastatic disease {2799}.

Acinic cell carcinoma

Acinic cell carcinoma is rare in the sinonasal tract and cases have been reported in the nasal cavity {996,1950, 2014,2244,2698} and maxillary sinuses {829,2860}. The signs and symptoms are non-specific but they include nasal obstruction and epiphora.

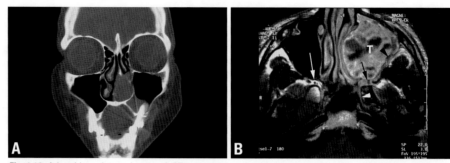

Fig. 1.16 Adenoid cystic carcinoma. **A** CT scan shows a nasal sinus mass focally extending into the bone. **B** The tumour (T) is inhomogenous and extends from the maxillary sinus into the infratemporal (black arrowhead) and the pterygopalatine fossa (black arrow). Perineural spread follows the Vidian cana (white arrowhead).

Mucoepidermoid carcinoma

Mucoepidermoid carcinomas are rare at this site, and should be distinguished from the more aggressive variants of squamous cell carcinoma, especially adenosquamous carcinoma {1039, 1291,2588}.

Epithelial-myoepithelial carcinoma

Epithelial-myoepithelial carcinoma is rare in the sinonasal tract. Cases have been reported to involve the nasal septum, nasal cavity and maxillary sinus {1011,1221,1450,2506}. Signs and symptoms are non-specific but have

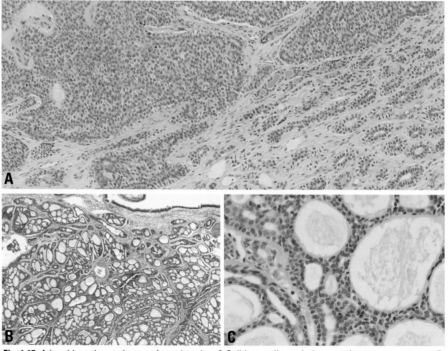

Fig. 1.17 Adenoid cystic carcinoma of nasal cavity. **A** Solid as well as tubular growth patterns are seen. **B** An intact surface mucosa overlying the cribriform and cystic patterns of a sinonasal adenoid cystic carcinoma. **C** A high power illustrating the relatively bland nuclear appearance with an intermediate to high nuclear to cytoplasmic ratio. Palisading is noted, along with small gland or tubule formation, in addition to the larger cyst-like spaces.

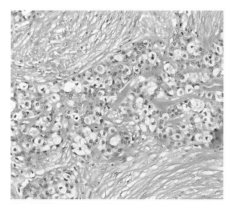

Fig. 1.18 Clear cell carcinoma.

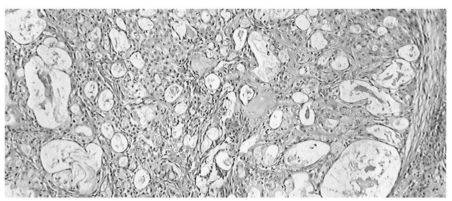

Fig. 1.19 Mucoepidermoid carcinoma. A low grade mucoepidermoid carcinoma has variable sized mucus filled cystic spaces lined by mucocytes and intermediate cells.

included the formation of polypoid masses and nasal obstruction.

Clear cell carcinoma

Clear cell carcinoma, N.O.S., of the sinonasal tract is rare {1757,1874} and it is important to exclude metastatic renal clear cell carcinoma {1664,2918}. Microscopically, these tumours consist of closely packed, polygonal clear cells arranged in sheets and theques. They contain glycogen but no mucin.

Other tumours

A variety of other salivary gland-type carcinomas have been rarely reported in the nasal cavity and paranasal sinuses. These include: malignant myoepithelioma {2918}, carcinoma ex pleomorphic adenoma {435}, polymorphous low-grade adenocarcinoma {1536} and basal cell adenocarcinoma {785}.

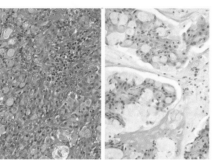

Fig. 1.20 Mucoepidermoid carcinoma. Solid epithelial growth pattern with occasional mucocytes (left); predominant cystic pattern with numerous mucocytes and a few intermediate cells (right).

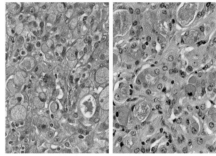

Fig. 1.21 Mucoepidermoid carcinoma. The mucin production (left) can be accentuated with a mucicarmine stain where both the intracytoplasmic and extracellular mucin is highlighted (right)

Table 1.2 Sinonasal glandular tumours*

Tumour types	No of cases	Percentage
Pleomorphic adenoma	73	23%
Oncocytic tumours	7	2%
Low-grade adenocarcinoma (including acinic cell carcinoma)	67	21%
Mucoepidermoid carcinoma	17	5%
Adenoid cystic carcinoma	54	17%
High grade adenocarcinoma	93	30%
Total	**311**	**100%**
* Modified from Heffner {1039}		

Neuroendocrine tumours

B. Perez-Ordonez

Neuroendocrine tumours are very rare in the nasal cavity, paranasal sinuses or nasopharynx. The recognizable types are typical carcinoid, atypical carcinoid and small cell carcinoma neuroendocrine type. It is unclear whether large cell neuroendocrine carcinoma that corresponds to the pulmonary counterpart occurs in these sites. There are also rare cases that do not fit these categories, and the diagnostic label "neuroendocrine carcinoma, not otherwise specified" may be applied.

Carcinoid tumour

ICD-O codes
Typical carcinoid   8240/3
Atypical carcinoid   8249/3

Typical and atypical carcinoids of the nasal cavity and paranasal sinuses are exceedingly rare, possibly because they are under-reported or have been included under other non-descriptive categories, such as "neuroendocrine carcinoma" {1676,2007,2384,2776}. They are otherwise similar to carcinoids in other sites.
Patients have ranged in age from 13-65 years, and present with nasal obstruction, epistaxis and/or facial pain. Most tumours arise in the nasal cavity but may extend into adjacent sinuses. A patient with two carcinoids - nasal and pulmonary - has been described {2384}. Another individual with the Multiple Endocrine Neoplasia Type I (MEN1) has been reported to have a carcinoid of the sphenoid sinus {2776}.
Paucity of cases and lack of significant follow-up preclude definitive statements about the prognosis. The tumours are at least locally aggressive.

Small cell carcinoma, neuroendocrine type (SCCNET)

Definition
Small cell carcinoma, neuroendocrine

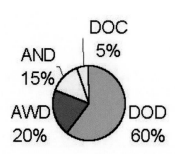

Fig. 1.22 Sinonasal small cell carcinomas, neuroendocrine type (SCCNET) are aggressive tumours with a mortality rate of > 60% despite multimodal therapy. (DOD, dead of disease; AWD, alive with disease; AND, alive no disease; DOC, dead other causes).

type is a high-grade carcinoma composed of small to intermediate sized cells resembling those of small cell carcinoma of pulmonary or extrapulmonary origin. Necrosis, large numbers of apoptotic cells, high mitotic rate, and lack of neurofibrillary stroma are microscopic hallmarks of this tumour.

ICD-O code   8041/3

Synonyms
Small cell carcinoma, small cell neuroendocrine carcinoma, oat cell carcinoma, poorly differentiated neuroendocrine carcinoma.

Epidemiology
SCCNET of the sinonasal tract is a rare tumour with no sex, racial, or geographic predilection and no known association

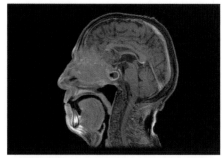

Fig. 1.23 MRI of a small cell carcinoma, neuroendocrine type (SCCNET) involving the superior nasal cavity, ethmoid and sphenoid sinuses, with extensive invasion of skull base and frontal lobe.

with smoking or radiation. The age range is from 26-77 years with a mean of 49 years.

Localization
SCCNET most commonly arise in the superior or posterior nasal cavity, and often extend into the maxillary or ethmoid sinuses. Primary tumours of the maxillary or ethmoid sinuses without nasal involvement can be seen in approximately 45% of cases. Secondary involvement of the nasopharynx is present in a minority of patients. Advanced tumours may invade the skull base, orbit, or brain.

Clinical features
The most common symptoms are epistaxis and nasal obstruction, followed by facial pain, palpable facial mass, and exophthalmos. Rare tumours have shown elevated serum levels of ACTH, calci-

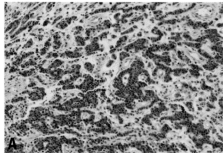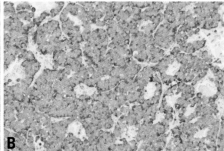

Fig. 1.24 Sinonasal carcinoid tumour. **A** Trabecular and insular patterns. **B** Diffuse and strong staining for neuron specific enolase (NSE).

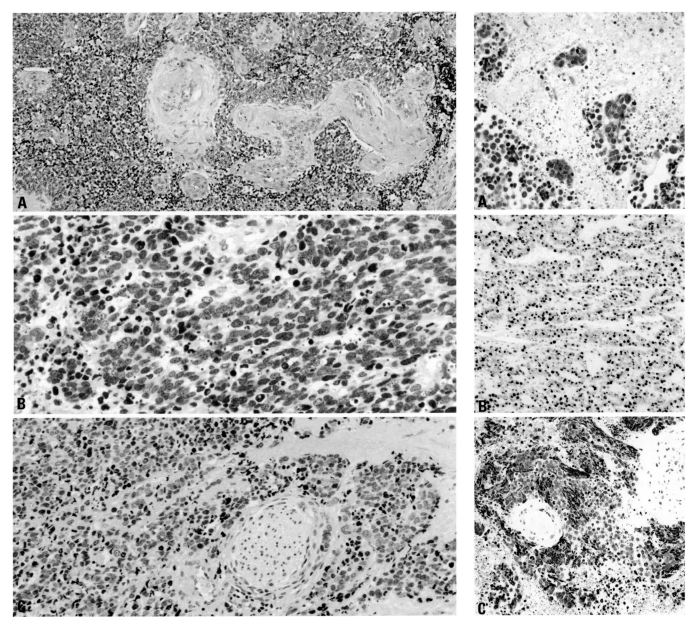

Fig. 1.25 Small cell carcinoma, neuroendocrine type (SCCNET) **A** Typical sinonasal SCCNET showing confluent sheets of tumour cells surrounding vessels of nasal mucosa. **B** Sinonasal SCCNET composed of small cells with high nucleo/cytoplasmic ratio and extensive apoptosis. The nuclei are hyperchromatic and lack visible nucleoli. **C** Sinonasal SCCNET with perineural invasion and numerous hyperchromatic apoptotic cells.

Fig. 1.26 Sinonasal SCCNET. **A** Patchy but strong staining for synaptophysin. Note the extensive tumour necrosis. **B** Diffuse and strong keratin expression. Note the characteristic perinuclear "dot". **C** Diffuse staining for CD56.

tonin, pro-gastrin releasing peptide (pro-GRP), or antidiuretic hormone with syndrome of antidiuretic hormone and hyponatremia {1259,1901,2042}.

Pathology

See Chapter 3 under "Neuroendocrine Neoplasms of the Larynx." An important differential diagnosis is olfactory neuroblastoma.

Prognosis and predictive factors

SCCNET are aggressive tumours with a poor prognosis and frequent local recurrence and distant metastasis despite multimodal therapy. Among twenty reported patients {849,1259,1358,1901, 2009,2042,2134,2153,2728,2742}, twelve (60%) died of disease, three (15%) were alive with no evidence of disease, four were alive with disease (20%), and one died of other causes. In a study of extrapulmonary small cell carcinomas {845}, which included seven cases involving the paranasal sinuses, the median survival of 14 patients with pri-

mary head and neck small cell carcinomas was only 14.5 months {845}. Follow-up data have shown a local recurrence rate of 45% and a distant metastasis rate of 35%. Common sites of metastases include cervical lymph nodes, lung, liver, bone marrow, and vertebrae.

Schneiderian papillomas

L. Barnes
L.L.Y. Tse
J.L. Hunt

The ectodermally derived ciliated respiratory mucosa that lines the nasal cavity and paranasal sinuses, so-called Schneiderian membrane, gives rise to three morphologically distinct types of papillomas. These are referred to individually as inverted, oncocytic, and exophytic papillomas or, collectively, as Schneiderian papillomas.

As a group, the Schneiderian papillomas are uncommon, representing only 0.4-4.7% of all sinonasal tumours {1423}.

Table 1.3 Distribution of Schneiderian papillomas

References	Total cases	Inverted	Oncocytic	Exophytic
Hyams {1158}	315	149	10	156
Michaels and Young {1714}	191	139	16	36
Buchwald et al. {302}	82	58	5	19
Sarkar et al. {2246}	35	24	9	2
Weiner et al. {2737}	105	82	2	21
Total	**728 (100%)**	**452 (62%)**	**42 (6%)**	**234 (32%)**

Inverted papilloma (Schneiderian papilloma, inverted type)

Definition
A papilloma derived from the Schneiderian membrane in which the epithelium invaginates into and proliferates in the underlying stroma.

ICD-O code   8121/1

Synonyms
Inverting papilloma, Schneiderian papilloma, papillomatosis

Epidemiology
Inverted papillomas are two to five times more common in males, and are found primarily in the 40-70 year age group. They are distinctly uncommon in children.

Etiology
Although a viral origin of inverted papillomas has long been suspected, viral inclusions have never been unequivocally demonstrated by light or electron microscopy. In addition, they are almost invariably negative when stained for human papillomavirus (HPV) by the immunoperoxidase technique. HPV genomes, however, have been demonstrated in inverted papillomas by in situ hybridization or the polymerase chain reaction, particularly HPV 6 and 11, sometimes HPV 16 and 18, and exceptionally, HPV 57. The frequency of finding the virus by these specialized techniques is highly variable, ranging anywhere from 0-100% {127}. In a collective review of 341 inverted papillomas evaluated for the presence of HPV by a variety of sophisticated molecular techniques, 131 (38%) were positive. Whether the virus is a passenger or etiologically related to the papilloma is unclear {1596}.

Epstein-Barr virus (EBV) DNA has been identified in 65% of inverted papillomas by polymerase chain reaction (PCR), raising the possibility that this virus might be involved in its pathogenesis {1596}. A subsequent study utilizing in-situ hybridisation found no evidence of EBV in the tumour cells, suggesting that the reported PCR positivity might be related to the presence of EBV-positive lymphocytes in the tissues {842}. There is no known association of inverted papilloma with allergy, inflammation, smoking, noxious environmental agents or occupation {1158}.

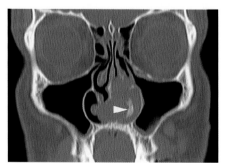

Fig. 1.27 Inverted papilloma. Coronal CT. The tumour bows the bone. The calcification (white arrowhead) may represent a sclerotic fragment of inferior turbinate.

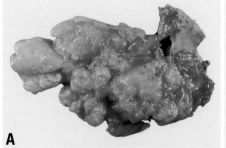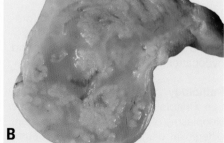

Fig. 1.28 Inverted papilloma. **A** Specimen removed intact. Note the opaque yellow-tan nodular polypoid appearance. **B** Cut surface of the lesion shown in A. Close inspection shows well-demarcated islands of epithelium which extend endophytically into the stroma.

Localization

Inverted papillomas characteristically arise from the lateral nasal wall in the region of the middle turbinate or ethmoid recesses, and often extend secondarily into the sinuses, especially the maxillary and ethmoid and, to a lesser extent, the sphenoid and frontal. Isolated lesions of the paranasal sinuses without nasal involvement however, do occur. Almost none arise primarily on the nasal septum {1297}.

Exceptionally, inverted papillomas may arise in sites other than the sinonasal tract. They have been recorded in the middle ear-mastoid {2757}, pharynx {2499}, nasopharynx {81}, and lacrimal sac {2217}. It has been suggested that ectopic migration of the Schneiderian membrane during embryogenesis could account for these aberrant papillomas in sites contiguous with the sinonasal tract {1158}. Whether all of these ectopic cases are bona fide inverted papillomas is uncertain.

Although overwhelmingly unilateral, rare cases of bilateral inverted papillomas have been described {211}. Such occurrence, however, should always arouse the suspicion of septal erosion and perforation from unilateral disease.

Clinical features

Signs and symptoms

Nasal obstruction is the most common presenting symptom. Other manifestations include nasal drainage, epistaxis, anosmia, headaches (especially frontal), epiphora, proptosis, and diplopia. Pain, on the other hand, is an uncommon initial complaint, occurring in only about 10% of all cases. When present, it should always arouse suspicion of secondary infection or malignant change.

On physical examination, inverted papillomas present as pink, tan, or grey; nontranslucent; soft to moderately firm, polypoid growths with a convoluted or wrinkled surface.

Imaging

Findings on imaging vary with the extent of disease. Early on, there may be only a soft tissue density within the nasal cavity and/or paranasal sinuses. Later, with more extensive disease, unilateral opacification and thickening of one or more of the sinuses is common, as are expansion and displacement of adjacent structures. Pressure erosion of bone may also be apparent and must be distinguished from the destructive invasion associated with malignancy, such as de novo carcinoma or carcinoma arising in and/or associated with an inverted papilloma.

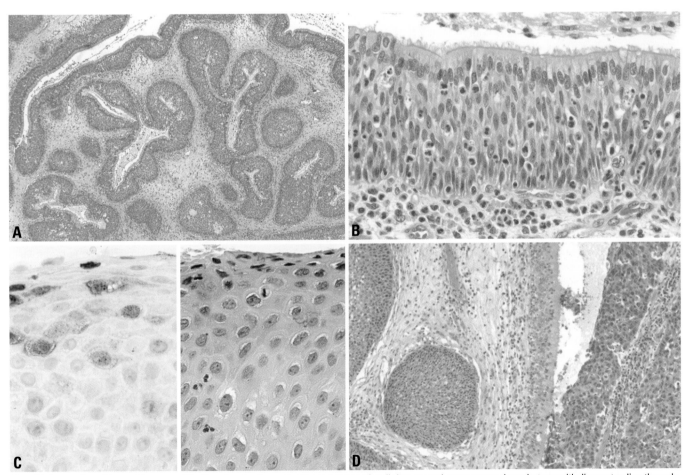

Fig. 1.29 Inverted papilloma **A** Low magnification showing hyperplastic aggregates of well-demarcated squamous and respiratory epithelium extending throughout the stroma. Note the absence of mucoserous glands. **B** Papilloma composed partially of hyperplastic, ciliated respiratory epithelium. Note the epithelial transmigration of neutrophils and the delicate basement membrane. **C** HPV nuclear and cytoplasmic reactivity can be seen in some inverted papillomas, usually in the same nuclei which exhibit features of "koilocytic" atypia (right). **D** Inverted papilloma and carcinoma. Note the inverted papilloma on the left and the normal ciliated respiratory epithelium of the sinonasal track in the middle of the illustration. The carcinoma at the right shows both in-situ and invasive components.

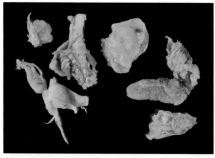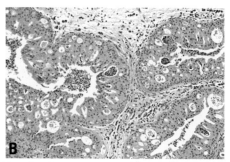

Fig. 1.30 Oncocytic Schneiderian papilloma. **A** Note the yellow-tan appearance and fine papillary excrescences in some of the fragments. Close inspection of the cut surface of the fragment in the top center part of the illustration shows an inverted component to the papilloma. **B** The epithelium is oncocytic and there are prominent intra-epithelial mucous cells, cysts and microabscesses.

Histopathology

Inverted papillomas are composed exclusively or almost exclusively of hyperplastic ribbons of basement membrane-enclosed epithelium that grow endophytically into the underlying stroma. Infrequently, a minor exophytic component may be seen. The epithelium is multilayered, usually 5-30 cells thick, and formed of squamous or ciliated columnar (respiratory epithelial) cells admixed with mucocytes. Nonkeratinizing squamous or transitional-type epithelium tends to predominate, and is frequently covered by a single layer of ciliated columnar cells. An occasional case may be composed almost entirely of respiratory epithelium. Gradations between these two extremes are not uncommon, resulting in a transitional epithelium reminiscent of that seen in the urinary tract. All of these epithelial types may be present in the same lesion, and their proportions may vary widely in different lesions or even in different areas of the same papilloma. Mitoses are not numerous and, if present at all, are seen primarily in the basal and parabasal epithelium.

Ten to 20% of inverted papillomas may show focal surface keratinisation, and 5-10% varying degrees of dysplasia {127}. These are not necessarily signs of malignancy, but they should alert the pathologist of the need of thorough evaluation of the papilloma. The stroma ranges from dense and fibrous to loose and myxoid, with or without an inflammatory component. The inflammatory cells, especially neutrophils, often transmigrate through the epithelium. Basement membrane thickening is not typically seen. Normal-appearing seromucinous glands are sparse to absent, because the neoplastic epithelium uses the ducts and glands

as scaffolds to extend into the stroma.

As inverted papillomas enlarge, they may obstruct the drainage of nearby sinuses. As a result, it is not uncommon to also find ordinary nasal polyps in inverted papilloma specimens. They can usually be identified grossly by their more myxoid appearance and the fact that they will transilluminate, whereas inverted papilloma will not.

Rarely, an inverted papilloma will exhibit focal surface changes reminiscent of a verruca vulgaris; that is, it shows focal papillary squamous epithelial hyperplasia with marked keratosis and/or parakeratosis, with a prominent granular cell layer, and often contains numerous vacuolated cells suggestive of koilocytes. Although this might be a viral effect, immunohistochemical stains for HPV are invariably negative. When this change is observed, the diagnosis of "inverted papilloma with focal verrucous hyperplasia" is appropriate and the patient should be followed closely for possible development of carcinoma, either verrucous carcinoma or squamous cell carcinoma.

Inverted papilloma and carcinoma

Inverted papillomas are occasionally complicated by carcinomas, especially squamous cell carcinoma and, to a much lesser extent, verrucous, mucoepidermoid, spindle and clear cell carcinomas, as well as adenocarcinomas. The incidence of malignant change in individual series of inverted papillomas has ranged from 2-27% {127}. In a collective review of 1390 inverted papillomas reported in the literature, 150 (11%) were associated with carcinoma and, of these, 61% of the carcinomas were synchronous and 39% metachronous {127}. For metachronous carcinomas, the mean interval from onset

of the inverted papilloma to the development of the carcinoma is 63 months (range, 6 months to 13 years) {1477}. Carcinomas complicating inverted papilloma vary from well to poorly differentiated and exhibit a broad range of behaviour. Some are in situ and of little consequence, whereas others are locally aggressive or may even metastasize. The carcinomas may actually arise within the papilloma, as evidenced by a gradation of histological changes ranging from dysplasia to carcinoma in-situ to frankly invasive carcinoma; whereas in others, the carcinoma is merely associated with a histologically bland inverted papilloma. Staining for CD44s may be helpful in identifying a malignant component. It is diffusely expressed in typical inverted papillomas, whereas its expression is reduced or absent in the associated carcinomatous component {1175}.

There is no correlation between the number of local recurrences of an inverted papilloma and the subsequent development of carcinoma. There is some evidence, however, to suggest that HPV 16 and 18 may be more carcinogenic than HPV 6 and 11 {1334}.

Preliminary data suggest that alterations in TP53, manifested by an increased protein expression or genetic mutation, can be used to predict which lesions are at risk for malignant change {715,765}.

Differential diagnosis

The differential diagnoses include nasal polyp with squamous metaplasia, respiratory epithelial adenomatoid hamartoma (REAH) and invasive carcinoma.

Nasal polyps with squamous metaplasia show thickening and hyalinization of the basement membrane, a prominent component of normal seromucinous glands and, often, a large number of stromal inflammatory cells. These features are typically absent in inverted papilloma. In addition, the surface epithelium of nasal polyps is thin, contains more mucocytes, and does not show the characteristic epithelial transmigration of neutrophils.

In contrast to inverted papilloma, REAH occurs primarily on the posterior nasal septum rather than the lateral nasal wall and/or paranasal sinuses {2766}. REAH is also composed of numerous glands lined by respiratory epithelial cells, surrounded by thick hyalinized basement membranes, features not seen in inverted papilloma.

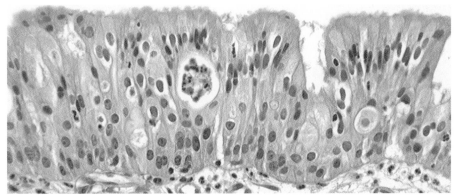

Fig. 1.31 Oncocytic papilloma. Stratified columnar epithelium with oncocytic features and small neutrophilic microabscesses are characteristic.

Invasive carcinoma can be distinguished from inverted papilloma by the presence of the following features: cellular pleomorphism, atypical mitoses, keratin pearls, loss of basement membranes, and stromal invasion associated with an inflammatory-desmoplastic response.

Prognosis and predictive factors
Though histologically benign, they have an unlimited growth potential and, if neglected, can cause considerable morbidity or even death by extending into contiguous structures. Attempts to remove these lesions intranasally by snare and avulsion have resulted in 'recurrence' (or persistence) rates of 0-74% (average, 60%) {1442}.
The preferred treatment for most lesions is a lateral rhinotomy and medial maxillectomy with meticulous removal of all mucosa in the ipsilateral paranasal sinuses. With this approach, the recurrence rate is usually <20% {1442}. Selected small tumours can be effectively removed by a less aggressive approach using endoscopic sinonasal surgery. Recurrences typically appear within 2-3 years of therapy but, in some instances, are delayed for many years. Attempts to correlate histological features with risk of recurrence have resulted in conflicting data {1158,1442,2417}. Even those with prominent mitotic activity and dysplasia do not invariably show an increased recurrence or malignancy. Nevertheless, dysplasia, especially if moderate to severe, demands thorough microscopic evaluation of all resected tissue to avoid overlooking small foci of carcinoma. The association between presence of HPV and the risk of recurrence is debatable {185,839}.

Oncocytic papilloma (Schneiderian papilloma, oncocytic type)

Definition
A papilloma derived from the Schneiderian membrane composed of both exophytic fronds and endophytic invaginations lined by multiple layers of columnar cells with oncocytic features. Intraepithelial microcysts containing mucin and neutrophils are characteristic.

ICD-O code   8121/1

Synonyms
Oncocytic Schneiderian papilloma, cylindrical cell papilloma, columnar cell papilloma, papillomatosis.

Epidemiology
Oncocytic papilloma is equally distributed between the sexes, and the majority of the patients are aged over 50 years.

Etiology
In contrast to exophytic and inverted papillomas, HPV has not been identified in oncocytic papillomas {127}.

Localization
Oncocytic papilloma almost always occurs unilaterally on the lateral nasal wall or in the paranasal sinuses, usually the maxillary or ethmoid. It may remain localized, involve both areas, or if neglected, extend into contiguous areas such as the orbit or cranial cavity.

Clinical features
Oncocytic papilloma presents as a fleshy, pink, tan, red-brown, or grey papillary or polypoid growth associated with nasal obstruction and intermittent epistaxis.

Histopathology
The oncocytic papilloma exhibits both exophytic and endophytic patterns of growth. The epithelium is multilayered, 2-8 cells thick, and is composed of tall columnar cells with swollen, finely granular cytoplasm reminiscent of oncocytes. The high content of cytochrome c oxidase and presence of numerous mitochondria ultrastructurally clearly establish their oncocytic character {129}. The nuclei are either small dark and uniform or slightly vesicular with barely discernible nucleoli. Cilia in varying stages of regression may be observed in a few of the outermost cells.
The epithelium characteristically contains numerous small cysts filled with mucin or neutrophils (microabscesses). The stroma varies from edematous to fibrous, and may contain modest numbers of lymphocytes, plasma cells, and neutrophils, but few eosinophils. Seromucinous glands are sparse to absent.

Oncocytic papilloma and carcinoma
Four to 17% of all oncocytic papillomas harbour a carcinoma {1158,1266,1611, 2723}. Most of these are squamous, but mucoepidermoid, small cell and sinonasal undifferentiated carcinomas have also been described.
As in inverted papilloma, the carcinoma complicating oncocytic papilloma may arise within the papilloma, as evidenced by a gradation of histologic changes ranging from dysplasia to in situ to invasive carcinoma, or it may only be associated with the papilloma. Prognosis depends on the histologic type, degree of invasion, and the extent of tumour. In some instances, the carcinoma is in situ and of little consequence to the patient, whereas others are locally aggressive and may metastasize.

Differential diagnosis
The intraepithelial mucin-filled cysts of an oncocytic papilloma are often mistaken for rhinosporidiosis. In rhinosporidiosis, the organisms are not limited to the epithelium but also involve stroma, and do not induce a diffuse oncocytic change.
Oncocytic papilloma is also occasionally confused with a low-grade papillary ade-

nocarcinoma. The presence of intact basement membranes and absence of infiltrative growth are features that indicate a benign lesion. In addition, the presence of intraepithelial mucin-filled cysts and microabscesses and the stratified oncocytic epithelium of a papilloma are rarely seen in a low-grade adenocarcinoma.

Prognosis and predictive factors

The clinical behaviour parallels that of the inverted papilloma. If inadequately excised, at least 25-35% will recur, usually within 5 years. Smaller tumours can be resected endoscopically.

Exophytic papilloma (Schneiderian papilloma, exophytic type)

Definition

A papilloma derived from the Schneiderian membrane composed of papillary fronds with delicate fibrovascular cores covered by multiple layers of epithelial cells.

ICD-O code   8121/0

Synonyms

Fungiform papilloma, everted papilloma, transitional cell papilloma, septal papilloma, squamous papilloma, papillomatosis, Ringertz tumour

Epidemiology

Exophytic papillomas are 2-10 times more common in men, and occur in individuals between 20 and 50 years of age (2-87 years) {1158,1908}.

Etiology

There is increasing evidence to suggest that exophytic papillomas may be etiologically related to HPV, especially types 6 and 11, rarely types 16 and 57b. In a collective review of exophytic papillomas evaluated for the presence of HPV by in situ hybridization and/or the polymerase chain reaction, about half of the cases were HPV positive {131}.

Localization

Exophytic papillomas arise on the lower anterior nasal septum with no significant lateralization. As they enlarge, they may secondarily involve, but only infrequently originate from the lateral nasal wall.

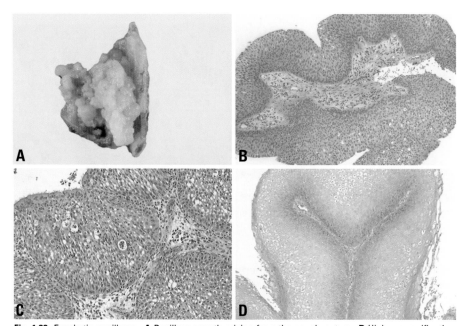

Fig. 1.32 Exophytic papilloma. **A** Papillary growth arising from the nasal septum. **B** Higher magnification showing the hyperplastic non-keratinizing squamous epithelium with scattered clear (mucous) cells. **C** Small neutrophilic abscess can be seen within the epithelium on occasion. **D** Koilocytic change (nuclear chromatin condensation, perinuclear halo and accentuation of the cell border) seen in exophytic papillomas.

Involvement of the paranasal sinuses is practically non-existent. Bilateral lesions are exceptional.

Clinical features

Epistaxis, unilateral nasal obstruction, and the presence of asymptomatic mass are the typical presenting symptoms. On physical examination, they appear as papillary or warty, grey, pink or tan, non-translucent growths attached to the nasal septum by a relatively broad base.

Histopathology

Most exophytic papillomas range up to about 2 cm. Microscopically, they are composed of papillary fronds with fibrovascular cores covered by epithelium, 5-20 cells thick, that vary from squamous to transitional (intermediate) to ciliated pseudostratified columnar (respiratory). Scattered mucocytes are common. Surface keratinization is absent or scant, unless the lesion has been irritated or if the papilloma is unusually large and hangs into the nasal vestibule, where it is exposed to the drying effect of air. Mitoses are rare and never atypical. Unless infected or irritated, the stroma contains few inflammatory cells.

Malignant change in exophytic papilloma is exceptional {301,1908}.

Differential diagnosis

Exophytic papillomas must be distinguished from the much more common, keratinizing cutaneous papillomas (e.g. verruca vulgaris) occurring in the nasal vestibule. The lack of extensive surface keratinization, presence of mucocytes, and presence of ciliated and/or 'transitional' epithelium help to confirm a diagnosis of exophytic papilloma. The presence of seromucinous glands and septal cartilage further indicate that the lesion is of mucosal rather than cutaneous origin.

Prognosis and predictive factors

Complete surgical excision is the treatment of choice. Inadequate excision rather than multiplicity of lesions probably accounts for the local recurrence of 22-50% {1158,1908}.

Respiratory epithelial adenomatoid hamartoma

B.M. Wenig

Definition
Benign nonneoplastic overgrowth of indigenous glands of the nasal cavity, paranasal sinuses and nasopharynx associated with the surface epithelium, and devoid of ectodermal neuroectodermal, and/or mesodermal elements.

Synonyms
Glandular hamartoma; seromucinous hamartoma.

Epidemiology
Hamartomas of the sinonasal tract and nasopharynx are uncommon. The majority of them are of pure epithelial type (respiratory epithelial adenomatoid hamartoma) {2766}, although pure mesenchymal hamartomas or mixed epithelial-mesenchymal hamartomas may also rarely occur {14,106,933,2766}. Respiratory epithelial adenomatoid hamartomas predominantly occur in adult patients with a decided male predominance; patients range in age from the 3rd to 9th decades of life, with a median age in the 6th decade {2766}.

Etiology
Respiratory epithelial adenomatoid hamartomas often arise in the setting of inflammatory polyps, raising a possible developmental induction secondary to the inflammatory process {2766}.

Localization
The majority occur in the nasal cavity, in particular the posterior nasal septum; involvement of other intranasal sites occurs less often and may be identified along the lateral nasal wall, middle meatus and inferior turbinate {2766}. Other sites of involvement include the nasopharynx, ethmoid sinus, and frontal sinus. Most are unilateral, but some may be bilateral.

Clinical features
Patients present with nasal obstruction, nasal stuffiness, epistaxis and/or chronic (recurrent) rhinosinusitis. The symptoms may occur over months to years. Associated complaints include allergies.

Macroscopy
Lesions are typically polypoid or exophytic with a rubbery consistency, tanwhite to red-brown appearance, measuring up to 6 cm in greatest dimension {933,2766}.

Histopathology
The lesions are dominated by a glandular proliferation composed of widely-spaced, small to medium-sized glands separated by stromal tissue. In areas, the glands arise in direct continuity with the surface epithelium, which invaginate downward into the submucosa. The glands are round to oval, and composed of multilayered ciliated respiratory epithelium often with admixed mucocytes. Glands distended with mucus can be seen. A characteristic finding is stromal hyalinization with envelopment of glands by a thick, eosinophilic basement membrane. Atrophic glandular alterations may be present in which the glands are lined by a single layer of flattened to cuboidal epithelium. Small reactive seromucinous glands can be seen. The stroma is oedematous or fibrous, and contains a mixed chronic inflammatory cell infiltrate.

Additional findings may include inflammatory sinonasal polyps, hyperplasia and/or squamous metaplasia of the surface epithelium unrelated to the adenomatoid proliferation, osseous metaplasia, rare association with inverted type Schneiderian papilloma, and rare association with a solitary fibrous tumour {2766}.

Prognosis and predictive factors
Conservative but complete surgical excision is curative.

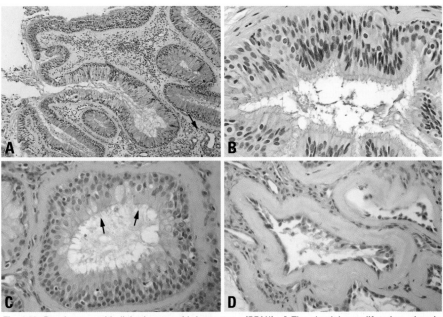

Fig. 1.33 Respiratory epithelial adenomatoid hamartoma (REAH). **A** The glandular proliferation arises in direct continuity with the surface epithelium with invagination downward into the submucosa. Clusters of seromucinous glands are seen (arrow). **B** Pseudostratified epithelium with cilia within the adenomatoid collections of a REAH hamartoma. **C** Cilia along the luminal border of the cells (arrows). **D** Atrophic changes in which the glands are lined by a single layer of flattened to cuboidal-appearing epithelium. Note the prominent thickened stromal hyalinization enveloping the glands.

Salivary gland-type adenomas

J.W. Eveson

Among glandular tumours of the sinonasal tract, about one-quarter of cases are benign, and practically all of them are salivary gland-type neoplasms {1039}. For details see Chapter 5 on 'Tumours of salivary glands'.

ICD-O codes
Pleomorphic adenoma	8940/0
Myoepithelioma	8982/0
Oncocytoma	8290/0

Pleomorphic adenoma
Most patients are between 20 and 60 years of age. Signs and symptoms are non-specific, and include unilateral nasal obstruction, epistaxis and a discernible mass. The tumour may resorb bone and extend into the maxillary sinuses. Most cases arise from the submucosa of the bony or cartilaginous nasal septum, but some arise in the lateral nasal wall {483,974,1210,1506}. The size varies from 0.5-5 cm {483} and tumours usually form polypoid, sessile swellings.
Microscopically, they are unencapsulated, and tend to be cellular with predominance of modified myoepithelial cells often of plasmacytoid hyaline type; stromal elements are sparse. Exceptionally, focal skeletal muscle differentiation can occur {1419}. If treated by wide surgical excision, recurrence is uncommon {483}.

Myoepithelioma
Myoepithelioma, including the spindle cell variant, of the sinonasal tract is very rare {188}.

Oncocytoma
Oncocytomas of the sinonasal tract are rare, and most arise from the nasal septum {1039}. They are usually small, but some extend posteriorly and can cause bone resorption {470,480,998}. The nasolacrimal duct may be involved, causing unilateral epiphora and purulent rhinorrhoea {555}. Those examples that have behaved aggressively {470} are more appropriately considered low-grade oncocytic adenocarcinomas rather than adenomas {449,605,1044}.

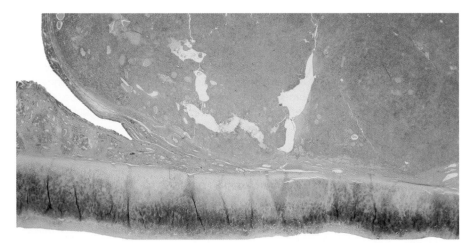

Fig. 1.34 Pleomorphic adenoma of nasal cavity. Tumour is circumscribed, and lies above the cartilage.

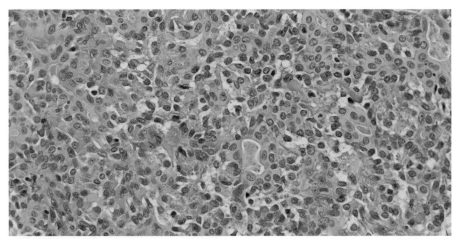

Fig. 1.35 Pleomorphic adenoma of nasal cavity. Tumour typically rich in modified myoepithelial cells.

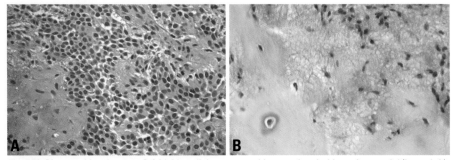

Fig. 1.36 Pleomorphic adenoma **A** A highly cellular tumour with myxochondroid matrix material (lower left). The cells are monotonous and plasmacytoid. **B** The myxochondroid matrix has a lacunar space (left), while short trabeculae of epithelial cells are seen within a more myxoid area.

Malignant soft tissue tumours

L.D.R. Thompson
J.C. Fanburg-Smith

Fibrosarcoma

Definition
A malignant tumour of fibroblastic/myofibroblastic phenotype.

ICD-O code 8810/3

Synonyms
Fibromyxosarcoma; chondromyxofibrosarcoma.

Epidemiology
The incidence of sinonasal tract fibrosarcomas is difficult to determine because the diagnosis is often one of exclusion. These tumours are rare, accounting for <3% of all non-epithelial tumours. However, they are considered the second most common soft tissue sarcoma after rhabdomyosarcoma in the head and neck {168,345,349,826,1041,1317, 2511}. They occur in all ages, with a peak in the 5th decade. There is a 3:2 female:male gender predilection {168, 345,826,1041,1317,2438,2511}.

Etiology
A few patients have developed fibrosarcoma within the field of prior irradiation.

Localization
Most fibrosarcomas originate in one or more paranasal sinuses, while origination confined to the nasal cavity alone is less common {168,345,826,1041,1317, 2438}. The "infantile-type" fibrosarcoma in the sinonasal tract is exceedingly uncommon in the sinonasal tract and occurs near the choana {349,1041, 1317}.

Clinical features
Nearly all patients have nasal obstruction, often associated with epistaxis, while pain, sinusitis, nasal discharge, swelling, anosmia, and proptosis are less common. The median duration of symptoms is quite short.

Macroscopy
The tumours are smooth, nodular, pedunculated, fungating or ulcerating. The lesions range in size between 2 and 8 cm, with the cut surface revealing a circumscribed but not encapsulated, fleshy, homogeneous white-tan to yellow-pink mass, variably firm dependent upon the collagen content. Necrosis and haemorrhage may be present in higher-grade tumours.

Histopathology
The tumours are unencapsulated, sometimes sharply circumscribed, although often infiltrative and occasionally ulcerating. Bone invasion is common. Surface epithelial invagination into the tumour can be prominent, simulating an inverted papilloma. Spindle cells are arranged in compact fascicles, intersected by various amounts of delicate thin to dense keloid-like collagen. The cell bundles are arranged at acute angles to one another, occasionally giving rise to a "herringbone" or "chevron" pattern, while in most areas there is a more subtle fasciculation. A prominent storiform pattern is not seen. There is a marked variability in the cellularity within and between tumours. The cells are fusiform with a centrally placed hyperchromatic, needle-like nucleus surrounded by tapering cytoplasm which is often indistinct, creating a syncytial appearance to the fascicles. Most sinonasal tract fibrosarcomas are low grade. Nuclear pleomorphism is usually slight to moderate, but occasionally prominent. Mitotic figures are found in variable numbers. Haemorrhage and necrosis can be found in the poorly differentiated forms, with areas of myxoid degeneration. Focal osteo-cartilaginous differentiation has been described {168, 345,826,1041,1317,2438}. Fibrosarcomas are immunoreactive with vimentin, and sometimes focally with actin {1041}.

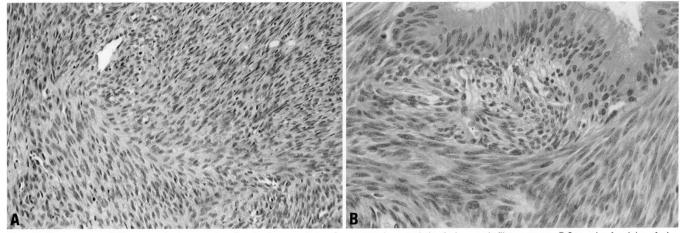

Fig. 1.37 Fibrosarcoma. **A** Short, angular intersections (herringbone or chevron) are most characteristic of a low grade fibrosarcoma. **B** Sweeping fascicles of minimally pleomorphic spindled cells can occasionally be seen. The overlying surface epithelium is unremarkable, including the presence of cilia.

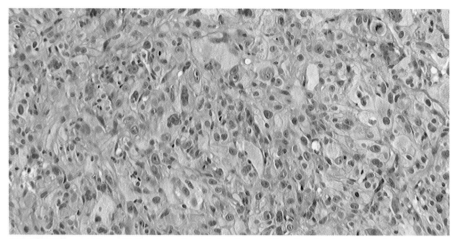
Fig. 1.38 Malignant fibrous histiocytoma. Remarkably pleomorphic cells with atypical mitotic figures.

Differential diagnosis

The differential diagnoses include malignant fibrous histiocytoma, spindle cell carcinoma, spindle malignant melanoma, malignant peripheral nerve sheath tumour, monophasic synovial sarcoma, rhabdomyosarcoma, glomangiopericytoma, desmoid fibromatosis, and nodular fasciitis {168,826,1041, 2332}.

Histogenesis

The (myo)fibroblast is considered the progenitor cell for these tumours.

Prognosis and predictive factors

Surgery is the treatment of choice, often followed by radiation therapy, yielding an overall long-term survival of 75% in low grade and localized tumours. The high incidence of recurrence (about 60%) is perhaps related to the complexity of the anatomy of the sinonasal tract and consequent difficulties of complete excision. Recurrence usually precedes metastasis, which occurs in about 15% of cases, most commonly to the lungs and bones and only rarely to lymph nodes. Poor prognostic factors include male gender, large tumour size, involvement of more than one contiguous site (nasal cavity and sinus, multiple sinuses), high histologic grade, and positive surgical margins {168,345,826,1041,1317,2438}.

Malignant fibrous histiocytoma

Definition

Malignant fibrous histiocytoma (MFH) is currently used as a diagnosis of exclusion for sarcomas composed largely of myofibroblasts or undifferentiated mesenchymal cells.

ICD-O code   8830/3

Synonyms

Fibroxanthosarcoma, malignant fibrous xanthoma, myxofibrosarcoma, myxoid malignant fibrous histiocytoma

Epidemiology

Although once considered the most common sarcoma of adults, the frequency of its diagnosis has diminished since the introduction of immunohistochemistry has allowed assignment of some pleomorphic sarcomas to specific sarcoma entities. Only 3% of MFH occur in the head and neck, with 30% of these arising in the sinonasal area {2187}. MFH rarely occurs in the nasopharynx {1032,1923}. Sinonasal MFH most commonly occurs in adults with a male predominance {2433}.

Etiology

Many sinonasal and nasopharyngeal MFH are a result of previous radiation, after a long latency period {1180,1345}.

Localization

The maxillary sinus is most commonly affected, followed by the ethmoid sinuses and nasal cavity, whereas the frontal and sphenoid sinuses and nasopharynx are affected far less commonly {279,536, 581,1032,1923,1936,2256,2426,2433}.

Clinical features

Symptoms include mass, swelling, facial pain, loose teeth, epistaxis, and nasal obstruction {279,1707,2015,2187,2426, 2433}.

Macroscopy

Tumours are generally smooth, nodular or pedunculated (polypoid), with a number being fungating or ulcerating. The cut surface reveals a fleshy, homogeneous white-tan to yellow-pink mass with necrosis and haemorrhage, measuring up to 8 cm in maximum dimension {714}.

Tumour spread and staging

Sinonasal MFH can directly extend into nasopharynx, orbit, and pituitary fossa {1032,1707} and commonly metastasizes to lungs, bones, liver, {1707,2426} and only rarely to lymph nodes {279,1032, 1707}.

Histopathology

Sinonasal MFH are generally infiltrative and ulcerative, but can occasionally be circumscribed. Pleomorphic MFH, the most frequent morphologic subtype of MFH in the sinonasal tract, is characterized by spindled to pleomorphic cells in a storiform growth pattern, with easily identified mitotic figures, including atypical forms, and necrosis. The cells are fusiform with tapering indistinct cytoplasm. Tumour giant cells with multiple nuclei may be found.

Immunohistochemistry

MFH are usually positive for vimentin and focally for actins. Importantly, MFH is a diagnosis of exclusion and is generally negative for desmin, skeletal muscle specific markers, S100 protein, HMB-45, epithelial markers and lymphoid markers.

Differential diagnosis

The differential diagnoses include fibrosarcoma, rhabdomyosarcoma, leiomyosarcoma, monophasic synovial sarcoma, malignant peripheral nerve sheath tumour, spindle cell carcinoma, spindle cell malignant melanoma and anaplastic large cell lymphoma.

Prognosis and predictive factors

Compared with other anatomical sites, MFHs of the head and neck generally have a slightly lower rate of recurrence and metastasis {133}.

Leiomyosarcoma

Definition
A malignant tumour of smooth muscle phenotype.

ICD-O code
8890/3

Epidemiology
Only a small number of sinonasal leiomyosarcomas have been reported {151,824,840,1144,1395,1416,1529, 2147,2240,2553}, accounting for <1% of all non-epithelial tumours. They occur in all ages, with a peak in the 6th decade (mean, 53 years) without a gender difference.

Etiology
There are a few reported cases with a prior history of radiation {824,1416,2147} or chemotherapy (cyclophosphamide specifically) {1416,2147}.

Localization
Involvement of both the nasal cavity and paranasal sinuses is more common than involvement of the nasal cavity alone {824,840,1144,1395,1416,1529,1745}.

Clinical features
Nearly all patients have nasal obstruction, frequently associated with epistaxis and pain, while nasal discharge, swelling, and blurred vision are less common. The duration of symptoms is usually long {824,840,1144,1395,1416, 1529,2147,2240,2553}. There is usually no lymphadenopathy. Plain radiographs show opacification of the nasal cavity or sinus(es), often suggesting sinusitis {1144,1395,1529,2553}.

Macroscopy
These tumours range in size up to 7 cm, with an average of about 4 cm. They are more likely infiltrative than circumscribed, and occasionally polypoid. The surface is typically ulcerated and crusted. These bulky tumours have a cut surface which reveals a soft to firm, greywhite and fleshy appearance. Haemorrhage, necrosis and cystic change are common.

Histopathology
Leiomyosarcomas are infiltrative neoplasms accompanied by surface ulceration. Bone or cartilage invasion is more frequent than surface or seromucinous gland invasion. Leiomyosarcomas are

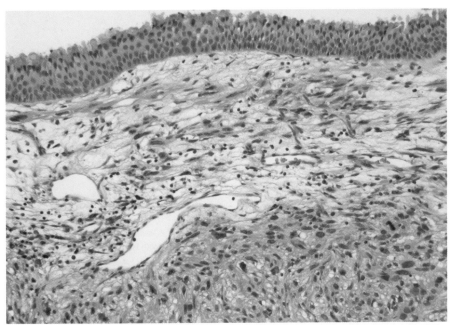

Fig. 1.39 Leiomyosarcoma. A spindle cell neoplasm with "cleared" cytoplasm, immediately adjacent to the nucleus, is seen below an intact surface mucosa. Mitotic figures are seen.

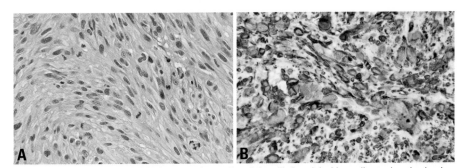

Fig. 1.40 Leiomyosarcoma. **A** A high power shows short, "cigar-like" nuclei with small cytoplasmic clearing adjacent to the nucleus. There are atypical mitotic figures. **B** Desmin reactivity in the remarkably pleomorphic tumour cells can help to confirm the smooth muscle differentiation.

composed of right-angle intersecting bundles of spindle cells. Palisading, storiform and "haemangiopericytoma-like" patterns can occur. The tumours are hypercellular, but coagulative tumour necrosis and haemorrhage can create a hypocellular appearance. The tumour cells have elongated, vesicular to hyperchromatic, lobulated or indented nuclei with blunt ends ("cigar-shaped"). The cytoplasm is fibrillary and eosinophilic, with frequent perinuclear vacuolation. Mitoses, both typical and atypical, are present to a variable degree {824,840, 1144,1395,1416,1529, 2147,2240,2553}.

Histochemistry and immunoprofile
Intracytoplasmic glycogen can be demonstrated with a PAS stain. Masson trichrome stain demonstrates red, longitudinally oriented parallel fibrils within the cytoplasm. Tumour cells are diffusely and strongly immunoreactive for vimentin, actin (smooth muscle or muscle-specific), desmin and h-caldesmon. There is generally no reactivity with keratin, CD34, CD117, S-100 protein or HMB-45 {1144,1395,2702}. The Ki-67 index is usually >15% {1144}.

Electron microscopy
Electron microscopy reveals variable features of smooth muscle cells, including myofilaments arranged in parallel arrays, dense bodies within the filaments, cell junctions, pinocytotic vesicles and basal lamina {1395,1529,1933}.

Differential diagnosis
The differential diagnoses include sinonasal glomangiopericytoma, periph-

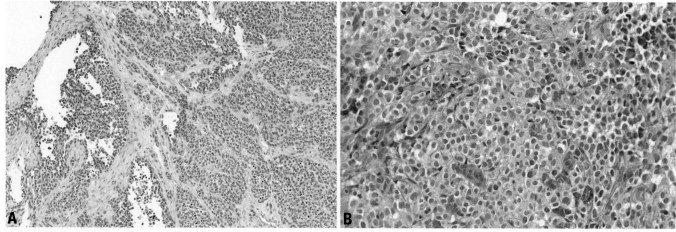

Fig. 1.41 Rhabdomyosarcoma **A** Nasal alveolar rhabdomyosarcoma, with typical alveolar pattern. **B** The tumour cells are ovoid and have hyperchromatic nuclei and scant eosinophilic cytoplasm.

eral nerve sheath tumour, fibrosarcoma, spindle cell carcinoma and melanoma {824,840,1144,1395,1416,1529,2147,22 40,2553,2603}.

Genetic susceptibility
There are isolated cases of children with leiomyosarcomas who have preexisting hereditary retinoblastomas {627}.

Prognosis and predictive factors
About half of the reported cases develop local recurrence, often within one year, and nearly 1/3 of these patients will subsequently develop metastasis (mostly to the lungs and liver). Complete surgical excision is difficult to achieve, and radiation and chemotherapy are used with variable results. {824,1416,2501}.
Poor prognostic factors include involvement of more than one contiguous site, large tumour size (>5 cm), high mitotic count (>20/10 high power field), tumour necrosis, and tumour stage {824,840, 1144,1395,1416,1529,2147,2240,2553}.

Rhabdomyosarcoma

Definition
A malignant tumour of skeletal muscle phenotype.

ICD-O code
8900/3
(Also see subtypes: 8910/3, 8912/3, 8920/3, 8901/3 in WHO Tumours of Soft Tissue)

Synonyms
Myosarcoma, malignant rhabdomyoma, rhabdosarcoma, embryonal sarcoma, rhabdomyoblastoma

Epidemiology
Approximately 40% of rhabdomyosarcomas occur in the head and neck {1978}, with about 20% in the nasal cavity, nasopharynx, and nasal sinuses {2745}. Rhabdomyosarcoma is the most common sarcoma in childhood. The embryonal subtype predominates in children, while the alveolar subtype predominates in adults {825,1273}. The pleomorphic subtype is rare {836,837}. There is an overall slight male predominance {825}.

Localization
The nasopharynx is more commonly involved than the sinonasal tract {326,724}. In adults, rhabdomyosarcoma is more common in the ethmoid sinuses, followed by the maxillary sinuses and nasopharynx {1856}.

Clinical features
Signs and symptoms include difficulty in breathing, epistaxis, facial swelling, visual disturbances, and sinusitis often of short duration. Tumours may appear as a large, polypoid sinonasal mass or may occasionally protrude as a gelatinous mass from the nares {825}.
CT and MRI imaging delineate the size and extent of the tumour {1453,2846}. The botryoid type shows grape-like rings and heterogeneous enhancement {980}.

Macroscopy
The embryonal subtype is generally poorly circumscribed, fleshy, pale and tan; the spindle cell variant is firm, fibrous, and tan-yellow with a whorled cut surface. The botryoid variant has a grape-like or polypoid appearance

{825}. The alveolar subtype is fleshy to firm tan-grey.

Tumour spread and staging
These tumours often spread to contiguous sites including base of the skull, temporal bones, and orbit {724,825}. About 40% metastasize to lymph nodes, bones, and lungs, and less commonly bone marrow, soft tissue, liver and brain {1441,1856}. The tumours are staged according to the Intergroup Rhabdomyosarcoma Study. Group I includes local disease, Group II residual disease or local spread, Group III incomplete resection or biopsy with gross residual disease, and Group IV metastatic disease at onset {613}. Most adult sinonasal and nasopharyngeal rhabdomyosarcomas are staged as Group III or IV at presentation {1856}.

Histopathology
Embryonal rhabdomyosarcoma has round to spindled cells with hyperchromatic nuclei. Larger rhabdomyoblasts with eosinophilic cytoplasm are usually identified, but cross striations are difficult to recognize. Myxoid stroma is common. The spindle cell variant, characterized by spindled cells in fascicular to storiform growth patterns, can be deceptively bland. The botryoid variant is polypoid with a submucosal hypercellular cambium layer, a myxoid hypocellular zone, and a deep cellular component.
Alveolar rhabdomyosarcoma typically has fibrous septa separating clusters of loosely cohesive groups of small to medium round tumour cells with hyperchromatic nuclei and scant eosinophilic cyto-

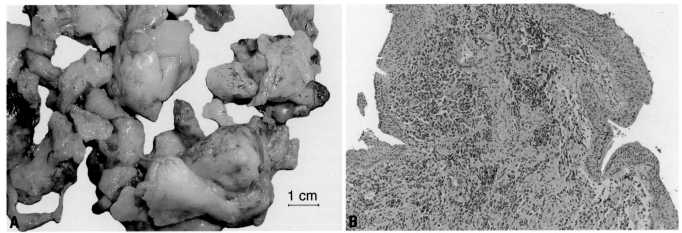

Fig. 1.42 Sinonasal rhabdomyosarcoma. **A** This macroscopic image demonstrates the similarity between a sinonasal polyp and a rhabdomyosarcoma. **B** Irregular islands of tumour in stroma may mimic carcinoma. Desmin and skeletal muscle markers can aid in the diagnosis of rhabdomyosarcoma.

plasm. Multinucleated giant cells with overlapping peripheral nuclei are often present. The solid variant grows in sheets and lacks septa. Rarely, the tumour can be composed exclusively or predominantly of clear cells. A mixed alveolar and embryonal pattern may occur.

Mitotic figures are usually easy to identify. Pleomorphism is occasionally observed focally. After treatment, there is often increased cytodifferentiation, with the cells exhibiting abundant eosinophilic fibrillary cytoplasm {2644}. Pleomorphic rhabdomyosarcoma is rare and uncommon in this location.

Immunohistochemistry
There is immunoreactivity for desmin, muscle specific actin, myoglobin, fast myosin, nuclear MyoD1 and nuclear myogenin (skeletal muscle myogenin,

myf4) {2619}. CD99 can be positive in 16% of cases {1084}.

Electron microscopy
Electron microscopy shows some degree of skeletal muscle differentiation ranging from well-formed Z-bands to incomplete sarcomeres with thick and thin filaments and ribosome-myosin complexes {724,837}.

Differential diagnosis
The differential diagnoses of embryonal rhabdomyosarcoma include sinonasal polyp with stromal atypia {1840} and various sarcomas. The differential diagnoses of alveolar rhabdomyosarcoma include various round blue cell tumours, including lymphoma, sinonasal undifferentiated carcinoma, small cell carcinoma of neuroendocrine type, mesenchymal chondrosarcoma, PNET/Ewing sarcoma,

olfactory neuroblastoma, and mucosal malignant melanoma.

Somatic genetics
Embryonal rhabdomyosarcoma shows allelic loss at 11p15 {271,925}. Alveolar rhabdomyosarcoma has a consistent translocation, usually t(2:13) (PAX3-FKHR), or less commonly t(1;13) (PAX7-FKHR) which can be performed on paraffin-embedded sections {141}.

Genetic susceptibility
Germline mutations of TP53 in Li-Fraumeni syndrome are found in some children with rhabdomyosarcoma.

Prognosis and predictive factors
Prognosis is determined by patient age, histologic subtype, and tumour clinical group {2123}. Younger patients have a more favourable prognosis than older

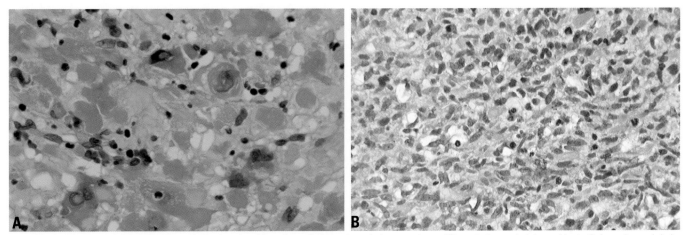

Fig. 1.43 A Alveolar rhabdomyosarcoma of nasal cavity. After chemotherapy, there is increased cytodifferentiation to rhabdomyoblasts. **B** An embryonal rhabdomyosarcoma demonstrates remarkably atypical spindle cells with small amounts of eosinophilic cytoplasm.

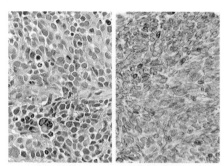

Fig. 1.44 Alveolar rhabdomyosarcoma showing scant cytoplasm surrounding atypical nuclei. There are small areas of eccentric eosinophilic cytoplasm (left). The tumour cells are strongly immunoreactive to desmin (right).

patients in all rhabdomyosarcoma subtypes. Currently, the 5-year survival is 44-69%, and 90% for clinical Group I disease {322,1084}. Adults have a poor prognosis, with 5-year survival of <10% {1841,1856}. Embryonal rhabdomyosarcoma has a better prognosis than alveolar rhabdomyosarcoma {2123}. Botryoid and spindle cell variants {346} have a better prognosis than embryonal rhabdomyosarcoma. Furthermore, alveolar rhabdomyosarcomas with PAX7/FKHR are thought to have better prognosis than PAX3/FKHR tumours {1298}.

Angiosarcoma

Definition
A malignant neoplasm of vascular phenotype whose constituent tumour cells have endothelial features.

ICD-O code   9120/3

Synonyms
Malignant haemangioendothelioma; malignant angioendothelioma; lymphangiosarcoma, haemangiosarcoma.

Epidemiology
Angiosarcoma is uncommon, accounting for less than 1% of all sinonasal tract malignancies {89,1603,1640,1848}. They occur in all ages, with a peak in the 5th decade, and a male predilection (male:female = 2:1). Females tend to be younger at presentation by up to a decade {823,1848,2633,2795,2812}.

Etiology
Radiation exposure {1556,1603,1848}, Thorotrast, arsenic and vinyl chloride are reported risk factors {2795}.

Localization
The maxillary sinus is most frequently affected. Other sites that may be involved primarily or secondarily include the nasal cavity and other paranasal sinuses {823,1848,2633,2795,2812}.

Clinical features
Patients present with recurrent epistaxis, profound pallor, a mass lesion, pain (including headache, otalgia, toothache), nasal obstruction, sinusitis, nasal discharge (often described as foul-smelling and blood tinged), paraesthesia and/or loose teeth. The duration of symptoms ranges from weeks to months, but is generally short (median, 4 months).

Lymph node and distant metastasis is not common at presentation.

Macroscopy
The tumours range up to 8 cm, with a mean of about 4 cm. They are nodular, polypoid and morulated, soft and friable, purple to red, often ulcerated with associated haemorrhage or clot and necrosis {823,1848,2633,2795,2812}.

Histopathology
Most sinonasal angiosarcomas are histologically low-grade. They infiltrate the adjacent tissues and bone, accompanied by necrosis and haemorrhage. They comprise tortuous anastomosing vascular channels that dissect the stroma, capillary-sized vessels and cavernous vascular spaces. The lining endothelial cells range from flat to plump spindly to epithelioid, and often form papillary tufts. Intracytoplasmic vacuoles (neolumen), often containing erythrocytes, are characteristic of the epithelioid variant. The degree of nuclear pleomorphism is variable. Mitotic figures, including atypical forms, are variably present {823,1848, 2633,2795,2812}.

Immunohistochemistry
Angiosarcomas are immunoreactive for CD34, CD31, Factor VIII R-Ag and vimentin, and focally keratin (especially the epithelioid variant) and actin {2812}.

Differential diagnosis
The differential diagnoses include granulation tissue, intravascular papillary

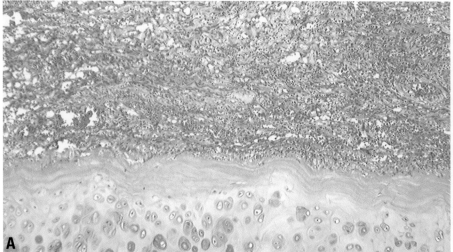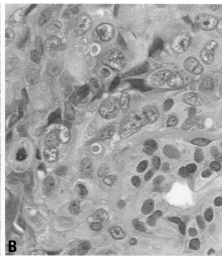

Fig. 1.45 Angiosarcoma. **A** A richly vascularized tumour abuts the cartilage. Many ramifying vascular channels are filled with erythrocytes. **B** A benign duct (right lower) is surrounded by a vascular neoplasm with "neolumen" formation and intraluminal erythrocytes. Note the mitotic figure.

endothelial hyperplasia, haemangioma, nasopharyngeal angiofibroma, angiolymphoid hyperplasia with eosinophilia, glomangiopericytoma, Kaposi sarcoma, malignant melanoma, carcinoma and large cell lymphoma {30,1388,1976, 2469,2764}.

Prognosis and predictive factors
Patients are usually treated by surgical resection with radiation and/or chemotherapy. Recurrences are common (50%), likely due to incomplete excision or possible multifocality. Metastasis is uncommon, and the predilection sites are the lung, liver, spleen, and bone marrow {1976}. The outcome is more favourable compared with the almost uniformly fatal outcome for cutaneous and soft tissue angiosarcomas {823, 1848,2633,2795,2812}

Malignant peripheral nerve sheath tumour

Definition
A malignant tumour of nerve sheath phenotype.

ICD-O code   9540/3

Synonyms
Neurogenic sarcoma, malignant schwannoma, neurofibrosarcoma.

Epidemiology
Malignant peripheral nerve sheath tumours (MPNSTs) comprise 2-14% of all

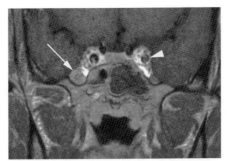

Fig. 1.46 Nerve sheath tumour of maxillary nerve. The nerve (arrow) at the entrance to foramen rotundum is enlarged compared to opposite side. This is similar to the appearance expected for perineural spread of malignancy. Note the carotid artery (arrowhead).

head and neck sarcomas {1231,1562}, arising de novo or less commonly in the setting of neurofibromatosis type 1 (NF1) {1059,1231,1795}. De novo MPNST peaks in the fourth decade, while those in the setting of NF1 occur at an earlier age. There is a female predominance for de novo sinonasal MPNST {1041}, and a male predominance in NF1-associated MPNST {774}.

Etiology
Radiation and possibly immunosuppression may be etiologic factors {1562}

Localization
They commonly arise from the ophthalmic and maxillary branches of the trigeminal (5th) cranial nerve, but can involve all of the sinonasal tract and nasopharynx {756,1153,1795,2018}.

Clinical features
Presenting symptoms include mass, pain, epistaxis, deviation or swelling of tonsils, nasal obstruction, and sinusitis {27,1319,1891,1964,2119}.

Macroscopy
MPNST is generally globoid to fusiform, pseudoencapsulated, cream-grey and firm, occasionally associated with surface ulceration. Infiltration into the surrounding soft tissues and bone is common. The tumours are often large (>5 cm) and may be attached to a nerve. Foci of cyst formation, necrosis and/or haemorrhage are frequent.

Tumour spread and staging
Local extension into contiguous structures along the path of the trigeminal nerve or through the foramen ovale are characteristic {1452}. MPNSTs metastasize to the lungs, bones, and/or liver, {1041} while the epithelioid variant tends to involve regional lymph nodes {1437}.

Histopathology
MPNSTs can either be spindled (95%) or epithelioid (5%) {1437}. At low magnification, both types show alternating areas of dense cellularity with less cellular myxoid areas. Geographic necrosis and perivascular accentuation of tumour cells are common. The tumour cells are fusiform and plump, arranged in tightly packed fascicles woven into a vague "herringbone" pattern, while in other areas the cells are wavy with fibrillar cytoplasmic extensions, arranged in a loose myxoid

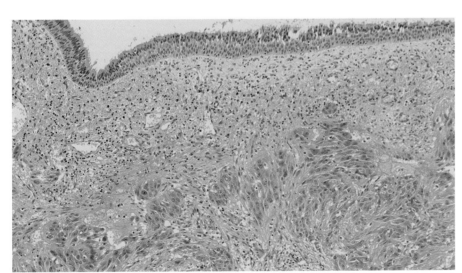

Fig. 1.47 Epithelioid malignant peripheral nerve sheath tumour (MPNST) of nasal cavity. Tumour composed of short fascicles of plump spindly or polygonal cells.

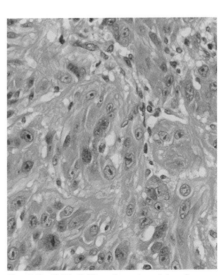

Fig. 1.48 Epithelioid malignant peripheral nerve sheath tumour of nasal cavity.

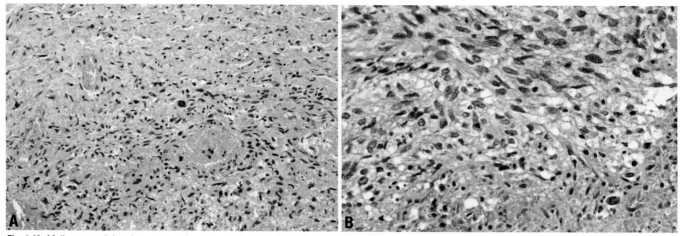

Fig. 1.49 Malignant peripheral nerve sheath tumour. **A** Increased cellularity with focal haemorrhage and hyperchromatic and atypical nuclei. **B** Highly cellular tumour with atypical spindle cell population with slightly 'wavy' nuclei. Note focal necrosis at the lower right corner.

background matrix. Focal palisading of nuclei may be present. The tumour cells are variably pleomorphic, with a high nuclear to cytoplasmic ratio and mitotic activity. Many sinonasal tract MPNSTs, in contrast to those occurring in other anatomic sites, are histologically and biologically low-grade {1041}. An origin from a nerve may or may not be apparent. MPNST with rhabdomyoblasts are known as malignant Triton tumours.

Immunohistochemistry
The spindle cell variant is usually focally positive for S100 protein and occasionally positive for glial fibrillary acidic protein (GFAP). However, up to 30% of MPNST may be negative for S100 protein {2784A}. The epithelioid variant is diffusely immunoreactive for S100 protein and may mimic malignant melanoma, {583,756,2603} but other melanoma markers are negative. In malignant Triton tumour, the rhabdomyoblasts are posi-

tive for desmin and other skeletal muscle markers.

Differential diagnosis
The differential diagnoses include synovial sarcoma, fibrosarcoma, spindle cell carcinoma, leiomyosarcoma and mucosal malignant melanoma {1041,2550, 2603}.

Precursor lesions
MPNST may arise from neurofibroma (especially in the setting of NF1) and only exceptionally from classic schwannoma.

Somatic genetics
Both NF1 alleles must be inactivated for MPNST to occur in NF1. Malignant progression from neurofibroma in NF1 is related to alterations of genes controlling cell cycle regulation, including TP53 {1459} and CDKN2A (which encodes p16) {1361,1895}.

Genetic susceptibility
MPNST of the sinonasal tract may be associated with NF1, typified by germline mutation of the NF1 tumour suppressor gene located on chromosome 17 {454}.

Prognosis and predictive factors
Surgery is the treatment of choice, although radiation and chemotherapy may have a palliative role. De novo sinonasal MPNSTs have a 5-year survival rate of about 90%, which is superior to that of 50-65% for MPNSTs arising in other anatomic locations {1041,1562,2715}. However, NF1-associated sinonasal MPNSTs have a 5-year survival rate of only about 15% {2119}. Poor prognostic factors include male gender, high tumour cellularity and high mitotic activity {1041}.

Borderline and low malignant potential tumours of soft tissues

L.D.R. Thompson
J.C. Fanburg-Smith
B.M. Wenig

Desmoid-type fibromatosis

Definition
A locally aggressive, cytologically bland tumour of (myo)fibroblastic phenotype.

ICD-O code
8821/1

Synonyms
Extra-abdominal desmoid, extra-abdominal fibromatosis, desmoid tumour, aggressive fibromatosis, juvenile desmoid-type fibromatosis, infantile fibromatosis.

Epidemiology
Although 15% of cases of desmoid-type fibromatosis occur in the head and neck, the sinonasal tract is uncommonly involved {6,903,2643}. All ages can be affected, especially children {903}. There is a male predilection {903}.

Localization
The maxillary sinus and turbinates are usually affected, and the involvement can occasionally be bilateral {514,826, 903}.

Clinical features
Symptoms include nasal obstruction, epistaxis, mass, facial pain, tooth displacement, and a non-healing tooth extraction site {514,826,903}.

Macroscopy
The lesion is tan-white, glistening, and rubbery to firm, and is often infiltrative. It measures up to 7 cm. Fibromatosis may be multicentric, especially in the setting of Gardner syndrome {562}.

Histopathology
This is an infiltrative growth with low to moderate cellularity, comprising broad fascicles of bland-looking spindle cells and collagen fibers often arranged in a uniform direction. Elongated blood vessels are frequently observed running parallel to each other.
The spindle cells have a myofibroblastic appearance, with low nuclear to cytoplasmic ratio and uniformly bland ovoid nuclei with indistinct nucleoli. Mitotic figures are infrequent and never atypical. The matrix is collagenized to focally myxoid, and keloid-like collagen may be present. The main differential diagnoses include hypertrophic scar and fibrosarcoma.
Diagnosis does not require immunohistochemistry, but vimentin and actins are positive. Desmin may be focally positive.

Genetic susceptibility
Fibromatosis can be part of Gardner syndrome {562}.

Prognosis and predictive factors
Fibromatosis can be locally aggressive and involve contiguous structures, with approximately 20% recurrence rate, but it does not metastasize {514,903,2643}. Recurrence generally occurs within the first few years and is related to inadequacy of surgical margins {514,903, 2643}.

Inflammatory myofibroblastic tumour

ICD-O code
8825/1

Inflammatory myofibroblastic tumour uncommonly occurs in the sinonasal tract {2429}. Please see corresponding section in 'Tumours of the hypopharynx, larynx and trachea'.

Glomangiopericytoma (Sinonasal-type haemangiopericytoma)

Definition
A sinonasal tumour demonstrating perivascular myoid phenotype.

ICD-O code
9150/1

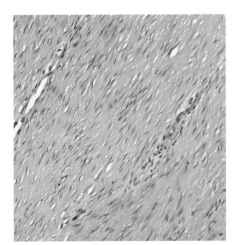

Fig. 1.50 Desmoid-type fibromatosis. Heavily collagenized stroma with spindle cells with bland nuclei and elongated vessels.

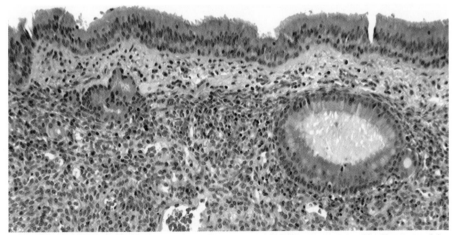

Fig. 1.51 Glomangiopericytoma. Characteristic diffuse growth within the submucosa, with effacement of the normal components of the submucosa and preservation of mucoserous glands. The overlying respiratory epithelium remains intact.

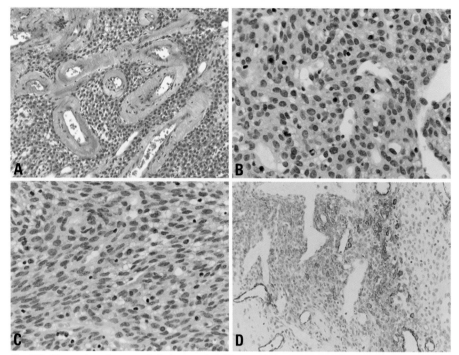

Fig. 1.52 Glomangiopericytoma. **A** A characteristic histomorphologic feature is the presence of prominent perivascular hyalinization. **B** Tumour cells are ovoid or polygonal. Note the delicate interspersed vascular spaces. **C** Streaming short spindly cells. Vascular spaces may not be obvious. **D** Immunostaining for muscle-specific actin is mainly in vessels and focally in tumour cells.

Synonyms

Sinonasal haemangiopericytoma; haemangiopericytoma-like tumour, sinonasal glomus tumour; haemangiopericytoma.

Epidemiology

Sinonasal glomangiopericytomas predilect to the nasal cavity and paranasal sinuses, where they comprise <0.5% of all neoplasms {343,482,2600}. There is a very slight female predominance. All ages can be affected (in-utero to 86 years), but the peak is in the 7th decade.

Localization

Tumours most frequently arise unilaterally in the nasal cavity alone, although extension into paranasal sinuses can occur. Isolated paranasal sinus involvement is uncommon. Rarely, large tumours may appear to arise bilaterally {216,343,482,638,649,681,1364,1779, 1846,2276,2600,2729}.

Clinical features

The majority of patients present with nasal obstruction, epistaxis, or non-specific findings, such as a mass, polyp, difficulty breathing, sinusitis, headache and nasal congestion, present for an average duration of <1 year. Imaging studies show nasal cavity or paranasal sinus opacification by a polypoid mass lesion, frequently accompanied by sinusitis, bone erosion and sclerosis {482,2600, 2729}.

Macroscopy

The generally polypoid tumours range up to 8 cm, with a mean size of about 3 cm. The tumours are beefy red to greyish pink, soft, edematous, fleshy to friable masses, often demonstrating haemorrhage.

Histopathology

This is a subepithelial well-delineated but unencapsulated cellular tumour, effacing or surrounding the normal structures. It is comprised of closely packed cells, forming short fascicles and sometimes exhibiting a storiform, whorled or palisaded pattern, interspersed with many vascular channels. The latter are in the form of capillary-sized to large patulous spaces that may have a "staghorn" or "antler-like" configuration. A prominent peritheliomatous hyalinization is characteristic. The neoplastic cells are uniform, elongated to oval, and possess vesicular to hyperchromatic, round to oval to spindle-shaped nuclei, and lightly eosino-philic cytoplasm. Mild nuclear pleomorphism and occasional mitotic figures may be present, but necrosis is not found. Extravasated erythrocytes, mast cells, and eosinophils are nearly ubiquitously present. Occasionally, tumour giant cells, fibrosis or myxoid degeneration may be seen.

Immunohistochemistry

Immunohistochemically, glomangiopericytoma is distinctly different from soft tissue haemangiopericytoma by yielding diffuse reactivity for actins, factor XIIIA and vimentin, and lacking strong diffuse staining for CD34. Bcl-2, FVIII-R Ag, CD99 and CD117 are negative {343, 638,1364,2070,2600}.

Differential diagnosis

The differential diagnoses include haemangioma, solitary fibrous tumour, glomus tumour, leiomyoma, synovial sarcoma and leiomyosarcoma.

Histogenesis

This tumour has been known as haemangiopericytoma-like tumour or sinonasal haemangiopericytoma, but it is clinically, morphologically and biologically distinct from soft tissue-type or dura-based haemangiopericytoma {446,544,773,936, 1723,1724,2276,2386,2689}. The proposed cell of origin is a modified perivascular glomus-like myoid cell.

Prognosis and predictive factors

Sinonasal glomangiopericytoma is indolent, with an overall excellent survival (>90% 5-year survival) achieved with complete surgical excision. Recurrence, which develops in up to 30% of cases, may occur many years after the initial surgery {216,343,638,649,2600}. Aggressive-behaving glomangiopericytomas (malignant glomangiopericytomas) are uncommon {216,343,482, 556,1779,2600}, and usually exhibit the following features: large size (>5 cm), bone invasion, profound nuclear pleomorphism, increased mitotic activity (>4/10 high power fields), necrosis, and proliferation index >10% {216,343,1364, 2600}.

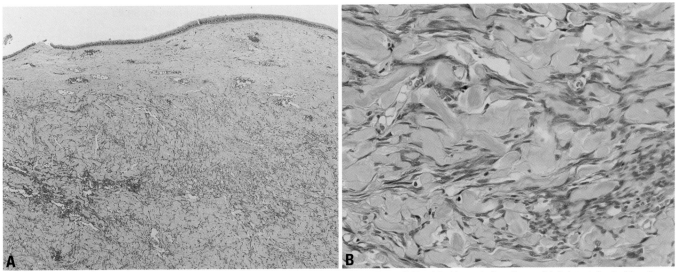

Fig. 1.53 Solitary fibrous tumour of nasal cavity. **A** Circumscribed tumour beneath epithelium. **B** Bland-looking spindly cells are tightly intertwined with collagen fibers.

Extrapleural solitary fibrous tumour

ICD-O code   8815/1

Solitary fibrous tumours are tumours of CD34-positive fibroblasts which often show a prominent haemangiopericytoma-like vascular pattern. They are exceedingly uncommon in the upper respiratory tract, where they comprise <0.1% of all neoplasms. All ages can be affected without a gender predilection. Tumours can affect the nasal cavity, nasopharynx or paranasal sinuses. Patients present with nasal obstruction, epistaxis or other nonspecific symptoms. The tumour is usually polypoid and firm. It is composed of a variably cellular proliferation of bland spindle-shaped cells with nondescript growth pattern associated with "ropy" keloidal collagen bundles and interlaced thin-walled vascular spaces. The latter may be prominent and exhibit a haemangiopericytoma-like pattern. Solitary fibrous tumours are immunoreactive for CD34 and bcl-2, and generally lack actin immunoreactivity. The diagnosis rests on a combination of architectural, cytomorphologic, and immunophenotypic features. The differential diagnoses include sinonasal glomangiopericytoma, fibrous histiocytoma, leiomyoma, schwannoma, synovial sarcoma, and fibrosarcoma. Complete surgical removal yields the best patient outcome. Occasional cases may potentially show a malignant behaviour {158,834,997,1706,2600,2800, 2914}. See WHO Classification of Tumours of Soft Tissue and Bone {775}.

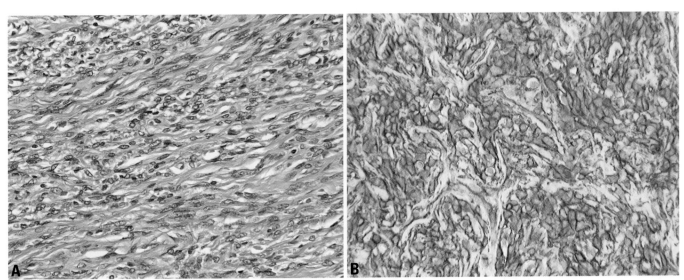

Fig. 1.54 Solitary fibrous tumour **A** Cytologically bland cells are arranged in streaming fashion, with collagen deposited between the cells. Haemorrhage is seen.. **B** A solitary fibrous tumour strongly and diffusely immunoreactive for CD34.

Benign soft tissue tumours

J.C. Fanburg-Smith
L.D.R. Thompson

Myxoma

Myxoma is a benign soft tissue tumour characterized by bland spindle shaped cells enbedded in hypovascular, myxoid stroma. For details see Chapter 6 (Odontogenic tumours).

Leiomyoma

Definition
A benign tumour of smooth muscle phenotype.

ICD-O code   8890/0

Synonyms
Angioleiomyoma; vascular leiomyoma; leiomyoblastoma

Epidemiology
Primary leiomyomas of the sinonasal tract are very rare {824,975,1144,1307, 1535,1796,2114,2635,2695}. There is a peak in the 6th decade, although men are younger than women by a decade at initial diagnosis. There is a female predilection, with a ratio of 3.5:1.

Etiology
Other than prior radiation, there are no known risk factors.

Localization
The turbinates are affected most frequently, {824,1144,1307,1535,1796, 2114,2635,2695} with isolated cases reported in the paranasal sinuses alone or in combination with the nasal cavity {1842}.

Clinical features
Nearly all patients have nasal obstruction, although nasal discharge, epistaxis, headaches and pain are also common {824,2114,2635,2695}.

Macroscopy
These tumours have an average size of 2 cm, but rare ones may be as large as 10 cm. They are sessile or polypoid, with a smooth, well circumscribed border.

Histopathology
Leiomyomas are located in the submucosa, separated from a typically intact mucosa. They are composed of spindled cells arranged in orderly fascicles, whorls and intersecting bundles. The cells have elongated, vesicular to stippled nuclei with blunt ends ("cigar-shaped"), surrounded by spindled, bipolar, fibrillar eosinophilic cytoplasm. They are highly differentiated, with little or no atypia, although rare cells may exhibit nuclear pleomorphism {2695}. Necrosis and invasion are absent, and mitotic activity is scarce. Mucinous degeneration, hyalinization or fibrosis, and adipocytes can be seen, but these features are usually focal and more likely seen in larger lesions {1144,1535,1796, 2695}. Vascular leiomyoma (angiomyoma) contains capillary, cavernous or venous vascular spaces, with the smooth muscle cells being associated with the vessel walls and represents the most common type of benign smooth muscle tumour in this region.

Immunoprofile
The tumour cells are diffusely and strongly immunoreactive for actins, desmin, h-caldesmon and vimentin. The Ki-67 index is usually <5% {1144}.

Differential diagnosis
The differential diagnoses include sinonasal glomangiopericytoma, haemangioma, peripheral nerve sheath tumour and leiomyosarcoma.

Prognosis and predictive factors
Complete excision is curative.

Haemangioma

Definition
A benign neoplasm of vascular phenotype.

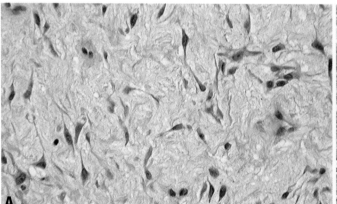
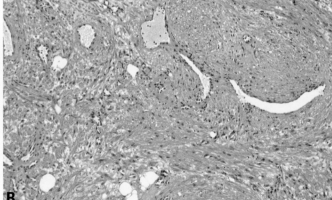

Fig. 1.55 A Myxoma. The stellate cells have thin processes which extend out into the background mucinous matrix. **B** Vascular leiomyoma. Spindle tumour cells are identified scrolling off thick muscle-walled vessels.

ICD-O code   9120/0

Synonyms
Lobular capillary haemangioma; pyogenic granuloma; capillary haemangioma; cavernous haemangioma; epulis gravidarum.

Epidemiology
Mucosal haemangiomas of the nasal cavity, paranasal sinuses and nasopharynx account for 10% of all head and neck haemangiomas and approximately 25% of all non-epithelial neoplasms of this anatomical region. The haemangiomas occur in all ages, although there is a peak in children and adolescent males, females in the reproductive years, and then an equal distribution beyond 40 years of age. Patients with cavernous haemangiomas tend to be men in the 5th decade {166,167,658,823,1037,1189, 1270,1738,2056,2333}.

Etiology
Lobular capillary haemangioma (pyogenic granuloma) has an association with injury and hormonal factors (pregnancy or oral contraceptive use) {2158}.

Localization
The septum is most frequently affected (specifically, the anterior septum in Little's area), followed by the turbinate (usually the tip) and the sinuses {658, 823,1037,1189,1270,1738,2056,2753}.

Clinical features
Patients present with unilateral epistaxis and/or an obstructive painless mass. Sinus lesions present as sinusitis, proptosis, mass, anaesthesia or pain. Symptoms are usually present for a short duration {658,823,1037,1189,1270,1738, 2056,2333,2753}.

Macroscopy
The tumours range up to 5 cm, with a mean size of <1.5 cm. Grossly, they appear as a red to blue submucosal soft, compressible, flat or polypoid lesion, often with an ulcerated surface. Cavernous haemangiomas are spongy on sectioning {658,823,1037,1189,1270, 1738,2056,2333,2753}.

Histopathology
Haemangiomas are usually localized and can be divided into capillary and cavernous types based on the size of the blood vessels. Haemangiomatosis is a more diffuse lesion often involving contiguous structures {823,1270,2126}.
Lobular capillary haemangioma is a circumscribed lesion comprising lobules of capillaries lined by plump endothelial cells and supported by prominent pericytes. The lobules are separated by a fibromyxoid stroma. The cellularity of the lobules may be quite high. Mitotic figures are often observed, but are never atypical. The surface epithelium often forms collarettes around the lesion {658, 823,1037,1189,1270,1738,2056,2333}. If the lesion is ulcerated and inflamed, the term 'pyogenic granuloma' has been applied.
Cavernous haemangiomas are frequently intraosseous or involve the turbinates or lateral nasal wall. They are composed of multiple, large thin-walled, dilated blood vessels separated by scant fibrous stroma {658,823,1037,1189,1270,1738, 2056,2333}.

Venous haemangiomas are composed of thick-walled veins with abundant smooth muscle, but rarely occur in this location.

Immunoprofile
The tumour cells are immunoreactive for Factor VIII related antigen, CD34, CD31 and Ulex europaeus I lectin. The proliferated blood vessels are enwrapped by actin-positive pericytes.

Differential diagnosis
Haemangiomas should be distinguished from granulation tissue, telangiectasia, vascular malformations, vascular polyps (haemorrhagic type), papillary endothelial hyperplasia, angiofibroma, bacillary angiomatosis, angiolymphoid hyperplasia with eosinophilia, glomus tumour, sinonasal glomangiopericytoma, lymphangioma, Kaposi sarcoma, and angiosarcoma. Haemangioma can be distinguished from granulation tissue by the lobular arrangement of the capillaries in the former and the more parallel arrangement of vessels in the latter. The distinction between a haemangioma and telangiectasia may be difficult but is facilitated in a patient with a known family history of hereditary haemorrhagic telangiectasia (Osler-Weber-Rendu syndrome) {658,823,1037,1189,1270,1738,2056, 2073,2333,2600}.

Prognosis and predictive factors
Haemangiomas are generally easy to remove, although larger tumours may be complicated by excessive bleeding. They should be removed in all ages, especially in children since aplasia of the nasal cartilages may cause eventual disfigurement. If the tumour is pregnancy-

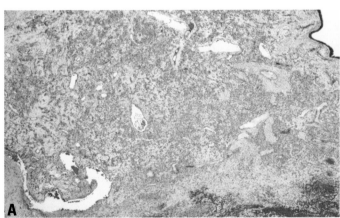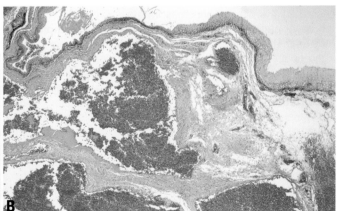

Fig. 1.56 Haemangioma. **A** A lobular arrangement around large patulous vessels is seen in this lobular capillary haemangioma. **B** Cavernous haemangioma with large, dilated vascular spaces and an intact surface epithelium.

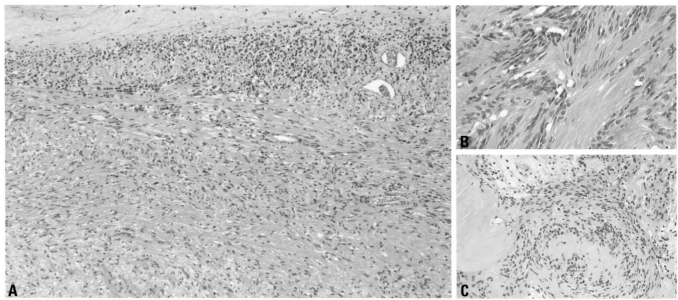

Fig. 1.57 Schwannoma. **A** A well circumscribed spindle cell neoplasm has focal degeneration with a lymphoid cuff. **B** Nuclear palisading around fibrillar cellular processes is characteristic for a peripheral nerve sheath tumour. **C** Hyalinized vessel next to a Verocay body with palisaded nuclei.

related, regression will often occur after parturition. Multiple recurrences are more common in children if the lesional bed is not completely eradicated.

Schwannoma

Definition
A usually encapsulated, benign tumour composed of differentiated, neoplastic Schwann cells.

ICD-O code   9560/0

Synonyms
Neurilemoma, neurilemmoma, benign peripheral nerve sheath tumour.

Epidemiology
Less than 4% of schwannomas involve the nasal cavity and paranasal sinuses {1091,2351}, and they occur in middle-aged adults with an equal gender distribution {2351}.

Localization
Sinonasal schwannomas arise from the branches of the trigeminal (5th) nerve and autonomic nervous system, and most commonly involve the ethmoid and maxillary sinuses, followed by the nasal cavity, sphenoid and frontal sinuses {1023,1091,2018,2351}. Cellular schwannoma tends to be located in the midline.

Clinical features
The presenting symptoms include obstruction, rhinorrhea, epistaxis, anosmia, headache, dysphagia, hearing loss, facial or orbital swelling, and pain {2018,2351}.

Macroscopy
Sinonasal schwannoma ranges in size up to 7 cm. It is a well-delineated but non-encapsulated globular, firm to rubbery yellow-tan mass. The cut surfaces show tan-grey, yellowish, solid to myxoid and cystic tissue, commonly with haemorrhage.

Tumour spread and staging
The tumour can expand into the orbit, nasopharynx, pterygomaxillary fossa and cranial cavity {2351}.

Histopathology
Schwannoma is composed of cellular Antoni A areas with Verocay bodies and hypocellular myxoid Antoni B areas. The cells are fusiform with elongated fribillary cytoplasm, and buckled to spindled nuclei which show little pleomorphism, although scattered large pleomorphic or bizarre cells can be present in some cases. Nuclear palisading is often evident in some foci. There are frequently small to medium-sized vessels with ectasia, thrombosis and perivascular hyalinization in the Antoni B areas. Extensive degenerative changes can occur, and

may result in only a thin rim of recognizable tumour. Cellular variants exhibit only the Antoni A pattern, but no fascicular growth or Verocay bodies.

Immunoprofile
The tumour cells are strongly and diffusely immunoreactive for S100 protein. CD34 only stains some more slender cells in the Antoni B areas. Neurofilament is absent. GFAP and keratins may be positive.

Prognosis and predictive factors
Schwannoma is a benign tumour with a very low recurrence potential. Malignant transformation is exceptional {1690}.

Neurofibroma

Definition
A benign tumour of peripheral nerve sheath phenotype with mixed cellular components, including Schwann cells, perineurial hybrid cells and intraneural fibroblasts.

ICD-O code   9540/0

Epidemiology
Neurofibromas are extremely rare in the sinonasal tract. In NF1-related neurofibromas, patients tend to be younger, with a male predominance {2745}. For the more common sporadic neurofibromas,

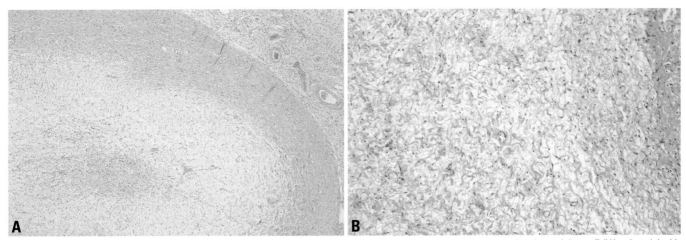

Fig. 1.58 Neurofibroma. **A** A central "circumscribed" area has cellular and hypocellular areas. There is nerve tissue noted at the periphery. **B** "Wavy" nuclei with bundles of collagen separated by a myxoid, degenerated stroma.

all ages may be affected, although patients tend to be older with an equal gender distribution.

Localization
The tumour arises from the ophthalmic or maxillary branches of the trigeminal (5th) nerve and is most commonly located in the maxillary and ethmoid sinuses and/or nasal cavity {288}. Plexiform neurofibroma may occur in the sinonasal area where it is found in the maxillary sinus {817}, usually associated with NF1.

Clinical features
Symptoms include epistaxis, rhinorrhoea, swelling, mass, obstruction, and pain {61,2018}.

Macroscopy
The tumour is firm, glistening, grey-tan, fusiform, and sometimes polypoid, in a submucosal location with an intact surface epithelium {61,1095}.

Histopathology
Neurofibromas are generally submucosal paucicellular lesions. They are composed of spindled cells with wavy, dark-staining nuclei and scanty cytoplasm, in a background of wavy collagen fibres, myxoid stroma and mast cells. The centre of the lesion usually shows residual neurites.

Immunoprofile
The tumour is diffusely immunoreactive for S100 protein, but the proportion of positive cells is lower than that in schwannoma. CD34 stains the admixed fibroblasts.

Genetic susceptibility
Sinonasal neurofibromas are generally not associated with NF1 {1091,1095, 2018}.

Prognosis and predictive factors
Neurofibromas are benign and have a very low recurrence rate. A small percentage of cases may undergo malignant transformation.

Meningioma

Definition
A benign neoplasm of meningothelial cells.

ICD-O code   9530/0

Epidemiology
Primary extracranial (ectopic, extracalvarial) meningiomas of the sinonasal tract are rare, comprising <0.5% of non-

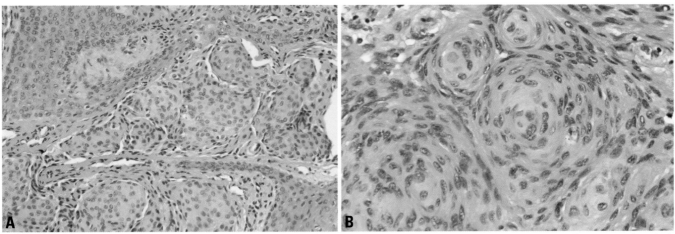

Fig. 1.59 Meningioma. **A** Meningothelial growth and "whorling". Note the squamous mucosa intimately associated with the meningioma. **B** "Whorling" of cytologically bland meningeal cells is prominent in this meningioma.

epithelial neoplasms {814,873,1109, 1781,2019,2221,2599}. They should be distinguished from intracranial meningiomas with extracranial/extraspinal extension into the sinonasal tract {721, 814,2599}. Any age can be affected, and there is a slight female predilection. Men tend to be younger than women by about a decade.

Localization

Sinonasal tract meningiomas involve both the nasal cavity and paranasal sinuses more frequently than either location alone. Most tumours are left-sided {814,873,1109,1781,2019,2221,2599}.

Clinical features

Symptoms include a mass (often polypoid), nasal obstruction, epistaxis, sinusitis, pain, headache, seizure, exophthalmos, periorbital edema, visual disturbance, ptosis, and facial deformity {814,873,1109,1781,2019,2221,2599}. Symptoms are present for an average of 4 years.

Macroscopy

The tumours range up to 8 cm, with a mean of about 3 cm. They may infiltrate bone and rarely ulcerate the mucosa. The cut surface is grey-white, tan or pink, gritty, firm to rubbery. Calcifications and fragments of bone are frequently visible.

Tumour spread and staging

Primary extra-cranial meningiomas have not been reported to metastasize {814, 873,2019,2599}.

Histopathology

Sinonasal meningiomas can exhibit a variety of histological patterns, most commonly meningotheliomatous, characterized by lobules of cells with whorl formation, indistinct cell borders, and bland nuclei with delicate chromatin {1329,2599}. Intranuclear pseudoinclusions and psammoma bodies are common. Other variants can also occur in the sinonasal tract, such as transitional, metaplastic (lipidized cells within tumour), and psammomatous type {1329}.

Immunoprofile

Meningiomas are immunoreactive for epithelial membrane antigen and vimentin, but usually negative for cytokeratin, although rare lesions can exhibit focal and weak cytokeratin immunoreactivity. They are frequently positive for progesterone receptor (50%) and occasionally for oestrogen receptor (25%). Glial fibrillary acidic protein and smooth muscle actin are negative.

Differential diagnosis

The differential diagnoses include carcinoma, melanoma, aggressive psammomatoid ossifying fibroma and follicular dendritic cell sarcoma/tumour {2599, 2771}.

Histogenesis

Meningiomas are derived from arachnoid cap cells located extra-cranially within the sheaths of nerves or vessels.

Prognosis and predictive factors

Complete surgical extirpation is sometimes difficult, and accounts for the up to 30% recurrence rate {1109,2019,2599}. The rare deaths are related to compromise of mid-facial structures or complications of surgery, rather than the aggressive nature of the tumour. Histologic features (such as hypercellularity, nuclear pleomorphism, necrosis), proliferation index and progesterone receptor status do not influence prognosis {1138,1139,1426,1666,2599}.

Malignant tumours of bone and cartilage

K. Saito
K.K. Unni

Chondrosarcoma, including mesenchymal chondrosarcoma

Definition
Chondrosarcoma is a malignant tumour of hyaline cartilage.

Mesenchymal chondrosarcoma is a malignant small round cell neoplasm with focal cartilaginous differentiation, and often with a pericytomatous vascular pattern.

ICD-O codes
Chondrosarcoma   9220/3
Mesenchymal chondrosarcoma
                                    9240/3

Synonym
Polyhistioma

Epidemiology
These tumours are rare in the facial skeleton. Chondrosarcomas account for <16% of all sarcomas of the nasal cavity, paranasal sinuses and nasopharynx {256,463,1367,4045}. Chondrosarcoma affects older adults, with a male predilection.

Mesenchymal chondrosarcoma is extremely rare, and affects young adults, with a female predilection.

Localization
Chondrosarcoma involves the alveolar portion of the maxilla, the maxillary sinus or the nasal septum. Mesenchymal chondrosarcoma involves the mandible and maxilla almost equally.

Clinical features
Patients with involvement of the nose present with nasal obstruction. Painful swelling is common with other sites of involvement.

Imaging
On plain radiographs, both tumours show osteolysis with stippled calcification, cortical destruction and possible soft tissue extension. Computerized tomograms and magnetic resonance images are useful in evaluating the extent of disease {463}.

Macroscopy
Chondrosarcomas are lobulated pale-blue glistening masses that may show cystic change. Mesenchymal chondrosarcomas have the fish-flesh appearance of high-grade sarcomas; chalky foci of calcification may offer a diagnostic clue.

Histopathology
Chondrosarcomas are often lobulated, and show round to oval cells in lacunae with a blue chondroid matrix that may show myxoid changes. Most are low-grade. Increased cellularity and permeation of the intertrabecular spaces of bone, if identified, are the most important features that distinguish chondrosarcoma from chondroma. Radiological corre-

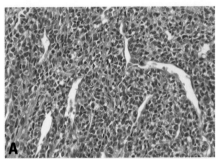
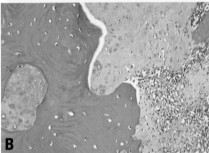
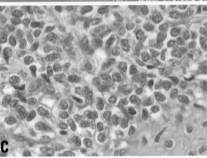

Fig. 1.62 Mesenchymal chondrosarcoma. **A** Small cells with scant cytoplasm arranged in a "haemangiopericytoma-like" pattern around open vascular channels without chondroid matrix identified in this field. **B** Normal Haversian bone is invaded by chondrosarcoma which blends with areas of undifferentiated mesenchymal cells (lower right). **C** The chondroid matrix shows lacunar spaces filled with the same nuclei identified in the mesenchymal component. Vague lacunar spaces surround the undifferentiated mesenchymal cells which display coarse nuclear chromatin in irregularly shaped nuclei. From P.D. Knott et al. {1343}.

lation is required for a definitive diagnosis {4045}.

Mesenchymal chondrosarcomas show a mixture of hyaline cartilage and small round to oval cells with hyperchromatic nuclei, frequently arranged in a pericytomatous vascular pattern. These cells

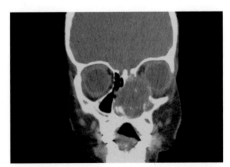

Fig. 1.60 Chondrosarcoma. CT shows a destructive lesion arising in nasal cavity invading into maxillary sinus. Note focal calcification.

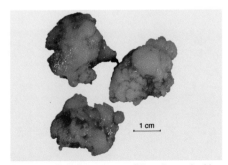

Fig. 1.61 Chondrosarcoma. Glistening pale blue fragments of cartilage.

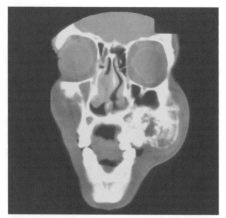

Fig. 1.63 CT of an osteosarcoma of the maxilla. The destructive lesion extends into soft tissue, producing a sunburst pattern of tumour bone.

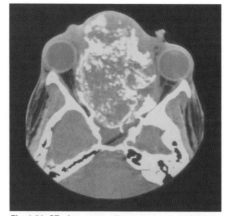

Fig. 1.64 CT of an unusual osteosarcoma arising in nose. The mineral present suggests cartilage differentiation.

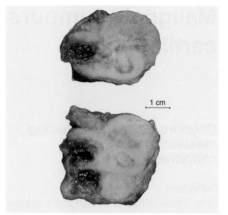

Fig. 1.66 Osteosarcoma. Gross specimen of osteosarcoma. The tumour is fleshy and surrounds the root of a tooth.

are frequently immunoreactive for CD99. The relative amounts of the two elements are quite variable. The chondroid lobules have the appearance of well-differentiated chondrosarcoma.

Prognosis and predictive factors

Chondrosarcomas are associated with an excellent prognosis if the lesions are completely resected. Approximately 20% of patients die of tumour, most often with uncontrolled local recurrence {2223,4045}

Mesenchymal chondrosarcoma is a high-grade tumour with an unpredictable prognosis. Patients with tumour of the facial skeleton do better than those with tumours of the remainder of the skeleton {2687}.

Osteosarcoma

Definition

Osteosarcoma is a primary malignant tumour of bone in which the neoplastic cells produce osteoid or bone.

ICD-O code   9180/3

Synonym

Osteogenic sarcoma

Epidemiology

Osteosarcomas of the jaws are very rare, with an incidence of 0.7 per million {868}. They are extremely rare in other head and neck sites. Patients are a decade older than those with extragnathic osteosarcomas {455,868,1366}. There is a modest male predilection.

Etiology

Over 10% of tumours are post-radiation, including Thorotrast exposure.

Localization

The maxilla and the mandible are affected almost equally. In the maxilla, the alveolar ridge and the antrum are predominantly involved, whereas in the mandible, the body is the main site.

Clinical features

Symptoms include swelling with or with-

out pain and loosening of teeth.

On plain radiograph, the tumour is usually lytic but may be sclerotic or mixed. In over half of the lesions, there is soft tissue extension. Computerized tomogram is better in demonstrating matrix mineralization and soft tissue extension {1457}.

Macroscopy

The tumours vary from the lobulated blue colour of cartilage to fleshy white to densely sclerotic masses.

Histopathology

Osteosarcomas of the jaws are generally better differentiated than extragnathic osteosarcomas. There is commonly chondroblastic differentiation, characterized by lobules of atypical-appearing chondrocytes in lacunae. There is a typical condensation of nuclei toward the periphery of the lobules, where sheets of spindle cells may be seen. The centre of the chondroid lobules shows bone formation in the form of trabeculae.

The remainder show osteoblastic or fibroblastic features. It is unusual to see benign giant cells within the tumour.

Prognosis and predictive factors

Some studies have shown that patients with osteosarcoma of the jaws have a better survival than those with extragnathic osteosarcomas {455,1366}. However, some other studies {206,868} have not confirmed this finding. Complete surgical resection is associated with better prognosis.

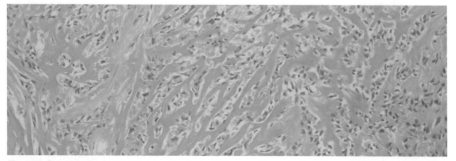

Fig. 1.65 Osteoblastic osteosarcoma with a typical filigree pattern of osteoid formation.

Benign tumours of bone and cartilage

G. Jundt
F. Bertoni
K.K. Unni
K. Saito
L.P. Dehner

Fibrous dysplasia

See Chapter 6 for details.

Giant cell lesion

Synonym
Giant cell granuloma.

Extragnathic giant cell lesion may rarely involve the paranasal sinuses {2161, 2243,2479,2648,2839}. Symptoms include pain, visual disturbances, exophthalmos, epistaxis, lacrimation, anaesthesia and swellings {728,1867,2322, 2839}.

Plain radiographs show nonspecific osteolytic defects. Their extent and possible impingement on brain or orbital contents is better visualized in cross sectional studies (CT, MRI) {2322,2839}. Brown tumour of hyperparathyrodism should be excluded.

Please refer to Chapter 6 for details.

Giant cell tumour of bone

Definition
An aggressive but benign neoplasm containing spindle-shaped stromal cells, mononuclear round to oval cells resembling histiocytes, and abundant evenly distributed osteoclastic giant cells.

ICD-O code   9250/1

Epidemiology
Giant cell tumour (GCT) accounts for about 5% of all bone tumours. Most cases occur in patients between 20 and 50 years {523,775,1146,1369}. CGT is slightly more common in women than in men {523,775,2831}.

Localization
In the skull, in the absence of Paget disease, the bones developing from endochondral ossification, i.e. sphenoid, ethmoid and temporal bone, are almost exclusively involved {207,496,870,875}.

Clinical features
Signs and symptoms
Clinical symptoms of GCTs depend on the site of occurrence. Sphenoidal lesions are associated with headache, diplopia and vision impairment or cranial nerve palsies (II, III, IV, V, VI and combinations). Temporal bone involvement causes deafness (conductive: middle ear and mastoid; sensorineural combined with vertigo: petrous bone), retroauricular pain, or swelling {676, 2328}. Duration of symptoms ranges from weeks to years {207}.

Imaging
On plain radiographs and CT, GCT presents with a nonspecific expansile and destructive osteolysis, generally lacking any matrix mineralization. The lesion shows contrast enhancement on CT {207,2177,2806}. A soft tissue mass in

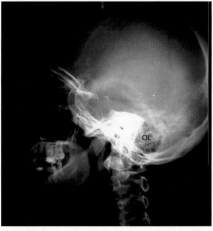

Fig. 1.67 Giant cell tumour. Large geographic osteolytic lesion (OL) at the base of the skull with an irregular dorsal margin.

the sphenoid sinus or the sella turcica, displacing the pituitary gland, is best seen on cross-sectional studies (CT, MRI) {983,2177,2556}.

Histopathology
The tumour is characterized by abundant multinucleated osteoclastic giant cells, with up to 50-100 nuclei, that are evenly distributed among sheets of stromal cells. In some areas, ovoid to plump spindled stromal cells are more prominent, and giant cells may be lacking. Regressive changes, including fibrosis, foam cell aggregates, haemosiderin deposits, and even necrosis may be present. Small foci of reactive woven bone are often seen. Mitoses are easily

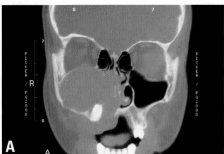
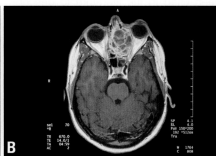
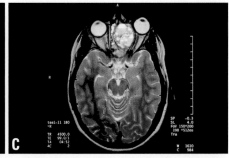

Fig. 1.68 Central giant cell lesion/granuloma. **A** Osteodestructive lesion of the right maxillary sinus extending into the nasal cavity, eroding the orbital floor and destroying the alveolar process of the maxilla with protrusion into the oral cavity.. **B** On T1 images the signal intensity is low. **C** Fluid levels are indicative for a pseudocystic (ABC-like) component.

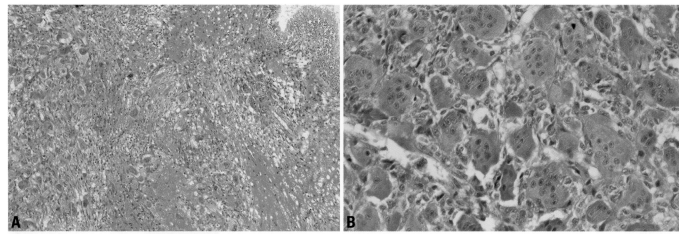

Fig. 1.69 Giant cell tumour. **A** Clustering of multinucleated giant cells. On the right are remnants of Rathke's pouch with ciliated columnar epithelium. **B** Densely packed giant cells with up to 20 nuclei. Intermingled are macrophages and oval stromal cells.

found in the mononuclear cells, but atypical ones do not occur and, if present, are a strong indicator for progression to malignant GCT {272}. Intravascular growth, particularly in the tumour periphery, may be noted, but has no prognostic relevance {207,775,2831}.

Histogenesis
The ovoid to plump spindled stromal cells represent the active proliferating tumour cell pool {2190}, capable of secreting cytokines and differentiation factors, including receptor activator of nuclear factor κ ligand (RANKL) {2207}. These factors attract monocytes, the second cell type in GCT, and promote fusion to osteoclasts, the third cell type in GCT. The monocytes and osteoclast-like giant cells represent a non-neoplastic tumour component {775,2831}.

Genetics
Cytogenetic studies reveal telomeric associations (TAS) as the most frequent chromosomal aberration {272}. Some GCTs show rearrangements in 16q22 or 17p13, similar to aneurysmal bone cyst, which is often associated with GCT. These rearrangements may indicate the possible presence of an aneurysmal bone cyst component {775}.

Prognosis and predictive factors
GCT of the skull is a locally aggressive lesion. Treatment consists of complete removal, if possible. Radiotherapy is also applied {207,1146}. Histologically malignant GCT of the skull has been rarely described, sometimes associated with Paget disease {365,1474}.

Chondroma

Chondromas of the sinonasal tract are extremely rare, and any cartilaginous tumour greater than 2 cm occurring in this site should be considered potentially malignant until proven otherwise.

ICD-O code   9220/0

Osteoma

Definition
A benign lesion composed of mature bone with a predominantly lamellar structure.

ICD-O code   9180/0

Synonyms
In the jaws and calvaria, the terms exostosis and osteoma have been used interchangeably {131}. The term 'osteoma' should be used in a restricted sense limited to lesions of the paranasal sinuses, facial bones and orbit, although it has been used in the literature to describe calvarian and mandibular ivory exostosis, surface (juxtacortical) osteoma of the long bones, torus palatinus and torus mandibularis.

Epidemiology
Among patients with sinonasal radiographs taken for a variety of reasons, up to 1% have been found to have osteomas. It may occur at any age, but especially in young adults. There is a 2:1 male predominance.

Localization
The osteomas may be single or multiple; central or on the bone surface, where they can be sessile or rarely pedunculated. They occur most commonly in the frontal and ethmoid sinuses. The maxillary and sphenoid sinuses are infrequently involved. In the jaws, the angle of the mandible is more frequently involved than the coronoid process or condyle.

Clinical features
Osteomas are often asymptomatic and incidentally discovered. However they can produce pain or symptoms related to the location. Multiple jaw osteomas are a frequent component of the Gardner syndrome (a form of familial adenomatous polyposis), being found in 70-90% of patients.
Osteomas are radiodense, sharply defined, well-circumscribed lesions occurring in either a central or peripheral location.

Macroscopy
The lesion is a well-circumscribed white bony mass, which is occasionally polypoid or exophytic.

Histopathology
Osteoma is characterised by compact cortical bone with scanty intervening fibrovascular stroma. In some cases, there is a peripheral rim of dense sclerotic lamellar bone surrounding trabeculae of lamellar or occasionally woven bone separated by fibrofatty vascular tissue.

Genetic predisposition
The presence of multiple osteomas is an

important clue that the patient may have Gardner syndrome.

Prognosis and predictive factors
No therapy is required unless the lesion causes cosmetic or functional problems. A local resection is the treatment of choice in such circumstances.

Chondroblastoma and chondromyxoid fibroma

ICD-O codes
Chondroblastoma   9230/0
Chondromyxoid fibroma   9241/0

Chondroblastomas and chondromyxoid fibromas are rare in the head and neck {177,988,1024,1120,1185,1348,1349, 1356,1466,2559,2683,2730}. See WHO Classification of Tumours of Soft Tissue and Bone {775}.

Osteochondroma (exostosis)

Definition
A pedunculated or sessile exophytic bony projection with a cartilaginous cap. The bony component is continuous with the underlying bone.

ICD-O code   9210/0

Epidemiology
Osteochondroma is one of the most common lesions of the long and flat bones. It may be solitary or multiple. In the facial bones, osteochondromas are very rare and almost invariably single. Osteochondromas of the facial skeleton have not been reported in the setting of multiple hereditary exostoses.
The mean age at diagnosis is 40 years, which is older than that of patients with tumours occurring outside the head and neck. Females are more commonly affected than males.

Localization
More than half of the lesions occur in the coronoid process of the mandible. The condyle can also be involved.

Clinical features
Osteochondroma involving the coronoid process or the condyle causes difficulty in opening the mouth or dysfunction of the temporomandibular joint. On plain radiographs, flaring of the cortex in continuity with the underlying bone and varying degrees of calcification and/or ossification are present. The cartilaginous cap is of variable thickness.

Macroscopy
A cartilaginous cap covers the bony protrusion.

Histopathology
The cap consists of hyaline cartilage, and the osteochondral junction resembles the growth plate. A well-defined zone of enchondral ossification matures into cancellous bone with marrow.

Prognosis and predictive factors
Excision is curative. No recurrence or malignant transformation has been reported in osteochondromas of the jaws.

Osteoid osteoma

ICD-O code   9191/0

Osteoid osteoma is a benign bone-forming tumour of limited growth potential, usually less than 1.5 cm, typically associated with nocturnal pain that is relieved by salicylates. It is very rare in the head and neck. It occurs in young patients (first three decades), with male predominance. On plain radiographs, dense cortical sclerosis surrounds a radiolucent nidus. Histologically, the nidus shows interconnected, ossified woven bone rimmed by osteoblasts. Fibrous tissue, vessels and multinucleated giant cells are identified in between the bony trabeculae. See WHO Classification of Tumours of Soft Tissue and Bone {775}.

Osteoblastoma

ICD-O code   9200/0

Definition
A rare, benign, bone-forming tumour in which osteoblasts rim woven bony trabeculae, forming a mass usually over 2 cm.

Epidemiology
Osteoblastoma is rare, and 90% of cases occur below the age of 30 years. It is more common in males.

Localization
In the head and neck, the most common site of involvement is the jaws, followed by the cervical vertebrae and the skull {1570}. The mandible is affected about two to three times more often than the maxilla. Most arise in the body of the mandible, rarely in the midline or coronoid process.

Clinical features
Osteoblastomas of the jaw cause swelling and toothache, and in the cervical spine, pain, scoliosis and nerve root compression. In contrast to osteoid osteoma, the pain is rarely nocturnal and not relieved by salicylates.

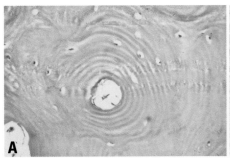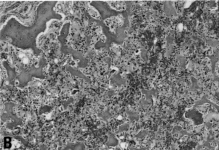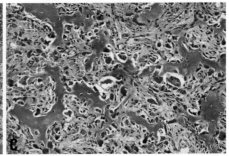

Fig. 1.70 A Osteoma of the right parietal bone. Mature lamellar bone with osteon-like structures. **B** Osteoid osteoma. Osteoblasts surround the trabeculae. **C** Nidus of an osteoblastoma, showing a single layer of osteoblasts lining the bony trabeculae.

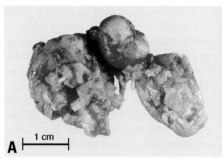
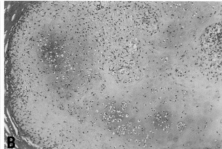

Fig. 1.71 Nasal chondromesenchymal hamartoma. **A** Multiple tumour fragments with a mucosal surface and nodules of cartilage. **B** Cartilaginous nodule, surrounded by cellular stroma.

On plain radiographs, osteoblastoma is a sharply circumscribed, oval-round lytic lesion. It may have a mixed lytic and sclerotic pattern, reflecting the degree of mineralization of the matrix. A reactive bony shell is detected at the periphery. Radiographic features indistinguishable from malignant lesions are reported in about one-third of cases.

Macroscopy
It is a red and gritty lesion often with cyst formation. The border between the tumour and the host bone is very sharp.

Histopathology
Woven bony trabeculae, rimmed by osteoblasts are haphazardly distributed within a richly vascularized fibrous stroma accompanied by osteoclast-like giant cells. Mitotic figures may be present, but without atypical forms. Degenerative nuclear atypia is occasionally present. When large plump osteoblasts with prominent nucleoli predominate, the tumour is often referred to as epithelioid osteoblastoma or aggressive osteoblastoma. However, these histologic features are not necessarily indicative of aggressive behaviour. Rarely, focal areas of hyaline cartilage may be identified, as well

as secondary aneurysmal bone cyst-like changes. At the periphery, there is no permeative growth pattern. The histologic features are identical to cementoblastoma. Tumours showing direct continuity with the root of a tooth are preferably termed a cementoblastoma.

Prognosis and predictive factors
Curettage or local excision is the treatment of choice. In the few cases with recurrence, a further conservative treatment will control the disease.

Ameloblastoma

Ameloblastomas are very rare in the sinonasal tract and nasopharynx {1554, 2257}. See Chapter 6 on odontogenic tumours for details.

ICD-O code   9310/0

Nasal chondromesenchymal hamartoma

Definition
A tumefactive process arising in the nasal cavity and/or paranasal sinuses

whose mixed chondroid, stromal, and cystic features are morphologically similar to the chest wall hamartoma.

Epidemiology
There are only 12 reported cases {45,1140,1284,1311,1678}. A pleuropulmonary blastoma was diagnosed in one of these children {1678}. One infant with the prenatal detection of hydrocephalus also had absence of the corpus callosum and hypoplasia of the cerebellar vermis. The age range is newborn to 16 years with most cases presenting in the first year of life, often before 3 months of age. There is a male predilection of approximately 3:1.

Clinical features
Signs and symptoms
Respiratory difficulty, the discovery of an intranasal mass and/or facial swelling are the most common presenting features. The respiratory distress is detected in the immediate neonatal period or develops later during feedings with accompanying cyanosis. A unilateral mass in the nasal cavity is the most consistent finding on physical examination.

Imaging
A mass density in the nasal cavity and/or the contiguous paranasal sinuses is noted on radiographic examination. Magnetic resonance or computed tomographic imaging discloses a dense mass with or without calcifications or a heterogeneous signal in a lesion with cystic features. Extension or involvement of the maxillary and/or ethmoid sinuses and erosion into the anterior cranial fossa are other accompanying changes.

Macroscopy
Multiple solid and cystic fragments of tis-

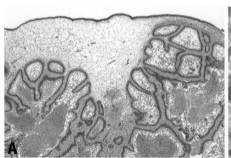
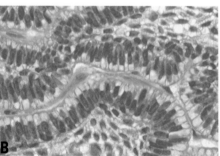
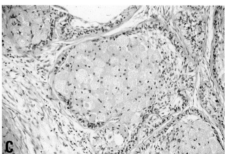

Fig. 1.72 Ameloblastoma. **A** An intact respiratory surface is subtended by a complex ameloblastic neoplasm with many lobules displaying a central stellate reticulum surrounded by the palisaded columnar ameloblastic epithelium. **B** Reverse polarity of the hyperchromatic columnar nuclei away from the basement membrane and towards the stellate reticulum. **C** Granular cell ameloblastoma showing islands of granular cells.

sues, some with identifiable foci of cartilage reflect the piecemeal nature of the resection in most cases. The precise site of origin of the mass has varied from the nasal septum, upper nasal cavity or floor of the anterior cranial fossa.

Histopathology

All tumours have had nodules of cartilage varying in size, contour and degree of differentiation. Some nodules resemble the chondromyxomatous nodules of a chondromyxoid fibroma, whereas others are well-differentiated cartilaginous nodules. At the periphery of the chondroid nodules, there is a loose spindle cell stroma or an abrupt transition to hypocellular fibrous stroma. Other areas can have a fibro-osseous appearance with a prominent cellular stromal component and small ossicles or trabeculae of immature woven bone resembling fibrous dysplasia. Yet another common pattern is a cellular stroma with hyalinized nodules with or without perivascular stromal cells displaying a pericytomatous pattern. Cellular myxoid foci are similar in some respects to cranial/nodular fasciitis. The aneurysmal bone cyst-like areas are surrounded by a stroma rich in multinucleated giant cells.

Immunoprofile

The cartilage, mature or immature, is immunoreactive for S-100 protein. The spindled stroma is immunoreactive for smooth muscle actin and vimentin.

Differential diagnosis

The differential diagnosis depends on the particular combination of microscopic features present in the biopsy or resection. Since cartilage is the dominant component, differential diagnoses include chondromyxoid fibroma and chondroblastoma {1858}. Other differential diagnoses may include aneurysmal bone cyst, fibrous dysplasia, cranial fasciitis and osteochondromyxoma {334}. Interestingly, the latter tumour may be congenital, may involve the paranasal

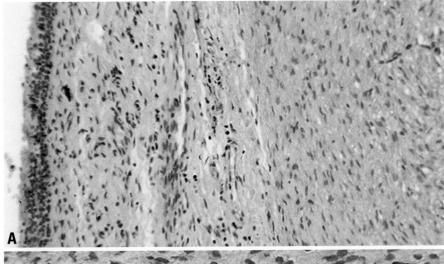

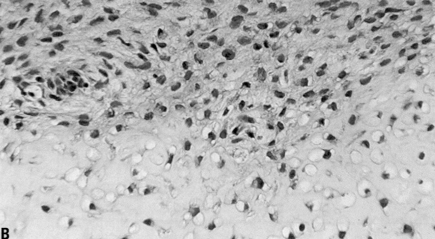

Fig. 1.73 Nasal chondromesenchymal hamartoma. **A** Loose spindle cell proliferation with a myxoid background. **B** The interface between the immature chondroid tissue and stroma resembles a chondromyxoid fibroma.

sinuses and is associated with the Carney complex in some cases. None of the patients with nasal chondromesenchymal hamartoma are known to have the Carney complex {1678}.

Prognosis and predictive factors

Information on the clinical behaviour is incomplete, but prognosis is apparently favourable. There is some capacity for continued local growth when the resection is incomplete.

Haematolymphoid tumours

A.C.L. Chan
J.K.C. Chan
M.M.C. Cheung
S.B. Kapadia

Non-Hodgkin lymphoma

Definition
Primary non-Hodgkin lymphomas (NHL) of the nasal cavity or paranasal sinuses are defined as lymphoid cell neoplasms in which the bulk of disease occurs in these anatomic sites.

Synonyms
Most cases described in the past as polymorphic reticulosis, malignant midline reticulosis, lethal midline granuloma or angiocentric immunoproliferative lesion, are now reclassifiable as extranodal NK/T cell lymphoma of nasal-type.

Epidemiology
Malignant lymphoma is the second most common malignancy of the nasal cavity and paranasal sinuses, following squamous cell carcinoma {1013}. It accounts for 14% of all cancers in these sites {1013}.
Although many different types of NHL can occur in the nasal cavity, the most common lymphoma type is extranodal NK/T cell lymphoma of nasal-type, especially in Asian populations {5,420}. The relatively high prevalence of this lymphoma type in Asians and Latin Americans also accounts for the higher overall incidence of nasal lymphomas in these populations as compared with Caucasian populations {58,2104}. Other

peripheral T-cell lymphomas, such as anaplastic large cell lymphoma, can also occur in the sinonasal region.

Lymphomas presenting in the paranasal sinuses are frequently B-cell lymphomas, with diffuse large B-cell lymphoma (DLBCL) being the most common {5,551,1837}. Other B-cell lymphomas that can involve the sinonasal regions include Burkitt lymphoma, follicular lymphoma, extranodal marginal zone B-cell lymphoma of MALT type, and mantle cell lymphoma {5}. Please also refer to the section of non-Hodgkin lymphomas in Chapter 4 on tumours of the oral cavity and oropharynx.
NHL of the nasal cavity and paranasal sinus is primarily a disease of adults, with male predominance. Patients with extranodal NK/T cell lymphoma of nasal-type have a male to female ratio of 3:1, and a median age of 53 years {420}. Patients with DLBCL are generally one decade older (median age 63 years), and the male to female ratio is 1.2:1 {5,420}. Children may rarely present with NHL of the nasal cavity and the paranasal sinuses, with Burkitt lymphoma being the most common type {2808}.

Etiology
The etiology is unknown, but extranodal NK/T cell lymphoma of nasal-type is strongly associated with Epstein-Barr virus (EBV) irrespective of the ethnic background of the patients {68,376, 1107,1263,1347,2671,2828}. There is only a weak association between B-cell lymphomas in the nasal cavity and the paranasal sinuses with EBV {376,511, 2617,2740}.
Immunosuppression (e.g. post-transplant, HIV infection) is associated with an increased risk of developing NHL, including in the nasal cavity and paranasal sinuses. Although the majority of the cases in immunosuppressed patients are DLBCL {511,2068}, extranodal NK/T cell lymphoma of nasal-type has also been reported {328}. Most of the NHL that arise in the setting of immuno-

suppression are also EBV-related {511}.

Localization
Lymphomas of the nasal cavity are often locally destructive, with obliteration of the nasal passages and maxillary sinuses. In particular, extranodal NK/T cell lymphoma can involve the adjacent alveolar bone, hard palate, orbit and nasopharynx in over half of the cases {1948}.
Lymphomas of the paranasal sinuses commonly show bony destruction and local extension to adjacent structures including the orbit, palate, nasal cavity, nasopharynx, and soft tissues in the cheek and infratemporal fossa {511, 1836,1837}. Maxillary sinus is the most commonly involved paranasal sinus.

Clinical features
Patients may present with nasal obstruction, epistaxis, nasal discharge, pain and nasal swelling or facial swelling. Locally advanced cases can cause destruction of midline facial structures. The nasal septum or palate may be perforated. Extension to the orbits can lead to proptosis and visual disturbance. Regional lymph node involvement may occur in some patients. Occasional patients have systemic symptoms including fever and weight loss. Haemophagocytic syndrome with pancytopenia occurs at presentation in a minority of patients with extranodal NK/T cell lymphoma of nasal-type {420,2533}.

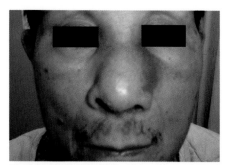

Fig. 1.74 Extranodal NK/T cell lymphoma of nasal cavity in a 69-year-old patient who presented with painful nasal swelling. MRI showed tumour involvement of the left nasal cavity, left ethmoidal and maxillary sinuses.

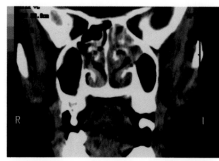

Fig. 1.75 CT scan of nasal NK/T cell lymphoma. The tumour involves the nasal cavity mainly on the left side, with extension to the medial part of the left maxillary sinus and the left ethmoidal sinuses.

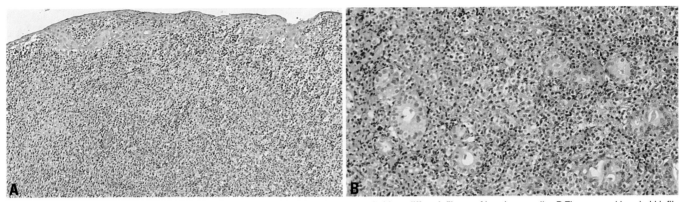

Fig. 1.76 Nasal NK/T cell lymphoma. **A** In this example, the mucosa is intact and expanded by a diffuse infiltrate of lymphoma cells. **B** The mucosal lymphoid infiltrate is destructive, resulting in separation and loss of mucosal glands.

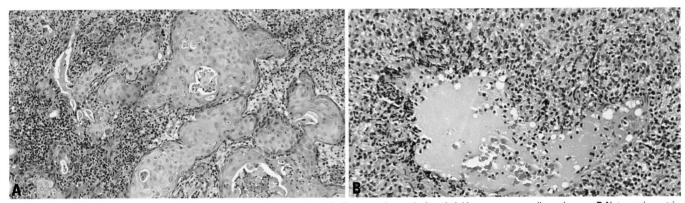

Fig. 1.77 Nasal NK/T cell lymphoma. **A** This case shows marked pseudoepitheliomatous hyperplasia, mimicking squamous cell carcinoma. **B** Note angiocentric and angiodestructive growth.

Tumour spread and staging

The majority (80%) of patients with extranodal NK/T cell lymphoma of nasal-type have localized disease at presentation (Stage IE/IIE) {420,1500,1505}. Bone marrow involvement at presentation is uncommon {2810}. Although extranodal NK/T cell lymphoma often shows localized disease at presentation, spread to other sites (such as skin, gastrointestinal tract, liver, lymph node, testis) during the course of disease is common.

Most of the patients (75%) with DLBCL of the nasal cavity and the paranasal sinuses present with low clinical stage (IE/IIE) {420,511}. In contrast to extranodal NK/T cell lymphoma, cervical lymph node involvement is more frequent at presentation (60%), and the common sites of relapse are lymph node, liver and lung {420}.

Extranodal NK/T cell lymphoma

ICD-O code   9719/3

Extranodal NK/T cell lymphoma of nasal-

type is characterized by a diffuse lymphomatous infiltrate expanding the nasal or paranasal sinus mucosa, with wide separation and destruction of the mucosal glands, which may undergo a peculiar clear cell change. Extensive coagulative necrosis and frequent apoptotic bodies are very common, as are ulceration, angiocentricity, angiodestruction and fibrinoid deposits in vessel walls. The lymphoma cells vary in size in different cases, ranging from small through medium-sized to large. Some nuclei have an irregular outline, while others can be round or oval. The cells have a moderate amount of pale cytoplasm, and cytoplasmic azurophilic granules can be identified in Giemsa-stained touch preparations. Some cases are associated with a rich inflammatory infiltrate, consisting of small lymphocytes, histiocytes, plasma cells and eosinophils. Occasionally pseudoepitheliomatous hyperplasia of the overlying squamous epithelium may occur, mimicking well differentiated squamous cell carcinoma.

Immunoprofile and genetics

The lymphoma most commonly exhibits an NK-cell immunophenotype of CD2+, surface CD3(Leu4)-, cytoplasmic CD3+, CD56+ {1196}. CD43 and CD45RO are commonly positive, but other T-cell markers (including CD5) and NK-cell markers (CD16, CD57) are usually negative. The tumours commonly exhibit a cytotoxic phenotype with expression of perforin, TIA1, and granzyme B {662,1773,1878, 1935}. Fas (CD95) and Fas ligand expression are frequent, and may account for the extensive necrosis {1877,1935}. Expression of the various NK cell receptors is variable. P-glycoprotein/MDR1 is often expressed (90%), and may explain the poor response to chemotherapy {2838}. The T-cell receptor genes are often in germline configuration {1196}. Practically all cases (>95%) are associated with EBV {68,376,1107,1263,1347,2671,2828}. The virus is best demonstrated in the tumour cells by in situ hybridization for EBER (EBV-encoded early RNAs) {376}. The EBV is in clonal episomal form, pro-

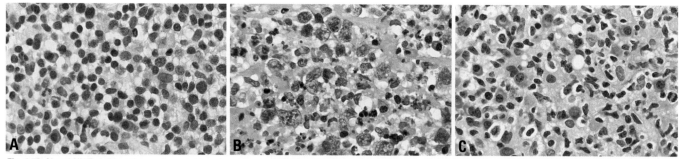

Fig. 1.78 Nasal NK/T cell lymphoma: the cytological spectrum. **A** Predominantly small cells that are slightly larger than small lymphocytes. Most cells show mild nuclear foldings. **B** Predominantly large cells. There are many intermingled apoptotic bodies. **C** This example is predominated by small lymphoid cells. The admixture of plasma cells may give the impression of a reactive inflammatory process (so-called polymorphic reticulosis). Note presence of mitotic figures.

viding additional evidence of the clonal nature of the lesion {1107,1693}.

Some cases are CD56 negative, but are still classified as extranodal NK/T cell lymphoma provided they express T-cell markers and cytotoxic markers, and are EBV positive. These cases may show clonally rearranged T-cell receptor genes and may represent a neoplasm of cytotoxic T-lymphocytes {426}. T-cell lymphomas which lack cytotoxic markers or evidence of EBV infection are diagnosed as peripheral T-cell lymphoma unspecified. Lymphoblastic lymphoma of probable NK-cell lineage (or so-called blastic NK-cell lymphoma) with expression of CD56 and TdT and no EBV association has also been described in the nasal cavity, but this is an entity distinct from the extranodal NK/T cell lymphoma of nasal-type {1352,1838}.

Differential diagnosis

Since the tumour cells of extranodal NK/T cell lymphoma can be masked by a prominent inflammatory infiltrate, the lesion can be mistaken as an infective, inflammatory or granulomatous lesion (including Wegener granulomatosis). It is not uncommon that a definitive diagnosis can only be reached after repeated biopsies. While Wegener granulomatosis sim-

ilarly presents with destructive nasal lesion, simultaneous pulmonary involvement may be present. There is serologic positivity for cytoplasmic anti-neutrophil cytoplasmic antibody (c-ANCA), and the main histologic findings are chronic inflammation with microabscesses and histiocytic infiltrate, in the absence of atypical lymphoid cells.

In those examples of extranodal NK/T cell lymphomas dominated by small cells with minimal atypia, a definitive diagnosis can be difficult to make. An angiocentric infiltrate with expansion of the mucosa and mucosal gland destruction, coupled with prominent necrosis, should raise suspicion for the diagnosis of extranodal NK/T cell lymphoma. Confirmation of the diagnosis can be made by demonstrating sheets of CD3+, CD56+ and EBER+ cells.

Some non-lymphoid CD56+ small round cell tumours (e.g. olfactory neuroblastoma, Ewing sarcoma/primitive neuroectodermal tumour, rhabdomyosarcoma) also enter in the differential diagnoses. However, these can be easily excluded by appropriate immunohistochemical stains {1532}.

Diffuse large B-cell lymphoma
ICD-O code   9680/3

In DLBCL of the nasal cavity or paranasal sinuses, the mucosa shows dense, diffuse and interstitial infiltration by large or medium-sized lymphoid cells. There may or may not be ulceration and necrosis. Occasional cases show angioinvasion. The tumour cells may resemble centroblasts or immunoblasts, or have a non-specific blastoid appearance. The nuclei are round, multilobated or irregularly folded, with multiple small membrane-bound nucleoli or single central prominent nucleolus. The tumour cells express pan-B markers (e.g. CD20, CD79a). Extramedullary myeloid sarcoma, plasmacytoma, undifferentiated carcinoma and amelanotic melanoma may resemble DLBCL, but these entities can be readily distinguished by appropriate immunohistochemical stains.

Histogenesis

Most cases of extranodal NK/T cell lymphoma of nasal-type are activated NK-cell neoplasms, while some appear to be neoplasms of cytotoxic T-cells {425}. DLBCL are mature B-cell neoplasms at either the germinal centre or post-germinal centre stage of differentiation.

Somatic genetics

A number of cytogenetic abnormalities

Table 1.4 Non-Hodgkin lymphomas in the nasal cavity or paranasal sinuses: differences in distribution according to cell lineage.

	Primary in nasal cavity		Primary in paranasal sinuses	
	NK/T- or T-cell lymphomas	B-cell lymphomas (mostly DLBCL)	NK/T- or T-cell lymphomas	B-cell lymphomas (mostly DLBCL)
Asian series {420,1837}	71%	29%	18%	82%
Western series {5}	54%	46%	25%	75%
DLBCL = diffuse large B-cell lymphoma				

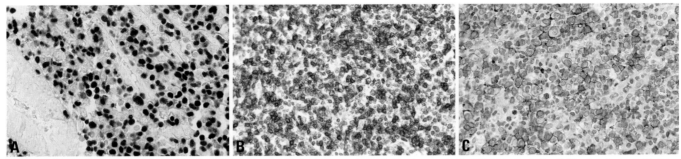

Fig. 1.79 Nasal NK/T cell lymphoma. **A** *In situ* hybridization for EBER shows nuclear labeling in practically all lymphoma cells. **B** The lymphoma cells show immunoreactivity for CD3ε. Surface CD3 as detected on frozen section is negative (not shown). **C** The lymphoma cells show membrane staining for CD56.

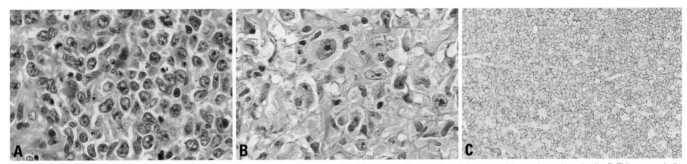

Fig. 1.80 Nasal large B cell lymphoma. **A** Centroblastic morphology, characterized by cells with round nuclei and membrane-bound nucleoli. **B** This example is dominated by very large pleomorphic cells with prominent nucleoli. **C** There is diffuse and uniform immunostaining for CD20.

have been reported in extranodal NK/T cell lymphoma of nasal-type, most commonly isochromosome 1q, isochromosome 6p, partial deletion of 6q, and aberration at 11q {2606,2811}. Comparative genomic hybridization and loss of heterozygosity studies have suggested frequent DNA loss at 1p, 6q, 11q, 12q, 13q, 17p, whole X, and frequent gain at 1p, 2q, 6p, 10q, 11q, 12q, 13q, 17q, 19p, 20q, Xp {1346,2382,2383}. Overall, the most frequent changes are del(6)(q21-25), del(17)(p12-p13), del(13)(q14-q34) and gain of 1p32-pter {422}. P53 protein overexpression occurs in 45-86% of cases {1496,2104,2105}, but P53 mutation is less common (24-48%) {1496,2105}. *TP53* mutation has been associated with large cell morphology and advanced stage {2105}. FAS gene mutation is frequently observed {2331,2534}. Aberrant methylation of promoter CpG region of P73 gene occurs in 94% of cases {2381}, and its detection by methylation-specific polymerase chain reaction may be helpful for monitoring residual disease or early relapse {2380}. There are no molecular data on DLBCL specifically occurring in the sinonasal tract.

Genetic susceptibility
Extranodal NK/T cell lymphoma of nasal-type has been reported in both the father and son of a family with known pesticide exposure {1354}.

Prognosis and predictive factors
Radiotherapy and/or systemic chemotherapy is the treatment of choice for localized disease. {420-422,1505, 1550}. Treatment of DLBCL follow protols for similar tumours elsewhere in the body, as some series showed that chemotherapy might be beneficial {1550,2091}.
The overall survival for extranodal NK/T cell lymphoma of nasal-type is only 30-50% {420-422,1312,1838}. In patients achieving complete remission, local relapse occurs in one-third to one-half of cases {421,1312}, and systemic failure is also common {421}. Factors associated with a worse outcome include: advanced stage, poor performance status, B symptoms, and bulky disease {422}. There is no conclusive evidence to suggest that the histologic grading of NK/T cell lymphoma can predict the clinical outcome. Expression of cutaneous lymphocyte antigen (CLA) may be associated with a worse prognosis, but this finding has yet to be confirmed {2863}.
The prognosis is slightly more favourable for DLBCL compared with extranodal NK/T cell lymphoma of nasal-type {420}. The overall survival for DLBCL is 35-60% {420,511,1550}. Prognostic factors have not been studied in detail in sinonasal DLBCL. A Western series reporting treatment results of lymphomas of the nasal cavity and the paranasal sinuses showed that the International Prognostic Index is the only significant predictor for freedom from progression rate {1550}.

Extramedullary plasmacytoma

Definition
A mass-forming lesion of monoclonal plasma cells that occurs outside the bone and bone marrow. By definition, patients with primary extramedullary plasmacytoma (EMP) do not have evidence of underlying multiple myeloma.

ICD-O code   9734/3

Epidemiology
The mean age of patients with EMP of the head and neck is 60 years (range 34-78 years), with a male predominance 4:1 {1267}.

Localization
Most frequent sites of envolement are nasal cavity, paranasal sinuses and nasopharynx {433,827,1267,1613,1972, 2347,2656,2746}.

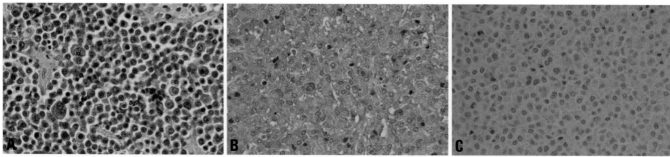

Fig. 1.81 Extramedullary plasmacytoma. **A** Poorly-differentiated plasmacytoma. Note mononuclear and multinucleated neoplastic plasma cells with prominent nucleoli. **B** Immunoperoxidase staining of plasmacytoma shows monoclonal kappa staining in cytoplasm of neoplastic plasma cells. **C** Immunoperoxidase staining shows absence of staining for lamda light chains in neoplastic plasma cells.

Clinical features

EMP tends to be solitary, with multiple tumours present in only 10% of cases at diagnosis. The presenting features of head and neck EMP are: soft tissue mass (80%), airway obstruction (35%), epistaxis (35%), local pain (20%), proptosis (15%), nasal discharge (10%), regional lymphadenopathy (10%), and cranial nerve palsy (5%). The mean duration of symptoms is about 4.5 months. The tumour ranges in size from 2-5 cm. The appearance varies from grey to red, soft to firm, and sessile or pedunculated. EMP bleeds easily and is usually smooth without mucosal ulceration. Cervical lymph nodes are enlarged in only 10% of patients {2500}. Occasional primary EMP may be associated with serum paraproteinaemia. An underlying multiple myeloma should always be excluded.

Macroscopy

EMP is lobulated, smooth or nodular, and has a fleshy or rubbery consistency.

Table 1.5 Sites of occurrence for head and neck extramedullary plasmacytomas

Site	Frequency
Nasal cavity	28%
Paranasal sinuses	22%
Nasopharynx	22%
Tonsil	7%
Larynx	5%
Pharynx	5%
Soft palate	3%
Salivary gland	2%
Thyroid	1%
Tongue	1%
Gingiva	1%
Cervical lymph node	1%
Miscellaneous sites, e.g. trachea, subcutaneous tissue	2%

Histopathology

There is a diffuse infiltrate of neoplastic plasma cells in the subepithelial tissue, accompanied by a scant vascularized stroma, and rarely blood lakes. There can be deposits of amyloid or immunoglobulin in the stroma.

The tumour can be well, moderately or poorly differentiated {18,1267}. Well-differentiated EMP is characterized by uniform normal-looking to mildly atypical plasma cells. Intracytoplasmic crystals can be abundant in some cases. Dutcher bodies are sometimes seen. Moderately-differentiated EMP comprises moderately atypical plasma cells that vary in size. Poorly-differentiated (anaplastic) EMP comprises large cells that are often barely recognizable as being plasma cells. The nuclei often show significant variation in size, and can be round or irregularly folded. The chromatin pattern ranges from vesicular to finely granular to coarsely clumped. Nucleoli can be prominent. The cytoplasm is amphophilic and eccentrically located, and a paranuclear hof (Golgi zone) may be present. Mitotic figures are frequent. Some tumour cells can be multinucleated.

Immunohistochemistry

Immunohistochemically, the plasma cells express cytoplasmic immunoglobulin with light chain restriction. CD20 is negative in most cases, and some cases express CD79a. PAX-5 is negative, while Oct-2 and Bob.1 are frequently positive. There is usually expression of CD38, CD138 and VS38, markers characteristically positive in but not specific for plasma cells. Epithelial membrane antigen is commonly positive, and rare cases can show cytokeratin immunoreactivity (often with a dot pattern). Leukocyte common antigen, CD31 or CD56 is sometimes positive.

Differential diagnosis

Well-differentiated EMP should be distinguished from reactive plasma cell proliferations, either non-specific or associated with specific disorders, such as rhinoscleroma or Rosai-Dorfman disease. Reactive plasmacytic proliferations show a polyclonal pattern of immunoglobulin staining.

Moderately or poorly-differentiated EMP can cause significant difficulties in distinction from large cell lymphoma, carcinoma, melanoma, extramedullary myeloid sarcoma and olfactory neuroblastoma. The occasional positive staining for cytokeratin can lead to a misdiagnosis of carcinoma. A high index of suspicion for EMP should be raised for any poorly differentiated neoplasm occurring in the upper aerodigestive tract. Features suggestive of the diagnosis include eccentrically placed nuclei, coarsely clumped "clock-face" chromatin in some nuclei, and amphophilic cytoplasm with a paranuclear hof. The diagnosis can be confirmed by immunohistochemistry or in-situ hybridization for immunoglobulin mRNA to look for monotypic light chain expression {18}.

Prognosis and predictive factors

The mainstay of treatment for primary EMP is radiotherapy. The prognosis of primary EMP is far more favourable than that associated with myeloma {1267}. Approximately 20% of patients with primary EMP will develop multiple myeloma, but it is not possible to predict which cases will progress.

Extramedullary myeloid sarcoma

ICD-O code   9930/3

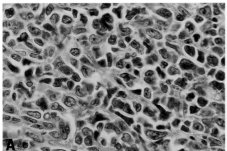 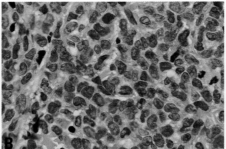 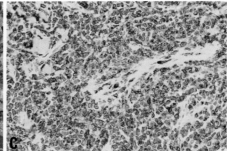

Fig. 1.82 Extramedullary myeloid sarcoma of nasal cavity. **A** In this case, some eosinophilic myelocytes (right field) are evident among primitive myeloid cells which show a fine cytoplasmic granularity. **B** This example comprises a uniform population of primitive myeloid cells (blasts). The nuclear membranes are delicate and the chromatin pattern is fine. Distinction from malignant lymphoma can be difficult on morphologic grounds. **C** The neoplastic cells show strong and uniform immunostaining for myeloperoxidase, supporting the presence of granulocytic differentiation (same case as B).

Extramedullary myeloid sarcoma, also known as granulocytic sarcoma, is a tumour mass of myeloblasts or immature myeloid cells occurring outside the bone marrow or bone. It can precede, co-exist with or follow the presentation of acute myeloid leukaemia. It can also arise as blastic transformation of an underlying chronic myeloproliferative disease or myelodysplastic syndrome.

The most common sites for occurrence of extramedullary myeloid sarcoma are lymph node and skin, but involvement of the nasal cavity and paranasal sinuses has also been reported {1701,2204}. The tumour mass comprises diffuse sheets of blast cells, which often show a single file pattern of infiltration in some areas. The blast cells have round or ovoid nuclei, very fine chromatin, small but distinct nucleoli, and a small to moderate amount of lightly eosinophilic cytoplasm. There can be better-differentiated cells with eosinophilic cytoplasmic granules. Intermingled eosinophilic myelocytes and metamyelocytes, if present, can provide an additional clue to the diagnosis. Giemsa-stained touch preparations are excellent for identification of cytoplasmic azurophilic granules as well as Auer rods, if present. Not uncommonly, extramedullary myeloid sarcoma is misdiagnosed as malignant lymphoma.

Immunohistochemistry
The tumour cells show chloroacetate esterase activity in approximately 75% of cases. Immunohistochemically, they express various myeloid markers (such as myeloperoxidase, CD13, CD33, CD117, CD68/KP1, neutrophil elastase and lysozyme), with myeloperoxidase being most sensitive and specific. Myeloid sarcoma with monocytic differ-

entiation shows a myeloperoxidase -, CD68/PGM1+ immunophenotype. The pan-T marker CD43 is commonly expressed and may lead to a misdiagnosis of T-cell lymphoma.

Histiocytic sarcoma

ICD-O code   9755/3

Histiocytic sarcoma, defined as a malignant proliferation of cells showing morphologic and immunophenotypic features of mature tissue histiocytes, is a rare tumour that can occasionally present in the nasal cavity {2043}. The large pleomorphic tumour cells have eccentrically-located round, ovoid, indented or grooved nuclei, and abundant eosinophilic cytoplasm that may show fine vacuolation. Phagocytosis is rare. Histologic distinction from large cell lymphoma is difficult, except that the cytoplasm tends to be voluminous and eosinophilic.

The diagnosis depends on the demonstration of histiocytic differentiation (granular staining for CD68 and lysozyme), in the absence of expression of pan-B markers (e.g. CD19, CD20, CD22, CD79a), pan-T markers (e.g. CD3), myeloid markers (e.g. MPO), Langerhans cell marker CD1a, and follicular dendritic cell markers (e.g. CD21, CD35). Since CD68 or lysozyme per se is not totally specific for histiocytic lineage, it is preferable to demonstrate additional haematolymphoid markers such as LCA/CD45, CD4,CD43 or CD163 to confirm the diagnosis. The frequent expression of CD43 may lead to a misdiagnosis of T-cell lymphoma. A small proportion of cases can express S100 protein.

Langerhans cell histiocytosis

ICD-O code   9751/1

Langerhans cell histiocytosis may occasionally present with nasal obstruction due to facial bone involvement {1183}. For details see Chapters 4 on tumours of the oral cavity and oropharynx' and 7 on tumours of the ear.

Juvenile xanthogranuloma

This histiocytic proliferation may mimic tumours of Langerhans cells. It commonly presents as skin nodules in infants and children, but rare extracutaneous cases involving the nasal cavity and paranasal sinuses have also been reported {568, 2245}. Some of the histiocytes have foamy cytoplasm, and frequently there are scattered Touton giant cells and spindly cells within the infiltrate of nondescript mononuclear cells. The histiocytes in juvenile xanthogranuloma express CD68 and factor XIIIa. In contrast to Langerhans cells, they are negative for S100 protein and CD1a.

Rosai-Dorfman disease

Rosai-Dorfman disease (sinus histiocytosis with massive lymphadenopathy) is an uncommon reactive condition of unknown etiology, characterized by proliferation of distinctive histiocytes that usually exhibit emperipolesis of lymphocytes. The tumour masses can mimic lymphoma or other malignancies both clinically and histologically. The patients are commonly children or young adults who present with massively enlarged

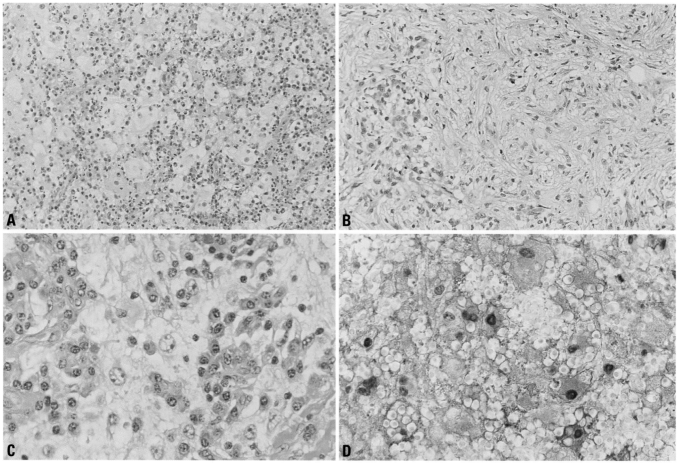

Fig. 1.83 Rosai-Dorfman disease of nasal cavity. **A** Low to medium magnification typically reveals alternating bands of dark-staining and light-staining cells. **B** The presence of spindly cells in a vague storiform growth pattern may lead to a misdiagnosis of fibrohistiocytic tumour. **C** The characteristic histiocytes are usually much larger than the typical histiocytes with round nuclei, distinct nucleoli, abundant light-staining cytoplasm, and indistinct cell borders. There are typically many admixed plasma cells. **D** Immunostaining for S100 protein selectively highlights the distinctive histiocytes. Both the nuclei and cell bodies are stained, while the phagocytosed lymphocytes become much more evident because of the negative staining.

cervical lymph nodes. Extranodal involvement is frequent (about 40% of cases), especially the upper aerodigestive tract {791,923,1378,2760}. The patients with upper aerodigestive tract disease present with nasal obstruction, sinusitis, epistaxis, facial pain or saddle nose deformity.

Histologically, low magnification examination reveals alternating pale and dark-staining areas. The pale areas show proliferation of a distinctive type of very large histiocytes with large round nuclei, distinct nucleoli, and voluminous lightly eosinophilic cytoplasm whose borders are often difficult to define. Some histiocytes show emperipolesis, with lymphocytes, plasma cells or neutrophils in the cytoplasm. These characteristic histiocytes can be few in number in extranodal sites. The lesion may be mistaken for rhinoscleroma. In some cases, a propor-

tion of histiocytes can exhibit atypical or irregular nuclei, and may lead to a misdiagnosis of malignancy such as histiocytic sarcoma or melanoma. The dark areas consist of large aggregates of plasma cells and small lymphocytes. Fibrosis is usually a prominent feature in extranodal disease, and the fibrotic bands can impart a nodular appearance. Together with spindling of some of the cells, the histologic features may strongly mimic those of fibrohistiocytic tumours or inflammatory pseudotumours. Immunohistochemically, the large histiocytes co-express S100 protein and the histiocytic marker CD68, and are negative for CD1a.

Most cases are treated by excision alone, with steroid, radiotherapy and chemotherapy having been given in a minority of cases. In general, the prognosis is excellent, most patients being free

of disease or with stable disease. However, some patients may develop recurrent disease in the original site or other body sites.

Neuroectodermal tumours

B.M. Wenig
P. Dulguerov
S.B. Kapadia

M.L. Prasad
J.C. Fanburg-Smith
L.D.R. Thompson

Ewing sarcoma (EWS) / Primitive neuroectodermal tumour (PNET)

Definition
A high-grade, primitive, round cell tumour of neuroectodermal phenotype. EWS and PNET represent a group of small round cell neoplasms with variable degrees of neuroectodermal differentiation, and are considered together in this section under the rubric of EWS/PNET.

ICD-O codes
Ewing sarcoma   9260/3
PNET   9364/3

Synonyms
Peripheral neuroepithelioma, peripheral neuroectodermal tumour, peripheral neuroblastoma

Epidemiology
Sinonasal Ewing sarcoma / primitive neuroectodermal tumour (EWS/PNET) is rare. This is mostly a tumour of children and young adults, with a peak in the 3rd decade {2211}. In children, approximately 20% of EWS/PNET occur in the head

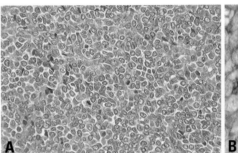
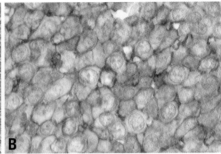

Fig. 1.84 Ewing sarcoma (EWS). **A** A "small blue round cell" tumour is comprised of intermediate sized cells with scant cytoplasm, although there are an increased number of mitotic figures. **B** While non-specific, the neoplastic cells are strongly and diffusely immunoreactive with CD99. The nuclei have very delicate nuclear chromatin, with margination to the periphery.

and neck, with about 20% of these arising in the sinonasal tract {2122}. On rare occasion, older adults may be affected {2611}. There is a very slight male predominance {2122}.

Localization
Sinonasal EWS/PNET most commonly occurs in the maxillary sinus {1518} and nasal fossa {1424,2069}.

Clinical features
Symptoms include pain, mass, and

obstruction {2069}. The tumour can be polypoid when arising from the nasal cavity {2069}. Bony erosion may or may not be present {2069}.

Macroscopy
EWS/PNET is a grey-white and glistening tumour with haemorrhage and often ulceration {2069}. It tends to be much smaller than that arising in other sites.

Tumour spread and staging
Intranasal tumours usually spread into

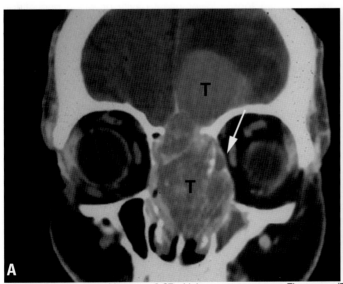
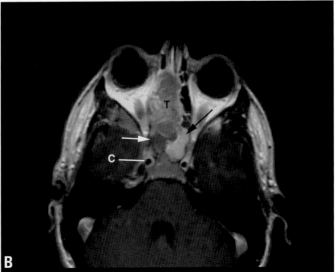

Fig. 1.85 Olfactory neuroblastoma. **A** CT with intravenous contrast. The tumour (T) extends through the floor of the anterior fossa. The lamina papyracea is bowed but the orbital fat (arrow) is normal indicating that the periorbita has not been breached. **B** T1 weighted image. The tumour (T) obstructs the sphenoid sinus. The right side shows secretions with low protein (white arrow). The left has higher protein and higher signal (black arrow). Carotid artery (C)

the paranasal sinuses {2069}. When metastases develop, they are mainly to the lungs and bone {2122}. Staging is according to the Clinical Groups of the Intergroup Rhabdomyosarcoma Study {2122}.

Histopathology
The tumour is composed of densely distributed, uniform, small to medium sized, round cells with a high nuclear to cytoplasmic ratio and fine chromatin. Mitotic activity is high, and coagulative necrosis is common. Some cases show more densely clumped chromatin or a greater degree of nuclear pleomorphism. Homer Wright rosettes are rare.

Immunoprofile
The immunophenotype includes reactivity for CD99 (MIC2, O13, HBA-71, p30/32, and 12E7), {2472} vimentin, and on occasion focally for keratins. Some cases express neural markers, such as synaptophysin, S100 protein, NSE, neurofilament protein, GFAP, and chromogranin. Fli-1 (one portion of the gene fusion product of EWS/FLI1) can be detected by immunohistochemistry.

Electron microscopy
Electron microscopy reveals, to a variable extent, interdigitating neuritic processes, neurofilaments, microtubules, neurosecretory granules and glycogen {1743,2069}.

Differential diagnosis
The differential diagnoses include malignant melanoma, melanotic neuroectodermal tumour, rhabdomyosarcoma, sinonasal undifferentiated carcinoma, lymphoma, olfactory neuroblastoma, and pituitary adenoma.

Histogenesis
A pluripotential fetal neuroectodermal cell is considered the progenitor.

Somatic genetics
Most EWS/PNET have a characteristic t(11;22) with EWS/FLI1 juxtaposition or other translocations involving EWS {2646}. Molecular analysis by PCR or FISH is helpful in diagnosis.

Genetic susceptibility
Sinonasal EWS/PNET has been reported in association with retinoblastoma {627, 1330}.

Prognosis and predictive factors
EWS/PNET has much better prognosis in the head and neck than in other anatomic sites {2122}. Size and stage are the most important prognostic factors. Tumours demonstrating the EWS/FLI1 fusion are reported to have a better prognosis than those with less common gene fusion types {552}. With improvements in imaging techniques and multimodality treatment, a 5-year survival of 60-70% can be achieved {23}.

Olfactory neuroblastoma

Definition
A malignant neuroectodermal tumour thought to originate from the olfactory membrane of the sinonasal tract.

Synonyms
Esthesioneuroblastoma, esthesioneurocytoma, esthesioneuroepithelioma, olfactory placode tumour.

ICD-O code   9522/3

Epidemiology
Olfactory neuroblastoma is an uncommon neoplasm representing approximately 2-3% of sinonasal tract tumours. The incidence has been estimated at 0.4 per million {2584}. Patients range in age from as young as 2 years to 90 years, and a bimodal age distribution has been noted in the 2nd and 6th decades of life {625,626,663,1159}. Both genders are affected equally. No racial predilection has been noted.

Etiology
There are no known etiologic agent(s) for human olfactory neuroblastoma. Injection of diethylnitrosamine in Syrian hamsters and N-nitrosopiperidine in rats has produced tumours histologically identical to human olfactory neuroblastoma {1078,2697}.

Localization
The most common site of origin is in the upper nasal cavity in the region of the cribriform plate. Included in the areas of the proposed origin are Jacobson's organ (vomeronasal organ), sphenopalatine (pterygoid palatine) ganglion, olfactory placode, and the ganglion of Loci (nervus terminalis). "Ectopic" origin in lower nasal cavity or within one of the paranasal sinuses (e.g., maxillary sinus) may occur. Olfactory neuroblastoma may

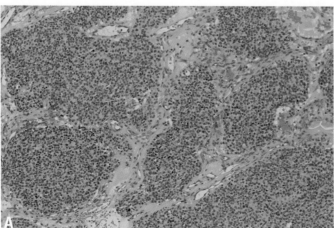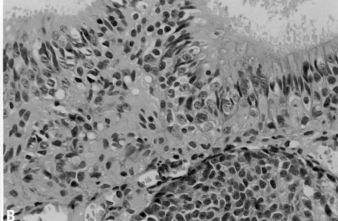

Fig. 1.86 Olfactory neuroblastoma. **A** Tumour lobules separated by a highly vascularized stroma. **B** Olfactory neuroblastoma accompanied by the hyperplasia of the olfactory epithelium.

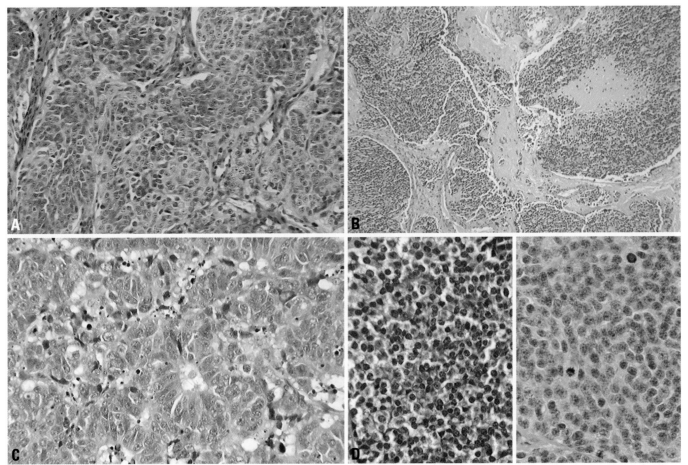

Fig. 1.87 Olfactory neuroblastoma. **A** Lobules of tumour separated by fibrovascular septa. **B** The lobules of tumour are separated by dense fibrovascular tissue. A large pseudorosette (Homer Wright) shows a central area of neurofibrillary matrix. **C** A high grade olfactory neuroblastoma showing a true Flexner-Wintersteiner rosette and increased mitotic figures. **D** The "small blue round cell" neoplasm has scant cytoplasm surrounding variably hyperchromatic nuclei. Granular nuclear chromatin can be seen. Mitotic figures are noted in higher grade lesions.

on occasion present as an intracranial (frontal lobe) mass with involvement of the superior aspect of the cribriform plate or rarely, occur intracranially with no intranasal component {987}.

Clinical features
Signs and symptoms
The main presenting symptoms are unilateral nasal obstruction (70%) and epistaxis (46%); less common manifestations include anosmia, headache, pain, excessive lacrimation and ocular disturbances. Typically, these tumours are slow-growing resulting in long-standing symptomatology, the mean delay between the appearance of the first symptom and the diagnosis being 6 months {626}.

Imaging
The radiologic features include the presence of a "dumbbell-shaped" mass extending across the cribriform plate. The extent of disease is best determined by pre- and postcontrast MR imaging in which there is intense signal in T2-weighted images with marked enhancement of T1-weighted images after gadolinium injection {2815}. Details of bone erosion (lamina papyracea, cribriform plate and fovea ethmoidalis) are better demonstrated by CT scan. Calcifications producing a speckled pattern on radiographic studies can be identified. Angiographic studies disclose a hypervascular neoplasm.

Macroscopy
The gross appearance includes a glistening, mucosa-covered, soft, polypoid, often highly vascularized mass varying from a small nodule measuring less than 1 cm to a large mass filling the nasal cavity and extending into paranasal sinuses, orbit and/or cranial cavity.

Histopathology
Characteristically, the tumours are localized to the submucosa, growing in circumscribed lobules or nests separated by a richly vascularized fibrous stroma. Less often the tumour shows a diffuse growth pattern. The overwhelming majority of tumours are not associated with an in-situ component. The neoplastic cells have uniform, small round nuclei with scant cytoplasm, dispersed ("salt and pepper") coarse to fine nuclear chromatin and inconspicuous nucleoli. Nuclear pleomorphism, mitotic activity and necrosis are usually absent. However, in higher-grade tumours, nuclear pleomorphism with prominent nucleoli, increased mitotic activity and necrosis may be present. The cells do not have distinct borders and are surrounded by a neurofibrillary matrix, which corresponds to tangles of neuronal cell processes. Rosettes of the Homer

Table 1.6 Hyams' histologic grading system for olfactory neuroblastoma

Microscopic Features	Grade 1	Grade 2	Grade 3	Grade 4
Architecture	Lobular	Lobular	±Lobular	±Lobular
Pleomorphism	Absent to Slight	Present	Prominent	Marked
Neurofibrillary matrix	Prominent	Present	May be present	Absent
Rosettes	Present*	Present*	May be present**	May be present**
Mitoses	Absent	Present	Prominent	Marked
Necrosis	Absent	Absent	Present	Prominent
Glands	May be present	May be present	May be present	May be present
Calcification	Variable	Variable	Absent	Absent

NF-neurofibrillary; *Homer Wright rosettes (pseudorosettes); **Flexner-Wintersteiner rosettes (true neural rosettes)

Wright type (pseudorosettes) and Flexner-Wintersteiner type (true neural rosettes) can be identified in up to 30% and less than 5% of tumours, respectively. The Homer Wright pseudorosettes represent the presence of cells in an annular arrangement surrounding central neurofibrillary matrix; distinct cell membranes are not present. Flexner-Wintersteiner rosettes are gland-like structures in which the annular arrangement of cells includes the presence of a distinct cell membrane. Perivascular pseudorosettes can be seen but are of no diagnostic utility. Uncommon findings include stromal calcifications, ganglion cells, melanin-containing cells and divergent differentiation. The latter may include the presence of glandular (adenocarcinoma-like), squamous, teratomatous and rhabdomyoblastic differentiation {1096,1734,2404}.

Grading

The microscopic grading {1159} includes four grades: Grade I is the most differentiated and includes lobular architecture with intercommunication of the neoplasm between lobules. The neoplastic cells are well-differentiated with uniform, small round nuclei with scant cytoplasm, dis-persed ("salt and pepper") nuclear chromatin and inconspicuous nucleoli. The cells do not have distinct borders; rather, the nuclei are surrounded by a neurofibrillary material suggesting cytoplasmic extension. Homer Wright rosettes are frequently seen. Varying amounts of calcification may be noted. Interlobular fibrous stroma is often extremely vascular. Mitotic activity and necrosis are absent. Grade II tumours share many of the histologic features described for Grade I lesions but the neurofibrillary element is less well defined, and the neoplastic nuclei show increased pleomorphism. Scattered mitoses can be seen. Grade III tumours may retain a lobular architecture with a vascular stroma. These hypercellular tumours are characterized by cells that are more anaplastic, hyperchromatic, and have increased mitotic activity as compared to Grade I or II tumours. Necrosis is seen. The neurofibrillary component may be focally present, but is much less conspicuous as compared to Grades I or II tumours. Flexner-Wintersteiner rosettes are uncommon. Calcification is absent. Grade IV tumours may also retain the overall lobular architecture, but the neoplastic element is the most undifferentiated and anaplastic of all the histologic grades. The cellular infiltrate is characterized by pleomorphic nuclei often with prominent eosinophilic nucleoli and an indistinct cytoplasm. Necrosis is commonly seen and there is increased mitotic activity, including atypical mitoses. Rosettes are uncommon. The neurofibrillary component is generally absent. Calcification is absent. Of note is that in any given tumour there may be histologic diversity with mixed (overlapping) features.

In general, the lower grade olfactory neuroblastomas are readily recognizable and diagnostic by light microscopy. Adjunct studies, particularly in the higher histologic grade tumours, may assist in the diagnosis. The advent of immunohistochemistry has diminished the role of histochemical stains, but silver stains such as Bodian, Grimelius and Churukian-Schenk may still be of assistance.

Immunoprofile

The most consistently expressed marker is neuron specific enolase (NSE). Reactivity is also present in a majority of cases for synaptophysin, neurofilament protein (NFP), class III beta-tubulin, and microtubule-associated protein. S-100

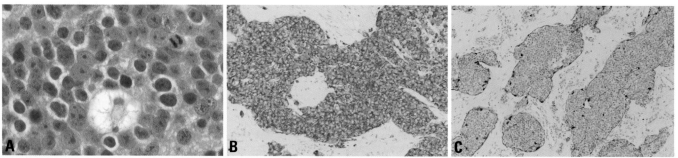

Fig. 1.88 Olfactory neuroblastoma. **A** A true Flexner-Wintersteiner rosette is surrounded by intermediate sized cells with scant cytoplasm and prominent nuleoli. A mitotic figure is present. **B** Immunostaining shows strong staining for synaptophysin. **C** Immunostaining shows the characteristic S100 protein+ sustentacular cells wrapping around the tumour islands.

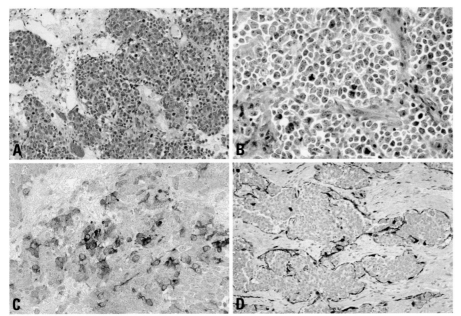

Fig. 1.89 Olfactory neuroblastoma Grade III / IV. **A** Tumour nests comprised of cell and with nuclear pleomorphism, increased mitotic activity and individual cell necrosis. **B** Higher magnification shows the presence of enlarged nuclei with moderate to marked pleomorphism, prominent nucleoli, absence of identifiable neurofibrilllary matrix, and increased mitotic figures, including atypical mitoses. **C** The immunohistochemical antigenic profile typically shows absence of cytokeratin and presence of NSE. **D** S100 protein is limited to sustentacular cells along the periphery of the neoplastic lobules.

protein staining typically is limited to the sustentacular cells situated along the periphery of the neoplastic lobules, although such cells may be sparse in the higher-grade tumours. In addition, immunoreactivity may be present for chromogranin, glial fibrillary acidic protein (GFAP), and Leu-7.

Cytokeratin is usually negative, but some cases can show some positive cells. Epithelial markers, including epithelial membrane antigen (EMA) and carcinoembryonic antigen (CEA) are absent. Leucocyte common antigen (LCA), HMB-45, desmin and CD99 are absent. Proliferation marker studies using Ki-67 and MIB-1 have shown a high proliferative index of 10-50% and flow cytometric analysis shows frequent polyploidy/aneuploidy {2560,2682}.

Electron microscopy

Electron microscopy evaluation is a useful adjunct in the diagnosis and includes the presence of dense core neurosecretory granules measuring 50-250 nm in diameter and neurite-like cell processes containing neurofilaments and neurotubules {1096,2567,2682}. In addition, Schwann-like cells and junctional complexes may be identified. When identified, olfactory rosettes show apical cilia

with a 9 + 2 microtubule pattern, microvilli, and junctional complexes.

Differential diagnosis

The differential diagnosis of olfactory neuroblastoma includes the group of small round cell malignant neoplasms that can occur in the sinonasal tract, i.e., sinonasal undifferentiated carcinoma, lymphoma, rhabdomyosarcoma, mucosal malignant melanoma and neuroendocrine carcinomas. This discussion will be limited to neuroendocrine carcinomas; for the others the reader may refer to the specific sections detailing these specific tumour types.

Neuroendocrine carcinomas (NEC) include, among different tumour types, the carcinoid tumour, atypical carcinoid tumour and small cell carcinoma. NEC of the sinonasal tract are extraordinarily rare, and in contrast to the larynx, the most common subtype is small cell carcinoma. By light microscopy, small cell carcinoma typically is a submucosal hypercellular proliferation growing in sheets, cords and ribbons; the distinct lobular pattern of olfactory neuroblastoma is absent. The cells are small and hyperchromatic with oval to spindle-shaped nuclei, absent nucleoli and minimal cytoplasm. Cellular pleomorphism,

high nuclear to cytoplasmic ratio, high mitotic activity, confluent necrotic areas and individual cell necrosis are readily apparent as well as lymphovascular and perineural invasion. Characteristically, crush artifacts of the neoplastic cells are seen. Squamous cell foci may occasionally be present; glandular or ductal differentiation is rarely seen. Although uncommon, neural-type rosettes similar to those seen in olfactory neuroblastoma can be seen in association with small cell carcinoma. The overall light microscopic findings should allow for differentiating small cell carcinoma from olfactory neuroblastoma in most cases, but immunohistochemical evaluation may be required in some cases. The immunohistochemical profile of small cell carcinoma includes variable reactivity for cytokeratin, chromogranin, synaptophysin, neuron specific enolase (NSE), S-100 protein and thyroid transcription factor-1 (TTF-1). Cytokeratin reactivity may include a punctate paranuclear or globoid pattern. The tumour usually is negative for cytokeratin, and the positive cases do not show a punctate paranuclear or globoid pattern. In contrast to olfactory neuroblastoma, NSE reactivity in small cell carcinoma is more likely to be focal than diffusely positive, and the S100 protein staining, if present, is dispersed throughout the cellular proliferation and not limited to sustentacular cells. Olfactory neuroblastoma is also negative for TTF-1.

Genetics

Studies on cytogenetic aberrations in olfactory neuroblastoma are sparse {2612,2521}. Studies have found partial gains of chromosome material on 8q, while the other findings are conflicting.

Inclusion of olfactory neuroblastoma within the Ewing sarcoma family of tumours {2428} or the primitive neuroectodermal tumours (PNET) {1865} has been proposed {2467} because of the identification, in certain cases, of translocation t(11;22), which is regarded as specific molecular abnormality for Ewing sarcoma {575}. Recent studies using immunohistochemistry, fluorescent in situ hybridization and reverse transcriptase PCR have failed to confirm this translocation in olfactory neuroblastoma {72, 1384,1709,2001}. Therefore, olfactory neuroblastoma should be considered an entity distinct from PNET and the Ewing sarcoma family of tumours.

Histogenesis

Proposed sources of origin of olfactory neuroblastoma include Jacobson's vomero-nasal organ, the sphenopalatine ganglion, the ectodermal olfactory placode, Loci's ganglion, autonomic ganglia in the nasal mucosa, and the olfactory epithelium. While a neuronal – neural crest origin is supported by the presence of neurofilaments in olfactory neuroblastoma {2634}, until recently {335}, few arguments linked olfactory neuroblastoma directly to the olfactory epithelium. The olfactory neuroepithelium is a unique neurosensory organ because olfactory neurons are continuously replaced throughout adult life by new ones {941,942}. Three types of cells are classically recognized in the olfactory epithelium: the basal cells, located against the basement membrane, the olfactory neurosensory cells, and the sustentacular supporting cells, the processes of which extend on the luminal surface. The globose basal cells constitute a stem cell compartment, which confers to this tissue its peculiar ability to regenerate not only physiologically but also when injured by trauma or environmental insults {1631,2690}. The globose basal cells express {1747} neural cell adhesion molecule (NCAM) {513} and mammalian homologue of Drosophila achaete-scute (MASH) gene {958}. These progenitor cells differentiate into olfactory neurosensory cells, which exhibit a progressive maturation from the basal membrane to the epithelial surface {1631,1884}. Each layer can be characterized by specific olfactory- and neuron specific markers. Immature olfactory cells express {1631,2690} GAP43, a 24 kD membrane-associated protein kinase C involved in polyphosphoinositide turnover {197}. As these cells mature, they send axons to the olfactory bulb and migrate towards the surface, they express olfactory marker protein (OMP) {1630} and NCAM, but not GAP43 {1631,1884,2690}.

Recently, olfactory neuroblastomas were found to express HASH, the human homologue of the MASH gene {335}, while staining negative for OMP. So far, HASH has only been demonstrated in medullary thyroid carcinoma and certain small cell lung carcinoma {111}. Further indirect evidence that olfactory neuroblastoma originates from olfactory stem cells can be derived from transgenic mice in which, the SV40T oncogene was

Table 1.7 Clinical staging for olfactory neuroblastoma {663,1243}

Stage	Extent of Tumour	5-Year survival
A	Tumour confined to the nasal cavity	75-91%
B	Tumour involves the nasal cavity plus one or more paranasal sinuses	68-71%
C	Extension of tumour beyond the sinonasal cavities	41-47%

inserted under the OMP gene promoter region {2307}: these mice did not develop olfactory neuroblastoma but adrenal and sympathetic ganglia neuroblastoma. Therefore, the currently available evidence links olfactory neuroblastoma with the basal progenitor cells of the olfactory epithelium.

Prognosis and predictive factors

Complete surgical eradication (craniofacial resection that includes removal of the cribriform plate) followed by full course radiotherapy is the treatment of choice {625,626,1777}. Limited success using chemotherapeutic modalities have been achieved for advanced unresectable tumours and/or for disseminated disease {2705}. High-dose chemotherapy, including platinum-based protocols and autologous bone marrow transplantation have resulted in long-term survival {634,1919,2064}. The overall 5-, 10- and 15-year survival rates have been reported to be 78%, 71% and 68%, respectively {634}. Initial multimodality therapy is associated with 5-year survival of 80% for low-grade tumours and 40% for high-grade tumours {1777}. The majority of the recurrences occur within the first two years {625}. The most frequent recurrence is local, with rates around 30%. Prognosis has traditionally been correlated to clinical staging with 5-year survival of 75-91%, 68-71% and 41-47% for Stage A, B and C tumours, respectively {663,1243}. More recently, complete tumour resection was found to be of more prognostic importance than clinical staging {1740}.

Other factors purportedly implicated in prognosis include histologic grading, proliferation rate and ploidy. Histologically lower grade tumours (Grades I and II) have been reported to have a better 5-year survival than higher-grade tumours (Grades III, IV) {1159}. High proliferation indices and high rate of ploidy/aneuploidy have been correlated

with increased morbidity (i.e., tumour recurrence, metastasis) and mortality (i.e., decreased survival) {2560,2682}.

The majority of tumours behave as locally aggressive lesions mainly involving adjacent structures (orbit and cranial cavity). Local recurrence and distant metastasis may occur years following the initial diagnosis. Approximately 15-70% of patients will experience local recurrence, 10-25% will have cervical lymph node metastasis, and approximately 10-60% will experience distant metastasis {131,663}. The more common sites of metastases include lymph nodes, lungs, and bone. All histologic grades have the capacity to metastasize.

Melanotic neuroectodermal tumour of infancy

Definition
Melanotic neuroectodermal tumour of infancy (MNTI) is a rare neoplasm of infants with a biphasic population of neuroblastic cells and pigmented epithelial cells.

ICD-O code
9363/0
[if benign]

Synonyms
Melanotic progonoma, retinal anlage tumour, melanotic ameloblastoma

Epidemiology
The tumour is very rare. It characteristically occurs in infants, with 80% of cases <6 months of age and 95% <1 year of age, with a 2:1 female predominance {1269}.

Localization
More than 85% of patients have a mass involving craniofacial sites: maxilla (70%), mandible (10%), skull (10%), neurocranial dura or brain (1%). Occasionally other sites, such as the epi-

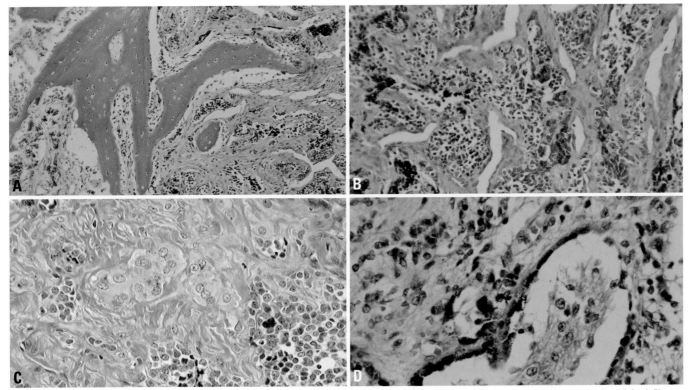

Fig. 1.90 Melanotic neuroectodermal tumour. **A** Section of maxilla shows tumour infiltration of bone. Note fibrous stroma containing neoplastic cellular infiltrate. **B** Dual population of neoplastic cells, including smaller blue neuroblastic cells and larger pigmented epithelial cells. **C** There is a trabecular, tubular, or alveolar arrangement of the biphasic cell population, with the larger pigmented cells surrounding groups of the smaller round, "blue" neuroectodermal cells. The trabeculae are separated by a dense collagenous stroma. **D** Note spatial relationship of larger pigmented epithelial cells surrounding smaller neuroblastic cells.

didymis (4%), skin (3%), uterus (1%), and mediastinum (1%) may be involved {1269,2026}.

Clinical features
Patients present with a rapidly growing pigmented mass, which is usually located in the anterior alveolar ridge of the maxilla. The duration of symptoms ranges from 2 weeks to 5 months (mean 2 months) {1269}. Infrequently, there are elevated levels of vanilmandelic acid, which normalize following adequate therapy.

Macroscopy
The tumours range from 1-10 cm (mean, 3.5 cm), and are smooth, firm to hard, and grey to blue-black {1269}.

Histopathology
This is a nonencapsulated mass composed of a dual population of small neuroblastic cells and larger melanin-containing epithelial cells in a vascularized dense fibrous stroma {1269,2026}. The epithelial cells show alveolar or tubular arrangement, and often surround nests of smaller neuroblastic cells. The latter possess small, round hyperchromatic nuclei and scant or fibrillary cytoplasm. The epithelial cells have larger, vesicular nuclei and abundant cytoplasm, most containing melanin granules. Mitoses and necrosis are rare or absent.

Immunoprofile
MNTI shows polyphenotypic expression of neural, melanocytic and epithelial markers, but without photoreceptor differentiation. Occasionally glial and rhabdomyoblastic differentiation may be seen. The larger cell (epithelial) component is immunoreactive for cytokeratin, HMB-45, vimentin, and sometimes epithelial membrane antigen {1269,2026}. Neuron-specific enolase, CD57/Leu-7 and dopamine-beta-hydroxylase are often positive in both the small neuroblastic cells and large cells. The small cells may express synaptophysin, glial fibrillary acidic protein focally, and desmin focally. The tumour cells are negative for chromogranin, desmin, CEA, retinol-binding protein, neurofilaments, alpha-fetoprotein, and S100 protein.

Electron microscopy
The small cells demonstrate neurosecretory granules and neuritic processes, and the large cells contain melanosomes and premelanosomes {517,571,1269}.

Differential diagnosis
The differential diagnoses include alveolar rhabdomyosarcoma, malignant lymphoma, EWS/PNET, metastatic neuroblastoma, immature teratoma and malignant melanoma. Primary melanoma, especially mucosal, is extremely rare in infants, should show S100 protein immunoreactivity, and lacks epithelial markers. Neuroblastomas may rarely be pigmented, but lack the dual cell population and usually show diffuse immunoreactivity for neuroendocrine markers.

Histogenesis
A neural crest origin is proposed {145, 517,571,1232,1269,2026}.

Prognosis and predictive factors
The treatment of choice is complete local excision {1269,1657,2092}. Radiotherapy and chemotherapy are to be avoided,

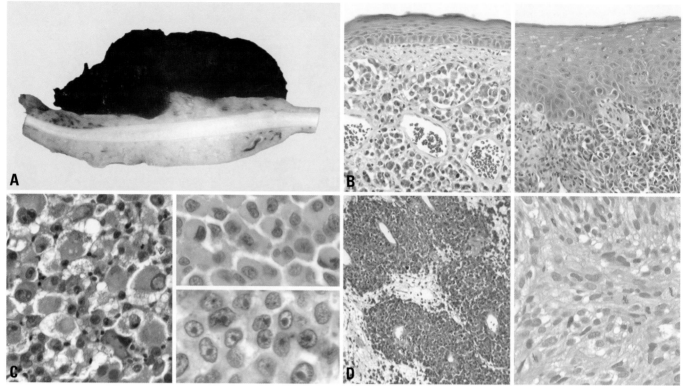

Fig. 1.91 Malignant melanoma. **A** This macroscopic view of a mucosal malignant melanoma of the septum demonstrates black pigment and the typical polypoid nature of the tumour. Note the well defined border at the base of the tumour. **B** The vast majority of tumours demonstrate a "Grenz" zone of separation between the surface and the malignant infiltrate (left), although pagetoid spread and surface epithelium involvement is appreciated (right). **C** Atypical plasmacytoid cells with eccentrically placed nuclei with prominent nucleoli and intranuclear cytoplasmic inclusions. A "Hof" zone is easily identified (left). Rhabdoid cells have abundant opaque eosinophilic cytoplasm arranged eccentrically from the atypical nuclei (right upper). Prominent, magenta nucleoli are common (right lower). **D** Characteristic peritheliomatous growth with areas of degeneration noted between the vessels (left). A storiform or cartwheel pattern with increased mitotic figures (right).

unless there is evidence of metastasis. Despite its rapid growth and tendency to destroy bone, MNTI pursues a benign clinical course in most cases {1269,2026}. However, if not totally excised, local recurrences occur frequently. About 7% of cases develop metastases to sites such as the lymph nodes, liver, bone, adrenal glands or soft tissue {2026}. The potential for recurrence or metastasis, however, cannot be predicted from the clinical or pathologic features.

Mucosal malignant melanoma

Definition
A malignant neoplasm derived from the melanocytes in the mucosa.

ICD-O code   8720/3

Synonyms
Melanosarcoma; melanoma

Epidemiology
Sinonasal mucosal malignant melanomas are rare, accounting for less than 1% of all melanomas {112,165}, and <5% of all sinonasal tract neoplasms {205,2603}. Both genders are equally affected, without a race predilection, although an increased incidence has been suggested in Japanese patients. Malignant melanomas typically affect older individuals in the 5-8th decade with a peak incidence in the 7th decade {165,260,273,386,484,500,560,807,930, 1076,2603}.

Etiology
Formaldehyde exposure and tobacco smoking have been suggested as possible etiologic factors {260,273,1318, 2603}.

Localization
The nasal cavity is affected most frequently, followed by a combination of the nasal cavity and paranasal sinuses. Large tumours may involve multiple

paranasal sinuses and present as extensive skull base tumours {260,273,386, 484,500,560,807,930,1324,2603}.

Clinical features
Symptoms include nasal obstruction, epistaxis, nasal polyp, pain, nasal discharge of variable duration, and melanorrhoea ("coal flecked" or brown nasal discharge) {273,386,930,1076,2603}.

Macroscopy
The lesions are large, bulky and polypoid tumours with a mean size of 2-3 cm, but may be larger with involvement of multiple paranasal sinuses. The vast majority are ulcerated. The cut surface varies from black and brown to light tan, depending upon the amount of melanin production {273,386,930,2603}.

Tumour spread and staging
At presentation, 70-80% of cases are localized, 10-20% have regional lymph node and <10% have distant metastasis {112,273,386,1324,2603}. However, dur-

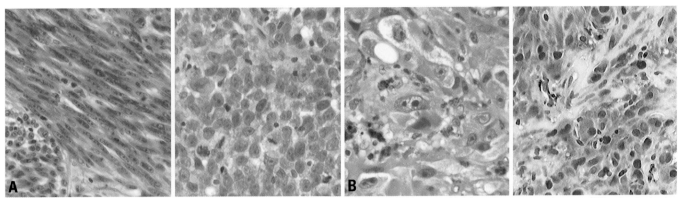

Fig. 1.92 Malignant melanoma. **A** Interlacing fascicles (left) and an undifferentiated to epithelioid pattern (right) can be seen in melanoma. **B** Focal melanin pigment noted in an epithelioid mucosal malignant melanoma (left) while an S-100 protein immunohistochemical study stains both the nucleus and cytoplasm.

ing the course of disease, an additional 20% may develop nodal metastasis and 40-50% may develop distant metastasis to lungs, brain, bone and/or liver {273,386,484,500,1324,2603}.

There is currently no universally accepted staging system. However, the most common and prognostically significant staging system in use is: stage I- localized tumours, stage II- tumours with lymph node metastases, and stage III- tumours with distant metastasis {1076}. Tumour thickness or depth of invasion cannot be accurately assessed due to the lack of a well-defined reference point for the surface in the respiratory mucosa, frequent ulceration, tissue fragmentation and poorly oriented specimen {273,386,2603}.

Histopathology
The tumours are comprised of epithelioid, spindled, plasmacytoid, rhabdoid, and/or multinucleated tumour cells. The cells are generally medium to large-sized {260,273,386,484,1472,2603}. They have a high nuclear to cytoplasmic ratio with pleomorphic nuclei containing prominent eosinophilic nucleoli and intranuclear cytoplasmic inclusions. Nuclear molding can be present. The cytoplasm is usually densely eosinophilic, and variably contains melanin pigment. Mitoses, including atypical forms, are frequent and easily identifiable. Vascular invasion and neurotropism may be identified in up to 40% of cases. An inflammatory infiltrate admixed with pigment-laden histiocytes is commonly identified within or adjacent to the tumour. Tumour cell necrosis is common, particularly in tumours displaying a peritheliomatous or pseudopapillary growth pattern. Other growth patterns include solid, alveolar or sarcomatoid.

Intraepithelial melanocytic atypia (melanoma in-situ) is sometimes seen in the overlying epithelium {260,273,386, 1472,1624,2603}. The tumours usually invade the subepithelial tissue and frequently extend into the bone, cartilage or skeletal muscle.

Immunoprofile
Malignant melanoma expresses S100 protein and vimentin {1472,1661}, and variably HMB45, tyrosinase, melan-A and microphthalmia transcription factor. Neuron specific enolase, CD117, CD99, synaptophysin, CD56, and CD57 have been reported to be occasionally positive, but epithelial membrane antigen, cytokeratins, and muscle markers are not expressed {260,273,484,1472,1661, 2603}.

Differential diagnosis
Sinonasal mucosal malignant melanoma may morphologically masquerade as a variety of benign and malignant neoplasms, such as "small blue round cell" neoplasms, pleomorphic neoplasms

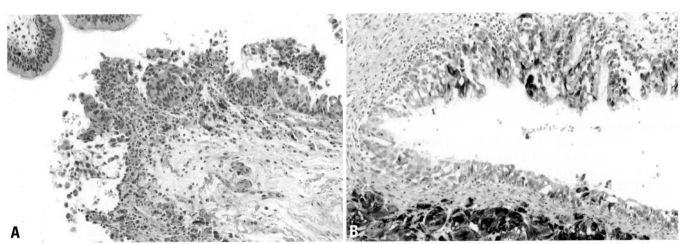

Fig. 1.93 Melanoma *in situ,* associated with primary mucosal melanoma of the maxillary sinus. **A** A portion of the respiratory epithelium is replaced by melanoma in situ and shows melanophages in the superficial lamina propria. **B** Anti-tyrosinase antibody (T311) strongly decorates the invasives tumour cells (bottom) as well as melanoma cells in the sinonasal respiratory epithelium.

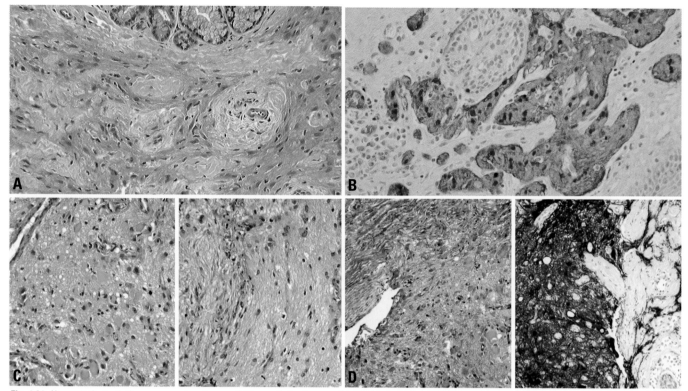

Fig. 1.94 Heterotopic central nervous system tissue. **A** Mucosal glands are subtended by reactive glial tissue composed of neuropil separated by dense, more brightly eosinophilic fibrous connective tissue. Astrocytes are not seen. **B** S-100 positivity in nuclei and cytoplasm of subepithelial glial cells. **C** The left side demonstrates a number of "gemistocytic-type" astrocytes within glial tissue, the right image shows classic neuroglial tissue without significant fibrosis or inflammatory cells. **D** Trichrome stain highlights the neural tissue red, while the reactive background fibrosis is blue (left). GFAP immunoreactivity is present in glial tissue, but not in the surrounding soft tissues (right).

(sinonasal undifferentiated carcinoma, anaplastic large cell lymphoma, angiosarcoma), or various sarcomas {260,273,386,1472,1661,2603}. Metastatic melanoma to the sinonasal tract, although highly uncommon, must always be excluded, as the prognosis is even poorer. Presence of intraepithelial atypical melanocytes favours primary melanoma {386,1624,2603}.

Histogenesis
Melanocytes, distributed throughout the upper respiratory tract are considered the progenitor of primary sinonasal mucosal malignant melanoma.

Genetic susceptibility
Patients with sinonasal mucosal malignant melanoma do not seem to be part of dysplastic nevus syndrome or xeroderma pigmentosum kindreds {273,2603}.

Prognosis and predictive factors
Surgery is the cornerstone of therapy, although wide free margins of resection are difficult to achieve. Radiation therapy has a palliative role {500,2078,2603}.

Local recurrence is frequent (67%-92%), may be repeated, and is a harbinger of adverse prognosis {273,386,560,1324, 2603}. Most tumours progress to regional and distant metastasis resulting in poor 5-year disease-specific survival that may range from 17- 47% {165,260,273, 386,560,1076,1324,2310,2603}. Other poor prognostic factors include advanced age, obstructive symptoms, tumour size >3 cm, location in paranasal sinuses and nasopharynx, vascular invasion into skeletal muscle and bone, high mitotic count, marked cellular pleomorphism and distant metastasis {165,273, 500,1324,2081,2310,2603}.

Heterotopic central nervous system tissue (nasal glioma)

Definition
A mass of heterotopic neuroglial tissue presenting in and around the nose.

Synonyms
Nasal glioma, nasal glial heterotopia

Epidemiology
Most patients present at birth, and 90% of cases are diagnosed by age of 2 years. There is no gender predilection.

Localization
The lesion is situated externally on or near the bridge of the nose in 60% of cases, within the nasal cavity in 30% of cases, and in both sites in 10% of cases. In the latter cases, communication of the intra- and extranasal components is through a defect in the nasal bone.

Clinical features
Extranasal heterotopic CNS tissue presents as a smooth noncompressible subcutaneous mass over the dorsum of the nose. The intranasal lesions usually present with nasal obstruction or nasal deformity. Heterotopic CNS tissue may occur at other sites, such as the paranasal sinuses, nasopharynx {2289}, pharynx, tongue, palate, tonsil and orbit, and may be referred to as "facial glioma". One-third of pharyngeal heterotopic CNS tissues are associated with cleft palate or choanal stenosis.

A helpful clinical sign is the absence of expansion or pulsation of the mass following compression of the ipsilateral jugular vein (negative Furstenberg test), due to lack of connection of the mass with the CSF pathway. Importantly, radiographic imaging scans (CT and MRI) reveal a soft tissue mass without an intracranial component or bony defect in the floor of the anterior cranial fossa.

Macroscopy
The lesion appears as a polypoid, smooth, soft, grey tan, non-translucent mass with encephaloid features. It usually measures 1-3 cm.

Histopathology
The lesion is non-encapsulated, composed of large or small islands of glial tissue with evenly spaced astrocytes and interlacing bands of vascularized fibrous connective tissue. The glial tissue merges with the collagen of the stroma or dermis. Mitoses are absent. At times, the astrocyte nuclei may appear enlarged or multinucleated. Long-standing or recurrent lesions tend to contain a considerable amount of fibrous tissue. Neurons are rare or absent. Rarely, choroid plexus, ependyma-lined clefts and pigmented retinal epithelium are seen, especially those of the palate and nasopharynx.

The glial tissue can be confirmed by immunoreactivity for glial fibrillary acidic protein (GFAP) or S100 protein {607,1273,1323,1991,2851}.

Differential diagnosis
The histologic differential diagnoses mainly include nasal encephalocele and, less frequently, a fibrosed nasal polyp. In contrast to heterotopic CNS tissue, encephaloceles are herniations of meningeal lined brain tissue that communicate with the intracranial ventricular system and subarachnoid space through a bony defect in the skull {1134}. Nasal encephalocele is composed of CNS tissue with easily found neurons. However, in nasal encephalocele of long-standing and in recurrences, the excessive fibrous tissue relative to the amount of glial cells and absence of neurons may make it impossible to distinguish from heterotopic CNS tissue.

Long-standing heterotopic CNS tissue may be mistaken for a fibrosed nasal polyp {1258}. The absence of glial tissue differentiates the latter from the former.

Histogenesis
It is a congenital malformation in which there is anterior displacement of mature cerebral tissue that has lost connection with the intracranial contents.

Prognosis and predictive factors
Adequate excision offers a cure in most cases, but incomplete excision can be accompanied by recurrence (15-30%). There is no local aggressive behaviour or malignant potential.

Ectopic pituitary adenoma

This lesion is described in Chapter 2 on tumours of the nasopharynx.

Germms cell tumours

A. Cardesa
M.A. Luna

Malignant germ cell tumours and terato-carcinosarcoma exhibiting histologic features similar to germ cell tumours of the gonads arise on rare occasions in the sinonasal tract. Immature teratomas and teratomas with malignant transformation are tumours of infancy and early childhood, whereas sinonasal yolk sac tumour and sinonasal teratocarcinosarcoma have only been documented in adults.

Immature teratoma

ICD-O code   9080/3

Immature teratomas are rare in the sinonasal tract and nasopharynx, and are composed of variable quantities of immature tissue elements, mostly neuroepithelial, that are interspersed with mature and immature tissues derived from the three embryonic germ layers. They are tumours of infancy and childhood {2317}.

Immature teratomas tend to be either solid-nodular or solid-cystic, while mature teratomas are usually cystic.

The tumour may contain cystic spaces lined by ciliated pseudostratified epithelium as well as primitive neuroepithelium with rosettes. Mitotic figures are frequently present in the immature areas; however, cellular atypia is not found. In infants and children, a teratoma with malignant transformation has to be excluded. In adults, thorough sampling of the specimen is mandatory to rule out teratocarcinosarcoma. Immature teratomas rarely behave in a malignant fashion {570}.

Teratoma with malignant transformation

ICD-O code   9084/3

Teratoma with malignant transformation is a neoplasm containing benign tissue elements of all three germinal layers and, in addition, a somatic malignancy. There is only a single reported case involving the sinonasal tract of a 13-month-old boy. The malignant component was a squamous cell carcinoma {1379}. The tumour was locally aggressive and recurred after surgery. There was no further recurrence 2 years after chemotherapy {1379}.

Sinonasal yolk sac tumour (endodermal sinus tumour)

ICD-O code   9071/3

This is a tumour that has the histological features of embryonic yolk sac, indistinguishable from yolk sac tumour (endodermal sinus tumour) of the gonads. Only two cases have been reported to arise in the sinonasal tract {1623}. Both patients were adults (aged 34 and 43 years). In one case, there was an admixed component of sinonasal nonkeratinizing carcinoma. The behaviour has been aggressive.

Sinonasal teratocarcinosarcoma

Definition
A complex malignant sinonasal neoplasm combining features of teratoma and carcinosarcoma. Benign and malignant epithelial, mesenchymal, and neural elements are typically present, including immature tissue with blastomatous features, while embryonal carcinoma, choriocarcinoma or seminoma is absent.

Synonyms
Malignant teratoma, blastoma, teratocarcinoma, teratoid carcinosarcoma

Epidemiology
Sinonasal teratocarcinosarcoma is very rare {755}. Approximately 60 cases have been published {755,1042,1619,1970, 2339,2578,2749}. Patients are exclusively adults, with age ranging from 18-79 years (mean 60 years). There is a marked male predominance {1042}.

Localization
It almost exclusively arises in the ethmoid sinus and maxillary antrum. One tumour has been reported to arise in the roof of the nasopharynx and another from the dorsum of the tongue {1042}.

Clinical features
Patients present with a short history of nasal obstruction and epistaxis {1042}. Imaging studies reveal a nasal mass, occasionally accompanied by opacification of the paranasal sinuses. Bone destruction may be seen.

Macroscopy
Tumours are usually bulky, soft to rubbery, and red-tan to purple.

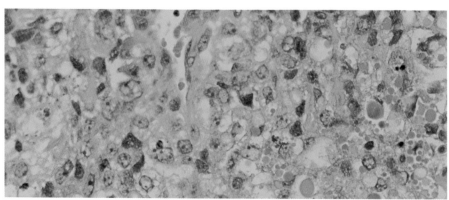

Fig. 1.95 Yolk sac tumour of nasal cavity. Typical features of yolk sac tumour, with many hyaline globules.

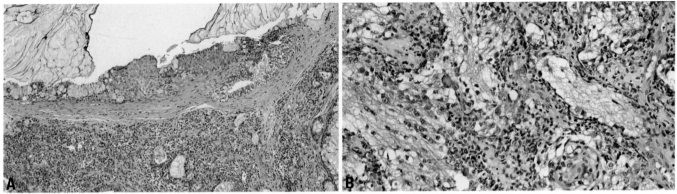

Fig. 1.96 Teratocarcinosarcoma. **A** Immature blastematous and glandular components are covered by a mixture of mature ciliated, mucinous and squamous epithelia. **B** Foci of neural differentiation showing fibrillary matrix and ganglion-like cells.

Histopathology

There are multiple tissue types derived from two or three germ layers, exhibiting variable degrees of maturity. In addition, there are intermingled carcinomatous and sarcomatous components {755, 2319}. The epithelial component is usually made up of keratinizing and nonkeratinizing squamous epithelium, pseudostratified columnar ciliated epithelium, and glandular structures lined by either cuboidal or columnar cells that may show mucous differentiation. Nests of immature squamous cells containing clear cells (fetal-appearing) are a common finding and an important diagnostic clue {1042}. The carcinomatous component is usually glandular, but sometimes squamous. Neuroepithelial elements with rosettes and neuroblastoma-like areas are present in most instances. The mesenchymal areas range from immature tissues (such as cartilage) to sarcomas (such as rhabdomyosarcoma and fibrosarcoma). There may be a proliferation of small round cells that are difficult to classify.

Immunoprofile

The undifferentiated/primitive component often shows positive immunoreaction for CD99 and occasionally synaptophysin and S-100 protein {1970}. The spindle cell component is consistently positive for vimentin, and sometimes desmin, myoglobin, and glial fibrillary acidic protein. The neuroepithelial component is positive for neuron-specific enolase and occasionally chromogranin, alfa-fetoprotein, and cytokeratin. The epithelial component is positive for cytokeratins, epithelial membrane antigen, and occasionally S-100 protein and glial fibrillary acidic protein.

Differential diagnosis

Inadequate sampling may lead to erroneous diagnoses of olfactory neuroblastoma, squamous cell carcinoma, undifferentiated carcinoma, adenocarcinoma, malignant salivary gland-type tumours and adenosquamous carcinoma {1042}.

Histogenesis

The tumour is unlikely to be of germ cell origin, but probably arises from a primitive cell in the olfactory/sinonasal membrane that not only reproduces the neuroectodermal features of olfactory neuroblastoma, but also has the capacity to differentiate into divergent types of somatic cells {1970}.

Prognosis and predictive factors

Teratocarcinosarcomas are highly malignant. They are locally aggressive, rapidly invading soft tissue and bone as well as the orbit and cranial cavities. They also have the potential to metastasize to regional lymph nodes and distant sites, mainly the lungs. The average survival is less than 2 years, with 60% of the patients not surviving beyond 3 years {1042}. Recurrences usually appear within 3 years.

Mature teratoma

Teratoma is the principal *benign germ cell tumour* of the sinonasal region and shows histologic features similar to its

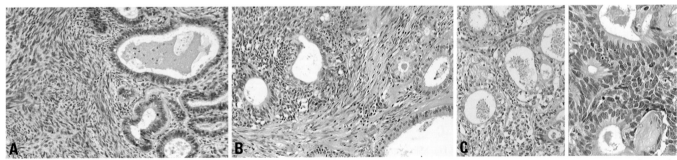

Fig. 1.97 Teratocarcinosarcoma. **A** The adenocarcinoma is intimately associated with the sarcomatous portion, arranged in a "teratoma-like" distribution. Cytologic atypia is present in both constituents of the neoplasm. **B** A primitive blastema-like component is immediately adjacent to a malignant glandular element that is juxtaposed with a malignant, cellular spindle cell constituent. **C** An adenocarcinoma with primitive blastema-like cells (left). The primitive cells can sometimes be arranged in a true rosette, similar to teratomas.

counterparts in the gonads and in other extragonadal locations.

Definition
Tumour composed of a variety of mature tissues that are foreign to the site of occurrence. There are typically tissues derived from two or three germ layers.

ICD-O code   9080/0

Synonyms
Teratoid tumour, benign teratoma.

Epidemiology
Teratomas of the head and neck account for only 6% of all teratomas {2558}. Mature teratomas in the sinonasal tract are even more uncommon {955}. Most cases occur in neonates and older infants, with equal sex distribution {955,1737}. Stillbirth, prematurity, fetal malpresentation, dystocia, and maternal polyhydramnios are frequent associations.

Localization
In the sinonasal tract, the maxillary antrum and nasal cavity are affected more often than the sphenoid sinus {1036,1408,1778,1805,2312}. The nasopharynx can also be the primary site of involvement.

Clinical features
Facial deformity, nasal obstruction, and a nasal mass are common manifestations. Occasional calcifications may be seen on imaging {955,1805}. Teratomas may be associated with other skull deformities, anencephaly, hemicrania, and palatal fissures {8}.

Macroscopy
The tumours are usually cystic, but can be solid or multilocular. They are commonly encapsulated masses that measure up to 7 cm.

Histopathology
Teratomas are composed of variable admixtures of mature skin, skin appendages, fat, glial tissue, smooth muscle, cartilage, bone, minor salivary glands, respiratory epithelium and gastrointestinal epithelium. Neural tissues are seen more often in sinonasal teratomas than in teratomas of other sites. Although the variegated histologic appearance of mature teratomas is usu-

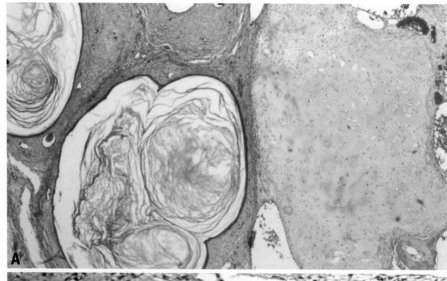

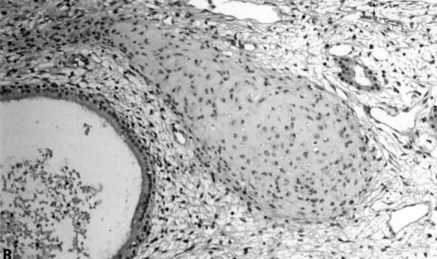

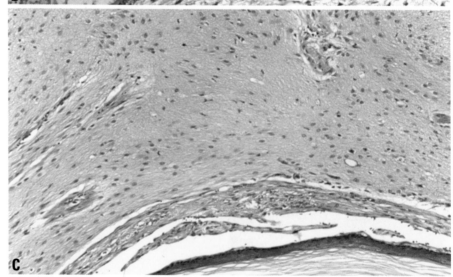

Fig. 1.98 Sinonasal mature teratoma. **A** Benign teratoma showing cysts lined by squamous epithelium and cartilage in stroma. **B** Cartilage and respiratory mucosa in mature teratoma. **C** Teratoma containing mature glial tissue.

ally diagnostic, heterotopic CNS tissue and meningocele should be considered in the differential diagnosis. The presence of immature elements or any other germ cell tumour excludes mature teratoma.

Histogenesis

The most popular theories are derivation from primordial germ cells or primitive somatic cells that escaped the influence of organizers and inducers {2558}.

Prognosis and predictive factors

Complete surgical excision is curative.

Dermoid cyst

Definition

A dermoid cyst is a developmental lesion histogenetically and histologically composed of ectoderm and mesoderm, but no endoderm.

ICD-O code   9084/0

Synonyms

Nasal dermoid sinus cyst, cystic dermoid.

Epidemiology

Dermoid cysts of the nose comprise 3% of all dermoids and about 10% of those of the head and neck region {2891}. There is a male predominance. More than half are detected in children 6 years old or less, and approximately a third are present at birth {582}.

Localization

Dermoid cysts of the head and neck are located more often in the subcutaneous tissue of the lateral supraorbital ridge and nose. In the nose, they occur most commonly in the bridge and always in the midline. The glabella, nasal tip, and columella are less common sites {582,2891}. A few cases have been described as originating in the paranasal sinuses {2622}.

Clinical features

Nasal dermoid cysts manifest as a midline nasal pit, fistula, or subcutaneous infected mass. They may cause broadening of the nasal bridge and occasionally cellulitis or purulent discharge. On palpation, the cysts are soft to fluctuant with a pale yellowish-pink colour noted beneath the thinned but intact epithelium; when keratin debris and sebum fill the lumen, they may have a doughy consistency {99,582,822,2891}. Most patients do not have other congenital malformations, but some do {2058}. Imaging studies are valuable in detecting a potential intracranial component and excluding an encephalocele {582, 2622,2891}.

Macroscopy

The cysts range up to 12 cm. The lumen contains cheesy, yellow-white material.

Histopathology

Dermoid cysts are lined with mature keratinizing squamous epithelium and frequently contain cutaneous appendages in the cyst wall. This lesion is differentiated from a teratoma by the limited variety of tissue types and the absence of endodermal components. Epidermal inclusion cysts may resemble dermoid cysts but do not contain adnexa and occur predominantly in adults {99,582,2622}.

Histogenesis

The most likely explanation for the ontogeny of dermoid cysts is the retention of ectodermal tissue along the lines of closure at junctions of bones, soft tissues, and embryonic membranes

Prognosis and predictive factors

Dermoid cysts are treated by complete surgical excision. Recurrence is uncommon (<7%) {582,2891}.

Secondary tumours

L. Barnes
L.L.Y. Tse
J. Hunt

Definition
Tumours that involve the nasal cavity and paranasal sinuses that originate from, but are not in continuity with, primary malignant neoplasms of other sites. Leukaemias and lymphomas are excluded.

Epidemiology
Metastases to the nasal cavity and paranasal sinuses are rare {1300,2085} and may occur in any age group. In a review of 82 cases, the median age of patients with metastatic tumours at diagnosis was 57 years (range 3 months to 76 years), and about 60% were males {202}.

Localization
The distribution of tumour among the paranasal sinuses and the most frequent tumour types to metastasize to these sites are shown in the Table 1.8 and 1.9. In 10-15% of cases, the metastases are limited to the nasal cavity.

Clinical features
Metastases to the sinonasal tract are haematogenous. They may be solitary or multifocal and ordinarily produce symptoms indistinguishable from those of a primary tumour. These include nasal obstruction, headache, facial pain, visual disturbances, exophthalmos, facial

Table 1.8 Most frequent sites of primary tumours that metastasize to the paranasal sinuses*

Primary Tumour	Frequency
Kidney	40%
Lung	9%
Breast	8%
Thyroid	8%
Prostate	7%
Miscellaneous	28%

*Data derived from reference {2085}

Table 1.9 Distribution of 168 tumours metastatic to paranasal sinuses*

Sinus	Frequency
Maxillary	33%
Sphenoid	22%
Ethmoid	14%
Frontal	9%
Multiple sinuses	22%

*Data based on reference {2085}

swelling, cranial nerve deficits and epistaxis (especially metastatic renal and thyroid carcinomas). In some instances, the metastasis may be the first manifestation of an otherwise clinically occult carcinoma, usually renal cell carcinoma.

Prognosis and predictive factors
Although the eventual outcome is usually poor, prognosis depends, in part, on whether the sinonasal metastasis is isolated or part of widespread disseminated disease. If the metastasis to the nasal cavity and sinuses is localized and treated aggressively, the average survival following discovery of the metastasis may be as long as 20-30 months {1300}.

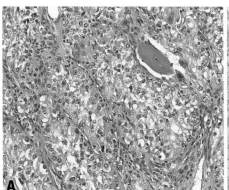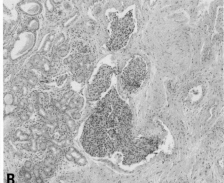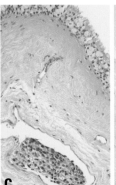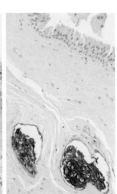

Fig. 1.99 Metastatic carcinoma. **A** Renal cell carcinoma metastatic to the maxillary sinus showing clear cells (due to accumulation of glycogen in the cytoplasm) and prominent sinusoidal vascularity. **B** Secondary prostatic adenocarcinoma. A malignant epithelial proliferation is identified within the large, patulous vessels in the sinonasal tract mucosa. **C** (Same case as B). The metastatic nature of the tumour (left) was confirmed when the prostate specific antigen (PSA) was strongly and diffusely immunoreactive in the cytoplasm of tumour cells within vascular spaces (right).

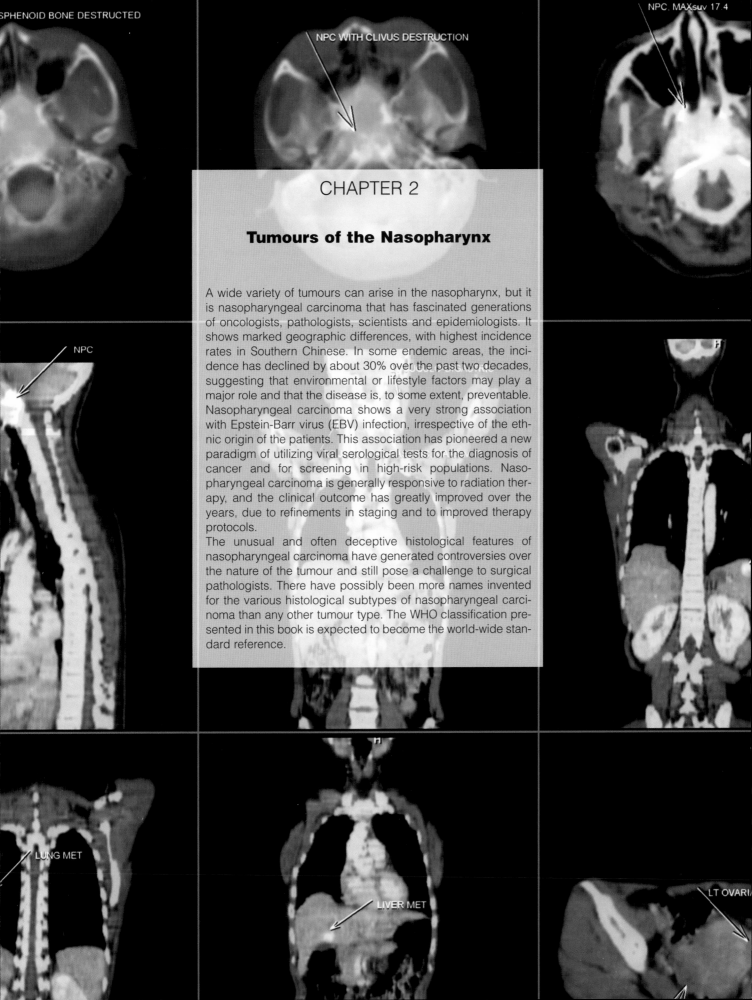

SPHENOID BONE DESTRUCTED

NPC WITH CLIVUS DESTRUCTION

NPC, MAXsuv 17.4

CHAPTER 2

Tumours of the Nasopharynx

A wide variety of tumours can arise in the nasopharynx, but it is nasopharyngeal carcinoma that has fascinated generations of oncologists, pathologists, scientists and epidemiologists. It shows marked geographic differences, with highest incidence rates in Southern Chinese. In some endemic areas, the incidence has declined by about 30% over the past two decades, suggesting that environmental or lifestyle factors may play a major role and that the disease is, to some extent, preventable. Nasopharyngeal carcinoma shows a very strong association with Epstein-Barr virus (EBV) infection, irrespective of the ethnic origin of the patients. This association has pioneered a new paradigm of utilizing viral serological tests for the diagnosis of cancer and for screening in high-risk populations. Nasopharyngeal carcinoma is generally responsive to radiation therapy, and the clinical outcome has greatly improved over the years, due to refinements in staging and to improved therapy protocols.

The unusual and often deceptive histological features of nasopharyngeal carcinoma have generated controversies over the nature of the tumour and still pose a challenge to surgical pathologists. There have possibly been more names invented for the various histological subtypes of nasopharyngeal carcinoma than any other tumour type. The WHO classification presented in this book is expected to become the world-wide standard reference.

NPC

LUNG MET

LIVER MET

LT OVARI

WHO histological classification of tumours of the nasopharynx

Malignant epithelial tumours
Nasopharyngeal carcinoma
    Nonkeratinizing carcinoma   8072/3
    Keratinizing squamous cell carcinoma   8071/3
    Basaloid squamous cell carcinoma   8083/3
Nasopharyngeal papillary adenocarcinoma   8260/3
Salivary gland-type carcinomas

Benign epithelial tumours
Hairy polyp
Schneiderian-type papilloma   8121/0
Squamous papilloma   8050/0
Ectopic pituitary adenoma   8272/0
Salivary gland anlage tumour
Craniopharyngioma   9350/1

Soft tissue neoplasms
Nasopharyngeal angiofibroma   9160/0

Haematolymphoid tumours
    Hodgkin lymphoma
    Diffuse large B-cell lymphoma   9680/3
    Extranodal NK/T cell lymphoma   9719/3
    Follicular dendritic cell sarcoma/tumour   9758/3
    Extramedullary plasmacytoma   9734/3

Tumours of bone and cartilage
    Chordoma   9370/3

Secondary tumours

---

[1] Morphology code of the International Classification of Diseases for Oncology (ICD-O) {821} and the Systematized Nomenclature of Medicine (http://snomed.org). Behaviour is coded /0 for benign tumours, /3 for malignant tumours, and /1 for borderline or uncertain behaviour.

TNM classification of carcinomas of the nasopharynx

TNM classification [1,2]

T-Primary tumour
TX   Primary tumour cannot be assessed
T0   No evidence of primary tumour
    Tis carcinoma in-situ
T1   Tumour confined to nasopharynx
T2   Tumour extends to soft tissues
T2a.   Tumour extends to oropharynx and/or nasal cavity without parapharyngeal extension*
T2b.   Tumour with parapharyngeal extension*
T3   Tumour invades bony structures and/or paranasal sinuses
T4   Tumour with intracranial extension and/or involvement of cranial nerves, infratemporal fossa, hypopharynx, orbit, or masticator space

N-regional lymph nodes**
NX   Regional lymph nodes cannot be assessed
N0   No regional lymph node metastasis
N1   Unilateral*** metastasis in lymph node(s), <6 cm in greatest dimension, above the supraclavicular fossa
N2   Bilateral metastasis in lymph node(s), <6 cm in greatest dimension, above the supraclavicular fossa
N3   Metastasis in lymph node(s), >6 cm and/or in the supraclavicular fossa
N3a.   >6 cm in dimension
N3b.   in the supraclavicular fossa#

Distant metastasis
M-   MX Distant metastasis cannot be assessed
M0   No distant metastasis
M1   Distant metastasis

Stage Grouping

Stage	T	N	M
Stage 0	Tis	N0	M0
Stage I	T1	N0	M0
Stage IIA	T2a	N0	M0
Stage IIB	T1	N1	M0
	T2a	N1	M0
	T2b	N0, N1	M0
Stage III	T1	N2	M0
	T2a, T2b	N2	M0
	T3	N0, N1, N2	M0
Stage IV A	T4	N0, N1, N2	M0
Stage IVB	Any T	N3	M0
Stage IVC	Any T	Any N	M1

*Parapharyngeal extension denotes postero-lateral infiltration of tumour beyond the pharyngobasilar fascia.
** The regional lymph nodes are the cervical nodes.
*** Midline nodes are considered ipsilateral nodes.
# Supraclavicular fossa is the triangular region defined by 3 points:
the superior margin of the sternal end of the clavicle,
the superior margin of the lateral end of the clavicle,
the point where the neck meets the shoulder. This includes caudal portions of Levels IV and V.

---

[1] {947,2418}.
[2] A help desk for specific questions about the TNM classification is available at www.uicc.org/index.php?id=508 .

Tumours of the nasopharynx: Introduction

J.K.C. Chan
B.Z. Pilch
T.T. Kuo
B.M. Wenig
A.W.M. Lee

The most common type of nasopharyngeal tumour is nasopharyngeal carcinoma, which is remarkable for the striking geographic differences in its incidence as well as the near consistent association with the Epstein-Barr virus (EBV). Nasopharyngeal carcinoma is also the prototype of a family of morphologically distinctive tumours – the lymphoepithelial carcinomas – that can arise in a variety of sites, such as other head and neck mucosal sites, salivary gland, lung and thymus, albeit uncommonly. Interestingly, in contrast to nasopharyngeal carcinoma, lymphoepithelial carcinomas occurring in these sites usually show a strong association with EBV only in Asians, but not in Caucasians.

Besides nasopharyngeal carcinoma, a broad range of neoplasms can arise in the nasopharynx, from epithelial to lymphoid, mesenchymal and neurogenic. Rarely, tumours derived from embryonic remnants either entrapped in their normal pathway of ascent or descent (ectopic pituitary tumour, craniopharyngioma) or dissociated from their normal regulatory influences (germ cell tumour) can occur. Since the nasopharynx is in close proximity to many different anatomic structures, tumours arising in the latter sites can also present clinically as a nasopharyngeal mass, for example, chordoma arising in the clivus.

Anatomy

The nasopharynx is the narrow tubular passage behind the nasal cavity. Its sloping roof and posterior wall are formed by the basi-sphenoid, basi-occiput and the first cervical vertebra. Anteriorly, it communicates with the nasal cavity via the choanae. The orifices of Eustachian tubes are in the lateral walls, and each is shielded superiorly and posteriorly by a comma-shaped elevation called the torus tubarius. Immediately above and behind the torus tubarius is a pharyngeal recess called the fossa of Rosenmüller. The nasopharynx tapers inferiorly, and continues as the oropharynx from the level of the soft palate.

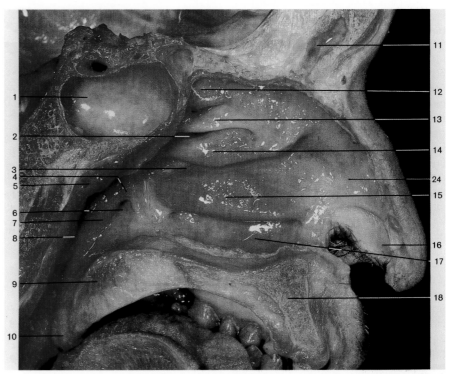

Fig. 2.1 Sagittal section of the head showing the nasopharynx, nasal cavity and paranasal sinuses. {3797}
1 - Sphenoidal sinus; 2 - Superior meatus; 3- Middle meatus; 4 - Tubal elevation; 5 - Pharyngeal tonsil; 6 - Pharyngeal orifice of Eustachian tube; 7 - Salpingopharyngeal fold; 8 - Pharyngeal recess; 9 - Soft palate; 10- Uvula; 11- Frontal sinus; 12 - Sphenoethmoidal recess; 13 - Superior nasal concha; 14 - Middle nasal concha; 15 - Inferior nasal concha; 16 - Vestibule; 17 - Inferior meatus; 18 - Hard palate; 24 - Atrium.

The nasopharynx constitutes part of the Waldeyer ring. Histologically, its mucosa is covered by respiratory-type ciliated epithelium, but variable amounts of squamous epithelium are common. The mucosa exhibits invaginations, forming crypts that abut the underlying stroma. The stroma is rich in lymphoid tissue that often includes reactive lymphoid follicles. The surface or crypt epithelium is commonly infiltrated by many small lymphoid cells, which expand and disrupt the epithelium to produce a reticulated pattern. Some seromucinous glands are present, but they are not as abundant as in the nasal mucosa.

Clinical features
Diagnostic procedures
Various imaging techniques, such as computed tomography and magnetic resonance imaging, are helpful for detection of the presence of a tumour, as well as in precise delineation of the extent of disease. Endoscopic examination with directed biopsy is the key in obtaining materials for a definitive histological diagnosis.

Tumour staging
The TNM staging system for nasopharyngeal tumours (see preceding section) is only applicable for epithelial tumours, and in fact has been developed specifically for nasopharyngeal carcinoma. For lymphomas, the Ann Arbor staging system is recommended {947}.

Classification of nasopharyngeal carcinomas
In the 1978 WHO classification, three histological subtypes of nasopharyngeal

carcinoma were recognized: squamous cell carcinoma (WHO type 1), nonkeratinizing carcinoma (WHO type 2), and undifferentiated carcinoma (WHO type 3) {2320}. In the 1991 WHO classification, the squamous cell carcinoma subtype (keratinizing squamous cell carcinoma) was retained, while the last two subtypes in the previous classification were combined under a single category of "nonkeratinizing carcinoma", which was further subdivided as being "differentiated" or "undifferentiated"; lymphoepithelioma-like carcinoma was considered a morphologic variant of undifferentiated carcinoma {2317}. The use of numerical designation of WHO types 1, 2 and 3 was eliminated. The wide ranging reported figures on the frequencies of various subtypes indicate that the boundaries between the categories are not always clear (such as less well differentiated forms of keratinizing squamous cell carcinoma versus nonkeratinizing carcinoma, and nonkeratinizing carcinoma versus undifferentiated carcinoma), sampling error is a significant problem due to the small size of the biopsies, and intra- and inter-observer reproducibility of the classification is sub-optimal {323,2318, 2497,2735}. In fact, squamous cell carcinoma and nonkeratinizing carcinoma have been viewed by some investigators as being merely variants of a fairly homogeneous group of tumours {2318,2577}. Notwithstanding these problems, the proportion of keratinizing squamous cell carcinoma among all nasopharyngeal carcinomas is probably higher in low-incidence compared with high-incidence areas.

The current WHO classification maintains the terminology of the 1991 classification, with the addition of one category: basaloid squamous cell carcinoma.

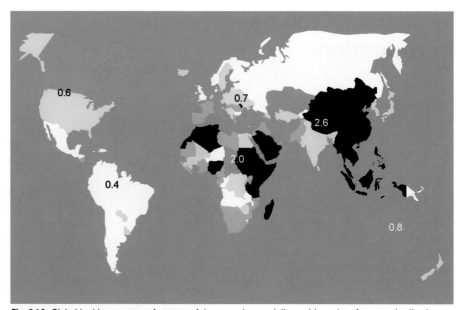

Fig. 2.1A Global incidence rates of cancer of the nasopharynx (all ages) in males. Age-standardized rates (ASR, world standard population) per 100,000 population and year. From: Globocan 2002 (http://www-depdb.iarc.fr/globocan/GLOBOframe.htm).

Nasopharyngeal carcinoma

J.K.C. Chan
F. Bray
P. McCarron
W. Foo
A.W.M. Lee
T. Yip
T.T. Kuo

B.Z. Pilch
B.M. Wenig
D. Huang
K.W. Lo
Y.X. Zeng
W.H. Jia

Definition

A carcinoma arising in the nasopharyngeal mucosa that shows light microscopic or ultrastructural evidence of squamous differentiation. It encompasses squamous cell carcinoma, nonkeratinizing carcinoma (differentiated or undifferentiated) and basaloid squamous cell carcinoma. Adenocarcinoma and salivary gland-type carcinoma are excluded.

ICD-O codes

Nonkeratinizing carcinoma
        8072/3
Keratinizing squamous cell carcinoma
        8071/3
Basaloid squamous cell carcinoma
        8083/3

Synonyms

Lymphoepithelioma, lymphoepithelioma-like carcinoma, lymphoepithelial carcinoma, Schmincke type lymphoepithelioma, Regaud type lymphoepithelioma, transitional cell carcinoma, intermediate cell carcinoma, anaplastic carcinoma, undifferentiated carcinoma with lymphoid stroma, vesicular nucleus cell carcinoma, squamous cell carcinoma (WHO-1), nonkeratinizing carcinoma (WHO-2), undifferentiated carcinoma (WHO-3).

Epidemiology

Global incidence and mortality

Nasopharyngeal carcinoma (NPC) shows a distinct racial and geographical distribution and a multifactorial etiology. Globally, there were approximately 65,000 new cases and 38,000 deaths in the year 2000 {730}. While rare in most parts of the world (onset rates commonly <1 per 105, or 0.6% of all cancers), there are certain populations for which the incidence is considerably higher, notably native and foreign-born Chinese, Southeast Asians (e.g. in Thailand, Philippines, and Vietnam), North Africans (e.g. in Algeria and Morocco), as well as native peoples of the Arctic region (e.g. in Canada and Alaska). Within these populations, there is a remarkable heterogeneity among ethnic lines {2872}. The highest incidence of NPC has long been observed in Hong Kong, where 1 in 40 men develop NPC before the age of 75 years {1981}.

Age and sex distribution

In high-risk groups, NPC incidence rises after the age of 30 years and peaks at 40-60 years, and thereafter declines {730}. The age distribution is similar in males and females, although rates in men are commonly 2-3-fold those observed in women {1981}.

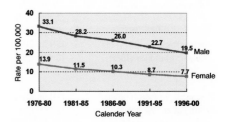

Fig. 2.3 Nasopharyngeal carcinoma in Hong Kong, 5-year trends in age-standardized incidence, 1976-2000.

Migration

In general, populations that migrate from high to low risk areas retain much of the elevated risk {304} seen in their country of origin, although this, and the extent to which the risk diminishes in successive generations, varies according to ethnicity. Such heterogeneity may be associated with several factors, possibly acting in combination - the degree of genetic predisposition, and the prevalence of certain risk factors related to lifestyle upon migration.

Time trends

Recent trends in NPC incidence in high-risk countries reveal convincing evidence of a decline in rates since the mid-1970s in Hong Kong {1446}. The speed of the decline points to the role of changing environmental risk factors. Rates in low-risk areas are, in view of the rarity of the disease, subject to a great deal of random variation, and trends are often difficult to interpret. In U.S. Whites and in England, rates are low and in slow decline. The evolution of trends in U.S. Blacks is unclear.

Etiology

The specific geographical and demographic distribution of nasopharyngeal carcinoma (NPC), the time trends, and patterns observed in migrants reflect the interplay of genetic susceptibility, infection by Epstein-Barr virus (EBV) and environmental factors (dietary and nondietary) in disease causation.

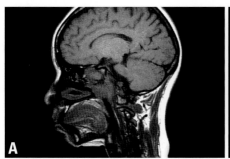
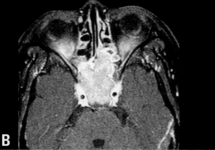

Fig. 2.2 Nasopharyngeal carcinoma. **A** and **B** Magnetic resonance imaging (MRI) of nasopharyngeal carcinoma (NPC): A 40-year old female patient presented with 2 months history of tinnitus, followed by neck masses, nasal symptoms, headache and diplopia. Physical examination showed left VI nerve palsy and bilateral upper-mid cervical lymph nodes. Endoscopy revealed tumour in the nasopharynx extending to posterior nasal cavity. Biopsy confirmed undifferentiated carcinoma. MRI showed NPC with extensive local infiltration of adjacent soft tissues, erosion of skull base / paranasal sinuses, and intracranial extension, together with bilateral retropharyngeal and cervical nodes.

Table 2.01 Reported EBV association in nasopharyngeal squamous cell carcinoma

Report	Technique of EBV demonstration	EBV positivity rate
Niedobitek e al 1991 {1892}	ISH for EBV DNA	Germany 0/7 China 0/1
Dickens et al 1992 {599}	DNA slot-blot hybridization	Hong Kong 5/8
Chen et al 1993 {405}	ISH for EBV DNA	Taiwan 9/9
Hording et al 1993 {1124,1125}	PCR for EBV DNA	Denmark 2/15
Della Torre et al 1994 {580}	PCR for EBV DNA	Italy 2/9
Pathmanathan et al 1995 {1988}	ISH for EBER, immunohisto-chemistry for LMP-1	Malaysia (Chinese patients) 31/31
Gulley et al 1995 {961}	ISH for EBER	USA 0/3
Kanavaros et al 1995 {1262}	ISH for EBER	Greece 0/13
Nicholls et al 1997 {1885}	ISH for EBER	Hong Kong 22/22 Chengdu, China 7/10 Birmingham, UK 3/7
Hwang et al 1998 {1157}	ISH for EBER	Taiwan 1/1
Zhang et al 1998 {2894}	ISH for EBER, IHC*	Southern China 10/10
Inoue et al 2002 {1176}	ISH for EBER	Japan 4/4

ISH = in-situ hybridization; PCR = polymerase chain reaction; EBV = Epstein-Barr virus
EBER = EBV-encoded early RNA, LMP-1 = latent membrane protein-1
*Immunohistochemistry (IHC) for early antigen-diffuse and 350/220 kd membrane glycoprotein of EBV

Epstein-Barr virus

The near constant association of EBV with NPC, irrespective of ethnic background, indicates a probable oncogenic role of the virus in the genesis of this tumour {1166,2107}. The evidence includes: (1) raised levels of antibodies, especially IgA, against EBV (most commonly viral capsid antigen and early antigen) in most patients with NPC compared with normal controls and patients with other cancer types; (2) higher titers of IgA antibodies against EBV in patients with large tumour bulk; (3) presence of EBV DNA or RNA in practically all tumour cells; (4) presence of EBV in a clonal episomal form, indicating that the virus has entered the tumour cell before clonal expansion; (5) presence of EBV in the precursor lesion of NPC, but not in the normal nasopharyngeal epithelium. The evidence was considered sufficient to classify EBV as carcinogenic by the International Agency for Research on Cancer (IARC) in 1997 {1166}. Nevertheless, it is likely that EBV infection takes place relatively late in the oncogenic process {1893}.

The EBV infection in NPC exhibits the type II latency pattern, that is, expression of EBV nuclear antigen-1 (EBNA-1) and latent membrane protein-1 (LMP-1), but not the immunogenic EBNA2-6. EBV encoded early RNAs (EBERs) are expressed in abundance. BZLF (Zebra) protein, which is expressed in lytic infec-

tion by EBV, is not detected. LMP-1, a viral protein with transforming properties, can induce epidermal hyperplasia, inhibit squamous differentiation, upregulate the adhesion molecule ICAM-1 and CD40, activate nuclear factor-κB (NF-κ-B), and induce expression of epidermal growth factor receptor.

Table 2.02 Common presenting symptoms and signs of nasopharyngeal carcinoma. Data from 722 consecutive patients treated at the Pamela Youde Nethersole Eastern Hospital, Hong Kong, during 1994 to 2001.

Presenting features	Frequency (%)
Symptoms	
Neck mass	42%
Nasal (post nasal drip, discharge, bleeding, obstruction)	46%
Aural (tinnitus, discharge, ear ache, deafness)	42%
Headache	16%
Ophthalmic (double vision, squint, blindness)	6%
Facial numbness	5%
Speech / swallowing problem	2%
Weight loss	4%
Physical signs	
Enlarged neck node(s)	72%
Bilateral neck nodes	35%
Neck nodes extending to supraclavicular fossa	12%
Cranial nerve palsy	10%
Deafness	3%
Dermatomyositis	1%

Environmental factors
Diet
In high incidence regions, high levels of volatile nitrosamines in preserved food have been implicated as the putative carcinogen for NPC development {2063}. In the 1960s, it was proposed that the increased incidence of NPC among Hong Kong boat dwellers compared to house dwellers may have been due to their staple diet of salted fish {1108}. From case-control studies on Chinese, consumption of Cantonese-style salted fish in the weaning period carries odds ratios ranging from 2-7.5 {2869,2870, 2913}. Animals fed salted fish may develop nasal tumours {1142,2871, 2913}. Other preserved or fermented foods in high incidence regions, consumed during weaning and early childhood, have also been incriminated as risk factors {2869,2903}. The importance of exposure in early life is supported by two studies showing that low-risk ethnic groups born in high-risk areas also have higher risk of NPC {1212,1213}. In low incidence regions like Northern China, the consumption of salted fish still carries an adjusted relative risk as high as 5.6 {304}.

Other environmental risk factors
Other purported risk factors include cigarette smoking {1900,2868,2875}, occupational exposure to smoke, chemical fumes and dusts, formaldehyde exposure {74,1090}, and prior radiation exposure {403}.

Localization
The most common site of origin is the lateral wall of the nasopharynx, especially the fossa of Rosenmüller, followed by the superior posterior wall. Cervical lymph node metastasis is a common occurrence.

Clinical features
Signs and symptoms
About half of the patients have multiple symptoms, but 10% are asymptomatic. Painless enlargement of upper cervical lymph node(s) is the most common presenting feature. Nearly half of the patients complain of nasal symptom(s), particularly blood stained post-nasal drip. Symptoms related to Eustachian tube obstruction (such as serous otitis media) also commonly occur. Headache and symptoms related to cranial nerve

involvement are features of more advanced disease.

In endemic areas, NPC is an important underlying malignancy in patients presenting with dermatomyositis, being found in 12% of patients {2005} although only 1% of patients with NPC have dermatomyositis {2573}.

Imaging

Magnetic resonance (MR) is the study of choice for assessing the loco-regional extent because of its superior sensitivity and multiplanar capability. Although CT is useful in depicting cortical bone erosion, MR is superior in revealing soft tissue infiltration and intracranial extension {442,1880} as well as marrow replacement permitting early recognition of bony involvement {442,1880}. Systemic imaging workup for patients with high metastatic risk include X-ray/CT of chest, ultrasonography/CT of liver, isotope bone scan and positron emission tomography coupled with CT (PET-CT).

Table 2.03 Structures involved by local infiltration of nasopharyngeal carcinoma at presentation. Source: Magnetic resonance studies of 308 patients from Pamela Youde Nethersole Eastern Hospital, Hong Kong.

Structures involved	Frequency
Adjacent soft tissues	
Nasal cavity	87%
Oropharyngeal wall, soft palate	21%
Parapharyngeal space, carotid space	68%
Pterygoid muscle (medial, lateral)	48%
Prevertebral muscle	19%
Bony erosion / paranasal sinus	
Nasal septum	3%
Pterygoid plate(s), pterygo-maxillary fissure, pterygo-palatine fossa	27%
Maxillary antrum	4%
Ethmoid sinus	6%
Sphenoid sinus, sphenoid bone, foramina lacerum, ovale, rotundum	38%
Clivus	41%
Petrous bone, petro-occipital fissure	19%
Jugular foramen, hypoglossal canal	4%
Pituitary fossa / gland	3%
Extensive/ intracranial extension	
Cavernous sinus	16%
Cerebrum, meninges, cisterns	4%
Infratemporal fossa	9%
Orbit, orbital fissure(s)	4%
Hypopharynx	2%

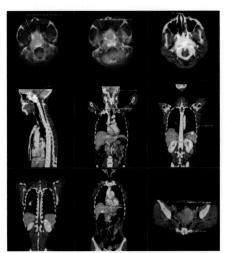

Fig. 2.4 Positron emission tomography coupled with computed tomography (PET-CT) of nasopharyngeal carcinoma. Physical examination and biochemistry did not show any sign suggestive of distant metastases. X-ray chest was normal. PET-CT revealed multiple distant metastases in lung, liver and spleen, in addition to extensive local infiltration and bilateral cervical lymph nodes.

Serological studies

Positive serology against Epstein-Barr virus (EBV) is found in close to 100% of patients with non-keratinizing NPC {976}. IgA against viral capsid antigen (VCA) and IgG/IgA against early antigens (EA) are the most extensively used diagnostic tool, with the reported detection rates for NPC varying from 69-93%. Newer antibody tests based on recombinant EBV antigens such as EBV nuclear antigens (EBNA), membrane antigen (MA), thymidine kinase (TK), DNA polymerase (DP), ribonucleotide reductase (RR), DNAase, and Z transactivator protein (Zta) have shown promise when used in combination {378,537}.

Another approach is to test for elevated levels of circulating EBV DNA or RNA (BamH1-W, EBERs or EBNA1) by quantitative PCR (Q-PCR) in the plasma or serum, with reported sensitivity in NPC up to 96% {35,1514,1549,2346}.

Relevant diagnostic procedures

All patients should have complete physical examination and endoscopic examination of the nasopharyngeal region. Biopsies are taken from the gross lesions. In the absence of a gross lesion, multiple biopsies should be taken from the lateral, superior and posterior walls of the nasopharynx for patients with high suspicion of NPC.

Macroscopy

The tumour can appear as a smooth bulge in the mucosa, a discrete raised nodule with or without surface ulceration, or a frankly infiltrative fungating mass. Sometimes no grossly visible lesion is seen.

Tumour spread and staging
Tumour spread

NPC is notorious for its highly malignant behaviour, with extensive loco-regional infiltration, early lymphatic spread, and disproportionately high incidence of haematogenous dissemination. Erosion of skull base and paranasal sinuses, intracranial spread (via eroded bone or basal foramina), infiltration of cranial nerves, and extension to more distant structures (infratemporal fossa, orbit, hypopharynx) occur as tumour invasion advances.

With the rich lymphatic plexus in the nasopharynx, lymphatic spread occurs early in the course of disease. In patients staged by MR, about 20% of patients have no enlarged nodes, and about half have retropharyngeal node involvement {2314}. The jugulo-digastric node is by far the most common palpable node at presentation, and involvement of the posterior cervical chain is more frequent than with other head and neck cancers. The strong association between the topographic level of lymphatic extension and the increased incidence of distant failure reflects that haematogenous dissemination occurs mainly via the draining of the lymphatic trunks at the lower end of the jugular chain into the great vessels. The most common sites of haematogenous deposits are, in descending order of frequency, bone, lung, liver, and distant nodes {2575}.

Staging

The current TNM staging system {947, 2418} is customized for NPC, as the natural

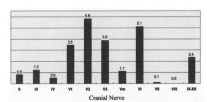

Fig. 2.5 The relative frequency of cranial nerve palsy due to nasopharyngeal carcinoma at the time of diagnosis. Source: 722 patients treated at the Pamela Youde Nethersole Eastern Hospital, Hong Kong, 1994-2001.

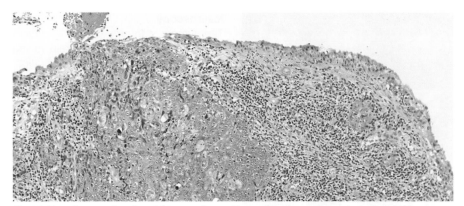

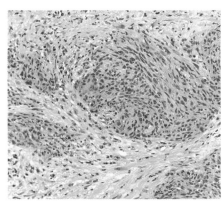

Fig. 2.6 Nasopharyngeal nonkeratinizing carcinoma. Tumour islands are obvious in the lymphoid stroma.

Fig. 2.7 Nasopharyngeal nonkeratinizing carcinoma. This example is accompanied by an abundant desmoplastic stroma.

behaviour and therapeutic considerations of NPC are so uniquely different from other head and neck cancers.

With accumulation of supporting data from different countries {448,490,1061, 1119,1444,1592,1966}, there is little doubt that the current staging system is superior to the past systems, both in terms of improved predictive accuracy and more balanced stage distribution.

Nonkeratinizing carcinoma
Histopathology
The biopsies vary in appearance from the presence of a frank tumour with surface ulceration to subtle involvement of the mucosa beneath an intact surface epithelium {2316,2318,2735}. The tumour comprises solid sheets, irregular islands, dyscohesive sheets and trabeculae of carcinoma intimately intermingled with variable numbers of lymphocytes and plasma cells. Subclassification into the undifferentiated and differentiated subtypes is optional, since their distinction is of no clinical or prognostic significance, and different areas of the same tumour or different biopsies taken at different time intervals from the same patient may exhibit features of one or the other subtype. When both subtypes are seen in a specimen, the tumour may be classified according to the prominent subtype, or as nonkeratinizing carcinoma with features of both subtypes.

The undifferentiated subtype, which is more common, is characterized by syncytial-appearing large tumour cells with indistinct cell borders, round to oval vesicular nuclei, and large central nucleoli. The cells often appear crowded or even overlapping. Sometimes, the nuclei

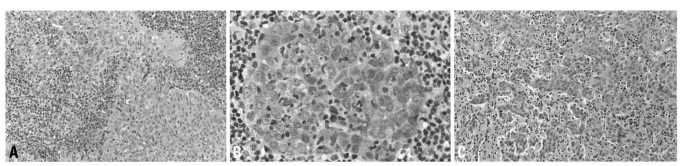

Fig. 2.8 Nasopharyngeal nonkeratinizing carcinoma. **A** This example of differentiated subtype is characterized by sheets of tumour separated by a dense infiltrate of lymphocytes and plasma cells. **B** Tumour island in a lymphoid cell-rich stroma. Some lymphocytes are also seen within the tumour. **C** This tumour shows an uncommon trabecular growth pattern.

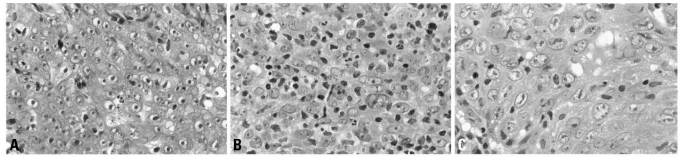

Fig. 2.9 Cytological spectrum of nasopharyngeal nonkeratinizing carcinoma, undifferentiated subtype. **A** The cells exhibit a syncytial quality, and possess vesicular nuclei, prominent nucleoli and amphophilic cytoplasm. **B** The syncytial-appearing cells have vesicular nuclei, distinct nucleoli and lightly eosinophilic cytoplasm. There are some intermingled lymphocytes. **C** Focally, there can be cells with more distinct cell borders and a moderate amount of eosinophilic cytoplasm.

can be chromatin-rich rather than vesicular. The scant cytoplasm is either amphophilic or eosinophilic. There can be small foci of primitive squamous differentiation, where groups of tumour cells exhibit a slightly greater amount of lightly eosinophilic cytoplasm and slightly more distinct cell borders.

The differentiated subtype differs from the undifferentiated subtype in showing cellular stratification and pavementing, often with a plexiform growth, reminiscent of transitional cell carcinoma of the bladder {2317}. The tumour cells show fairly well-defined cell borders and sometimes vague intercellular bridges, and there may exceptionally be occasional keratinized cells. Compared with the undifferentiated subtype, the cells are often slightly smaller, the nuclear-cytoplasmic ratio is lower, the nuclei can be more chromatin-rich, and nucleoli are usually not as prominent.

A desmoplastic stroma is uncommon. Areas of coagulative necrosis are sometimes present, and can be extensive. The density of lymphocytes and plasma cells is highly variable. At one extreme, there are no or few lymphocytes within the tumour islands, although some lymphoid cells are present in between, which probably merely represent the native lymphoid tissue in the nasopharyngeal mucosa. At the other extreme, abundant lymphocytes and plasma cells infiltrate the tumour islands, breaking them up into tiny clusters or single cells and obscuring the epithelial nature of the tumour; the term "lymphoepithelial carcinoma" may be applied for such cases. In metastatic sites, the lymphocyte density in the tumour may or may not be maintained. In some cases, scattered epithelioid granulomas are present, and may be so prominent as to mask the small islands of carcinoma {404}. Many admixed eosinophils are seen in about one-fourth of cases {830,1463,1555}. Some cases show a prominent infiltrate of neutrophils even in the absence of ulceration.

There are a number of inconstant features. The carcinoma cells can assume a plump or slender spindle shape focally or extensively, with formation of streaming fascicles. The nucleoli of the spindly cells are often not as prominent as the syncytial-appearing cells. In some cases, isolated or groups of tumour cells

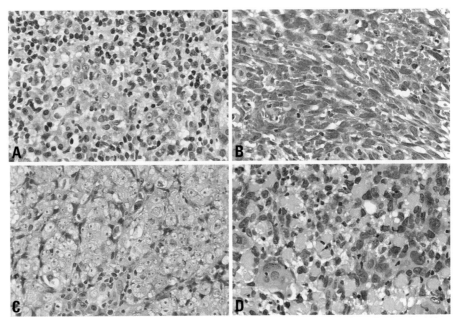

Fig. 2.10 Nasopharyngeal nonkeratinizing carcinoma, undifferentiated subtype. **A** So-called lymphoepithelial carcinoma, characterized by lymphoid cells apparently breaking up the tumour into tiny aggregates, rendering it difficult to appreciate the epithelial nature of the neoplasm. **B** This case comprises spindly cells with dark-staining nuclei and inconspicuous nucleoli. **C** Among the carcinoma cells with vesicular nuclei, there can be tumour cels with a shrunken appearance and dark-staining nuclei. **D** Some examples show many amyloid globules among the tumour cells. Some globules are intracellular, and displace the nucleus of the tumour cells to one pole.

may appear shrunken, with dark smudged nuclei and dense amphophilic or eosinophilic cytoplasm; it is unclear whether such changes reflect a degenerative phenomenon in a subpopulation of tumour cells, or a biopsy artefact. There can be Pagetoid spread of the carcinoma into the surface or crypt epithelium. In approximately one-tenth of cases, there are interspersed spherical amyloid globules {2084}. The amyloid globules are usually smaller than a tumour cell,

and can be present intracellularly (sometimes causing indentation of the tumour cell nucleus), scattered among the carcinoma cells, or in the adjacent stroma. They are derived from keratins, and are probably of tumour origin. In the uncommon papillary variant, there are papillary fronds comprising delicate stromal cores covered by stratified tumour cells morphologically no different from those of the usual nonkeratinizing nasopharyngeal carcinoma. Rare cases can show cyto-

Table 2.04 Frequency of histological subtypes of nasopharyngeal carcinoma.

Current WHO classification	High incidence population		Intermediate incidence	Low incidence population	
	Hong Kong*	Singapore {2318}	Tunisia {323}	Japan {2497}	U.S.A. {2735}
Keratinizing squamous cell carcinoma	1%	17%	8%	13%	25%
Nonkeratinizing carcinoma	99%	83%	92%	87%	75%
- Undifferentiated	92%	42%	76%		
- Differentiated	7%	41%	16%		
Basaloid squamous cell carcinoma	<0.2%	NA	NA	NA	NA

NA = Not available; *Queen Elizabeth Hospital, 2001-2003

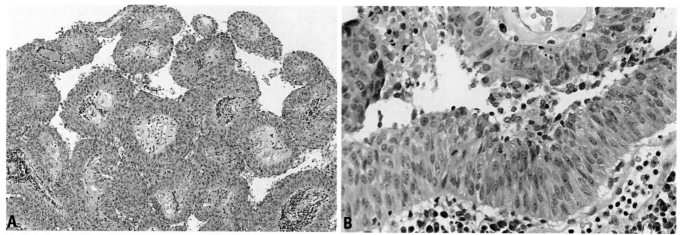

Fig. 2.11 Nasopharyngeal nonkeratinizing carcinoma with papillary architecture. **A** The tumour forms exophytic papillae with fibrovascular cores. **B** The lining cells show features of differentiated nonkeratinizing carcinoma.

plasmic clear cell change, but this is such an uncommon feature that the alternative diagnosis of lymphoma or salivary gland-type carcinoma should always be considered. Exceptionally, there is accumulation of extracellular edema fluid or mucosubstance, breaking up the tumour islands to produce a complex reticulated pattern. Nasopharyngeal carcinoma may contain intracytoplasmic mucin in very rare cells. It has also rarely been reported to occur in combination with a component of adenocarcinoma {1200, 1389}. Nasopharyngeal carcinoma may present initially with cervical lymph node metastases. The lymph nodes can be involved extensively or subtly (such as submergence of the tumour in the lymphocyte-rich paracortex). The tumour takes the form of islands and strands, being intermingled with variable numbers of lymphocytes, plasma cells and eosinophils. Some tumour cells can resemble Reed-Sternberg cells or lacunar cells. Coupled with a dense lymphoid infiltrate, a misdiagnosis of Hodgkin or non-Hodgkin lymphoma is sometimes made {330,1470}. A desmoplastic stroma may be present. In approximately one fifth of cases, there are epithelioid granulomas, and in half of these cases, the granulomas show caseous necrosis {1470}. Nasopharyngeal carcinoma may also metastasize as a wholly or partly cystic lesion containing necrotic material.

Immunoprofile
Practically all tumour cells show strong staining for pan-cytokeratin (AE1/AE3, MNF-116); this uniform staining contrasts with the usually focal staining observed in undifferentiated carcinomas of other sites, such as the lung and thyroid. The staining for high molecular weight cytokeratins (such as cytokeratin 5/6, 34ßE12) is strong, and staining for low molecular weight cytokeratins (such as CAM5.2) is often weaker and sometimes patchy. Cytokeratins 7 and 20 are both negative {801}. In undifferentiated nonkeratinizing carcinoma, the cytokeratin immunostain highlights the scanty wisps of cytoplasm that wrap around the large nucleus and extend outward as short narrow processes. As a result of the cell nests being broken up by infiltrating lymphocytes, a distinctive reticulated or meshwork pattern is produced. In differentiated nonkeratinizing carcinoma, the tumour cells, with a broader rim of cytoplasm, are obviously polygonal on immunostaining for cytokeratin.

Immunoreactivity for epithelial membrane antigen in nasopharyngeal carcinoma is often only focal {816}. In most cases, the tumour exhibits strong nuclear staining for p63, a basal cell marker that normally highlights the basal and parabasal cells of the overlying stratified squamous epithelium.

The lymphoid cells represent a mixture of T cells and B cells, usually with the former predominating, especially within and around the tumour islands {854,883, 1070,1962,2912}. At least a proportion of the T cells are activated cytotoxic cells. The plasma cells are polyclonal. There are variable numbers of scattered S100

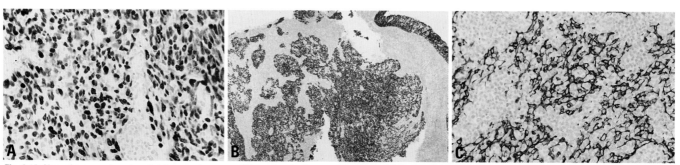

Fig. 2.12 Nasopharyngeal nonkeratinizing carcinoma, undifferentiated subtype. **A** In-situ hybridization for EBER shows that all tumour cells exhibit nuclear labeling. **B** Immunostaining for pan-cytokeratin highlights the surface epithelium as well and irregular clusters and sheets of positive cells (carcinoma) in the stroma. **C** Immunostaining for cytokeratin usually reveals a meshwork pattern of staining.

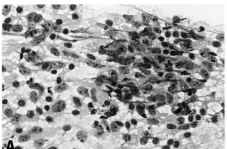
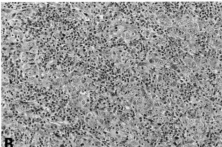
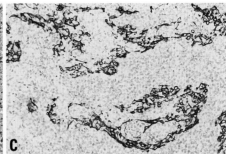

Fig. 2.13 Metastatic nasopharyngeal carcinoma in lymph node. **A** Fine needle aspiration smear shows tight clusters of tumour cells among small lymphocytes. **B** In histological sections, examination under medium magnification often reveals areas where cohesive tumour growth is evident. **C** The epithelial nature of the tumour is readily confirmed by immunostaining for cytokeratin, whereby a meshwork pattern of staining is often observed.

protein-positive dendritic cells. Some studies have reported the following features to be associated with a better prognosis: high density of dendritic cells; high number of infiltrating lymphocytes; and low number of granzyme B-positive cytotoxic cells {854,883,1903,1962,2912}.

Epstein-Barr virus detection
Nonkeratinizing nasopharyngeal carcinoma is associated with Epstein-Barr virus (EBV) in practically 100% of cases, irrespective of the ethnic background of the patient. EBV latent membrane protein-1 (LMP1) is usually positive in only 30-40% of cases, and the immunostaining is often patchy and weak, and thus is not a reliable method to demonstrate the presence of EBV {16,961,1988,2061}. The simplest and most reliable way to demonstrate EBV is in-situ hybridization for EBV encoded early RNA (EBER), which is present in abundance in cells latently infected by EBV. Practically all the tumour cells should show nuclear labelling {1137,1157,1176,2061,2233, 2638,2684}. In-situ hybridization for EBER can aid in the diagnosis of nasopharyngeal carcinoma if there are difficulties in distinguishing between carcinoma and reactive epithelial atypia. A positive result also strongly suggests a nasopharyngeal origin (although not entirely specific) for a metastatic nonkeratinizing carcinoma of unknown primary. On the other hand, it is less reliable to use polymerase chain reaction to look for EBV in the tumour, because even a few bystander EBV-positive lymphocytes can give rise to a positive result {2638}.

Cytopathology
Nasopharyngeal aspirate or brush is used in some centres to produce cytologic preparations for diagnosis of nasopharyngeal carcinoma. However, since the diagnostic sensitivity of nasopharyngeal cytology is limited (70-90%) {387,1001}, nasopharyngeal biopsy is the preferred method for obtaining a definitive histological diagnosis {387}. On the other hand, fine needle aspiration cytological examination of enlarged cervical lymph nodes is invaluable in reaching a diagnosis of metastatic nasopharyngeal carcinoma, either for initial diagnosis or staging {380,1355}. The aspirate smears show, in a background of lymphocytes and plasma cells, irregular clusters of large cells with overlapping vesicular nuclei and large nucleoli. The cytoplasm of these cells is often fragile and barely visible. There are commonly many naked nuclei {1760}. The presence of dispersed large tumour cells among the lymphoid cells may result in a pattern strongly reminiscent of Hodgkin lymphoma {1355}. The diagnosis can be readily confirmed by immunostaining for cytokeratin and in-situ hybridization for EBER either on the cell smears or cell block preparations.

Electron microscopy.
Although squamous differentiation is primitive or not evident in most cases of nasopharyngeal carcinoma at the light microscopic level, there is usually convincing evidence of squamous differentiation at the ultrastructural level. At least some carcinoma cells contain small bundles of tonofilaments or tonofibrils, in addition to well-formed desmosomes {1470, 1513,2082,2568}.

Differential diagnosis
Crush artefacts are common in nasopharyngeal biopsies, making it difficult to determine whether the observed distorted cells represent carcinoma or merely lymphoid cells. Such biopsies should be scrutinized in the better-preserved areas for tumour cell clusters. If there are uncertainties, immunostaining for cytokeratin is of great help in reaching a diagnosis of nasopharyngeal carcinoma. In the non-neoplastic nasopharyngeal mucosa, cytokeratin immunostaining highlights the sharply delineated surface and crypt epithelium, with no positive cells in the stroma other than those in seromucinous glands. Mucosa involved by nasopharyngeal carcinoma typically shows irregular clusters of cytokeratin-positive cells in the stroma.

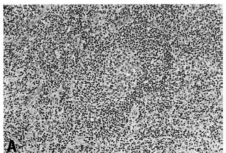
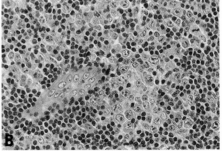

Fig. 2.14 Nasopharyngeal mucosa. **A** Germinal centre cells mimicking nasopharyngeal carcinoma. **B** Nasopharyngeal lymphoid hyperplasia mimicking nasopharyngeal carcinoma. In the left field, the venule with no obvious lumen can also be mistaken for a cluster of carcinoma cells.

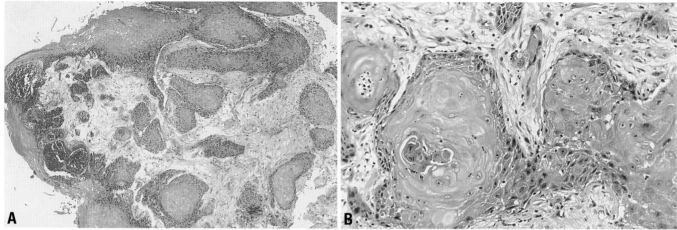

Fig. 2.15 Nasopharyngeal keratinizing squamous cell carcinoma, well differentiated. **A** The tumour shows invasion into the stroma. **B** Irregular islands of carcinoma infiltrate an abundant desmoplastic stroma. The tumour cells show obvious squamous differentiation and keratinization.

A number of benign cellular changes can mimic nonkeratinizing carcinoma. (1) Clusters of germinal centre cells may be mistaken for carcinoma because of the presence of large cells with vesicular nuclei and the absence of a well-defined mantle zone. The identification of admixed centrocytes (smaller "atypical" cells with irregular-shaped or angulated nuclei) and tingible-body macrophages points toward the lymphoid nature of the large cells, which can be confirmed by immunostaining (leucocyte common antigen positive, cytokeratin negative) {2317}. (2) A tangentially sectioned crypt harbouring cells with reactive changes that include nuclear enlargement can produce a pattern simulating an island of carcinoma lying in a lymphoid cell-rich stroma. In contrast to nasopharyngeal carcinoma, the nuclei are not as large and thus not so crowded, and the nucleoli are not as prominent. A negative in-situ hybridization for EBER would render a diagnosis of nasopharyngeal carcinoma most unlikely {2318}. (3) The nasopharyngeal mucosa can sometimes exhibit reactive lymphoid hyperplasia, accompanied by an increased number of immunoblasts in the lymphoid stroma, raising a suspicion for carcinoma. In contrast to the latter, the large cells are non-cohesive and have well-defined amphophilic cytoplasm. The diagnosis can be confirmed by a lack of cytokeratin immunoreactivity as well as positive immunostaining for lymphoid markers in the large cells {323}. (4) The lymphoid tissue-associated venules lined by plump endothelial cells with vesicular nuclei may be mistaken for clusters of carcinoma cells. The presence of distinct basement membrane around the groups of cells, lack of large nucleoli, and negative staining for cytokeratin would be against the diagnosis of carcinoma.

Distinction between nonkeratinizing carcinoma and large cell lymphoma can at times be difficult. In the nasopharyngeal mucosa or metastatic deposit in lymph node, dispersed growth of the carcinoma cells and accompanying eosinophil infiltration may lead to a misdiagnosis of Hodgkin lymphoma {330,394,2880}. Features favouring a diagnosis of carcinoma include the presence of cohesive cell groups in some foci (best appreciated at medium magnification) and the generally poorly defined cell borders; the diagnosis can be readily confirmed by immunostaining for cytokeratin. Nasopharyngeal carcinoma with marked cellular spindling can mimic a high-grade sarcoma. In most cases, the diagnosis can be reached by identifying in some foci a component of typical nasopharyngeal carcinoma, and can be further confirmed by cytokeratin immunoreactivity.

Post-treatment biopsies

After treatment by radiation therapy, it may take weeks (up to 10 weeks) for the nasopharyngeal carcinoma to disappear histologically {1401}. The radiated carcinoma cells usually show evidence of radiation injury in the form of enlarged and bizarre nuclei, accompanied by an increased amount of cytoplasm that is often finely vacuolated. If biopsy is positive, repeat biopsies should be taken every two weeks – remission is defined by two subsequent negative biopsies {1401,1402,1886}.

Radiation-induced changes in the normal nasopharyngeal mucosa can be mistaken for malignancy. The surface or crypt epithelium can exhibit enlarged, hyperchromatic or even bizarre nuclei, but such changes can be recognized to be benign because they are limited to some but not all cells (random cytologic atypia) and the normal nuclear-cytoplasmic ratio is maintained. Mucosal epithelial atypia usually does not persist beyond one year. If there are uncertainties as to whether the atypical cells represent residual carcinoma or irradiated normal cells, positive in-situ hybridization for EBER would strongly favour the former interpretation. There can also be bizarre stromal cells (radiation fibroblasts) with large smudged nuclei or large vesicular nuclei with prominent nucleoli; these atypical cells can persist for many years. These cells can be distinguished from residual or recurrent carcinoma by their occurrence as single cells and by the amphophilia of the cytoplasm. The stroma frequently contains ectatic blood vessels showing variable degrees of radiation injury such as enlarged prominent endothelial cells and abundant fibrinoid deposits.

Some patients with nasopharyngeal carcinoma develop local recurrence. The nasopharyngeal biopsies should be interpreted in the same way as for patients without a prior history of nasopharyngeal carcinoma. The recurrence can be morphologically identical to the original tumour, or may show a slightly greater degree of squamous differentiation. Some recurrences, especially those occurring after a long interval (>5 years), may represent new primaries rather than a genuine relapse of the original tumours {1445}. Radiation-induced tumours in the nasopharynx typically develop after a long latency period, and usually take the form of keratinizing squamous cell carcinomas or sarcomas (especially osteosarcomas) {403,600}.

Keratinizing squamous cell carcinoma
Histopathology
This is an invasive carcinoma showing obvious squamous differentiation at the light microscopic level, in the form of intercellular bridges and/or keratinization over most of the tumour, morphologically similar to keratinizing squamous cell carcinomas occurring in other head and neck mucosal sites {2317}. The degree of differentiation can be further graded as: well differentiated (most common), moderately differentiated and poorly differentiated. The tumour typically grows in the form of irregular islands, accompanied by an abundant desmoplastic stroma infiltrated by variable numbers of lymphocytes, plasma cells, neutrophils and eosinophils {1555}. The tumour cells are polygonal and stratified. The cell borders are distinct and separated by intercellular bridges. The cells in the centres of the islands or facing the surface often show a greater amount of eosinophilic glassy cytoplasm, sometimes with identifiable cytoplasmic tonofibrils, indicative of cellular keratinization. Occasionally keratin pearls are formed {2735}. The nuclei often show hyperchromasia, and the degree of nuclear pleomorphism ranges from mild to marked. The surface epithelium is frequently involved, apparently representing carcinoma in-situ.

Keratinizing squamous cell carcinoma can arise de novo or as a radiation-associated carcinoma occurring many years after radiation therapy for nonkeratinizing nasopharyngeal carcinoma {403,2316, 2735}. Compared with nonkeratinizing carcinoma, keratinizing squamous cell carcinoma shows a greater propensity for locally advanced tumour growth (76% versus 55%) {2136} and a lower propensity for lymph node metastasis (29% versus 70%) {1859}. While some studies suggest that this subtype of nasopharyngeal carcinoma has lower responsiveness to radiation therapy and a worse prognosis compared with nonkeratiniz-

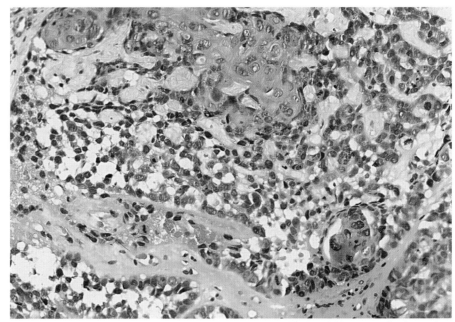

Fig. 2.16 Basaloid squamous cell carcinoma of the nasopharynx. The basaloid tumour cells show a festooning growth pattern, and are interspersed by tumour cells with squamous differentiation.

ing carcinoma {1122,1859,2136,2318}, others have not found this subtype to differ in biological behaviour {363,778}.

Immunoprofile and Epstein-Barr virus detection
Keratinizing squamous cell carcinoma shows immunoreactivity for pan-cytokeratin, high molecular-weight cytokeratin, and focally epithelial membrane antigen. For radiation-induced keratinizing squamous cell carcinoma, there is no association with EBV {403}. However, for de novo keratinizing squamous cell carcinomas, data on the EBV status are conflicting. In general, the patients have lower or negative IgA titres against EBV compared with nonkeratinizing carcinomas {1486,1860,2549}. Molecular studies of EBV in the tumour tissues have yielded conflicting results. Summarizing the literature, it appears that EBV is almost always positive in areas endemic for nasopharyngeal carcinoma, EBV is often positive in intermediate incidence areas, while EBV is positive in only a proportion of cases in low incidence areas {405, 580,599,961,1124,1125,1157,1176,1262 ,1885,1892,1988,2894}. Keratinizing squamous cell carcinomas tend to carry lower copy numbers of EBV compared with nonkeratinizing carcinomas {2108}. On in situ hybridization, the nuclear signals of EBER are usually confined to the less differentiated cells (basal cells that

surround the individual tumour islands), but not in the cells showing obvious squamous differentiation.

The role of human papillomavirus in keratinizing squamous cell carcinoma remains uncertain {1125}.

Differential diagnosis
The frank invasive growth, nuclear atypia and obvious squamous differentiation usually permit a straight-forward diagnosis of keratinizing squamous cell carcinoma to be made. However, in some cases, particularly those arising after radiation therapy for nonkeratinizing nasopharyngeal carcinoma, distinction between a very well differentiated keratinizing squamous cell carcinoma and squamous metaplasia/hyperplasia can be extremely difficult, since the nuclear atypia can be very subtle and focal, and invasion may not be obvious in the former. Assessment of invasion is further hampered by the abundant fibrinous deposits in the stroma related to prior radiation, and the usual desmoplastic stroma may be lacking. To arrive at a definitive diagnosis, sometimes multiple biopsies are required to identify convincing stromal invasion as well as focal mild nuclear atypia.

Basaloid squamous cell carcinoma
Several cases of basaloid squamous cell carcinoma, morphologically identical to the same tumour more commonly occur-

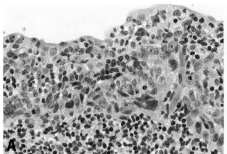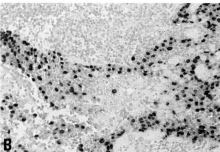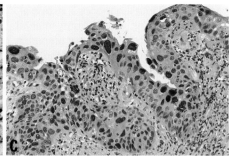

Fig. 2.17 Pure nasopharyngeal carcinoma-in-situ. **A** The surface epithelium consists of disarrayed cells with enlarged and crowded nuclei which vary in size, compatible with carcinoma in-situ. This patient was not given any treatment, and has remained disease-free at 7 years. **B** In-situ hybridization for EBER shows that the atypical epithelial cells are positive. **C** In this unusual example, the cells that comprise the surface epithelium exhibit marked nuclear pleomorphism and hyperchromasia. This example of radiation-associated carcinoma-in-situ has subsequently evolved into an invasive keratinizing squamous cell carcinoma.

ring in other head and neck sites (See chapter on hypophyarnx, larynx and trachea for details), have been reported to occur as primary tumours of the nasopharynx {116,117,1790,1997,2714}. Among the 6 cases with information, the M:F ratio is 2:1, and patients' ages ranged from 27-79 years (mean 55 years). Four cases had stage T3 or T4 disease; and two had lymph node metastasis. None had distant metastasis at presentation. On follow-up, three patients had no evidence of disease at 34-52 months; three were alive with disease at 19-46 months. The tumour appears to show a lower clinical aggressiveness compared with basaloid squamous cell carcinoma occurring in other head and neck sites. Among 4 cases tested for EBV, all three Asian cases were positive, while one Caucasian case were negative {1790,2714}.

Precursor lesions

In biopsies of nasopharyngeal carcinoma, an in-situ or intraepithelial component is identified in only 3-8% of cases, but it is often difficult to determine whether the invasive carcinoma has originated from the overlying in situ carcinoma or has merely invaded the surface epithelium {364,1504,1989,2852,2911}. Pure nasopharyngeal carcinoma in-situ, as confirmed by multiple biopsies to rule out an invasive component, is very rare {419,1989,2911}. These findings suggest that most nasopharyngeal carcinomas do not originate from nasopharyngeal carcinoma in-situ, or the evolution from the latter to the former occurs over a short time scale such that the latter is rarely detected.

Histologically, pure nasopharyngeal carcinoma-in-situ is characterized by atypical epithelial change confined to the surface or crypt epithelium, and lacking an invasive component. The epithelium is usually slightly thickened, and consists of cells with variable loss of polarity, nuclear enlargement, nuclear crowding

and distinct nucleoli. Sometimes there can be scattered amyloid globules. Some attempts have been made to grade the spectrum of intraepithelial neoplastic changes (dysplasia/carcinoma-in situ, or nasopharyngeal intraepithelial neoplasia) in the nasopharynx, but reproducibility and difficulties in recognizing the lower grade lesions remain an issue. So far, all cases of nasopharyngeal carcinoma in-situ studied have been positive for EBV (EBER), confirming that EBV infection precedes the acquisition of invasiveness by nasopharyngeal carcinoma {419,1971,2813}. Analysis of the EBV termini shows the virus to be in a clonal form, providing indirect support for the clonality of the epithelial proliferation {1989}. Thus in situ hybridization for EBER may aid in the distinction between carcinoma-in-situ and non-specific reactive atypia of the nasopharyngeal epithelium.

There are only limited data on the natural history of untreated pure nasopharyngeal carcinoma in-situ (or dysplasia). A proportion of patients develop invasive cancer on follow-up {1971,1989}.

Histogenesis

Nasopharyngeal carcinoma arises from the surface or crypt epithelium of the nasopharyngeal mucosa. In some cases, the tumour appears to arise from the basal layers of the stratified squamous epithelium, a finding further supported by the strong immunoreactivity for p63 in both the tumour and normal basal cells.

Somatic genetics

Nasopharyngeal carcinoma (NPC) is believed to result from accumulation of multiple genetic alterations and Epstein-Barr virus (EBV) latent infection in the

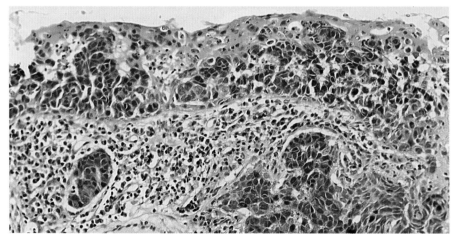

Fig. 2.18 Nasopharyngeal carcinoma with an intraepithelial component. The invasive carcinoma is accompanied by an abnormal surface epithelium comprising similar cells.

nasopharyngeal epithelial cells {611, 1542}. EBV genome is detected in all undifferentiated NPC cells and in high-grade dysplastic lesions of the nasopharynx, but rarely found in the adjacent normal nasopharyngeal epithelial cells or in the low-grade dysplastic lesions {361,1989}. The expression of EBV latent genes (e.g. EBNA1, LMP-1, LMP-2) may alter multiple signal transduction pathways and thus contribute to the transformation of the nasopharyngeal epithelium {611}.

Cytogenetics and comparative genomic hybridization (CGH)

Only few well-characterised karyotypes of NPC have been described. Despite the many complex rearrangements found, rearrangement and deletion on chromosome 3 have been consistently noted in this cancer {1141,2707,2813}. The spectral karyotyping (SKY) analyses have defined the common chromosomal regions of loss including 3p12-p21, 11q14-qter as well as the common regions of gain including 7p15-p14, 7q11.2-q21, 8q21.1-q22, 12q22-q24.1 and 20q were frequently detected {2813}. CGH studies have identified multiple recurrent chromosomal aberrations including loss on chromosomes 3p, 9p, 9q, 11q, 13q, 14q and 16q and gains of 1q, 3q, 12p, and 12q. Common regions of loss are 3p14-21, 14q24-qter, 11q21-qter while common regions of gains are 3q21-26 and 12q13-15 {413,716,1148}. Array-based CGH analyses and fluorescence in-situ hybridization (FISH) analyses have identified a cryptic amplification at 3q26 {964,1149}.

Molecular genetic alterations

In concordance with CGH results, loss of heterozygosity (LOH) studies have revealed high frequencies of deletion on chromosomes 3p, 9p, 9q, 11q, 13q, 14q and 16q. Multiple minimally deleted regions are identified at 3p14–24.2, 11q21–23, 13q12–14, 13q31–32, 14q24–32, and 16q22–23 {1545}. The characteristic LOH on 3p, 9p, and 14q in almost all tumours suggests that the putative tumour suppressor genes located in these regions probably play important roles in the genesis of NPC. Moreover, deletions on 3p and 9p have been shown to be early events in NPC tumorigenesis {360,361}. Inactivation of the P16 tumour suppressor gene on 9p21 by homozygous dele-

tion and methylation has been shown to be the most common molecular alteration in NPC tumourigenesis {1541, 1543}. Loss of P16 may result in cell cycle deregulation, while aberrations of the two major cell cycle regulators, P53 and RB, are rare {2453,2504}. Some studies have also found a high frequency of promoter hypermethylation of RASSF1A, a tumour suppressor gene on 3p21.3, in 70-80% of all cases of primary tumours {1403,1544}. The tumour suppressor function of RASSF1A may involve the DNA repair system and the RAS-dependent growth control. Other NPC-associated genes in the minimally deleted regions include TSLC1 at 11q23, EDNRB at 13q22, E-CADHERIN and RB2/130 at 16q {457,1542,1546,2642}. Epigenetic inactivation of multiple cancer-associated genes is common in NPC. Aside from P16 and RASSF1A, high frequencies of aberrant methylation are detected in EDNRB (90.5%), RARB2 (80%), DAP-kinase (76%), RIZ1 (60%) and E-CADHERIN (52%) {390,1403, 1546}. Widespread hypermethylation of CpG islands over the genome imply a "methylator" phenotype in this cancer.

Expression profiles / Proteomics

In NPC, P53 mutation is rare, but DN-P63, a P53 homologue, is consistently over-expressed and may block P53-mediated transactivation and apoptotic network in cancer cells {506,2453}. Frequent aberrant expression of the cyclin D1, P27 and BCL-2 may also be involved in dysregulation of cell proliferation and apoptosis pathway {100,1415, 1566}. Overexpression of the hypoxia

associated proteins, HIF-alpha, CA IX, and VEGF, is common and associated with poor prognosis {1150}. High MET protein expression level correlates with poor survival in late-stage NPC {2094}.

Genetic susceptibility

There is strong evidence that genetic predisposition is involved in the genesis of NPC. Epidemiological studies strongly support the existence of susceptible populations in the world: the prevalence of NPC is highly variable in different ethnic groups {1979}; migrants from high-risk areas continue to exhibit high risk of NPC {952,1501}, familial clustering of NPC is frequently observed {2893}.

HLA

There is an association between HLA phenotype and NPC risk. The association between HLA-A2 and NPC was first reported among Chinese in Singapore {2364}. Subsequent studies have confirmed the association of HLA A2-B46 haplotype with NPC in many different countries {382,1089,1223,1565,1567, 2365,2366}. In addition, increased risk of NPC has been found in individuals harbouring HLA B17 in southern China {1567,2874}, Singapore {382} and Malaysia {381}. Haplotypes A2-B17 {2895}, A2-B38 {1565}, and A2-B16 {2827} are also shown to be associated with increased risk of NPC. These findings are further supported by linkage or association studies that provide evidence for a NPC predisposing gene in close linkage with the HLA locus {1565, 1567,1947}. There is a negative association with NPC risk for alleles A11, B13

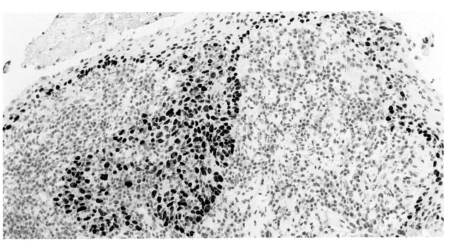

Fig. 2.19 Nasopharyngeal carcinoma. Both the carcinoma cells and normal basal cells are immunoreactive for p63.

and B22 {916}. On the other hand, an association between HLA and NPC has not been found in NPC patients in Alaskan Eskimos, Indians {1427}, North Africans {208,1071,1762} and Caucasians {313,314,1769}.

GSTM1 and CYP2E1

Polymorphism of some metabolic enzyme genes has been reported to influence susceptibility to NPC. Glutathione S-transferase M1 (GSTM1) detoxifies benzopyrene and other carcinogens in tobacco smoke. Studies on association between absence of GSTM1 and increased risk for NPC are conflicting {415,1857}.

The cytochrome P450 2E1 (CYP2E1) enzyme catalyzes the metabolic activation of low-molecular weight nitrosamines such as those detected in NPC-associated foods. A variant form of the gene that is detectable by Rsa I digestion (the c2 allele) has been shown to exhibit higher enzymatic activity. If dietary nitrosamines from preserved foods indeed play a direct role in NPC development, exposed individuals possessing different CYP2E1 genotypes may experience differential levels of NPC risk. In a population-based case-control study from Taiwan, individuals possessing the c2/c2 genotype experienced a 2.6-fold risk relative to those with one or two copies of the wild-type allele {1088}. This finding adds to the evidence that nitrosamine-containing preserved foods are important nasopharyngeal carcinogens.

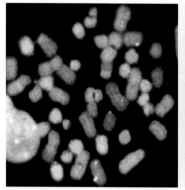
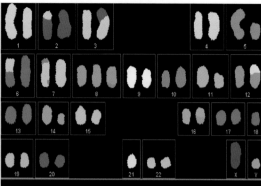

Fig. 2.20 Nasopharyngeal carcinoma. Spectral karyotyping (SKY) analysis of a nasopharyngeal carcinoma cell line C66-1 exhibiting multiple structural rearrangements.

PIGR and TCR

The mechanism of the entry of EBV into the nasopharyngeal epithelium has not yet been conclusively elucidated, but a receptor on nasopharyngeal epithelial cells, namely polymeric immunoglobulin receptor (PIGR), has been proposed to be involved. It has been reported that one single nucleotide polymorphism (SNP) (1739C->T), located on exon 7 of the gene, is significantly associated with increased risk of NPC {1102}. The SNP is a missense mutation altering the amino acid alanine to valine, and it occurs adjacent to the endoproteolytic cleavage site of the PIGR extracellular domain. It is hypothesized that the homozygous 1739C state may result in the altered efficiency to release IgA-EBV complex and hence increase the possibility of nasopharyngeal epithelial cells to be infected by EBV.

Since T cell receptor (TCR) may mediate immunity against EBV infection, effort has been made to test the association between polymorphism of TCR and NPC. A study has shown NPC susceptibility to be associated dominantly with a 20-kb fragment (P=0.02, RR=8.2) {412}.

Chromosome 4p

With construction of a human genome genetic linkage map and development of methods and algorithms, linkage analysis has become the robust tool to connect phenotypes with genotypes. A whole genome scan for linkage with NPC has been performed on 32 high risk NPC Cantonese pedigrees {729}. The marker D4S405 on chromosome 4p12–p15 yielded a maximum multipoint lod score of 3.06, a heterogeneity adjusted lod score (HLOD) of 3.21, and a non-parametric linkage score of 2.75 (P=0.005),

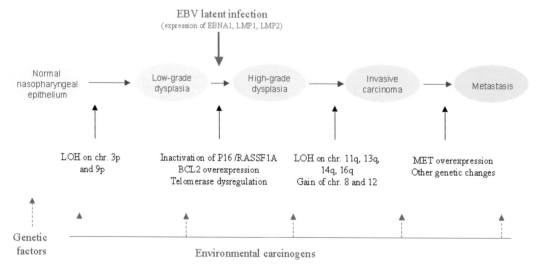

Fig. 2.20A Multistep evolution of nasopharyngeal cancer.

suggesting that a disease susceptibility gene may be linked with D4S405. Fine mapping and haplotype analysis has localized the NPC predisposing gene to chromosome region 4p15.1–q12.

In summary, NPC development may involve susceptibility gene mutations (major genes) and gene polymorphisms (minor-effect genes). In some familial cases, inherited genetic alterations (major gene transmission) could be the first "hit", and EBV infection may contribute to the second "hit". Therefore, familial cases usually have a much younger age of onset. However, some other familial cases and probably most sporadic cases may get the first "hit" from both inherited genetic alterations (minor-effect genes, such as HLA, CYP2E1) and somatic genetic changes. In the high prevalence areas like south China, most of the NPC cases belong to this type and they usually have older age of onset than the familial cases with a major gene transmission {2890}.

Prognosis and predictive factors

The mainstay of treatment for NPC is radiation therapy. Progressive improvement of treatment results for NPC has been reported both from endemic and non-endemic areas. The average 5-year survival steadily increased from around 35% for patients treated in the 1940–60 {1755,1785,2096}, to 55-60% in the 1970–90s {1061,1592,2096,2693}. A recent study of patients without distant metastases treated during 1996–2000 showed that a 5-year disease-specific survival (DSS) of 81% and overall sur-

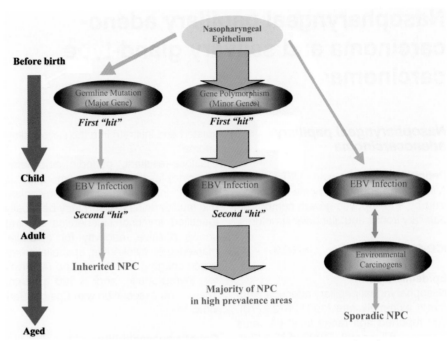

Fig. 2.22 A putative model for the development of the three forms of nasopharyngeal carcinoma.

vival 75% can now be achieved {1448}. The presenting stage is the most important prognostic factor. A recent study using the 2002 TNM staging System shows that the 5-year DSS for Stage I is 98%, Stage II A-B 95%, Stage III 86%, and Stage IVA-B 73%. In addition, tumour volume may prove to be useful for predicting local control {447,2520}.

The importance of host factors varies among different series. In general, younger age (less than 40 years) and female gender are associated with better prognosis {2574}. Interestingly, the influence of age is mainly on local failure, while that of gender is on distant failure. The values of EBV antibodies for predicting prognosis and monitoring disease progression are rather limited {567, 2855}. High baseline titers often persist even in patients in remission. Although rising titers to VCA, EA and Zta are associated with disease relapse, the elevation is often not consistently high or early enough for disease monitoring.

Circulating plasma/serum EBV DNA is a more promising prognostic factor. High plasma/serum EBV DNA titers are associated with advanced stages {1549}; both pre-treatment and post-treatment titers correlate significantly with survival {362,1547}. The titer is substantially elevated in patients with active disease (especially distant metastasis), and drops to very low titers upon remission

{362,1548,1882,2346}.

Aneuploid status or high pre-treatment tumour proliferative fractions, as determined by DNA flow cytometry, correlate significantly with poor survival {2854}. Other biological factors that might have prognostic significance include tumour angiogenesis, c-erbB2 {2209}, p53 {1658}, nm23-HI {965}, interleukin-10 {828}, and vascular endothelial growth factor {2095}.

Treatment factors affect the ultimate survival. Significant improvements in treatment results have been attributed to refinement of radiotherapy technique {1454}, dose escalation {2561,2576}, accelerated fractionation {1447,2717}, addition of chemotherapy (concurrent + sequential) {29,1515,2180}, and combination of new strategies {2803}.

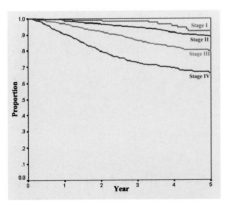

Fig. 2.21 Nasopharyngeal carcinoma. Actuarial disease-specific survival for different stages of nasopharyngeal carcinoma (Source of data: Hong Kong Nasopharyngeal Cancer Study Group on 2687 patients staged with the UICC/AJCC 5th Edition at public centres in Hong Kong during 1996-2000).

Nasopharyngeal papillary adeno-carcinoma and salivary gland-type carcinomas

T.T. Kuo
J.K.C. Chan
B.M. Wenig
J.W. Eveson

Nasopharyngeal papillary adenocarcinoma

Definition
A low-grade adenocarcinoma characterized by an exophytic growth comprising papillary fronds and glandular structures.

ICD-O code   8260/3

Epidemiology
Nasopharyngeal papillary adenocarcinoma is extremely rare {1902,2672,2770}. The reported age range is 11-64 years (median 37 years) {1902,2672,2770}. Gender distribution is nearly equal {1902,2672,2770}.

Localization
The tumour most commonly involves the roof, lateral wall and posterior wall of the nasopharynx {2770}.

Clinical features
Nasal obstruction is the main presenting symptom. The diagnosis can be readily confirmed by endoscopic biopsy.

Macroscopy
The tumours are soft or gritty and exophytic, with a papillary, polypoid, or cauliflower appearance. The tumours measure up to 4 cm (median size 2.5 cm) {2770}.

Tumour spread and staging
The tumours usually remain confined within the nasopharynx except one reported case with extensive local invasion {1902}.

Histopathology
Nasopharyngeal papillary adenocarcinoma arises from the surface epithelium {2770}. The tumour comprises arborizing delicate papillary fronds and crowded glands. The lining columnar or pseudostratified cells have bland, round to oval nuclei and tiny nucleoli. Mitotic figures are rare; necrosis may be focally identified. Psammoma bodies may be found in some cases. The tumours are unencapsulated and infiltrate into the surrounding stroma.

Diastase-resistant, periodic acid-Schiff intracytoplasmic positive material is present; intraluminal and intracytoplasmic mucicarmine staining may be focally identified. Immunohistochemical staining shows positive reactivity for epithelial markers (i.e., cytokeratin, epithelial membrane antigen), but there is no reactivity for thyroglobulin and S-100 protein. There is no association with Epstein-Barr virus.

Genetic susceptibility
A case has been reported in a patient with Turner syndrome {1902}.

Prognosis and predictive factors
This is an indolent low-grade malignant neoplasm with no metastatic potential. It has an excellent prognosis if a complete excision can be achieved {2770}.

Salivary gland-type carcinomas

These are very rare in the nasopharynx {2448}. Men are affected nearly three times more frequently than women {1389}. The age range is from 15-74 years with a median age of 50 years. The most frequent types are, in order of frequency, adenoid cystic carcinoma, mucoepidermoid carcinoma and adenocarcinoma not otherwise specified {2273}. Carcinomas at this site frequently present at an advanced stage and often with invasion of the base of the skull, intracranial extension and involvement of the cranial nerves.

Adenoid cystic carcinomas {336,1449,2273,2718} are typically insidious in onset, and symptoms may include middle ear effusion, epistaxis, diplopia and symptoms due to cranial nerve palsy (such as pain, paraesthesia, anaesthesia). The microscopic features are similar to those of adenoid cystic carcinoma elsewhere. The 5 and 10 year survival are 78% and 49.5% respectively, and 35% of patients will develop metastasis to bone or lung {2718}.

Mucoepidermoid carcinomas {1321, 1389,2273} are microscopically similar to those in other sites but rarely psammoma bodies can be seen.

Other rare salivary gland-type carcinomas of the nasopharynx include epithelial-myoepithelial carcinoma {1174}, myoepithelial carcinoma {1899}, acinic cell carcinoma {1890} and polymorphous low-grade adenocarcinoma {1469,2763}.

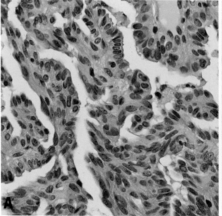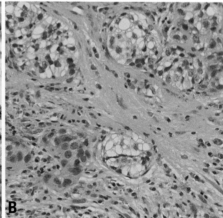

Fig. 2.23 A Nasopharyngeal papillary adenocarcinoma. The tumour comprises complex papillae and glands lined by columnar to spindly cells with bland-looking nuclei. **B** Mucoepidermoid carcinoma of nasopharynx. There are solid islands of squamoid cells and clear cells.

Benign epithelial tumours

M.A. Luna
A. Cardesa
L. Barnes
L.L.Y. Tse

J.L. Hunt
B.M. Wenig
L.P. Dehner
J.J. Buchino

Hairy polyp

Definition
A presumed developmental anomaly that clinically manifests as a polyp covered by skin with hair and sebaceous glands.

Synonyms
Teratoid polyp, dermoid polyp.

Epidemiology
Hairy polyps occur in newborns and older infants. There is an unexplained female predominance (female to male ratio 6:1) {1296}.

Localization
The lateral wall of the nasopharynx, the superior nasopharyngeal aspect of the soft palate, and the tonsils are classic locations for hairy polyps {1296}. They also have been infrequently reported in the middle ear {1310}. No cases have been reported in the sinonasal tract.

Clinical features
The usual clinical presentation is a pedunculated mass in the oropharynx or nasopharynx of a newborn or older infant. In the middle ear, the hairy polyps cause recurrent otitis media that is not responsive to the usual treatment. There are individual reports of associated cleft palate or multiple congenital anomalies, including the Dandy-Walker malformation {88}.

Histopathology
The surface of the polyp is composed of skin with a delicate hyperkeratotic layer and pilosebaceous units. The core is formed by fibroadipose tissue often with foci of cartilage, muscle and bone. Hairy polyps are distinguished from teratomas by a lack of endodermal components.

Histogenesis
It has been argued that these polyps are congenital anomalies of the first branchial cleft or choristomas {1045}.

Prognosis and predictive factors
Complete surgical excision is curative.

Schneiderian-type papilloma

Definition
A benign tumour that arises from the surface epithelium of the nasopharynx and resembles Schneiderian papillomas of the sinonasal tract {81,1924}.

ICD-O code   8121/0

Synonyms
Fungiform papilloma, inverted papilloma, transitional papilloma, nasopharyngeal papilloma.

Epidemiology
Schneiderian-type papillomas of the nasopharynx are distinctly uncommon. They occur in older individuals (mean 62 years, range 45-79) and are 2-3 times more common in males {2499}.

Etiology
Anatomically, the posterior choanae represent the boundary between the ectodermally-derived (Schneiderian membrane) and endodermally-derived respiratory mucosa that, respectively, line the sinonasal tract and nasopharynx. It is thought that aberrant embryologic displacement of normal Schneiderian mucosa might account for these lesions in the nasopharynx.

Clinical features
Most do not exceed two cm in greatest dimension. They are often incidental findings or, at most, result in nasal airway obstruction. The more common Schneiderian papilloma of the sinonasal tract with secondary involvement of the nasopharynx must be excluded before accepting the lesion as primary in the nasopharynx.

Histopathology
They are similar to those occurring in the nasal cavity and paranasal sinuses (see section on sinonasal papillomas). Most are of the inverted type (ICD-O code 8121/1).

Prognosis and predictive factors
Transnasal or transoral excision is the treatment of choice. Local recurrences are not uncommon. At least one case has been associated with a separate focus of nasopharyngeal squamous cell carcinoma {2499}.

Squamous papilloma

Squamous papillomas are uncommon in the nasopharynx, and they are morphologically similar to those found in the larynx. See chapter on 'Tumours of the hypopharynx, larynx and trachea'.

Ectopic pituitary adenoma

Definition
A benign pituitary gland neoplasm occurring separately from, and without involvement of the sella turcica (i.e., with normal anterior pituitary gland).

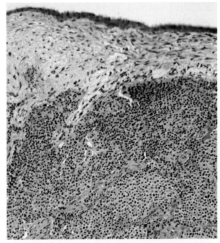

Fig. 2.24 Ectopic pituitary adenoma. Ectopic pituitary adenoma of the nasopharynx appearing as a submucosal and unencapsulated cellular tumour; the nasopharyngeal surface epithelium is intact and seen on top.

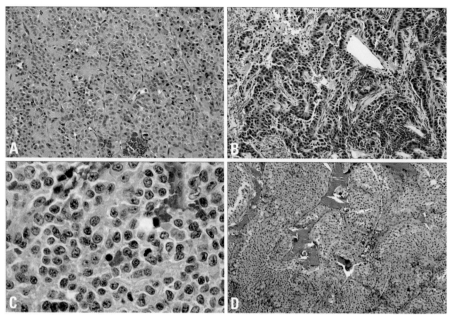

Fig. 2.25 Ectopic pituitary adenoma. **A** Organoid growth pattern. **B** Growth in the form of ribbons. **C** Scattered mitotic figures are seen in a tumour that otherwise shows uniform neoplastic cells with minimal pleomorphism and dispersed chromatin. **D** Extension into bone may be present.

ICD-O code   8272/0

Synonyms
Extrasellar pituitary adenoma; extrasellar adenohypophysial tissue; extracranial pituitary adenoma; sphenoidal pituitary adenoma; adenomatous pharyngeal pituitary.

Epidemiology
Ectopic pituitary adenomas of the upper aerodigestive tract are rare, and predominantly occur in adults but have been identified over a wide range of ages, from 16 – 84 years, with a reported mean and median age at presentation of 49 years and 58 years respectively {1425, 2752}. Females are affected more often than men {1425,2752}.

Etiology and pathogenesis
The etiology of ectopic pituitary adenomas is unknown. Extrasellar involvement by a pituitary adenoma can result from downward extension of a sellar-based pituitary tumour or occur as an adenomatous tumour arising from ectopic pituitary tissues. The latter may occur from two sources, including embryologic rests along the course of the cephalic invagination of Rathke's pouch (infrasellar) or anterior pituitary cells attached to the supradiagphragmatic portion of the pituitary stalk. This discussion will be limited to infrasellar-derived ectopic pituitary adenomas.

Localization
In the upper aerodigestive tract, ectopic pituitary adenoma most commonly occurs in the sphenoid bone and sinus {55,1425,1538,2627} and nasopharynx {417,488,2752}. Other sites of occurrence include the nasal cavity {1131, 2129,2752}, ethmoid sinus {2752}, and temporal bone {2129}.

Clinical features
The clinical presentation of ectopic pituitary adenomas is primarily related to its space- occupying effects, and include airway obstruction, chronic sinusitis, headache, epistaxis, cerebrospinal fluid leakage and visual field defects {237, 417,1425,1667,2627,2752}. Clinical evidence of hormonally active tumours can be identified in over half of the cases {1425} and include Cushing disease {235,309,1261,1538,2274,2396}, acromegaly {491,685,2725} hyperparathyroidism {1538}, hyperthyroidism {488}, amenorrhea {1051}, and hirsutism {2752}. Radiographic imaging is helpful in localizing the lesion and determining the relationship to the sella turcica {2396}. Of note is the fact that the extent of tumour and erosion of bone do not completely correlate with severity of clinical signs and symptoms {1425}.] Furthermore, erosion of the sella turcica does not exclude an ectopic origin {1425}.

Macroscopy
Grossly, it is a polypoid and pedunculated mass ranging in size from 0.7-7.5 cm {1538}. It is usually solitary; rare examples may occur synchronously in separate sites {237}.

Histopathology
Ectopic pituitary adenomas are submucosal and unencapsulated cellular tumours with solid, organoid and trabecular growth patterns; tumour nests are separated by fibrovascular stroma. The neoplastic cells have round to oval nuclei with dispersed nuclear chromatin, inconspicuous to small nucleoli, and granular cytoplasm that can be eosinophilic, amphophilic or clear. Extracellular stromal hyalinization may be prominent. Nuclear pleomorphism, mitotic activity and necrosis are uncommon. The surface epithelium is intact and unremarkable. The tumour effaces the normal structures in the submucosa although residual seromucous glands can be identified.

Immunoprofile
Ectopic pituitary adenomas show strong cytoplasmic immunoreactivity for cytokeratin, synaptophysin, chromogranin, neuron specific enolase, and may stain for a variety of pituitary hormones including adrenocorticotropic hormone (ACTH), prolactin, thyroid stimulating hormone (TSH), follicle stimulating hormone (FSH), growth hormone (GH), and luteinizing hormone (LH). Tumours may demonstrate immunoreactivity with only a single pituitary hormone (monohormonal pituitary adenoma), multiple hormones (plurihormonal pituitary adenoma) or no pituitary hormone (null cell pituitary adenoma).

Electron microscopy
Intracytoplasmic secretory granules of varying numbers can be identified.

Prognosis and predictive factors
Surgical resection is the treatment of choice for smaller, accessible tumours {1425}; complete surgical eradication is usually curative {2752}. However, complete surgical resection may not be possible for larger, invasive tumours. When resection is incomplete or cannot be accomplished due to size and extent of

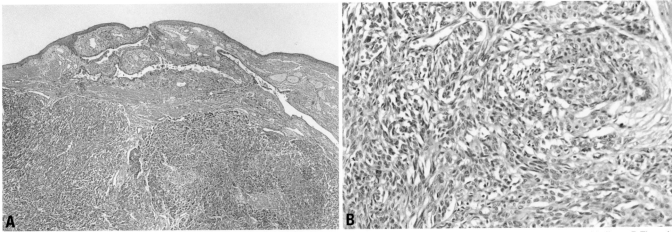

Fig. 2.26 Salivary gland anlage tumour. **A** The cellular tumour nodules communicate in the form of glandular structures with the surface epithelium. **B** There is merging of spindle cells into abortive tubules.

the tumour, postoperative radiotherapy is indicated {55,1425,2627,2666}. Dopamine agonist drugs (e.g., bromocriptine) have been effective in reducing the size (not permanently) in prolactin-secreting adenomas and the mitotic rate of other pituitary adenomas {1425}. Somatostatin analog treatment with octreotide has been shown to reduce tumour size and may, in the proper setting of a pituitary adenoma with high somatostatin receptor content, be administered in lieu of surgery in patients whose tumours are too large to be adequately resected {2093}. A rare example of malignant transformation of an ectopic pituitary adenoma has been reported {1131}.

Salivary gland anlage tumour

Definition
A benign tumour with mixed epithelial and mesenchymal elements, recapitulating the early stages in the embryology of the salivary gland between the 4th and 8th weeks of development.

Synonym
Congenital pleomorphic adenoma

Epidemiology
Fewer than 20 cases have been reported in the literature {229,233,296,572,1007, 1168,1720,1763}. Most patients are diagnosed in the immediate neonatal period or by the age of 6-weeks. Males exceed females by a 13:3 ratio.

Clinical features
Almost all patients present with respiratory and feeding difficulties. Bleeding has rarely been reported. Clinical examination reveals a midline pedunculated erythematous polyp {229}.

Macroscopy
A firm, smooth to lobulated mass measuring between 1.3 and 3 cm in greatest dimension is the typical gross appearance. The surface is usually glistening. The remnants of a stalk may or may not be apparent. A vague nodularity is appreciated on its greyish-tan to reddish cut surface. Cysts and interstitial haemorrhage may occur.

Histopathology
A non-keratinizing squamous mucosa overlies multiple contiguous cellular nodules. The nodules are separated by fibrous and myxoid stroma containing duct-like structures and nests of solid or cystic squamous epithelium. In areas, the duct-like structures are connected to the surface epithelium. The epithelial units within the internodular stroma blend into the cellular nodules, which are comprised of fusiform cells forming short fascicles or trabecular structures, interspersed with poorly formed tubules with or without lumens. The fusiform cells have eosinophilic cytoplasm with indistinct cell borders. The nuclei are bland and uniform, and mitotic activity is quite low. The interstitium can show haemorrhage, and rarely bone formation {296}.

Immunoprofile
The cellular nodules display a mixed pattern of reactivity for vimentin, cytokeratin and actin and are generally non-reactive for S-100 protein and glial fibrillary acidic protein. Nascent tubules and ducts within the stromal nodules show a luminal pattern of positivity for epithelial membrane antigen. The differentiated epithelial components are reactive for pancytokeratin and cytokeratin 7; epithelial membrane antigen positivity is restricted to the tubular structures. Salivary gland amylase is expressed consistently.

Prognosis and predictive factors
Complete excision is curative in virtually all cases.

Craniopharyngioma

ICD-O code   9350/1

Exceptionally, craniopharyngioma can arise in the nasopharynx or involves the nasopharynx through downward invasion from a suprasellar location. The morphological features are identical to the suprasellar counterpart {316,1609,1612, 2062,2083,2525}.

Nasopharyngeal angiofibroma

L.D.R. Thompson
J.C. Fanburg-Smith

The spectrum and clinicopathological features of nasopharyngeal soft tissue tumours are similar to those of other sites in the upper aerodigestive tract, except for angiofibroma, which typically presents in the nasopharynx.

Definition

A benign, highly cellular and richly vascularized mesenchymal neoplasm that involves the nasopharynx in males.

ICD-O code   9160/0

Synonyms

Juvenile nasopharyngeal angiofibroma; angiofibroma; fibroangioma; fibroma

Epidemiology

Nasopharyngeal angiofibroma represents <1% of all nasopharyngeal tumours {190,267,512,1434,1503,1861, 2654}. Boys and adolescent to young men are almost exclusively affected, with a peak in the 2nd decade of life. If a female is affected, testicular feminisation has to be excluded. Fair-skinned and red-haired males are more commonly affected.

Etiology

There is no known etiology although testosterone-dependent puberty-induced tumour growth may be ameliorated by blockade of estrogen or progesterone receptors within the tumour {717, 1861}.

Localization

This tumour arises in the posterolateral nasal wall or the nasopharynx. There is often extensive infiltration into the surrounding tissues {190,267,512,1434, 1503,1861,2654}.

Clinical features

Patients usually present with nasal obstruction and/or recurrent, spontaneous epistaxis, nasal discharge, facial deformity (including proptosis), diplopia, exophthalmos, sinusitis, otitis media, tinnitus, rhinolalia, deafness, headaches,

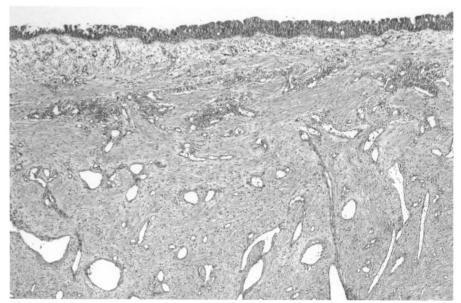

Fig. 2.27 Nasopharyngeal angiofibroma. The intact respiratory epithelium overlies a richly vascular neoplasm which has variably-sized vessels surrounded by a cellular fibroblastic stroma with collagen.

dyspnoea, and rarely, anosmia or pain {190,267,512,1434,1503,1861,2654}.

Imaging

Routine radiographs reveal a soft tissue density in the nasopharynx in conjunction with anterior bowing of the posterior wall of the maxillary sinus as well as distortion and posterior displacement of the pterygoid plates (Holman-Miller sign). Bony margins may be eroded, but are distinct. Computed tomography allows for accurate determination of the extent of the disease as well as the best possible surgical approach. Angiography allows for identification of the feeding vessel(s) and pre-surgical embolization. Tumour blush on angiogram is characteristic {1434,2654}. Due precautions have to be taken in obtaining biopsies from the lesion because of the risk of life-threatening bleeding.

Macroscopy

The tumours range in size up to 22 cm, with a mean of about 4 cm. They are polypoid with a rounded or multinodular contour, with red, grey-tan cut surfaces

{190,267,512,1434,1503,1861,2654}.

Tumour spread and staging

The tumour expands in all directions from the nasopharyngeal region, following the path of least resistance: anteriorly into the nasal cavity and maxillary sinuses, laterally into the pterygoid region, temporal fossa and infratemporal fossa (resulting in a cheek or intraoral buccal mass); superiorly into orbit and middle cranial fossa; or to the opposite side. This type of extensive involvement is seen in up to 30% of cases, explaining the potential aggressive nature of this benign neoplasm {190,267,512,1434,1503,1861, 2654}.

A number of staging systems have been suggested, {384,767,2111,2309} with a modification based on size and location used most frequently.

Histopathology

There is a vascular proliferation set in a fibrous stroma. The vessels are mostly thin-walled, slit-like ("staghorn") or dilated with calibres ranging from capillary size to large, patulous vessels. The muscular layer can be absent, focal and pad-like, or circumferential. Endothelial cells may be plump but are usually attenuated. The fibrous stroma consists of plump spindle, round, angular, or stellate shaped cells and a varying amount of fine and coarse collagen fibres; background myxoid degeneration is common (especially in embolized specimens). The nuclei of the stromal cells are generally cytologically bland, but they may be multinucleated or show some degree of pleomorphism in the more cellular areas. Mast cells may be seen, but other inflammatory elements are usually absent (except when there is surface ulceration) {190,267,512,1434,1503,1861,2654}.

Long-standing lesions show increased fibrosis and diminished vasculature. Treatment with hormones results in increased collagenization of the stroma with fewer, but thicker-walled vessels. In specimens excised after embolization, the tumour often shows areas of infarction, and emboli can be seen in some blood vessels. Sarcomatous transformation is an exceedingly uncommon event, usually following radiation therapy {2431}.

Immunoprofile

Occasional elastic fibres can be identified in the vessel walls, although they are generally absent in the stroma. The vessel wall cells are immunoreactive with vimentin and smooth muscle actin (SMA), whereas the stromal cells are immunoreactive with vimentin only, except in areas of increased fibrosis, where focal SMA may be identified. Desmin may be focally immunoreactive in larger vessels at the periphery of the tumour. Stromal and endothelial cells are variably reactive with androgen and estrogen/progesterone receptors. Factor VIII R-Ag, CD34 and CD31 highlight the endothelium, but not the stromal cells. The stromal cells are negative for S-100 protein {190,1503}. Platelet derived growth factor B and insulin-like growth factor type II are both over-expressed {1812}.

Electron microscopy

Ultrastructurally, the stromal cells contain lobulated nuclei, intranuclear inclusions, variable amounts of rough endoplasmic reticulum and thin filaments, hemidesmosomes, focal basal lamina and prominent pinocytotic vesicles, suggesting a hybrid mesenchymal cell (myofibroblast) {2565}.

Differential diagnosis

The differential diagnosis includes lobular capillary haemangioma (pyogenic

Table 2.05 System for staging nasopharyngeal angiofibroma {384,767,2309}.

Stage	Description
Stage I	Tumour limited to the nasopharynx with no bone destruction
Stage II	Tumour invading the nasal cavity, maxillary, ethmoid, or sphenoid sinuses with no bone destruction
Stage III	Tumour invading the pterygopalatine fossa, infra-temporal fossa, orbit or parasellar region
Stage IV	Tumour with massive invasion of the cranial cavity, cavernous sinus, optic chiasm, or pituitary fossa

granuloma), nasal inflammatory polyps with fibrosis or atypical stromal cells, antrochoanal polyps, and peripheral nerve sheath tumour.

Histogenesis

It has been proposed that the tumour arises from a fibrovascular nidus that lies dormant until puberty, when testosterone stimulates tumour growth {1861}.

Genetic susceptibility

There are isolated reports of an association with familial adenomatous polyposis {757,885}.

Prognosis and predictive factors

This benign tumour is characterized by local aggressive growth, with recurrences in about 20% of patients (>50% in older series), most commonly intracranially, and usually within the first 2 years after diagnosis. Patients may be managed with selective angiographic embolization or hormonal therapy prior to definitive surgical resection. Radiation therapy has been successfully implemented to manage large, intracranial, or recurrent tumours, but surgery is still the therapy of choice {190,267,512,1434, 1503,1861,2654}.

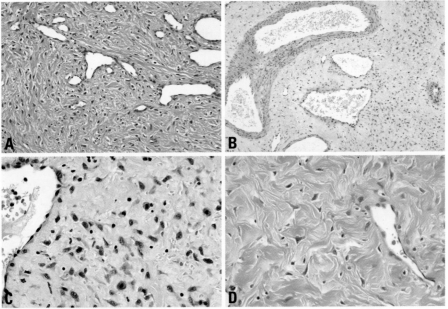

Fig. 2.28 Nasopharyngeal angiofibroma. **A** Thin walled vessels surrounded by dense, "keloid-like" collagen. Stellate fibroblasts are noted. **B** Smooth muscle-walled vessels, patulous vessels and capillaries are all surrounded by the characteristic collagenized stroma. **C** A large thin-walled vessel is associated with fibrous connective tissue, inflammatory cells and stellate fibroblasts. **D** Heavily collagenized stroma demonstrates only a few stellate fibroblastic cells.

Haematolymphoid tumours

A.C.L. Chan
J.K.C. Chan
M.M.C. Cheung

Hodgkin lymphoma

Hodgkin lymphoma only rarely shows primary involvement of the nasopharynx {1274,1602,1756,1763,1922}. The patients usually present with nasal obstruction or otitis media, and frequently have low stage (stage I/II) disease. Most of the tumours are of mixed cellularity and nodular sclerosis subtypes. The majority of cases involving the nasopharynx are associated with Epstein-Barr virus {1274,1756}. Please refer to 'Hodgkin lymphoma' in 'WHO classification of tumours: Tumours of haematopoietic and lymphoid tissues' for details.

Non-Hodgkin lymphoma

Definition
Primary non-Hodgkin lymphoma (NHL) of the nasopharynx is defined as a lymphoid cell neoplasm in which the bulk of disease occurs in this site.

Epidemiology
Nasopharyngeal NHL accounts for 2.5% of all extranodal NHLs {809}. Most cases have been reported in the literature in combination with either NHL of the nasal

cavity or NHL of the Waldeyer ring, rendering it difficult to extract the specific details on nasopharyngeal NHL {420,1704,2250,2849}. In some cases, there is simultaneous involvement of both the nasopharynx and nasal cavity, precluding determination of the site of origin of the NHL.

In the West, nearly all cases of nasopharyngeal NHL are of B-cell lineage (most commonly diffuse large B-cell lymphoma, DLBCL) {1704}. The situation is different in Asia, where B-cell lymphomas account for only 50-60% of cases {420,2849}, due to a higher frequency of extranodal NK/T cell lymphomas and peripheral T-cell lymphomas.

Most patients with nasopharyngeal NHL are adults. Patients with extranodal NK/T cell lymphoma of nasal-type have a male to female ratio of 3:1, and a median age of 53 years {420}. Patients with B-cell lymphomas are generally one decade older (median age of 63 years), and the male to female ratio is only 1.2:1 {420}. Burkitt lymphoma occurs more frequently in children and young adults {2826}.

Etiology
The etiology is unknown, except that extranodal NK/T cell lymphoma of nasal-type is strongly associated with Epstein-

Barr virus (EBV) (>95%) irrespective of the ethnic background of the patients {1195}. The association of nasopharyngeal DLBCL with EBV is weak {376}.

Clinical features
The patients present with nasal obstruction, epistaxis, hearing impairment, dysphagia, headache or neck mass, similar to the presenting symptoms of nasopharyngeal carcinoma. A small proportion of patients have concurrent cervical lymphadenopathy, a feature seen more frequently in DLBCL than extranodal NK/T cell lymphoma.

Tumour spread and staging
The majority (80%) of patients have localized disease (Stage IE/IIE) at presentation {420,1500,1505,1550}. Extranodal NK/T cell lymphoma tends to disseminate to various sites, such as skin, gastrointestinal tract, liver, lymph node and testis, during the course of disease. There is a propensity for DLBCL to spread to the cervical lymph nodes {420}.

Histopathology
DLBCL and extranodal NK/T cell lymphoma of nasal-type occurring in the nasopharynx are morphologically and

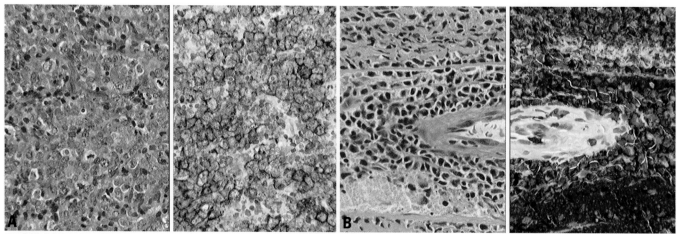

Fig. 2.29 Primary non-Hodgkin lymphoma of the nasopharynx. **A** Diffuse large B-cell lymphoma. A diffuse infiltrate of large lymphoid cells with high nuclear-cytoplasmic ratio and mitotic figures (left). There is strong CD20 immunoreactivity, confirming the B-cell immunophenotype (right). **B** Extranodal NK/T-cell lymphoma. The neoplastic cells infiltrate the vascular wall (left), and show immunoreactivity for CD3ε (right).

immunophenotypically similar to those seen in the nasal cavity. Other types of NHL, for example, Burkitt lymphoma, follicular lymphoma, mantle cell lymphoma, extranodal marginal zone B-cell lymphoma of MALT type, and peripheral T-cell lymphoma unspecified may also affect the nasopharynx, but at a much lower frequency {420,1704,2849}. Please refer to the sections of 'non-Hodgkin lymphoma' in 'Tumours of the nasal cavity and paranasal sinuses' and 'Tumours of the oral cavity and oropharynx' for details.

Differential diagnosis

Distinction between nasopharyngeal carcinoma and DLBCL can be difficult at times because the carcinoma cells in nasopharyngeal carcinoma can appear discohesive due to submergence in a dense lymphoplasmacytic infiltrate, while DLBCL can sometimes form tight cell clusters. Positive immunostaining for cytokeratin would support the former diagnosis, and expression of lymphoid markers (including CD20) would support the latter. Infectious mononucleosis involving the nasopharynx can also mimic DLBCL {2547}, but can be suspected or recognized by the young age of the patient, presence of a range of large cells with apparent maturation to plasmablasts and plasma cells, lack of frank cytologic atypia, and polyclonal immunoglobulin staining in the large cells.

Extranodal NK/T cell lymphoma with small cell predominance can be difficult to recognize as being a malignant neoplasm. Histologic features suggestive of the diagnosis include extensive effacement of architecture, marked coagulative necrosis, angiocentric growth, and wide separation of the mucosal glands. The diagnosis is supported by the demonstration of sheets of CD56+, CD3ε+, EBER+ cells. In the rare case of herpes simplex infection involving the nasopharynx, there can be a dense lymphoid infiltrate with extensive CD56 expression, causing confusion with extranodal NK/T cell lymphoma. In contrast to NK/T cell lymphoma, these CD56+ cells express CD4 and CD5, and there is no association with EBV. The diagnosis is confirmed by identifying the herpes simplex virus-infected multinucleated giant cells with ground glass nuclei with or without nuclear inclusions, which can be further

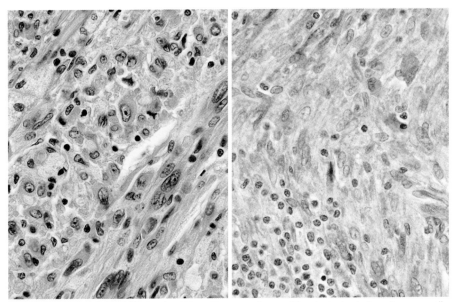

Fig. 2.30 Nasopharyngeal follicular dendritic cell sarcoma/tumour. The atypical spindly cells are usually sprinkled with small lymphocytes (left). They are immunoreactive for CD21 (right).

confirmed by immunostaining for herpes simplex virus {2523}.

Prognosis and predictive factors

Radiotherapy is the treatment of choice for extranodal NK/T cell lymphoma , often in combination with additional treatment modalities {421}. Chemotherapy and/or radiotherapy is usually given for patients with DLBCL.

The overall survival rate for extranodal NK/T cell lymphoma of nasal-type is only 30-50% {421,422,1312,1838}. Factors associated with worse outcome include: advanced stage, poor performance status, B symptoms and bulky disease {422}. B-cell lymphomas show a slightly more favourable outcome {420}.

Follicular dendritic cell sarcoma / tumour

Follicular dendritic cell sarcoma/tumour is a rare tumour showing morphologic, immunophenotypic and ultrastructural features of follicular dendritic cells. Primary involvement of the nasopharynx is rare {189,359}, and may arise from an underlying hyaline-vascular Castleman disease {359}. Please refer to the section of 'Follicular dendritic cell sarcoma/tumour' in 'Tumours of the oral cavity and oropharynx' for details.

Extramedullary plasmacytoma

ICD-O code   9734/3

Approximately 22% of head and neck extramedullary plasmacytomas occur in the nasopharynx, which is the second most common site after the sinonasal tract. See corresponding section in 'Tumours of the nasal cavity and paranasal sinuses' for details.

Other haematolymphoid tumours

Castleman disease, extramedullary myeloid sarcoma and Rosai-Dorfman disease (sinus histiocytosis with massive lymphadenopathy) can occasionally affect the nasopharynx {359,2631,2637, 2760}. Please refer to Chapter 1 on 'Tumours of the nasal cavity and paranasal sinuses' for details.

Tumours of bone and cartilage

K.K. Unni
K. Saito

The spectrum and clinicopathological features of nasopharyngeal tumours of bone and cartilage are similar to those of other sites in the upper aerodigestive tract, except for chordoma, which typically presents in the nasopharynx.

Chordoma

Definition
A low-grade malignant tumour that recapitulates the notochord.

ICD-O code   9370/3

Epidemiology
Chordomas account for approximately 4% of malignant bone tumours {2655}. About a third involve the base of the skull, and a small proportion may involve the nasopharynx and/or paranasal sinuses. There is a male predilection. The patients are predominantly adults, but children can also be affected.

Clinical features
Patients usually present with non-specific symptoms, such as headache, nasal obstruction, and symptoms related to cranial nerve involvement. Rarely, they present with nasal polyps {325}.
Imaging studies show lytic destruction of the basisphenoid centred in the clivus. The tumour frequently extends into the middle cranial fossa and nasopharynx. Calcification is occasionally seen.

Histopathology
Chordomas typically show a lobulated growth pattern. Polygonal or ovoid tumour cells are arranged in cords, lobules and sheets in a myxoid background. The nuclei are typically round and uniform, but may exhibit considerable pleomorphism. The cytoplasm is abundant and eosinophilic, and at times clear. Vacuolated cells (physaliferous cells) are present to a variable degree. The tumour cells are immunoreactive for cytokeratins, epithelial membrane antigen and S100 protein.

The main differential diagnoses are epithelial neoplasms (such as mucinous carcinoma, salivary gland tumours, poorly differentiated carcinoma) and chondrosarcoma. The lobulation, physaliferous cells and diffuse strong S100 protein immunoreactivity distinguish chordoma from carcinoma. Chondrosarcoma is negative for cytokeratin.

Prognosis and predictive factors
Chordoma is a low-grade tumour and distant metastases are rare. Chordomas involving the nasopharynx are often treated by radiation therapy because complete surgical resection is practically impossible because of the anatomy {709}.

Secondary tumours

L. Barnes
L.L.Y. Tse
J.L. Hunt

Definition
Tumours that metastasize to the nasopharynx from other primary malignancies. Direct invasion from tumours of adjacent sites, leukemias and lymphomas are excluded.

Epidemiology
Metastases to the nasopharynx are extremely rare {1685}. The majority of patients are over the age of 50 years. Reported primary tumours and tumour sites include malignant melanoma (cutaneous) 9 cases, kidney (3 renal cell, 1 Wilms), lung (4 cases), and one case each of breast, colon and cervical cancer {1685}.

Clinical features
Patients may be asymptomatic or present with nasal obstruction, epistaxis, unilateral serous otitis media secondary to blockage of the eustachian tube, or otalgia. Large bulky metastases can extend into the nasal cavity or deform the soft palate.
A long disease-free interval between treatment of the primary tumour and the appearance of metastasis in the nasopharynx may confuse the diagnosis, raising the possibility of a new primary neoplasm of the nasopharynx. However, this is not uncommon for malignant melanoma and renal cell carcinoma.

Pathogenesis
Most metastases to the nasopharynx are haematogenous, possibly arising in some instances through Batson's paravertebral venous plexus.

Prognosis and predictive factors
Metastasis is an ominous sign associated with a poor prognosis.

CHAPTER 3

Tumours of the Hypopharynx, Larynx and Trachea

Squamous cell carcinoma is, by far, the most important tumour of the hypopharynx, larynx and trachea. It is clearly related to the abuse of tobacco and alcohol and, as such, could be drastically reduced if individuals would only alter their lifestyles. Precursor lesions have been identified and the genetic-molecular events underlying their origin and progression into clinically apparent carcinomas are gradually being elucidated. The terminology of these precursor lesions, however, is still evolving and no single classification has been universally accepted. The three most commonly used classifications and their equivalent terms are presented.

WHO histological classification of tumours of the hypopharynx, larynx and trachea

Malignant epithelial tumours

Squamous cell carcinoma	8070/3
Verrucous carcinoma	8051/3
Basaloid squamous cell carcinoma	8083/3
Papillary squamous cell carcinoma	8052/3
Spindle cell carcinoma	8074/3
Acantholytic squamous cell carcinoma	8075/3
Adenosquamous carcinoma	8560/3
Lymphoepithelial carcinoma	8082/3
Giant cell carcinoma	8031/3
Malignant salivary gland-type tumours	
Mucoepidermoid carcinoma	8430/3
Adenoid cystic carcinoma	8200/3

Neuroendocrine tumours

Typical carcinoid	8240/3
Atypical carcinoid	8249/3
Small cell carcinoma, neuroendocrine type	8041/3
Combined small cell carcinoma, neuroendocrine type	8045/3

Benign epithelial tumours

Papilloma	8050/0
Papillomatosis	8060/0
Salivary gland-type adenomas	
Pleomorphic adenoma	8940/0
Oncocytic papillary cystadenoma	8290/0

Soft tissue tumours

Malignant tumours

Fibrosarcoma	8810/3
Malignant fibrous histiocytoma	8830/3
Liposarcoma	8850/3
Leiomyosarcoma	8890/3

Rhabdomyosarcoma	8900/3
Angiosarcoma	9120/3
Kaposi sarcoma	9140/3
Malignant peripheral nerve sheath tumour	
Synovial sarcoma	9040/3
Borderline tumours / LMP	
Inflammatory myofibroblastic tumour	8825/1
Benign tumours	
Schwannoma	9560/0
Neurofibroma	9540/0
Lipoma	8850/0
Leiomyoma	8890/0
Rhabdomyoma	8900/0
Hemangioma	9120/0
Lymphangioma	9170/0
Granular cell tumour	9580/0

Haematolymphoid tumours

Tumours of bone and cartilage

Chondrosarcoma	9220/3
Osteosarcoma	9180/3
Chondroma	9220/0
Giant cell tumour	9250/1

Mucosal malignant melanoma	8720/3

Secondary tumours

---

[1] Morphology code of the International Classification of Diseases for Oncology (ICD-O) {821} and the Systematized Nomenclature of Medicine (http://snomed.org). Behaviour is coded /0 for benign tumours, /3 for malignant tumours, and /1 for borderline or uncertain behaviour.

TNM classification of carcinomas of the larynx

TNM classification [1,2]

T – Primary tumour

TX	Primary tumour cannot be assessed
T0	No evidence of primary tumour
Tis	Carcinoma in situ

Supraglottis

T1	Tumour limited to one subsite of supraglottis with normal vocal cord mobility
T2	Tumour invades mucosa of more than one adjacent subsite of supraglottis or glottis or region outside the supraglottis (e.g., mucosa of base of tongue, vallecula, medial wall of pyriform sinus) without fixation of the larynx
T3	Tumour limited to larynx with vocal cord fixation and/or invades any of the following: postcricoid area, pre-epiglottic tissues, paraglottic space, and/or with minor thyroid cartilage erosion (e.g. inner cortex)
T4a	Tumour invades through the thyroid cartilage and/or invades tissues beyond the larynx, e.g., trachea, soft tissues of neck including deep/extrinsic muscle of tongue (genioglossus, hyoglossus, palatoglossus, and styloglossus), strap muscles, thyroid, oesophagus
T4b	Tumour invades prevertebral space, mediastinal structures, or encases carotid artery

Glottis

T1	Tumour limited to vocal cord(s) (may involve anterior or posterior commissure) with normal mobility
T1a	Tumour limited to one vocal cord
T1b	Tumour involves both vocal cords
T2	Tumour extends to supraglottis and/or subglottis, and/or with impaired vocal cord mobility
T3	Tumour limited to larynx with vocal cord fixation and/or invades paraglottic space, and/or with minor thyroid cartilage erosion (e.g. inner cortex)
T4a	Tumour invades through the thyroid cartilage, or invades tissues beyond the larynx, e.g., trachea, soft tissues of neck including deep/extrinsic muscle of tongue (genioglossus, hyoglossus, palatoglossus, and styloglossus), strap muscles, thyroid, oesophagus
T4b	Tumour invades prevertebral space, mediastinal structures, or encases carotid artery

Subglottis

T1	Tumour limited to subglottis
T2	Tumour extends to vocal cord(s) with normal or impaired mobility
T3	Tumour limited to larynx with vocal cord fixation
T4a	Tumour invades through cricoid or thyroid cartilage and/or invades tissues beyond the larynx, e.g., trachea, soft tissues of neck including deep/extrinsic muscle of tongue (genioglossus, hyoglossus, palatoglossus, and styloglossus), strap muscles, thyroid, oesophagus
T4b	Tumour invades prevertebral space, mediastinal structures, or encases carotid artery

N – Regional lymph nodes##

NX	Regional lymph nodes cannot be assessed
N0	No regional lymph node metastasis
N1	Metastasis in a single ipsilateral lymph node, 3 cm or less in greatest dimension
N2	Metastasis as specified in N2a, 2b, 2c below
N2a	Metastasis in a single ipsilateral lymph node, more than 3 cm but not more than 6 cm in greatest dimension
N2b	Metastasis in multiple ipsilateral lymph nodes, none more than 6 cm in greatest dimension
N2c	Metastasis in bilateral or contralateral lymph nodes, none more than 6 cm in greatest dimension
N3	Metastasis in a lymph node more than 6 cm in greatest dimension

Note: Midline nodes are considered ipsilateral nodes.

M – Distant metastasis

MX	Distant metastasis cannot be assessed
M0	No distant metastasis
M1	Distant metastasis

Stage Grouping

Stage 0	Tis	N0	M0
Stage I	T1	N0	M0
Stage II	T2	N0	M0
Stage III	T1, T2	N1	M0
	T3	N0, N1	M0
Stage IVA	T1,T2,T3,	N2	M0
	T4a	N0, N1, N2	M0
Stage IVB	T4b	Any N	M0
	Any T	N3	M0
Stage IVC	Any T	Any N	M1

---

[1] {947,2418}.
[2] A help desk for specific questions about the TNM classification is available at www.uicc.org/index.php?id=508
[3] ## The regional lymph nodes are the cervical nodes.

TNM classification of carcinomas of the hypopharynx

TNM classification [1,2]
TNM classification of carcinomas of the hypopharynx {947,2418}

T – Primary tumour

TX   Primary tumour cannot be assessed
T0   No evidence of primary tumour
Tis   Carcinoma in situ
T1   Tumour limited to one subsite of hypopharynx and 2 cm or less in greatest dimension
T2   Tumour invades more than one subsite of hypopharynx or an adjacent site, or measures more than 2 cm but not more than 4 cm in greatest dimension, without fixation of hemilarynx
T3   Tumour more than 4 cm in greatest dimension, or with fixation of hemilarynx
T4a   Tumour invades any of the following: thyroid/cricoid cartilage, hyoid bone, thyroid gland, oesophagus, central compartment soft tissue*
T4b   Tumour invades prevertebral fascia, encases carotid artery, or invades mediastinal structures.

*Note: Central compartment soft tissue includes prelaryngeal strap muscles and subcutaneous fat.

N – Regional lymph nodes##

NX   Regional lymph nodes cannot be assessed
N0   No regional lymph node metastasis
N1   Metastasis in a single ipsilateral lymph node, 3 cm or less in greatest dimension
N2   Metastasis as specified in N2a, 2b, 2c
N2a   Metastasis in a single ipsilateral lymph node, more than 3 cm but not more than 6 cm in greatest dimension
N2b   Metastasis in multiple ipsilateral lymph nodes, none more than 6 cm in greatest dimension
N2c   Metastasis in bilateral or contralateral lymph nodes, none more than 6 cm in greatest dimension
N3   Metastasis in a lymph node more than 6 cm in greatest dimension
Note: Midline nodes are considered ipsilateral nodes.

M – Distant metastasis

MX   Distant metastasis cannot be assessed
M0   No distant metastasis
M1   Distant metastasis

Stage Grouping

Stage	T	N	M
Stage 0	Tis	N0	M0
Stage I	T1	N0	M0
Stage II	T2	N0	M0
Stage III	T1, T2	N1	M0
	T3	N0, N1	M0
Stage IVA	T1,T2,T3	N2	M0
	T4a	N0, N1, N2	M0
Stage IVB	T4b	Any N	M0
	Any T	N3	M0
Stage IVC	Any T	Any N	M1

---

[1] {947,2418}.
[2] A help desk for specific questions about the TNM classification is available at www.uicc.org/index.php?id=508
[3] ## The regional lymph nodes are the cervical nodes.

Tumours of the hypopharynx, larynx and trachea: Introduction

L. Barnes
L.L.Y. Tse
J.L. Hunt
M. Brandwein-Gensler
M. Urken

P. Slootweg
N. Gale
A. Cardesa
N. Zidar
P. Boffetta

With emphasis now on accurate staging and conservative surgery to retain as many functions as possible, especially in the larynx, the pathologist has emerged as an invaluable member of the health care team. Precise and detailed examination of resected head and neck specimens regarding the site of origin of the tumour, structures involved, tumour grade, adequacy of resection margins, and the presence of lymph node metastasis, extranodal spread of tumour, perineural involvement, and vascular invasion are just a few of many features that are important to the clinician who must decide on the total therapeutic regimen for the patient.

Definitions / anatomy

Larynx

The larynx extends from the tip of the epiglottis to the inferior border of the cricoid cartilage. Anteriorly, its boundaries are the lingual epiglottis, the thyrohyoid membrane, the anterior commissure, thyroid cartilage, cricothyroid membrane and the anterior arch of the cricoid cartilage. The posterior boundaries include the posterior commissure mucosa (which covers the cricoid cartilage) the arytenoid region, and the interarytenoid space.

The larynx is divided into three compartments - supraglottis, glottis, and subglottis. The supraglottis is composed of the epiglottis, aryepiglottic folds, false vocal cords (vestibular folds), ventricles and saccules. The tip of the epiglottis and the aryepiglottic folds form the superior and lateral supraglottic margins. The inferior limit is a horizontal plane passing through the lateral margin of the ventricle at its junction with the superior surface of the true vocal cord (vocal fold) {947}. The ventricle is the "pocket" between the true and false vocal cords. The lateral superior ventricular extension, or "cul-de-sac", is variably sized, and referred to as the saccule. The epiglottis is further divided into suprahyoid and infrahyoid components by a plane at the level of the hyoid bone.

The glottis extends, superiorly, from a horizontal plane passing through the lateral margin of the ventricle, at its junction with the superior true vocal cord, to an imaginary horizontal plane 10 mm inferiorly from the lateral margin of the ventricle {947}. The glottis consists of the true vocal cords, plus their undersurfaces, and the anterior and posterior commissures. The subglottis extends from 10 mm below the true vocal cords to the inferior margin of the cricoid cartilage. Most tumours that clinically appear as

"subglottic", actually arise from the undersurface of the true vocal cord and are still considered glottic. The term "transglottic" does not refer to a specific anatomic site. It designates those tumours that cross the ventricle vertically, to involve both the supraglottis and glottis, and occasionally subglottis {1679}. The growth and spread of laryngeal tumours is determined by the site of origin and the anatomic barriers of the different laryngeal compartments {1941}. Three of these are especially important: anterior commissure tendon (Broyles' ligament), paraglottic space and the preepiglottic space.

The anterior commissure tendon is a band of fibrous tissue 1 mm in width and 10 mm in length that extends from the vocal ligaments to the midline of the inner surface of the upper thyroid cartilage {286}. It is significant not only because it contains lymphatic and blood vessels, but also because it is devoid of perichondrium at the attachment to the thyroid cartilage, thereby acting as a conduit for tumour spread into the adjacent soft tissue or the prelaryngeal (Delphian) lymph node.

The paraglottic space is a potential space deep to the ventricles and saccules filled with adipose and loose connective tissue. It is bounded by the

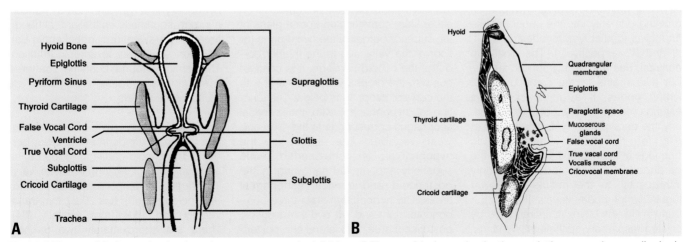

Fig. 3.1 A Diagram of the larynx showing the various components and subdivisions. **B** Diagram of the larynx showing the paraglottic space and surrounding landmarks. Reprinted from Ref. {131}. Courtesy of Marcel Dekker Inc.

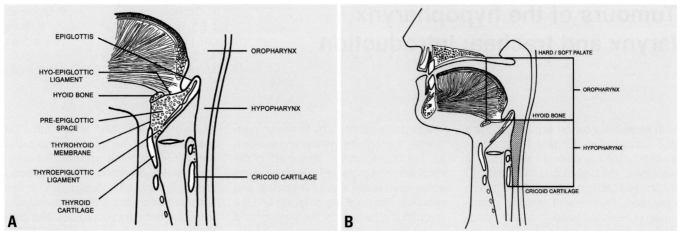

Fig. 3.2 A Diagram of the larynx and pre-epiglottic space. **B** Diagram and boundaries of the oropharynx and hypopharynx, with relationship to oral cavity and larynx, respectively.

conus elasticus inferiorly, the thyroid cartilage laterally, the quadrangular membrane medially and the pyriform sinus posteriorly. The pre-epiglottic space, also filled with adipose and connective tissue, is triangular shaped. It is bounded anteriorly by the thyroid cartilage and thyrohyoid membrane, posteriorly by the epiglottis and thyroepiglottic ligament, and superiorly by the hyoepiglottic ligament which forms its base. Both paraglottic and pre-epiglottic spaces contain lymphatics and blood vessels, but no lymph nodes. Suprahyoid epiglottic tumours are distinct from the more common infrahyoid tumours in that they are superior to the pre-epiglottic space, and often spread to the base of the tongue. Tumours that invade the pre-epiglottic and paraglottic spaces may spread without impedance through the loose connective tissue and eventually invade the extralaryngeal tissues. The supraglottic larynx is well endowed with lymphatics draining primarily into the upper, middle and lower jugular lymph nodes (levels II, III and IV, respectively). The glottis, in contrast, has a limited lymphatic supply, but also drains to the same group of lymph nodes. If a glottic carcinoma extends more than one centimeter inferiorly, the paratracheal lymph nodes are at risk for metastasis. The lymphatic drainage of the subglottis is mainly to the paratracheal lymph nodes and, only infrequently, to the middle and lower jugular lymph nodes (levels III and IV). Early in life, the larynx is entirely lined by ciliated respiratory epithelium. With time, this epithelium is gradually replaced by non-keratinizing stratified squamous

epithelium. The adult larynx is lined entirely by squamous epithelium, with the exception of the ventricles and the subglottis – which continue to be lined by respiratory epithelium. Infrequently, one may see small patches of persistent ciliated respiratory epithelium in an otherwise typical adult supraglottis. The nonkeratinized squamous mucosa of the true vocal cords is normally about 5-10 cells thick. Although mucoserous glands are abundant in the supraglottis and subglottis, they are essentially absent in the true vocal cords.

Hypopharynx

The pharynx is a hollow muscular tube extending from the skull base to the lower border of the cricoid cartilage. It is arbitrarily divided into three regions: nasopharynx, oropharynx, and hypopharynx. The hypopharynx (also known as laryngopharynx) lies behind the larynx and partially surrounds it on either side, commencing from a plane of the superior border of the hyoid bone (or floor of the vallecula) to the inferior border of the cricoid cartilage. It is continuous with the oropharynx above and with the cervical esophagus below. The junction of hypopharynx with the cervical esophagus corresponds to the sixth cervical vertebra. The lumen of the hypopharynx is cone-shaped, wide superiorly and rapidly narrowing in the postcricoid and cervical esophageal areas. The hypopharynx has three components: right and left pyriform sinuses, postcricoid area, and lateral and posterior pharyngeal walls. The pyriform sinuses are extralaryngeal gutters nestled

against the thyroid lamina. Each pyriform sinus is shaped like an inverted pyramid with the apex pointed toward the lower limit of the cricoid cartilage. The superior border corresponds to the pharyngoepiglottic fold. Each sinus has three walls, medial, lateral and anterior. The postcricoid area forms the anterior wall of the hypopharynx and connects the two pyriform sinuses. It extends from the level of the arytenoid cartilages to the inferior border of the cricoid cartilage {947}. The lateral pharyngeal wall merges with the pyriform sinus. The posterior pharyngeal wall extends from the level of the superior surface of the hyoid bone to the inferior border of the cricoid cartilage.

The hypopharynx is richly supplied with lymphatics. The major drainage is along the jugular chain (levels II, III and IV), retropharyngeal lymph nodes and the node of Rouviére at the skull base. The hypopharynx is typically lined by nonkeratinizing squamous epithelium, although areas of parakeratin or orthokeratin can be seen secondary to chronic irritation. The lamina propria contains scattered lymphoid aggregates as well as mucoserous glands.

Trachea

The trachea extends from the lower border of the cricoid cartilage to the carina and averages 11 cm long in adults, varying roughly in proportion to an individual's height {1660}. It is 20-27 mm transversely and 16-20 mm sagitally {64}. There are approximately two tracheal cartilaginous rings per centimeter of trachea, with a total of about 18-22.

Although usually referred to as rings, the cartilages are incomplete posteriorly, and form about two-thirds of a circle. The tracheal cartilages are connected to each other by fibroelastic annular ligaments. Sometimes the first tracheal ring may be fused to the cricoid cartilage. The trachea is continuous with the larynx superiorly and the bronchi inferiorly. Anteriorly, it is intimately associated with the thyroid gland and posteriorly with the esophagus. The trachea is lined entirely by ciliated respiratory epithelium and contains abundant mucoserous glands in the lamina propria. Posteriorly, the non-cartilaginous or membranous portion of trachea contains prominent smooth muscle. The submucosal lymphatics drain toward the posterior part of the trachea and connect with the paratracheal lymph nodes. They also anastomose with subcarinal, peribronchial and esophageal lymph nodes {64}.

Neck dissections

A neck dissection is a tissue mass containing the cervical lymphatics. In its classical form, it extends from the submandibular soft tissues to the supraclavicular fatty tissue, laterally bordered by the platysma, and medially by the internal jugular vein. The lymph nodes in this area are divided into 6 different compartments, referred to as levels {2183}.

Level I is subdivided in two compartments, the submental area (level IA) that lies between both anterior bellies of the digastric muscle and the hyoid bone dorsally, and the submandibular area (level 1B) that lies between the anterior belly of the digastric muscle medially and the mandibular bone laterally. Dorsally, this area is bordered by the tendon between the anterior and posterior belly of the digastric muscle that is attached to the

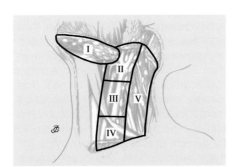

Fig. 3.3 Schematic drawing to show the various lymph node levels in the neck. Drawing by John A.M. de Groot.

hyoid bone, and the stylohyoid muscle. Thus, the triangle of soft tissue enclosed anteriorly and laterally by the mandible and dorsally by the hyoid is subdivided into one median compartment, the submental area and 2 lateral compartments, the submandibular areas.

Level II represents the upper jugular (cervical) group of lymph nodes. This area extends from the base of the skull superiorly to the level of the inferior border of the hyoid bone inferiorly. The lymph nodes in this area mainly cluster in the vicinity of the internal jugular vein and are laterally covered by the body of the sternocleidomastoid muscle.

Level III represents the middle jugular (cervical) group of lymph nodes. These lymph nodes are located around the middle third of the internal jugular vein that superiorly begins where the upper jugular compartment ends; the lower border lies at the inferior border of the cricoid cartilage.

Level IV comprises the lymph nodes located around the lower third of the internal jugular vein extending from the inferior border of the cricoid cartilage superiorly to the clavicle inferiorly.

Level V is the lymph nodes collectively taken together as the posterior triangle group. This is a triangular area lying between the anterior border of the trapezius muscle posteriorly, the posterior border of the sternocleidmastoid muscle anteriorly and the clavicle caudally. It is subdivided into a superior compartment, level VA that contains the spinal accessory lymph nodes and a lower compartment (level VB) that contains the transverse cervical and the supraclavicular lymph nodes. A horizontal plane through the inferior border of the anterior cricoid arch separates both sublevels.

Level VI is the anterior compartment. This compartment has the hyoid bone as its cranial and the suprasternal notch as its caudal border. Both lateral borders are the common carotid arteries. This area is rectangular and lies between the area defined as level I above and the sternum below.

Four different types of neck dissections are recognized {2183}.

A radical neck dissection consists of lymph nodes from level I through V. The internal jugular vein, sternocleidomastoid muscle, and spinal accessory nerve also form part of it. A modified radical neck dissection comprises all lymph nodes

from levels I-V while preserving one or more of the non-lymphoid structures that should be specified, e.g. modified radical neck dissection with preservation of spinal accessory nerve.

If less than level I-V is removed, the neck dissection is referred to as selective, while specifying the levels that are included. The use of terms such as supra-omohyoid neck dissection is less preferable due to ambiguities about the extent of the surgical procedure.

Extended radical neck dissection is the fourth type. This term refers to any type of neck dissection that consists of a radical neck dissection together with additional structures either lymphatic or non-lymphatic that have to be identified specifically. These structures may be additional lymph node compartments, nerves, or blood vessels.

Examination of a neck dissection should be done with the following questions in mind: (1) does the specimen contain lymph nodes with metastatic deposits, (2) if so, how many lymph nodes with metastases are present, specified for each level (3) what is the size of the largest positive lymph node, necessary for staging, and (4) is there extracapsular tumour spread?

Dissection of the specimen starts with determination of the type of neck dissection and identification of the various lymph nodes levels and any additional non-lymphoid structures that may have been removed. As the anatomical boundaries that are used by the surgeons to identify the lymph node levels are not present in the specimen, these cannot be used by the pathologist. Optimal processing of a neck dissection therefore requires that the surgeon submit the specimen with all lymph node levels properly labelled.

Epidemiology

Age and sex distribution

Laryngeal and hypopharyngeal squamous cell carcinoma (SCC) occur most frequently in the sixth and seventh decades, but some cases have been described in children {123,1934}. They are more common in men {344,2113} though the male:female ratio is decreasing in some countries; women are becoming increasingly affected because of increased prevalence of smoking over the last two decades {584}.

Tracheal SCC occurs predominantly

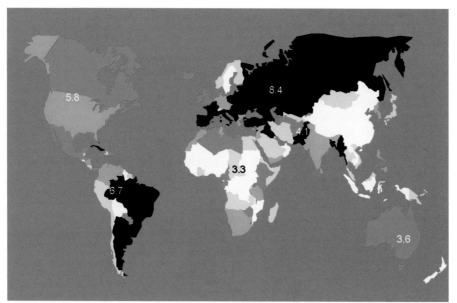

Fig. 3.5 Global incidence rates of cancer of the larynx (all ages) in males. Age-standardized rates (ASR, world standard population) per 100,000 population and year. From: Globocan 2000 {730}.

between 40 and 60 years of age, men are affected at least twice as often as women {1040}.

Incidence

SCC comprises about 95% of laryngeal malignancies. The majority originate from the supraglottic and glottic regions, although there are geographic variations in the relative ratio between these two sites. The incidence in men is high (10/100,000 pa or more) in southern and central Europe, southern Brazil, Uruguay and Argentina and among Blacks in the United States. The lowest rates (<1/100,000 pa) are recorded in South-East Asia and central Africa. The incidence in women is below 1/100,000 pa in most populations. An estimated 140,000 new cases occurred worldwide in 1990, 86% of these patients were men {1980,1981}. The incidence is slightly more common in urban that in rural areas {344,2113}.

There are also geographic differences in the topographic distribution of the laryngeal SCC {126}. In France, Spain, Italy, Finland and the Netherlands, supraglottic SCC predominates, while in the United States, Canada, England and Sweden glottic SCC is more common. In Japan, SCC is approximately equally distributed between the two sites.

Interpretation of incidence rates of hypopharyngeal cancer is probably complicated by absence or misclassifi-

cations within subsites of the pharynx. Recorded incidence is highest among men (>2.5/100,000 pa) in India, Brazil and Central and Western Europe, and is lowest (<0.5/100,000 pa) in East Asia, Africa and Northern Europe. Incidence among women is low (<0.2/100,000 pa) in most populations except India, where rates up to 1/100,000 pa are recorded {1981}. This is probably due to the fact that tobacco is more often chewed than smoked in India.

Tracheal carcinoma is rare with approximately one tracheal carcinoma per 75 laryngeal carcinomas. It accounts for less than 0.1% of cancer deaths {1040}. SCC is the most frequent malignant tumour of the trachea representing 56-73% of all tracheal carcinomas {1040}.

Trends

The incidence of laryngeal and hypopharyngeal SCC is increasing in much of the world, both in men and in women. This increase is related to changes in tobacco and alcohol consumption {344}.

Primary prevention of laryngeal and hypopharyngeal SCC could be achieved by cessation of smoking and reduction of alcohol consumption {344}.

Etiology

Tobacco and alcohol - Larynx

Most cases of laryngeal cancer in Western countries are related to smoking and alcohol abuse {90}. The combined

effect follows a multiplicative rather than additive model {285,772,1607,1608, 1800,1943,2647,2885}. The increased relative risk (RR) for alcohol consumption differs by site, and is higher for the supraglottis and hypopharynx and lower for the glottis and subglottis {2647}. The impact of increased RR (10x) for smoking is stronger for glottic than supraglottic SCC {2647}. Studies in several populations have shown a direct dose-related response between smoking and SCC and the benefits of cessation. Smoking black tobacco cigarettes entails a stronger risk than smoking blond tobacco {2235}. Other smoking habits that increase the RR of laryngeal SCC include: smoking at a young age, long duration, high number of cigarettes per day, and deep smoke inhalation {195,1035}. The influence of tobacco on RR of laryngeal SCC is confirmed even for non-drinkers {308,2833}. Case controlled studies from Italy and Switzerland show an increased RR of 2.46 for heavy drinkers and laryngeal SCC. The RR for current smokers who do not drink is 9.38 {238}. Avoiding cigarettes and alcohol could prevent about 90% of laryngeal and hypopharyngeal SCC {718}.

Tobacco and alcohol - Hypopharynx

Studies from India have also reported an association between chewing tobacco-containing products {968} and hypopharyngeal SCC. Tobacco and alcohol are also the main risk factors for hypopharyngeal SCC. The effect of alcohol is stronger and the impact of tobacco is weaker than for laryngeal SCC.

Asbestos and occupational exposure

There is controversy regarding occupational asbestos exposure and increased risk for developing laryngeal SCC {247, 1255,1982,2484}. A recent review has not supported a causative role for asbestos exposure {283}. However, there is evidence supporting other occupational exposures and increased risk of laryngeal SCC, such as polycyclic aromatic hydrocarbons, metal dust, cement dust, varnish, lacquer, etc {1608}. After adjustment for alcohol and tobacco consumption, the increased risk ranged from 1.8 for cement dust to 2.7 for polycyclic aromatic hydrocarbons. Significant associations are also found with ionizing radiation, diesel exhausts, sulphuric acid mists and mustard gas {1608,2821}.

Human papillomavirus (HPV)

There is conflicting evidence implicating HPV16, in 3-85% of laryngeal SCC {1523}. The prevailing opinion is that HPV has a minor causative role, if any, in laryngeal carcinogenesis {853,1253, 1510,1523,1999,2330}. Additionally, HPV DNA has been detected in 12-25% of individuals with clinically and histologically normal larynges {1912,2172}, suggesting that the occasional demonstration of HPV in laryngeal SCC may be incidental.

Diet and nutritional factors

A protective effect is probably exerted by high intake of fruits and vegetables {238, 565,1405,1910,1951,2003,2885,2901}. Specific evidence regarding carotenoids and vitamin C, is inadequate for a conclusion {2821}. Maté drinking has been suggested to be a risk factor in studies from Brazil and Uruguay {90}.

Gastroesophageal reflux

Gastroesophageal reflux has been related to increased risk of laryngeal SCC, especially among patients who lack other major risk factors {80,812,1782, 2724}. Gastroesophageal reflux may act as a promoter in the presence of tobacco and alcohol {812}.

Genetic susceptibility

There is no evidence of strong genetic factors in laryngeal carcinogenesis; however, polymorphisms for enzymes implicated in the detoxification of alcohol and tobacco, such as alcohol and aldehyde dehydrogenases, are likely to represent weak susceptibility factors, with relative risks in the order of 1.5-2 {200,1590}. Bloom syndrome is an inheritable condition with a predisposition towards laryngeal and hypopharyngeal SCC.

Pathology overview and principles

Compartmentally, the supraglottis is distinct from the glottis and subglottis. The supraglottis is embryologically derived from the buccopharyngeal anlage (branchial arches III and IV) while the glottis is derived from the laryngotracheal anlage (branchial arches V and VI). The fascial compartmentalization, as well as the lymphatic drainage is distinct for the supraglottis and glottis and is the oncologic basis for the supraglottic horizontal laryngectomy. Dye injected into the supraglottis remains confined and

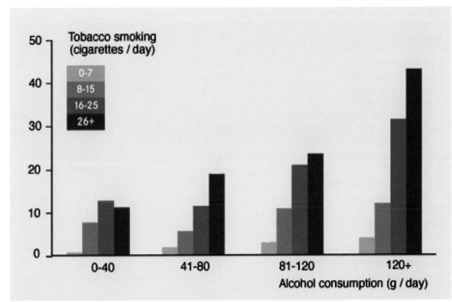

Fig. 3.6 Multiplicative increase in relative risk of laryngeal cancer as a consequence of both alcohol drinking and active smoking (colour coding approximates progressive doubling of risk as exposure increase). From A.J. Tuyns et al. {2647}.

does not travel to the ventricular or glottic tissues. Likewise, glottic dye injections do not pass superiorly to the ventricle or inferiorly to the mucosa overlying the cricoid cartilage. In fact, the mucosa overlying the lamina propria of the glottis (Reinke's space or laryngeal bursa) may burst from fluid distention rather than allowing injected dye to extend into the ventricle or cross the anterior commissure. These studies also confirm that the larynx is divided into right and left compartments {2087}.

The anatomic site of occurrence of tumour within the larynx can influence 1) the type of presenting symptoms, 2) stage at presentation, 3) treatment, and 4) prognosis. The vast majority of malignancies of the supraglottis and glottis are SCC. However the relative distribution of SCC per laryngeal compartment varies worldwide. Non-squamous tumours comprise a small subset of laryngeal malignancies, and are more likely encountered in the supraglottis and infraglottis than the glottis.

Glottic tumours present with hoarseness and are typically small when detected. In contrast, the supraglottis is a clinically silent area and, as such, tumours in this site are often large at the time of diagnosis. Epiglottic tumours may present with a change in vocal quality (a muffled or "hot potato voice"), airway obstruction, dysphagia and/or cervical metastasis.

Tumours at the base of the epiglottis may escape visualization at indirect laryngoscopy ("Winkelkarzinom" or "cancer in the corner"). Primary ventricular tumours are rare and often remain obscured on laryngeal examination, merely forming a bulge beneath the false vocal cord. Tumours of the pyriform sinus are usually large when discovered and typically present as odynophagia or referred otalgia. If the tumour involves the medial wall or the apex of the pyriform sinus, vocal cord dysfunction may result.

Content of surgical pathology report, including cervical lymph nodes

The surgical pathology report of a laryngectomy specimen should indicate the type of procedure (hemi-, supraglottic-, or total laryngectomy), and whether any additional tissues are attached (neck dissection, thyroid gland, parathyroid gland). Additional features that should be addressed include 1) site of origin, size and extent of the tumour; 2) histologic type and grade; 3) presence of perineural, lymphovascular, cartilaginous and/or extralaryngeal invasion and 4) status of the resection margins {3,290}.

The neck dissection should include the details as stated above (see 'Anatomy - Neck dissections').

Surgical pathology report of a hypopharyngectomy specimen should indicate whether the tumour is arising from the

Table 3.1 Histologic diagnoses for 479 patients with laryngeal malignancies*

Histology	N	%
Carcinoma-in-situ	46	9.6%
Squamous cell carcinoma	383	79.9%
Verrucous carcinoma	5	1.0%
Spindle cell carcinoma	8	1.7%
Lymphoepithelial carcinoma	1	0.2%
Subtotal	443	92.5%
Neuroendocrine carcinoma	4	0.8%
Adenoid cystic carcinoma	2	0.4%
Mucoepidermoid carcinoma	3	0.6%
Chondrosarcoma	8	1.7%
Liposarcoma	3	0.6%
Lymphoma	6	1.2%
Plasmacytoma	1	0.2%
Malignant granular cell tumour	1	0.2%
Secondary papillary thyroid carcinoma	7	1.5%
Fibrosarcoma, low-grade	1	0.2%
Total	**479**	**100.0%**

*Mount Sinai Medical Center, 1994-2003

right or left pyriform sinus, postcricoid area or posterior-lateral pharyngeal wall. If it originates in the pyriform sinus, as most do, it should be noted whether the tumour is arising from the medial or lateral wall, extends to the apex of the sinus or involves the larynx.

For tracheal resection, indicate the length of segment excised and whether the tumour is intra- or extraluminal.

Clinical features and diagnostic procedures

A detailed history and physical examination with attention to specific symptoms will often point to the site and extent of the tumour. There are four critical variables that guide the clinician toward the most appropriate course of therapy: pathologic diagnosis, local extent of tumour, status of regional lymph nodes and presence or absence of distant metastasis.

Imaging studies should always preceed endoscopy since the latter procedure often results in edema and a decrease in the accuracy of image studies. Direct endoscopy is not only necessary to obtain a biopsy but also important to further evaluate the extent of the disease and rule out additional primary tumours. Distant metastasis frequently distinguishes surgical from non-surgical candidates. Accordingly, tests for hepatic function and imaging studies of lung and bones are invaluable.

Second primary tumours

Second primary tumours (SPT) are defined as additional primary malignancies that are distinctly separate from the index tumour (IT). Synchronous SPT are diagnosed at the same time, or within six months of the IT. If the SPT is discovered after six months, it is classified as metachronous. The median prevalence of synchronous SPT for the upper aerodigestive tract (UADT) is 9% {1027}. The annual risk for SPT, is rather constant and varies between 1.5% {453} and 5.1% {1309} among patients with UADT SCC.

The definition of SPT has been further expanded based on molecular markers of clonality or genetic profiling. This includes comparing patterns of loss of heterozygosity (LOH) and specific p53 mutations at various hotspots among IT, SPT and adjacent mucosa. There are drawbacks to comparing only LOH patterns: 1) LOH at various loci can be so frequent, as to be coincidentally present in two tumours, and 2) Progression in genomic loss can be seen with tumour recurrence. This issue is addressed to some extent by p53 mutational analysis, however, identical mutations can occur at various hotspots in 5% of tumours. Some studies have revealed both similarities and discordances in genetic profiling between paired IT and SPT {248}. Concordant genetic profiles of IT and adjacent mucosa support the concept of mucosal field cancerization as a clonal

expansion phenomenon in proximity to the IT. So SPT can arise either as related (clonal) events via lateral mucosal spread of premalignant cells, or as genetically unrelated events. Furthermore, there appears to be an indirect relationship between the distance from the IT to SPT, and the time interval between both, and genetic clonality. Thus synchronous multicentric tumours may be explained by the migration or the distant settling of tumoral cells, whereas distant SPT or metachronous tumours would be better explained by the concept of field cancerization. Newly proposed definitions for "true" SPT, local recurrence, second field tumour and metastasis have been proposed based on molecular profiling {248}. "True" SPT are genetically distinct with discordant genetic profiles compared with the IT. If two metachronous carcinomas yield concordant genetic profiles, then the latter tumour is a locoregional recurrence of the former. A "second field tumour" (SFT) distinguishes a second, genetically discordant neoplasm adjacent to the IT, not as a local recurrence but due to the second tumour arising within the same "condemned mucosa" of the IT.

The likelihood and site for developing SPT are influenced by the site of the IT. For UADT IT, the most frequent site for SPT is within the UADT {453,1027,1309, 1473,1898}; usually an oral SPT associated with intraoral IT. With respect to the larynx, the risk of developing SPT is higher in patients with supraglottic tumours than in those with glottic tumours {1473, 1898}. Patients with glottic carcinomas are more likely to develop SPT along the respiratory axis (usually lung carcinoma), whereas patients with supraglottic carcinomas are more likely to develop SPT along the aerodigestive axis. No doubt this relates to the specific environmental promoters. The risk of developing SPT clearly correlates with tobacco and alcohol abuse. This risk is more than doubled in patients using tobacco and alcohol, as compared to those patients without exposure {1473}. There is a direct dose-dependent relationship between tobacco and alcohol exposure and risk of SPT development {453,1473}. The risk of developing a SPT after laryngeal IT increased proportionally to the number of cigarettes smoked per day at the time of the diagnosis {1106}.

Susceptibility towards the development

of SPT can be demonstrated via mutagen sensitivity tests, such as bleomycin-induced chromatid breaks of cultivated lymphocytes {461,462}. Increased mutagen sensitivity is significantly associated with an increased risk of SPT, with higher risk for both smoking-related and all SPTs (relative risks 2.62 and 2.77, respectively) {2450}. A significantly higher number of chromatid breaks are seen in patients with multiple cancers (mean 1.20) than in patients with a single cancer (mean 0.96) {461,462}. Radiation exposure is also carcinogenic, yet might also have a protective effect on the development of SPT. For patients with laryngeal IT, the latency period for SPT development in irradiated regions was significantly longer than that in non-irradiated patients, suggesting that radiotherapy (RT) may delay the development of SPT {1898}. In patients with laryngeal IT treated by primary RT, the incidence of laryngeal SPT was lower (4.3%) as compared to those patients with laryngeal IT treated primarily surgically, (9.2%), again implying a protective effect {1684}.

Prognosis and predictive factors

Small glottic or supraglottic SCC can be treated conservatively by laser excision, limited resection, or primary radiotherapy (RT), with curative potential, and overall good survival {1605}. RT failures can be salvaged by conservative, potentially curative voice-sparing surgery. Glottic or supraglottic carcinomas that fix the vocal cord(s) can be treated either by primary resection, with possible adjuvant RT, or organ sparing protocols (neoadjuvant chemotherapy with curative RT). If the carcinoma persists or recurs, overall survival is not compromised by delayed, salvage, total laryngectomy.

The TNM tumour classification consistently correlates, on multivariate survival analyses, with disease-free and overall survival. Among TNM stage IV patients, extensive cartilage invasion and/or bulky tumour volume are predictors of poor response to chemoradiotherapy; these patients are best treated with primary resection and possible adjuvant RT {1883}. Clinical comorbidities have been demonstrated to significantly affect survival over TNM prognosticators {2041}. The Washington University Head and Neck Comorbidity Index incorporates seven conditions (congestive heart disease, cardiac arrhythmia, peripheral vascular disease, pulmonary disease, renal disease, cancer controlled, and cancer uncontrolled) weighted according to severity, and is a significant predictor of survival.

Generally, histological grading has limited impact on survival. By contrast, the pattern of tumour invasion at the advancing host/tumour interface has been demonstrated, by itself or in combination with other histological variables, to have predictive value for laryngeal carcinoma {290}. Thus within T1/T2 laryngeal SCC, biopsy assessment of the pattern of invasion, may be utilized to predict which patients may respond to primary RT, versus which patients are better treated by primary resection. In multivariate analysis, overexpression of p53 is predictive of improved overall survival {1103}. p53 overexpression and elevated PCNA (proliferating cell nuclear antigen) index have been demonstrated to be significant independent predictors of successful organ preservation {249}.

Hypopharyx

SCC is optimally treated with surgery and adjuvant RT. Prognosis is inversely related to TNM stage and extracapsular spread. {148,1370}.

Trachea

SCC is the most common primary tracheal malignancy, which is usually treated with RT. Poor prognosticators include mediastinal and distant metastases and poor patient performance status {393,1217}.

Squamous cell carcinoma

A. Cardesa
N. Gale
A. Nadal
N. Zidar

Definition
Squamous cell carcinoma (SCC) is the most common malignancy of the larynx, pharynx and trachea. It occurs mainly in adult males who abuse tobacco and alcohol, and is characterized by squamous differentiation.

ICD-O code   8070/3

Synonym
Epidermoid carcinoma

Epidemiology
See Introduction page 113-114.

Etiology
See Introduction page 114-115.

Localization
The most common sites for laryngeal SCC vary according to geography, with the supraglottic and glottic regions being the most common locations. Hypopharyngeal SCC originates most frequently in the pyriform sinus, followed by the posterior pharyngeal wall, and the postcricoid area {1053,2661}.
Tracheal SCC occurs frequently in the lower third, and less frequently in the upper and middle thirds {1040}.

Clinical features
Signs and symptoms
Clinical features depend on the localization of SCC. The most common early symptom in glottic carcinoma is hoarseness. Symptoms of supraglottic, and hypopharyngeal tumours include dysphagia, change in quality of voice, foreign body sensation in the throat, haemoptysis, odynophagia and neck mass. Dyspnoea, and stridor are especially common in subglottic tumours {749}. Tracheal SCC usually presents clinically with dyspnoea, wheezing or stridor, acute respiratory failure, cough, haemoptysis, and/or hoarseness {2143}.

Macroscopy
Laryngeal and hypopharyngeal SCC may present as a flat plaque with a well-

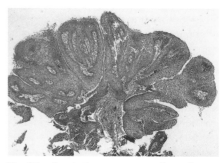
Fig. 3.9 Exophytic squamous cell carcinoma. Exophytic bulbous, rounded projections with areas of invasion into the stroma.

defined, raised edge, or exhibits a polypoid exophytic appearance, which may relate to prognosis. The surface of the tumour is sometimes ulcerated {1711}. Tracheal SCC usually presents as a polypoid mass projecting into the lumen, rarely does it grow as a circumferential or an annular mass {1040}.

Tumour spread and staging
SCC may spread directly to contiguous structures, or via lymphatic and blood vessels to lymph nodes and more distant sites.

Direct spread to contiguous structures
Supraglottic SCC tends to spread into the pre-epiglottic space, pyriform sinus or towards the base of the tongue, but it rarely invades the glottis and thyroid cartilage. Glottic SCC tends to remain localized for a long period; in late stages of the disease, it may extend to the opposite true vocal cord, to the supraglottis and subglottis; it may also extend through the thyroid cartilage and invade the soft tissue of the neck. The subglottic SCC may spread to the thyroid gland, hypopharynx, cervical esophagus and tracheal wall. SCC that crosses the ventricles and involves the supraglottis and glottis, is termed transglottic SCC {1679}. Hypopharyngeal SCC frequently involves the larynx.

Stomal recurrence
Stomal recurrence, defined as recurrent SCC at the mucocutaneous junction of

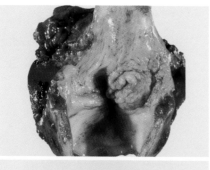

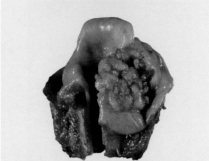
Fig. 3.7 Laryngeal squamous cell carcinoma (SCC) of the right ventricular fold (upper) and in the right pyriform sinus (lower).

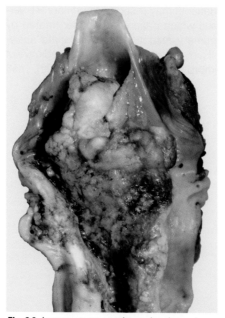
Fig. 3.8 Laryngectomy specimen showing a large hypopharyngeal squamous cell carcinoma occupying both postcricoid region as well as the right pyriform sinus.

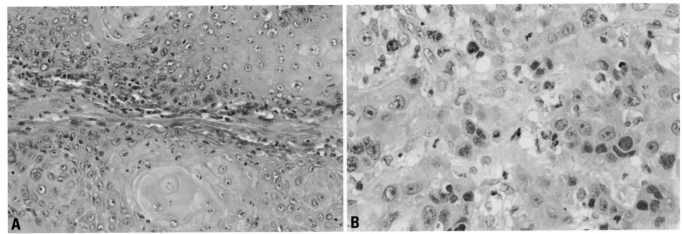

Fig. 3.10 Squamous cell carcinoma (SCC). **A** Well differentiated SCC. **B** Poorly differentiated SCC.

the tracheostoma, is a well recognized, but infrequent complication after total laryngectomy. Patients with subglottic and postcricoid involvement and advanced stage of the primary SCC are at risk to develop this complication.

Local and distant metastases
Laryngeal, hypopharyngeal and tracheal SCC are likely to metastasize to the regional lymph nodes. The location and frequency of lymph node metastases depends upon the site of the primary tumour. Extracapsular spread (ECS) refers to carcinoma penetrating the lymph node capsule and infiltrating extracapsular tissue. Extracapsular spread is further divided into macroscopic and microscopic ECS {337}; macroscopic ECS is evident to the naked eye and appears as matted lymph nodes. Microscopic ECS is only evident on histologic examination and is usually limited to the adjacent perinodal fibroadipose tissue.
Clinically relevant haematogenous metastases are infrequent but may occur in late stages of the disease. The most common site for spread is the lung, and less commonly, liver and bones {2435}. In patients with blood-borne metastases, regional lymph node metastases are usually also present or have been treated.

Staging
Tumours of the larynx and hypopharynx are staged by the TNM system (AJCC and UICC) {947,2418}. Tracheal tumours are not included in the TNM system. In the definition of the N classification, the specified 3.0 cm and 6.0 cm measurements include the total tumour mass in

the area (lymph node mass) and not just the individual lymph node size {2801}.

Histopathology
Squamous differentiation, often seen as keratinization with variable "pearl" formation, and invasive growth are the prerequisite features of SCC. Invasion is manifested by disruption of the basement membrane, and extension into the underlying tissue, often accompanied by stromal reaction. Angiolymphatic and perineural invasion are additional signs of malignancy.
The tumours are traditionally graded into well-, moderately-, and poorly differentiated SCC. Well differentiated SCC resembles closely normal squamous epithelium. Moderately differentiated SCC contains distinct nuclear pleomorphism and mitotic activity, including abnormal mitoses; there is usually less keratinization. In poorly differentiated SCC, immature cells predominate, with numerous typical and atypical mitoses, and minimal keratinization. Although keratinization is more likely to be present in well- or moderately-differentiated SCC, it should not be considered an important histological criterion in grading SCC. Most SCC are moderately differentiated, so grading by differentiation is really of limited prognostic value, as compared to pattern of invasion.

Invasive front
Tumour growth at the invasive front can show an expansive pattern, an infiltrative pattern, or both. Expansive growth pattern is characterised by large tumour islands with well-defined pushing margins and is associated with a better prog-

nosis. Infiltrative growth pattern is characterized by scattered small irregular cords or single tumour cells, with poorly defined infiltrating margins and is associated with a more aggressive course {290}. Some guidelines recommend categorizing tumours into cohesive, and non-cohesive fronts, (Reporting Guideline for the Royal College of Pathologists).

Stromal reaction
Invasive SCC is almost always accompanied by stromal reaction that consists of desmoplasia with deposition of extracellular matrix and proliferation of myofibroblasts {2907}. Neovascularization is frequently seen.

Immunoprofile
SCC expresses epithelial markers such as cytokeratins. The patterns of expression of cytokeratin subtypes may change during malignant transformation and relate to the histologic grade, degree of keratinization, and the likelihood of metastases. Low-grade SCC expresses medium-high molecular weight (MW) cytokeratins, but not low MW cytokeratins, similarly to normal squamous epithelium. In contrast, high-grade SCC tends to lose the expression of medium-high MW cytokeratins, and express low MW cytokeratins {1617}. High-grade SCC may express vimentin {2668}.

Electron microscopy
SCC exhibits desmosomes and attached tonofilaments {880}.

Differential diagnosis
The diagnosis of SCC is usually not prob-

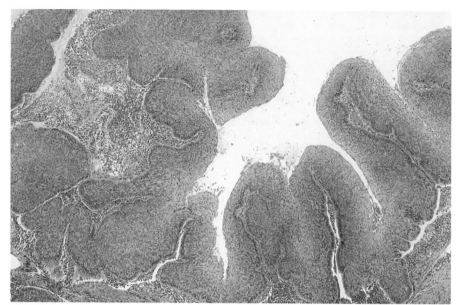

Fig. 3.11 Exophytic squamous cell carcinoma. Small fibrovascular cores are seen in the centre of papillary projections of squamous cell carcinoma.

lematic. However, the exophytic variant of SCC must be distinguished from papillary and verrucous SCC. The exophytic SCC is composed of broad-based neoplastic fronds, and in contrast to papillary SCC, lacks prominent branched fibrovascular cores {171,2602}. Verrucous SCC is composed of papillary projections and bulbous invaginations, lacking cytological atypia.

Well-differentiated SCC must also be distinguished from pseudoepitheliomatous hyperplasia, a benign hyperplastic epithelial condition composed of irregular elongated rete pegs extending deeply into the stroma. It typically occurs in association with chronic infections (tuberculosis, mycosis), trauma, and classically, granular cell tumours. The cytological features of malignancy are not found in pseudoepitheliomatous hyperplasia.

Distinguishing SCC from radiation changes can be difficult. Radiation can result in ulceration, epithelial and stromal atypia, inflammation and vascular changes. The seromucinous glands may be atrophic. Squamous metaplasia and hyperplasia of ducts, can mimic SCC. Preservation of ductal lumens and lobular architecture aid in making this distinction.

Moderately or poorly differentiated SCC must be distinguished from various subtypes of SCC. The differential diagnosis also includes other malignant tumours,

such as adenocarcinoma, neuroendocrine carcinoma, melanoma and lymphoma. The correct diagnosis is best achieved by the use of appropriate immunohistochemistry.

Precursor lesions
Precursor lesions are defined as altered epithelium with an increased likelihood for progression to SCC {847,852,1253, 1581}. Epithelial dysplasia is the term used traditionally to describe these microscopic alterations, although other terms have been proposed (see section on epithelial precursor lesions). Pathologists are frequently asked to assess epithelial dysplasia, because it is believed to be an important indicator of malignant potential. The likelihood of malignant change directly relates to the severity of dysplasia. However, it is clear that malignancy can develop from any grade of dysplasia or even from morphologically normal epithelium.

Histogenesis
SCC originates from the squamous mucosa or from ciliated respiratory epithelium that has undergone squamous metaplasia.

Somatic genetics
Cytogenetics and comparative genomic hybridization (CGH)
The most frequent chromosomal alterations detected by CGH are +3q, +5p,

+8q, +11q13, +17q, and –3p. Additional alterations, such as +1q, +7p, +7q +9q, +14q, +18p, and -4p, -5q, -11qter, and -18q are also frequent {1074,1145}. These alterations are very similar to those reported with conventional karyotyping analysis of early passage cells from laryngeal carcinomas {1219}. Predictive models based on hierarchical branching and distance-based trees indicate +3q21-29 as the most important early chromosomal alteration, followed in importance and chronology by –3p {1145}. High-level amplifications are found at 3q24-qter and, less frequently 11q13, 18p, 18q11.2, 8q23-24, and 11q14-22. Some of these amplifications are at loci containing known oncogenes (*CCND1* for 11q13) {1074}.

Metastazising tumours show a higher number of DNA copy losses than non-metastazising tumours. Losses at 8p, 9q, and 13 are more frequent in metastatic than in primary tumours {1381}.

Molecular genetic alterations
Neoplastic transformation implies modulation of a large number of genes {1810} as well as telomerase re-activation as indicated by hTERT expression {1588}.
CCND1 is amplified and overexpressed mostly in advanced cases {811,1207}. *MYC* and *EGFR* are amplified in 6-25% of cases although amplification is not related to overexpression {612,794,811}. Loss of *RB1* expression is seen in less than 20% of tumours {1208,2546} although LOH at 13q14 is present in 60% or more of tumours, suggesting the existence of other(s) tumour suppressor gene(s) neighbouring *RB1* {2857}.
TP53 mutations are found in 13-50% of laryngeal tumours. The excess of G to T transversions and the codons more frequently affected are both attributed to the carcinogenic effect of tobacco smoking {1939,2027}. *TP53* alterations are found in premalignant lesions indicating participation early in the neoplastic transformation process {847,1809}. However, neither *TP53* overexpression nor CDKN1A expression are reliable markers for *TP53* mutations. Instead, CDKN1A expression is clearly related to squamous differentiation {1811}. *TP73L*, a *TP53* homologue with oncogenic potential, maps to 3q27-28, a region with frequent gains. In primary carcinoma, low-copy number *TP73L* amplification has been detected by fluorescent in-situ

hybridization (FISH) {2837}.

The role of HPV infection in laryngeal carcinoma may be overestimated {1810}. The use of PCR-based techniques for the detection of HPV-DNA has yielded variable results (for a review see {1523}). In fact, the virus has even been demonstrated in more than 12-25% of non-neoplastic samples examined {2008}.

CDKN2A can be inactivated by mutation, homozygous deletion, and promoter hypermethylation {1208,2168}. CDKN2A mutations can occur in cases with mRNA and/or protein overexpression {1209}.

Significant levels of MMP13 mRNA are detectable in some laryngeal tumours, restricted to those that retain features of squamous differentiation. MMP13 expression is coordinated with MMP2 and MMP14 overexpression, two molecules that can efficiently activate MMP13. Both MMP13 expression and MMP14 overexpression are associated with advanced tumours, indicating a more aggressive behaviour {348}. CDH1 expression is lower in metastatic tumours {798}. In addition, gene expression silencing of CDH1 by promoter hypermethylation is more frequent in metastatic (77%) than in primary laryngeal tumours (40%) {95}.

Prognosis and predictive factors

The overall 5-year survival rate is 80-85% in glottic SCC, 65-75% in supraglottic SCC, about 40% in subglottic SCC {126}, 62.5% in hypopharyngeal SCC {2434}, and 47% in tracheal SCC {2143}.

Clinical predictive factors
Stage
TNM remains the most significant predictor of survival.

Localization
Tumour localization is important {754}. The best prognosis has been reported for glottic SCC, and the worst prognosis for hypopharyngeal, subglottic and tracheal SCC.

Other factors that can have an impact on the presentation and outcome of SCC include age, {428,2374}, comorbidity (concurrent diseases) {402} and performance status {428}.

Histopathological predictive factors
Resection margins
The complete excision of tumour is the most important principle of oncologic surgery. Negative resection margins are generally associated with decreased recurrence and improved survival {1557, 2403}. Although controversial, a distance of a few millimeters may be adequate in selected glottic SCC {2462,2738}. For supraglottic, advanced glottic, and hypopharyngeal SCC, resection margins have not been precisely defined but distances of at least 5 mm or greater are desired {841}.

Proliferation
Proliferation fraction determined immunohistochemically with antibodies against Ki67 and proliferating cell nuclear antigen (PCNA) have been reported to correlate strongly with the degree of differentiation in SCC {1372,2906} and the presence of lymph node metastases {798}. However, proliferation fraction is not an independent prognostic factor {1372}.

Lymphovascular and perineural invasion
The penetration of tumour cells into lymphatic and/or blood vessels is associated with an increased propensity for lymph node and/or distant metastases. It tends to occur in aggressive SCC and is associated with recurrence and poor survival {2853}. Similarly, perineural invasion is associated with increase local recurrence, regional lymph node metastases and decrease survival {708,2853}.

Extracapsular spread in lymph node metastases
Lymph node metastasis is the single most adverse prognostic factor in head and neck SCC {750}. Recent studies have shown that the presence of extracapsular spread in lymph nodes is strongly associated with both regional recurrence and distant metastases, resulting in decreased survival {750, 1094,2507}.

DNA ploidy
The prognostic significance of DNA ploidy has been studied extensively and the results are controversial. Some studies have shown that aneuploid tumours are associated with a higher rate of lymph node metastases and decreased survival {652,2545,2805} while others have not confirmed this {139,574}. Conflicting results have also been reported regarding the predictive value of DNA ploidy and treatment response {2545, 2774}.

Genetic predictive criteria
The prognostic value of p53 abnormalities is generally inconclusive for laryngeal carcinoma {79,1809,1914}. CCND1 amplification is related to poor prognosis independent of stage {192}. Simultaneous CDK4 and CCND1 overexpression is associated with poor prognosis {615}. In patients with locally advanced laryngeal cancer, CDKN2A mutations have prognostic significance in predicting adverse outcome {183}

Verrucous carcinoma

A. Cardesa
N. Zidar

Definition
Verrucous carcinoma (VC) is a non-metastasizing variant of well-differentiated squamous cell carcinoma (SCC) characterized by an exophytic, warty, slowly growing neoplasm with pushing margins.

ICD-O code   8051/3

Synonym
Ackerman tumour {12}

Epidemiology
VC occurs predominantly in men in the 6th and 7th decades of life {1671}.

Etiology
VC has been related to tobacco smoking. Human Papillomavirus (HPV) genotypes 16 and 18, and rarely 6 and 11, have been identified in some, but not all, VC {250,289,777,1233,1283}.

Localization
Larynx is the second most common site of VC in the head and neck (after oral cavity) and accounts for 15-35% of all VC {1350} and 1-4% of all laryngeal carcinomas {777,1671,1956}. Most arise from the anterior true vocal cords, though it may occur in the supraglottis, subglottis, hypopharynx and trachea {1350,1671}

Clinical features
Hoarseness is the most common presenting symptom; other symptoms include airway obstruction, weight loss,

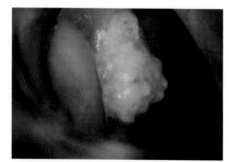

Fig. 3.12 Endoscopic view of a verrucous carcinoma. Wart-like, whitish outgrowth of the vocal cord.

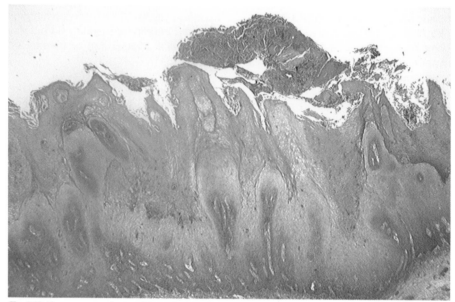

Fig. 3.13 Verrucous carcinoma. A large lesion with abundant keratosis arranged in "church-spire" configuration. There is a broad, pushing border of infiltration.

dysphagia, and throat pain {1671,1956}. Enlarged lymph nodes are common and reactive rather than neoplastic {978}.

Macroscopy
VC presents as a sharply circumscribed, broad based exophytic warty tumour which is usually firm, and tan to white.

Histopathology
VC consists of thickened club-shaped papillae and blunt intrastromal invaginations of well-differentiated squamous epithelium with marked keratinization and thin fibrovascular cores. The squamous epithelium lacks cytologic criteria of malignancy, and by morphometry, the cells are larger than those seen in SCC {489}. Mitoses are rare, and observed in the basal layers. DNA synthesis (S-phase) is also limited primarily to the basal layers {737}. VC invades the stroma with a pushing, rather than infiltrating border. Dense lymphoplasmacytic host response is common. Intraepithelial microabscesses are seen, and the abundant keratin may evoke a foreign body reaction.
The surrounding mucosa shows progres-

sive transition from hyperplasia to VC. A downward dipping of epithelium often "cups" the VC periphery, and is the ideal site for deep biopsy {174,1192}.
Hybrid tumours are VC containing foci of conventional SCC. The incidence of hybrid tumours in the larynx is approximately 10% {1956}. It is important to recognize this variant of VC, as it has the potential to metastasize {131,174}.

Differential diagnosis
The differential diagnosis of VC includes exophytic SCC, hybrid VC, papillary SCC, keratinizing squamous cell papilloma and verruca vulgaris. VC lacks cytological atypia, this distinguishes it from exophytic SCC, hybrid VC and papillary SCC. The pushing margins of VC are smooth, in distinction to the irregular shaped invasive islands of SCC. Papillomas have thin, well-formed papillary fronds, with limited keratinization, as compared to the markedly keratinized papillae of VC. Verruca vulgaris of the larynx {722} characteristically contains layers of parakeratotic squamous cells with large keratohyaline granules, identical to their counterpart on the skin.

Prognosis and predictive factors

VC is characterized by a slow, locally invasive growth causing extensive local destruction if left untreated. Pure VC does not metastasize {746,1956}. In contrast, hybrid VC has the potential for metastasis and, accordingly these patients should be managed as similarly staged patients with SCC {1956}. VC has an excellent prognosis; the reported five-year survival rate for laryngeal VC is 85-95% {751,1350}. Patients with VC may be treated by excision (by laser or surgery), or by radiotherapy. Although surgery is more effective, radiotherapy is an acceptable alternative for patients who are poor surgical candidates {978,1350, 1671,1956,2582}. Some reports have suggested that VC may undergo anaplastic transformation following radiotherapy. Critical review of these cases however has shown many to be unrecognized hybrid VC or other carcinomas that were inappropriately labelled as VC.

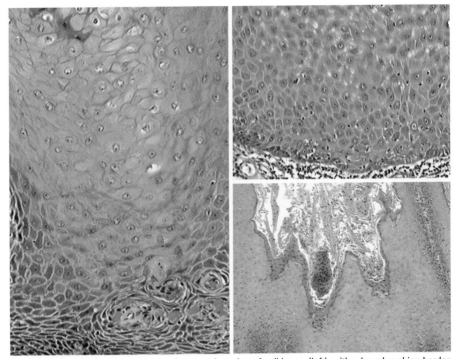

Fig. 3.14 Larynx verrucous carcinoma. Increased number of cell layers (left), with a broad pushing border of infiltration without cytologically atypical cells (right upper). Keratosis, including parakeratotic crypting is present (right lower).

Basaloid squamous cell carcinoma

A. Cardesa
N. Zidar
C. Ereño

Definition
Basaloid squamous cell carcinoma (BSCC) is an aggressive, high-grade, variant of SCC composed of both basaloid and squamous components.

ICD-O code   8083/3

Synonyms
Basaloid carcinoma, adenoid cystic-like carcinoma.

Epidemiology
BSCC occurs in both sexes, but predominantly in men 60-80 years of age {132, 1578,2128,2709}.

Localization
The pyriform sinus and supraglottic larynx are the usual sites of involvement {684,688,1337,1578,1774,2128,2709}. It has also been described in the trachea {1992,1997,2232}.

Clinical features
BSCC may present with neck mass, hoarseness, pain, sore throat, dysphagia, cough, otalgia, bleeding, and/or weight loss {117,1997,2128}.

Etiology
Tobacco and alcohol abuse have been proven to be strong risk factors {117, 132,1997,2128}.

Macroscopy
BSCC appears as a centrally ulcerated mass with extensive submucosal induration that may be confused with a minor salivary or soft tissue tumour {132,1578, 1997,2128}.

Histopathology
BSCC has two components, i.e. basaloid and squamous cells. Basaloid cells are small, with hyperchromatic nuclei without nucleoli, and scant cytoplasm. They are closely packed, growing in a solid pattern with a lobular configuration, and in some cases, there is prominent peripheral palisading. Comedo-type necrosis is frequent. Distinctive features of BSCC, not found in SCC, are small cystic spaces containing PAS- and Alcian blue-positive material, and stromal hyalinization {117,2709}. BSCC is always associated with a SCC component which can be either in-situ carcinoma, or invasive keratinizing SCC. The latter is usually located superficially; it may also present as a focal squamous differentiation within the basaloid tumour islands. The junction between the squamous and basaloid cells may be abrupt {117,132}. Rarely, BSCC is associated with a spindle cell component {1791}. Metastases may demonstrate basaloid carcinoma, squamous carcinoma, or both {688,1578, 2128}.

Immunoprofile
BSCC expresses cytokeratins and epithelial membrane antigen but the percentage of positive cells is highly variable. To avoid false-negative results, a cocktail of cytokeratin antibodies (i.e. CAM 5.2, AE1/3) is recommended {132}. The antibody 34ßE12, directed against high MW cytokeratins is most sensitive for the detection of basaloid cells {117,1774}. In the distinction between BSCC and adenoid cystic carcinoma, absence of myoepithelial cells and the presence of dot-like vimentin expression in BSCC can be helpful. S-100 protein reactivity is not helpful in the differential diagnosis, and if observed, usually corresponds to intermingled dendritic cells. BSCC is negative for chromogranin, synaptophysin, and glial-fibrillary acid protein {117,132,1337}.

Electron microscopy
Desmosomes and tonofilaments have been observed in basaloid and squamous cells. There are no neurosecretory

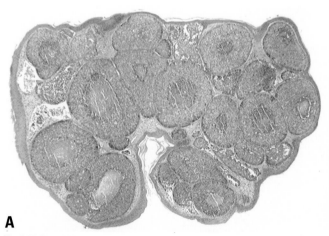
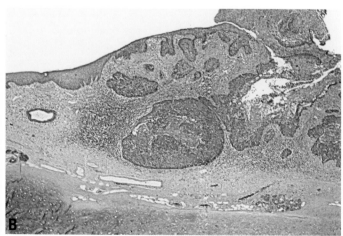

Fig. 3.15 Basaloid squamous cell carcinoma of the larynx. **A** Polypoid tumour with an intact squamous epithelium, subtended by lobules of basaloid cells with areas of central comedonecrosis. **B** Panoramic view of a tumour that arises from the surface epithelium and is composed of basaloid and squamous nests of cells situated above the epiglottic cartilage.

granules, myofilaments, or secretory granules in BSCC {1082,2709}.

Differential diagnosis

This includes neuroendocrine carcinoma, adenoid cystic carcinoma, and adenosquamous carcinoma. Neuroendocrine carcinoma typically lacks squamous differentiation, and is strongly positive for neuroendocrine markers. Adenoid cystic carcinoma, especially the solid variant, may resemble BSCC but adenoid cystic carcinoma has a myoepithelial component {132, 1337} and lacks in most instances squamous differentiaton. Furthermore, palpable metastatic cervical lymph nodes, quite common in BSCC, are very rare in adenoid cystic carcinoma {2128}. Adenocarcinoma and adenosquamous carcinoma can be distinguished from BSCC by the presence of true ductoglandular differentiation, and intracellular mucin.

Histogenesis

The suggested precursor of the BSCC is a totipotent primitive cell located in the basal cell layer of the surface epithelium, or in the proximal ducts of minor salivary glands {2128,2709}.

Prognosis and predictive factors

BSCC is an aggressive, rapidly growing tumour characterised by an advanced stage at the time of diagnosis and a poor prognosis. Metastases to the regional lymph nodes have been reported in two thirds of patients {117,1337,1997,2128}, and distant metastases involving lungs, bone, skin and brain, in 35-50% of patients {117,1337,2128}. Although controversial, it is generally believed that BSCC is more aggressive than SCC when matched stage for stage {117,736,1337,1578,2709,2787,2798}.

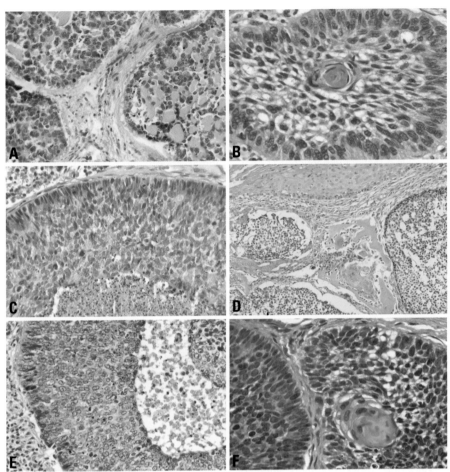

Fig. 3.16 Basaloid squamous cell carcinoma (BSCC). **A** Abundant intercellular hyaline globules conferring a cribriform-like pattern. **B** Nest of basaloid cells with peripheral palisading of the nuclei and a central keratin pearl. **C** Peripheral palisading of hyperchromatic columnar nuclei and areas of central necrosis. **D** Hyaline stromal deposits between nests of basaloid and squamous cells. **E** Central comedo-type of necrosis in a basaloid nest. **F** Peripherally palisaded nuclei with hyperchromatic nuclei in cells with high nuclear to cytoplasmic ratio. Abrupt keratinization is noted in the centre of this lobule.

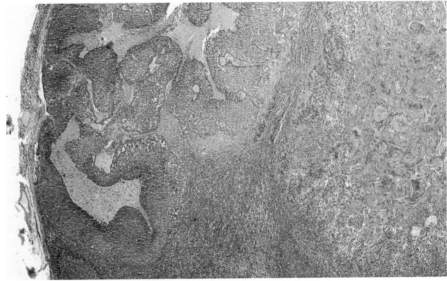

Fig. 3.17 Metastastatic basaloid squamous cell carcinoma in a regional lymph node, displaying both basaloid (left) and squamous (right) components.

Papillary squamous cell carcinoma

A. Cardesa
N. Zidar
A. Nadal
C. Ereño

Definition
Papillary squamous cell carcinoma (PSCC) is a distinct variant of SCC characterized by an exophytic, papillary growth, and a favourable prognosis.

ICD-O code   8052/3

Epidemiology
PSCC occurs predominantly in males in the 6th and 7th decades {501,743,2602}.

Etiology
Smoking and alcohol abuse are etiologic factors {501,2602}. Although HPV has been suggested as an etiologic factor, {929} reported prevalence of HPV has varied from 0-48% {171,501,2488}. Its role in the etiology of PSCC is therefore unsettled.

Localization
The larynx and the hypopharynx are among the most common sites of involvement {501,687,743,2488,2602}. Laryngeal PSCC is most often found in the supraglottis, slightly less often in the glottis, and rarely in the subglottis {131, 687,1187,2602}.

Clinical features
Hoarseness and airway obstruction are

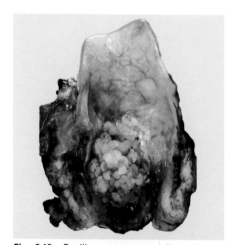

Fig. 3.18 Papillary squamous cell carcinoma (PSCC). Exuberant papillary neoplastic outgrowth in the glottic-supraglottic region.

the most common presenting symptoms. Other features include dysphagia, sore throat, cough, and haemoptysis.

Macroscopy
PSCC presents as a soft, friable, polypoid, exophytic, papillary tumour. It frequently arises from a thin stalk, but broad-based lesions have also been described.

Tumour spread and staging
Metastases to the regional lymph nodes may be present, but distant metastases are rare {743}. Lung metastases have been observed in a few patients with laryngeal PSCC {2488}.

Histopathology
The tumour is characterized by a predominant papillary growth pattern {2602}. These papillae have thin fibrovascular cores covered by neoplastic, immature basaloid cells or more pleomorphic cells. Commonly, there is minimal keratosis. Foci of necrosis and haemorrhage are frequent. Multiple PSCC or precursor lesions may occur. Stromal invasion consists of a single or multiple nests of tumour cells with dense lymphoplasmacytic inflammation at the tumour-stromal interface. If no stromal invasion is found, the lesion should be called atypical papillary hyperplasia or PSCC in-situ.

Differential diagnosis
This includes squamous papilloma, verrucous carcinoma, and exophytic SCC. Though squamous papilloma and verrucous carcinoma share similar architecture with PSCC, the latter is easily recognized by atypia of the squamous epithelium {743}. Most PSCC strongly express p53 immunohistochemically {2488}. The distinction between exophytic and papillary SCC can be difficult as the criteria for diagnosing exophytic SCC are not clearly delineated {171,2602}. In general, the papillary stalks of PSCC are much better defined than in exophytic SCC.

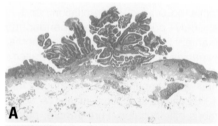

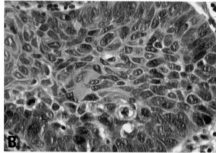

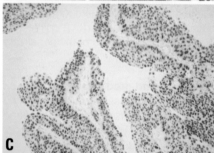

Fig. 3.19 PSCC. **A** Low power view of the tumour revealing the characteristic papillary finger-like pattern of growth. **B** Markedly pleomorphic cells showing focal intercellular bridge formation. **C** Strong nuclear immunoreactivity for p53.

Precursor lesions
PSCC may evolve from pre-existing papillary mucosal hyperplasia or squamous cell papilloma. Precursor lesions may be solitary or multiple {171,2488}.

Prognosis and predictive factors
Patients with PSCC are generally believed to have a better prognosis than those with SCC though reports in the literature are controversial {131,171,1187, 2488,2602}. The better prognosis is probably related to limited invasion.

Spindle cell carcinoma

A. Cardesa
N. Zidar

Definition

Spindle cell carcinoma (SPCC) is a biphasic tumour composed of a squamous cell carcinoma, either in-situ and/or invasive, and a malignant spindle cell component with a mesenchymal appearance, but of epithelial origin.

ICD-O code   8074/3

Synonyms

Sarcomatoid carcinoma, carcinosarcoma, collision tumour, pseudosarcoma,

Epidemiology

SPCC occurs predominantly in males in the 7th decade of life {1490,2604}.

Etiology

SPCC has been linked to cigarette smoking and alcohol consumption {1490, 2604} and may develop after radiation exposure {1482,1490,2604}.

Localization

Larynx is among the most common sites in the head and neck {204}. Less frequently it arises in the hypopharynx {62}. In the larynx, the glottis is most frequently involved {1490}.

Clinical features

Patients usually present with hoarseness, dysphagia, and/or airway obstruction {1490}.

Macroscopy

It usually exhibits a polypoid appearance of variable size. The surface is frequently ulcerated. It may rarely appear as an ulcerative infiltrative lesion.

Tumour spread and staging

SPCC metastasizes to the regional lymph nodes in up to 25% of cases; but distant dissemination is less common (5-15 %) {1420,1490,2604}.

Histopathology

The spindle cell component usually forms the bulk of the tumour, which can assume several patterns. Resemblance

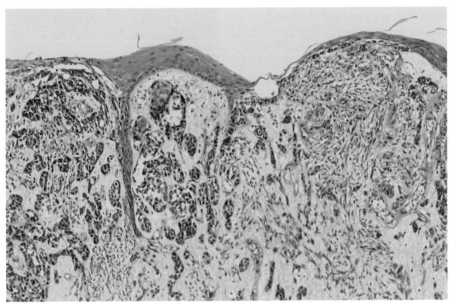

Fig. 3.20 Spindle cell carcinoma. The spindle cell component coexists with basaloid-squamous components seen to arise from the epithelial surface.

to fibrosarcoma or malignant fibrous histiocytoma is most common {1490,2604}. Occasional cases can appear less malignant and resemble a reactive fibroblastic proliferation or radiation-induced stromal atypia {62}. Foci of osteosarcomatous, chondrosarcomatous, or rhabdosarcomatous differentiation may be present, particularly in patients with previous radiotherapy (RT) {1420,1490,2604}. Evidence for squamous epithelial derivation can be seen as either in-situ carcinoma or as invasive SCC. Carcinoma-in-situ can be obscured by extensive ulceration. Infiltrating SCC may be focal, requiring multiple sections for demonstration {1482}. Sometimes, only spindle cells are present; in such cases, SPCC can be mistaken for a true sarcoma. (see below). Metastases usually contain SCC alone or both SCC and spindle cell component, and rarely, only the spindle cell component {2457,2604}.

Immunoprofile

Tumour cells can express both epithelial and mesenchymal markers {1700,2882}. Cytokeratin expression can be demonstrated in spindle cells in 40–85% of cases {671,1700,2407,2535,2610,2882}. The most useful epithelial markers are AE1AE3, CK1, CK18 and epithelial membrane antigen (EMA) {2604}. Spindle cells express vimentin and often other mesenchymal filaments, such as smooth muscle actin, muscle specific actin, and desmin.

Electron microscopy

SPCC often displays features of epithelial differentiation in spindle cells, such as desmosomes and tonofilaments {175, 1056,2535,2882}.

Differential diagnosis

The diagnosis of SPCC generally requires the demonstration of both malignant spindle cells and squamous cell carcinoma, either in-situ or invasive. When a SCC component is inconspicuous, then the spindle cells should be investigated for evidence of epithelial differentiation. However, even in the absence of SCC and negative epithelial markers, SPCC cannot be entirely ruled out. In the larynx and hypopharynx sarcomas are very rare, and SPCC is still more likely. SPCC can also be confused with reactive or benign spindle cell proliferations, such as nodular fasciitis, and inflammatory myofibroblastic sarcoma, and low-grade myofibroblastic sarcoma, and myoepithelial carcinoma.

Histogenesis

There is mounting molecular evidence that SPCC is a monoclonal epithelial neoplasm {954,2596,2620}, with a divergent (mesenchymal) differentiation {172,954, 1490,2596,2620}, rather than a collision tumour, or biphasic derivation, or "pseudosarcoma" {126}.

Prognosis and predictive factors

Favourable prognostic features are: low-stage, polypoid rather than endophytic growth, a glottic site of origin, relatively shallow depth of sarcomatoid process, and absence of prior radiation {172}. Although controversial, limited immunoreactivity for polyclonal cytokeratin has been associated with significantly improved survival rates {1944,2604}. The reported 5-year survival is between 65 and 95% {168,2604}.

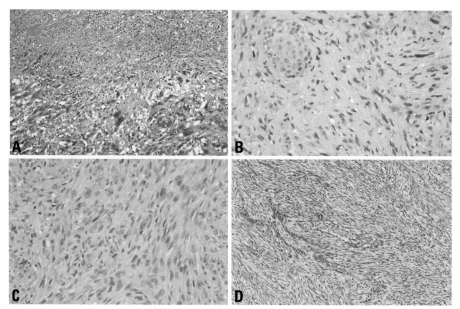

Fig. 3.21 Spindle cell carcinoma. **A** The ulcerated surface is subtended by a highly pleomorphic spindle cell population with atypical mitotic figures. **B** Transition between squamous cell carcinoma and spindle cell component. **C** Pure spindle cell component with marked cellular atypia mimicking a leiomyosarcoma. **D** Spindle cell component surrounding small nests of squamous cells mimicking synovial sarcoma.

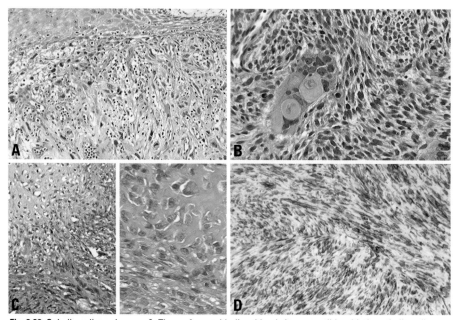

Fig. 3.22 Spindle cell carcinoma. **A** The surface epithelium blends imperceptibly with the spindle cell component. **B** Abrupt areas of squamous differentiation within a spindle cell carcinoma. **C** Metaplastic cartilage, including malignant transformation (left) and metaplastic osteoid, including malignant transformation (right) can be seen in spindle cell carcinoma. **D** Strong and diffuse immunoreactivity for keratin is seen in a majority of spindle cell carcinomas.

Acantholytic squamous cell carcinoma

A. Cardesa
N. Zidar
L. Alos

Definition
This is an uncommon histopathologic variant of squamous cell carcinoma (SCC), characterised by acantholysis of the tumour cells, creating pseudolumina and false appearance of glandular differentiation.

ICD-O code   8075/3

Synonyms
Adenoid squamous cell carcinoma, pseudoglandular SCC, SCC with gland-like features, angiosarcoma-like SCC, pseudovascular adenoid squamous cell carcinoma.

Etiology
No special etiological factor has been discovered for the mucosal acantholytic SCC {2876}.

Localization
It rarely arises in the supraglottic larynx {1079} and hypopharynx {157}, but is more frequent in sun-exposed areas of the head and neck {1847}.

Clinical features
There are no special clinical features.

Macroscopy
There are no special gross features.

Tumour spread and staging
As with SCC

Histopathology
This neoplasm is composed of SCC, but with foci of acantholysis in tumour nests, creating the appearance of glandular differentiation. The pseudolumina usually contain acantholytic and dyskeratotic cells, or cellular debris, but they may be empty {157,742}. They are more frequent in the deeper portions of the tumour. There is no evidence of true glandular differentiation or mucin production. The SCC component predominates, and is usually moderately differentiated. Clear and spindle cells may also be present. The stroma is usually desmoplastic, with a lymphoplasmacytic response {157, 742}. The acantholysis may also form anastomosing spaces and channels mimicking angiosarcoma.

Immunoprofile
Acantholytic SCC expresses epithelial markers, such as cytokeratins, and epithelial membrane antigen {742}.

Electron microscopy
The tumour cells exhibit hemidesmosomes and attached tonofilaments, and no glandular features thus supporting the squamous origin {2876}.

Differential diagnosis
Acantholytic SCC must be differentiated from adenosquamous carcinoma, adenoid cystic carcinoma, and mucoepidermoid carcinoma. This is achieved by demonstrating a lack of true gland formation, absence of myoepithelial cells and negative mucin staining. Vascular markers can be used to distinguish it from angiosarcoma. Cytokeratin, however, might be positive also in some angiosarcomas {939}.

Histogenesis
Acantholytic SCC is derived from the surface squamous epithelium.

Prognosis and predictive factors
Prognosis is similar to SCC, however some reports suggest a more aggressive behaviour {157,742,899,2876}.

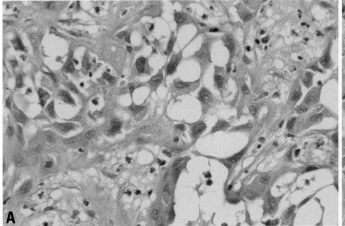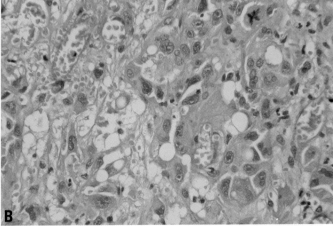

Fig. 3.23 Acantholytic squamous cell carcinoma. **A** Marked acantholysis of squamous cells giving rise to anastamosing empty spaces with pseudoglandular appearance. **B** Acantholytic channels, intermingled with dilated capillary blood vessels, mimicking angiosarcoma.

Adenosquamous carcinoma

A. Cardesa
N. Zidar
L. Alos

Definition
This rare aggressive neoplasm originates from the surface epithelium and is characterized by both squamous cell carcinoma (SCC) and true adenocarcinoma.

ICD-O code   8560/3

Epidemiology
There is a male predisposition, with a tendency to develop in the 6th and 7th decades.

Etiology
Cigarette smoking and alcohol consumption have been implicated {1294}. The role of gastroesophageal reflux has not been well established.

Localization
The larynx is the most frequent site, {15,43,831,876,1294}; the hypopharynx is occasionally involved {1646,2237}.

Clinical features
Patients present with hoarseness, sore throat, dysphagia, and/or haemoptysis {1294}.

Macroscopy
It can present as an exophytic or polypoid mass, or as a poorly defined mucosal induration, frequently with ulceration {876,1294}.

Histopathology
The main feature is both true adenocarcinoma and SCC. The two components occur in close proximity, but they tend to be distinct and separate, not intermingled as in mucoepidermoid carcinoma. The SCC component can present either as in-situ or as an invasive SCC {43}. The adenocarcinomatous component tends to occur in the deeper parts of the tumour. It consists of tubular structures that give rise to "glands within glands". Mucin production is typically present, either intraluminal or intracellular, and can appear as signet ring cells. However, mucin is not a requirement for the diagnosis in the presence of true

Table 3.2 Differential diagnosis between adenosquamous carcinoma and mucoepidermoid carcinoma of the head and neck

Adenosquamous carcinoma	Mucoepidermoid carcinoma
Squamous carcinoma in-situ	No squamous carcinoma in-situ
Origin from squamous epithelium	Origin from seromucinous ducts
Keratin pearls	Limited keratin pearls
Glands at lower invasive parts	Glands widely intermingled
No lobular arrangement	Lobular arrangement
No intermediate cells	Large, clear "Intermediate cells"

glanduloductal formation. Metastases may display both components; one usually predominates.

Immunoprofile
There is positive staining for high-molecular weight cytokeratin in both components. The glandular component expresses CEA and low MW cytokeratins: specifically, CK7 is positive, and CK20, is negative {43,1646}.

Electron microscopy
Features of both squamous and adenocarcinomatous differentiation are found {231,1190}.

DNA ploidy
A high prevalence of aneuploidy has been demonstrated {43}.

Differential diagnosis
This includes mucoepidermoid carcino-

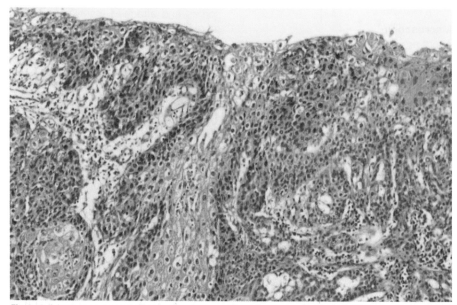

Fig. 3.24 Adenosquamous carcinoma. A squamous cell carcinoma in-situ (upper-left) appears in continuity with gland-like formations (bottom-right).

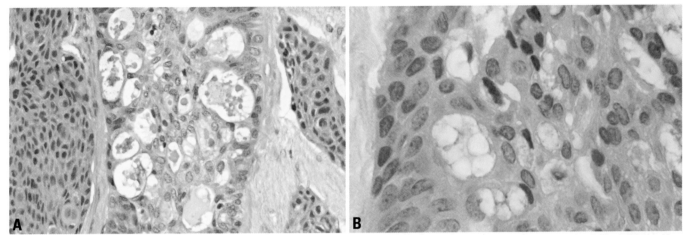

Fig. 3.25 Adenosquamous carcinoma of the larynx. **A** Blended adenocarcinoma and squamous cell carcinoma within a single tumour mass. **B** Mucin-filled epithelial cells are part of areas of squamous differentiation.

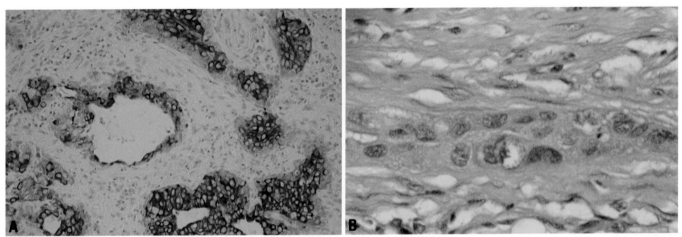

Fig. 3.26 Adenosquamous carcinoma. **A** Positive imunohistochemical reaction for CK7 in areas with glandular differentiation. **B** Mucicarmine positive secretion in the cytoplasm of a single signet ring cell showing a markedly atypical nucleus.

ma, acantholytic SCC, and SCC invading seromucinous glands, and necrotizing sialometaplasia. The most important differential diagnosis is from mucoepidermoid carcinoma as adenosquamous carcinoma has a poorer prognosis (see Table 3.02) {231}.

The presence of mucin in true glandular spaces helps to distinguish adenosquamous carcinoma from acantholytic carcinoma. SCC invading or entrapping mucoserous glands can mimic adenosquamous carcinoma, especially in biopsy specimens. In such cases, preservation of lobular gland architecture, and lack of significant atypia can distinguish SCC from adenosquamous

carcinoma. Adenosquamous carcinoma is distinguished from necrotizing sialometaplasia, a benign condition that lacks the cytological features of malignancy.

Adenosquamous carcinoma will always have a surface (mucosal) component (dysplasia, in-situ carcinoma), whereas this feature is not seen in mucoepidermoid carcinoma.

Histogenesis

Adenosquamous carcinoma originates from basal cells of surface epithelium that are capable of divergent differentiation {1844,1873,2285,2677}.

Prognosis and predictive factors

Adenosquamous carcinoma is reported as being more aggressive than SCC {876,1844,2237,2611}. Many present as high stage tumours. However, stage for stage comparison with SCC has not been well established. In a recent review, 75% of patients had regional lymph node metastases, and 25% of patients had distant metastases {1294}, most commonly to the lungs {731,1294}. The reported 5-year survival rate is 15-25% {831,876,1294}, Half of the patients die of disease after a mean of 23 months (range 12-35 months) {43}.

Lymphoepithelial carcinoma

W.Y.W. Tsang
J.K.C. Chan

Definition
Lymphoepithelial carcinoma (LEC) is an undifferentiated carcinoma with a prominent, reactive lymphoplasmacytic infiltrate, morphological indistinguishable from nasopharyngeal carcinoma.

ICD-O code   8082/3

Synonyms
Lymphoepithelioma {2317}; undifferentiated carcinoma of the nasopharyngeal type {2317}; lymphoepithelioma-like carcinoma {2741}; undifferentiated carcinoma with lymphoid stroma

Epidemiology
LEC of the larynx, hypopharynx and trachea are very rare, and account for less than 0.5% of all cancers in these sites {1722}. There is a male predominance of 4:1, and the mean age is 60 years. In contrast to nasopharyngeal carcinoma, almost all reported cases have occurred in Caucasians {621,1601}.

Etiology
Smoking and alcohol abuse are noted {621}. Epstein-Barr virus (EBV) is uncommonly demonstrated {621,1601,1637, 2741}.

Localization
They occur with equal incidence in the larynx and hypopharynx. About two-thirds of the laryngeal tumours are found in the supraglottic region {1601,1637}.

Clinical features
Patients present with hoarseness, neck mass, sore throat, cough, otalgia, dysphagia or haemoptysis.

Macroscopy
The tumour forms a mass that may show deep or superficial ulceration.

Tumour spread and staging
Many patients have cervical lymph node metastasis at presentation or early in the course. Distant metastasis (liver, lung, mediastinum, and skin) develops in about one-third of patients {1601,1637}.

Histopathology
Some LEC show a pure growth pattern, indistinguishable from LEC of other sites. (see Chapter 2 on Tumours of the Nasopharynx). In about half of the cases, there is a component of squamous cell carcinoma that accounts for 10-75% of the entire tumour {1601}. The overlying epithelium can show carcinoma-in-situ.

Prognosis and predictive factors
LEC of the larynx and hypopharynx are aggressive, with a propensity for regional lymph node and distant metastasis. A mortality rate of 30% at median follow up of 21 months has been reported {1601}.

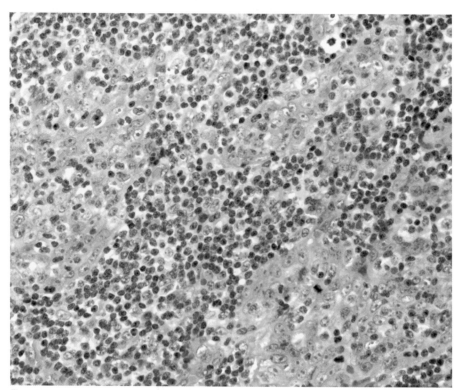

Fig. 3.27 Lymphoepithelial carcinoma. Islands of undifferentiated carcinoma cells intimately admixed with numerous small lymphocytes and plasma cells.

Giant cell carcinoma

L. Barnes
L.L.Y. Tse
J.L. Hunt

Definition
An undifferentiated carcinoma composed of many bizarre multinucleated giant cells, often containing neutrophils or cellular debris in the cytoplasm. It is similar to giant cell carcinoma of the lung {474,768,890,989,2722}.

ICD-O code
8031/3

Synonyms
Large cell carcinoma, pleomorphic carcinoma, undifferentiated carcinoma, anaplastic carcinoma.

Epidemiology
Giant cell carcinomas of the larynx are extremely rare {744}.

Etiology
Smoking and alcoholic consumption have been implicated.

Localization
The tumours have all occurred in the larynx, with no site of predilection {744}.

Clinical features
Progressive dysphonia and dyspnoea are the most common complaints.

Macroscopy
The tumours are indistinguishable from squamous cell carcinoma (SCC).

Histopathology
The hallmark is the presence of numerous, non-cohesive, bizarre giant cells that contain prominent, frequently multiple nuclei with coarse chromatin and large nucleoli. The cytoplasm is abundant, eosinophilic, sometimes vacuolated, and often contains neutrophils or cellular debris. Additionally, the tumour contains a background population of smaller anaplastic tumour cells. Giant cell carcinoma may exist in a pure or mixed form, in association with SCC, adenocarcinoma, or spindle cell carcinoma {474,768}.

Histogenesis
The histogenesis remains uncertain, and

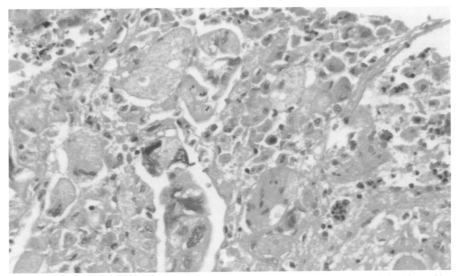

Fig. 3.28 Giant cell carcinoma. Clusters of pleomorphic giant cells in a background with admixed foamy histiocytes and inflammatory cells.

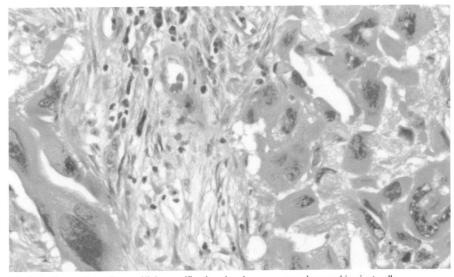

Fig. 3.29 Giant cell carcinoma. High magnification showing numerous pleomorphic giant cells.

it has been questioned whether giant cell carcinoma is a specific entity {768}.

Prognosis and predictive factors
The reported cases have shown a poor prognosis {744}.

Malignant salivary gland-type tumours

J.W. Eveson

In a large series of laryngeal tumours from one institution, 72% of salivary gland-type neoplasms were malignant {1039}. The majority were mucoepidermoid and adenoid cystic carcinomas.

ICD-O codes

Mucoepidermoid carcinoma
                8430/3
Adenoid cystic carcinoma
                8200/3

Mucoepidermoid carcinomas

Laryngeal mucoepidermoid carcinomas (MEC) are rare, only about 100 cases have been reported {1573}. They comprise one third of malignant laryngeal salivary-type tumours {1606}. They are much more common in men and most cases present between the ages of 45 and 75 years (peak incidence in the 6th decade) but cases have been reported in children {1750}. The most common site is the supraglottis {1937}. They present with progressive hoarseness and dysphagia or dysphonia. Nearly half of the cases present with, or develop, cervical lymph node metastases {217,533}.

Tumours size is variable. Microscopically they are similar to MEC elsewhere. The behaviour tends to be unpredictable. However, it is acknowledged that a significant number of tumours originally diagnosed as high-grade MEC may have been adenosquamous carcinomas that generally have a poorer prognosis.

Adenoid cystic carcinoma

Adenoid cystic carcinoma (ACC) is very uncommon in the larynx and forms only 0.07-0.25% of all laryngeal carcinomas {732,2475}, accounting for 1% of all ACC {2446}. Only 120 reported cases were identified in a literature review {642}. Most occur between the fourth and sixth decades {1039}. The majority are subglottic (60%) or supraglottic (35%) and the true cords are involved in only 6% of cases {1573}. The microscopic features and outcome of laryngeal ACC are the same as in other sites {469,1942}.

Other salivary-type tumours

A variety of other carcinomas have been reported in the seromucous glands of the larynx. However, they are very rare and

Table 3.3 Salivary gland-type neoplasms of the larynx*.

Tumour types	No of cases	%
Pleomorphic adenoma	3	5
Oncocytic tumours	12	21
Cystadenoma	1	2
Mucoepidermoid carcinoma	11	19
Adenoid cystic carcinoma	11	19
Adenosquamous carcinoma	19	33
Total	57	

*Modified from Heffner {1039}

are usually presented as single case reports: acinic cell carcinoma {734,1250, 2146,2454}, malignant myoepithelioma {1167}, carcinoma ex pleomorphic adenoma {180,232,1729,2220}, epithelial myoepithelial carcinoma {1726}, salivary duct carcinoma {745,910}, papillary adenocarcinoma {2182}, mucinous adenocarcinoma {2640} and clear cell carcinoma {1855,2020,2306}.

Neuroendocrine tumours

L. Barnes

Neuroendocrine neoplasms of the larynx are a heterogeneous group of tumours that vary from benign to highly malignant. Similar to the lung, they can be divided into several types. As a group, they are uncommon with only about 500 cases recorded in the literature as of 1998 {738}. The atypical carcinoid is the most frequent, constituting 54% of all neuroendocrine tumours in this site, followed by the small cell carcinoma, neuroendocrine type (34%), paraganglioma (9%) and the typical carcinoid (3%) {125,648,897, 2420,2816}.

Cells similar if not identical with Kultchitsky cells of the bronchi are found in the larynx. These, as well as pluripotential endobronchial stem cells, are the putative cells of origin of the typical carcinoid, atypical carcinoid, and small cell carcinoma, neuroendocrine type. Paragangliomas of the larynx are derived from paraganglia normally found in the larynx and are discussed in chapter 8.

Typical carcinoid

Definition
An epithelial tumour of low-grade malignancy composed of round to spindle cells with histologic, immunohistochemical and ultrastructural evidence of neuroendocrine differentiation.

ICD-O Code   8240/3

Synonyms
Carcinoid, mature carcinoid, well differentiated (Grade I) neuroendocrine carcinoma.

Epidemiology
The typical carcinoid (TC) is the least common of the neuroendocrine neoplasms of the larynx with only 42 cases recorded as of 2005 {2420}. It is three times more common in men and most patients are between 45-80 years of age (average 64 years) at diagnosis {738, 2419}.

Table 3.4 Classification of neuroendocrine tumours of the larynx.

Terminology	Synonyms
A. Typical carcinoid	Carcinoid, well differentiated (Grade I) neuroendocrine carcinoma
B. Atypical carcinoid[1]	Malignant carcinoid, moderately differentiated (Grade II) neuroendocrine carcinoma, large cell neuroendocrine carcinoma[1]
C. Small cell carcinoma, neuroendocrine type[2]	Small cell neuroendocrine carcinoma, poorly differentiated (Grade III) neuroendocrine carcinoma
D. Combined small cell carcinoma, neuroendocrine type, with non-small cell carcinoma (squamous cell carcinoma, adenocarcinoma,etc.)	Combined small cell carcinoma, composite small cell carcinoma
E. Paraganglioma	Non-chromaffin paraganglioma

[1]Some atypical carcinomas may fulfill the diagnostic criteria of large cell neuroendocrine carcinoma of lung
[2]Not all small cell carcinomas of the larynx will show neuroendocrine differentiation

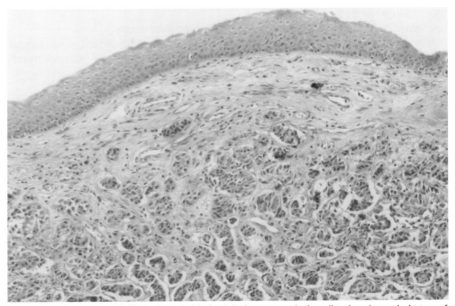

Fig. 3.30 Typical carcinoid. Typical carcinoid of epiglottis composed of small trabeculae and clusters of cells lying in the lamina propria. The overlying squamous mucosa is intact and free of atypia and/or dysplasia.

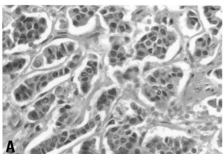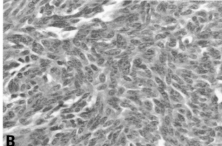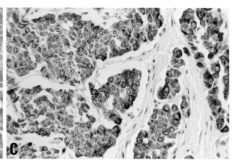

Fig. 3.31 Typical carcinoid. **A** Observe the uniform cells without nucleoli. Mitoses and necrosis are not seen. **B** Typical carcinoid with spindle cell component. The spindle cells are uniform and free of mitoses. There is no nuclear molding or necrosis. **C** The cells are strongly positive for chromogranin.

Localization

Most occur in the supraglottic larynx in the vicinity of the aryepiglottic fold, arytenoid or false vocal cord.

Clinical features

Symptoms, ranging from three weeks to four years in duration, include dysphagia, hoarseness and a sore throat. At least one patient developed the carcinoid syndrome after the tumour metastasized to the liver {738}.

Macroscopy

The tumours have ranged from 0.5 – 3.0 cm. (average 1.6 cm.) in greatest dimension and present as a submucosal or polypoid mass {738}.

Histopathology

TCs are composed of round and/or spindle cells that grow in small nests, trabeculae, large sheets, glands and/or rosettes. The cytoplasm is pink and the nuclei have finally stippled or dense chromatin. Nucleoli and mitoses are sparse to absent (less than 2 mitoses/10 HPFs). Necrosis and pleomorphism are not seen. The stroma is highly vascular and often focally fibrotic or hyalinized.

Rarely, carcinoids, either typical or atypical, may be oncocytic or oncocytoid. The distinction depends on the presence (oncocytic) or absence (oncocytoid) of mitochondria on ultrastructural examination. A few may contain mucin and, exceptionally, even amyloid.

Immunohistochemistry

TCs are positive for cytokeratin, epithelial membrane antigen (EMA), carcinoembryonic antigen (CEA), synaptophysin, chromogranin, neuron specific enolase (NSE), and protein gene product 9.5. They are also variably positive for a variety of peptides, including serotonin, calcitonin, bombesin and somatostatin.

Electron microscopy

TCs contain abundant membrane-bound, electron-dense neurosecretory granules varying in size from 90-230 nm {2762}. Cellular junctional complexes are observed as well as numerous mitochondria if the TC is of the oncocytic type.

Differential diagnosis

See under atypical carcinoid.

Prognosis and Predictive factors

Since radiation and chemotherapy are ineffective, surgery is the treatment of choice. The extent of resection should be as conservative as possible, as long as complete removal is achieved. A neck dissection is not warranted.

Although the series is small, data indicate that 33% of patients with TCs of the larynx have experienced distant metastases (liver, bones) {648,2419}. At least one patient developed the carcinoid syndrome and another died of disease five years after treatment. While this suggests that TCs of the larynx may be more aggressive than those of the lung, some of these tumours on critical review are probably best classified as atypical carcinoids.

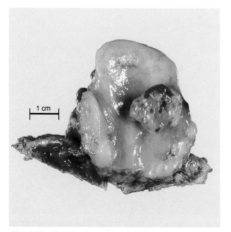

Fig. 3.32 Atypical carcinoid, polypoid and focally haemorrhagic, arising from the epiglottis.

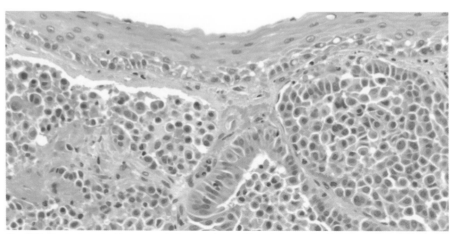

Fig. 3.33 Atypical carcinoid composed of trabeculae and broad sheets of cells. The cells are larger and more pleomorphic than those seen in a typical carcinoid.

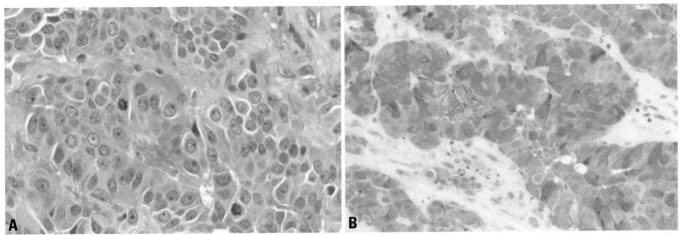

Fig. 3.34 Atypical carcinoid. **A** Same case as shown in Figure 3.33. Higher magnification shows large cells with prominent nucleoli and mitoses. **B** Tumour cells are strongly positive for calcitonin.

Atypical carcinoid

Definition
An epithelial tumour composed of round to spindle cells with histologic, immuno-histochemical and ultrastructural evidence of neuroendocrine differentiation exhibiting more mitoses and cellular atypia than a typical carcinoid.

ICD-O code   8249/3

Synonyms
Malignant carcinoid, moderately differentiated (Grade II) neuroendocrine carcinoma, large cell neuroendocrine carcinoma.

Epidemiology
The atypical carcinoid (AC) is 15 times more common than the TC and is the most frequent neuroendocrine neoplasm of the larynx. It is 2-3 times more common in men and has been described in patients from 36-83 years of age (average 61 years) {2769,2816}. Most are heavy smokers.

Localization
Over 90% arise in the supraglottic larynx in the vicinity of the aryepiglottic fold, arytenoid or false vocal cord.

Clinical features
Hoarseness, dysphagia, pain in the throat and a neck mass are the usual symptoms. An associated paraneoplastic syndrome is exceptional.

Macroscopy
The tumours present as a tan, gray, pink or haemorrhagic submucosal or poly-poid mass 0.2 – 4.0 cm. in greatest dimension (average 1.6 cm) {2769, 2816}.

Histopathology
ACs are infiltrative tumours that grow in a variety of patterns, including small nests, sheets, trabeculae, glands and/or a combination of these patterns. Cysts with intracystic papillary-like projections of tumour cells may also be seen. In contrast to TCs, the cells are larger and the nuclei are often vesicular and contain prominent nucleoli. Mitoses (usually 2-10/10 HPFs) necrosis, cellular pleomorphism and angiolymphatic invasion are common. Some tumours may even fulfill the diagnostic criteria of large cell neuroendocrine carcinoma of the lung (10 or more mitoses per 10 high power fields and prominent necrosis). Mucinous changes, amyloid, spindle cells and oncocytic-oncocytoid cells may also be observed.

Immunohistochemistry
The tumours may stain for synaptophysin (100%), cytokeratin (96%), chromogranin A (94%), calcitonin (80%), CEA (75%), somatostatin (50%), serotonin (21%), and adrenocorticotrophic hormone (17%) {2816}.

Electron microscopy
Membrane-bound, electron-dense neurosecretory granules ranging from 70-420 nm are prominent {2769}. Cellular junctional complexes, rough endoplasmic reticulum, mitochondria, Golgi complexes and infrequent bundles of tonofilaments may also be seen.

Differential diagnosis
AC may be confused for a TC, paraganglioma, malignant melanoma, and medullary thyroid carcinoma. The AC is distinguished from the TC by the presence of larger cells, prominence of nucleoli, mitoses, necrosis, pleomorphism and angiolymphatic invasion. AC is positive for cytokeratin, CEA and calcitonin, whereas the paraganglioma is negative for these markers. Malignant melanoma is positive for HMB-45 and tyrosinase and negative for synaptophysin and cytokeratin. Separating AC from metastatic medullary thyroid carcinoma (MTC) may be more problematic since both tumours are positive for synaptophysin, calcitonin and CEA. Clinical and imaging studies to detect the presence or absence of a mass in the larynx or thyroid may offer some assistance. Although the serum calcitonin level is almost invariably elevated in metastatic MTC and usually negative in AC, rare cases of laryngeal AC associated with elevated levels of serum calcitonin have been reported {2409}. Reliance on this test to distinguish between these two tumours is, therefore, not absolute. Knowledge of the serum CEA level (especially if markedly elevated), however, may be helpful. This test is almost universally elevated in MTC, but thus far, has not been reported in association with AC. More recently, thyroid transcription factor – 1 (TTF) has been useful in separating these two tumours. MTC is strongly and diffusely positive for this marker while the AC is typically negative or only focally, weakly positive.

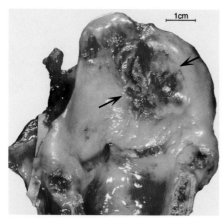

Fig. 3.35 Small cell carcinoma, neuroendocrine type, involving the epiglottis. The tumour (arrows) is ulcerated and indistinguishable from a squamous cell carcinoma From L. Barnes et al. {131}, with permission from Marcel Dekker, Inc. New York.

Prognosis and Predictive factors
ACs are aggressive tumours, with 5- and 10-year accumulative survival rates of 48% and 30%, respectively. Metastases to cervical lymph nodes have observed in 43% of patients, to skin and subcutaneous tissues in 22%, and to other distant sites in 44% (particularly lungs, liver, and bones {2816}.

Similar to TCs, ACs are usually resistant to radiation and chemotherapy. Surgery is preferred and, depending on the site of the tumour, requires a partial or total laryngectomy. Because of the high incidence of cervical lymph node metastasis, a neck dissection, even when the lymph nodes are clinically negative, is warranted {752}.

Factors adversely affecting prognosis include metastatic disease at presentation, positive tumour margins, angiolymphatic invasion, and tumours larger than one centimeter {2769,2816}. Determination of DNA ploidy has no prognostic significance {1097}.

Small cell carcinoma, neuroendocrine type

Definition
A highly malignant epithelial tumour composed of small round, oval or spindle cells with evidence of neuroendocrine differentiation.

Synonyms
Small cell carcinoma, small cell neuroendocrine carcinoma, poorly differentiated (Grade III) neuroendocrine carcinoma, oat cell carcinoma, anaplastic small cell carcinoma, small cell neuroendocrine carcinoma of intermediate type.

ICD-O Code   8041/3

Epidemiology
Although the second most common neuroendocrine tumour of the larynx, small cell carcinoma, neuroendocrine type (SCCNET), is still an unusual neoplasm accounting for only 0.5% of all laryngeal carcinomas. It is three times more common in men and is distinctly unusual in patients below 40 years of age {897}. Most are heavy smokers.

Localization
Although the tumour may arise in any

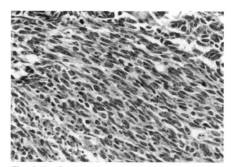

Fig. 3.37 Small cell carcinoma, neuroendocrine type. High magnification showing small spindle cells with hyperchromatic nuclei devoid of nucleoli. Note the nuclear molding and small foci of necrosis - apoptosis.

region of the larynx, the supraglottis is, by far, the most common site.

Clinical features
Symptoms and signs are those associated with other laryngeal neoplasms and depend on the site of origin. Hoarseness and dysphagia are the usual complaints. Almost half of patients have cervical lymph node metastases at presentation. Exceptionally the tumour may be associated with a paraneoplastic syndrome. Among these include Cushing, Eaton-Lambert, and Schwartz-Bartter syndromes {752}.

Macroscopy
The tumours often present as ulcerated submucosal lesions and, as a consequence, may be indistinguishable from ordinary squamous cell carcinoma.

Histopathology
The tumour is composed of sheets or rib-

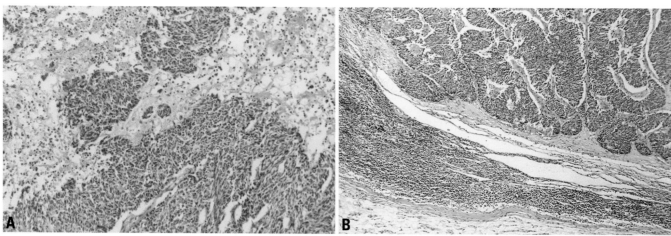

Fig. 3.36 Small cell carcinoma, neuroendocrine type. **A** Low magnification. Note the necrosis. **B** Small cell carcinoma, neuroendocrine type with lymph node metastases.

bons of closely packed cells with inconspicuous cytoplasm and round, oval and/or spindle nuclei with dense chromatin and absent nucleoli. Mitoses, necrosis, apoptosis, and lymphatic, vascular, and perineural invasion are common as well as nuclear molding and DNA-coating of the walls of blood vessels. Rare rosettes may be seen. The mucosa is often ulcerated but the marginal epithelium is free of dysplasia. Exceptionally, SCCNET may be associated with a squamous or adenocarcinoma (see "Combined carcinoma" below).

Immunophenotype
The immunoprofile is essentially similar to that of the TC and AC. Some may also express thyroid transcription factor – 1.

Ultrastructure
Membrane-bound, electron-dense neurosecretory granules ranging from 50-200 nm are scant compared to the TC and AC {2762}.

Differential diagnosis
The differential diagnosis includes TC, AC, basaloid squamous cell carcinoma, malignant lymphoma, and a metastasis from a primary SCCNET of the lung. Compared to TC and AC, SCCNET is composed primarily of short spindle cells without nucleoli and exhibits more nuclear molding, necrosis and mitotic activity. In addition, SCCNET may be positive for thyroid transcription factor – 1 while the AC is usually negative {1097}. Basaloid squamous cell carcinoma

(BSCC) is a biphasic tumour composed of basal and squamous cell components that characteristically grow in a lobular pattern with central comedonecrosis. In addition, BSCCs often exhibit prominent nucleoli, cyst-like areas and hyalinosis and are negative for neuroendocrine markers and TTF. Malignant lymphomas are positive for leukocyte common antigen and negative for neuroendocrine markers. A metastasis from a primary SCCNET of the lung is based primarily on negative imaging studies of the lung.

Prognosis and predictive factors
SCCNET is an aggressive tumour with early regional and distant metastasis. Almost half of patients will present with positive cervical lymph nodes and about 60-90% will develop distant metastases, especially to the lungs, liver and bones. The 2- and 5-year survival rates are 16% and 5%, respectively {897}. Because many patients have disseminated disease at the time of diagnosis, radical surgery (laryngectomy with neck dissection) is rarely indicated. Instead a therapeutic protocol using a combination of local radiation and chemotherapy, similar to that for pulmonary SCCNET, is advocated.

Combined small cell carcinoma, neuroendocrine type

Small cell carcinoma, neuroendocrine type (SCCNET) associated with a squamous or adenocarcinomatous compo-

nent are referred to as combined or composite carcinomas. They are unusual, representing less than 10% of all SCCNETs of the larynx. Only 14 cases have been described as of 2004. Most, if not all, have been associated with a squamous cell carcinoma, either in-situ or invasive {1201}. Treatment and prognosis is otherwise similar to that of a "pure" SCCNET.

Epithelial precursor lesions

N. Gale
B.Z. Pilch
D. Sidransky
W.H. Westra
J. Califano

Definition

Precursor lesions are defined as altered epithelium with an increased likelihood for progression to squamous cell carcinoma (SCC). The altered epithelium shows a variety of cytological and architectural changes that have traditionally been grouped under the term dysplasia. However, other classifications, e.g. squamous intraepithelial neoplasia (SIN) and squamous intraepithelial lesions (SIL, Ljubljana classification) have also proven to be useful {222,504,846,1054, 1055,1253,1254,1711,2317}. Rarely, malignant transformation can develop even from morphologically normal epithelium. Atypia is not considered synonymous with dysplasia. Atypia has been used in the context of inflammatory and regenerative changes particularly referring to cytologic features. In this text, the term atypia refers to cytological change that may or may not be pre-malignant. Various classifications have evolved to describe the spectrum of histological changes in relation to their malignant potential {222,504,846,1054,1055,1253, 1254,1711,2317}.

Epidemiology

The entire spectrum of laryngeal and hypopharyngeal precursor lesions are mostly seen in the adult population and affect men more often than women. This gender disparity is especially pronounced after the sixth decade {245}. Mean ages for the first precursor lesion diagnosis are reported from 48.0-56.5 years {243,1253}. The incidence varies worldwide with the magnitude and manner of carcinogen exposure.

Etiology

Precursor lesions are strongly associated with tobacco smoking and alcohol abuse, and especially a combination of these two {221,566,766,1607,1608, 1800,2564}. The risk of developing these lesions increases with duration of smoking, the type of tobacco and the practice of deep inhalation.
Additional etiological factors are: indus-

Table 3.5 Classification schemas that histologically categorize precursor and related lesions

2005 WHO Classification	Squamous Intraepithelial Neoplasia (SIN)	Ljubljana Classification Squamous Intraepithelial Lesions (SIL)
Squamous cell hyperplasia		Squamous cell (simple) hyperplasia
Mild dysplasia	SIN 1	Basal/parabasal cell hyperplasia*
Moderate dysplasia	SIN 2	Atypical hyperplasia**
Severe dysplasia	SIN 3***	Atypical hyperplasia**
Carcinoma in-situ	SIN 3***	Carcinoma in-situ

* Basal/parabasal cell hyperplasia may histologically resemble mild dysplasia, but the former is conceptually benign lesion and the latter the lower grade of precursor lesions.
** 'Risky epithelium'. The analogy to moderate and severe dysplasia is approximate.
*** The advocates of SIN combine severe dysplasia and carcinoma in-situ.

trial pollution, specific occupational exposures, nutritional deficiency, and hormonal disturbance {766,1253,1255, 1256,1608,1982}.
The role of human papillomavirus (HPV) infection in laryngeal carcinogenesis remains unsolved {2412}. The prevalence of HPV in laryngeal carcinoma varies significantly among various studies, ranging from 0% to 54.1% {2517}. Although the overall prevalence of HPV infection found in 9 studies of precursor lesions {97,276,793,853,927,928,1522, 2065,2172} was 12.4%, HPV DNA was detected in a clinically and histologically normal larynx in 12-25% of individuals {1912,2172}. Thus, definite evidence of an etiologic role of HPV in precursor lesions, at least at present, is lacking, and HPV infection in precursor lesions may represent an incidental HPV colonization rather than true infection of the laryngeal mucosa.

Localization

Precursor lesions appear mainly along the true vocal cords. Two thirds of vocal cord lesions are bilateral {243}. They can extend over the free edge of the vocal cord to the subglottic surface. An origin in, or extension along the upper surface

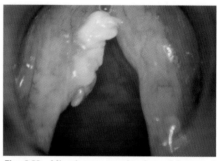

Fig. 3.38 Microlaryngoscopic view of laryngeal leukoplakia. Both vocal cords are moderately thickened; an exophytic, well-circumscribed, white plaque is seen in the left vocal cord.

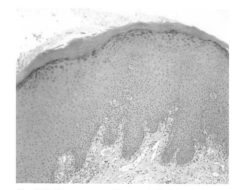

Fig. 3.39 Squamous cell hyperplasia (simple hyperplasia). There is an increased number of ordinary-arranged, otherwise normal cells in the spinous layer. A keratin layer is present on the surface.

of the vocal cord is less common {1253,1332}. The commissures are rarely involved {243}. Hypopharyngeal precursor lesions are rarely identified as the common presentation is established malignancy {2661}. No good data exist regarding tracheal precursor lesions.

Clinical features

Most patients with precursor lesions give a history of a few months or more of symptoms, but may be asymptomatic {243}. Symptoms depend on the location and severity of the disease and include fluctuating hoarseness, throat irritation, sore throat, and/or chronic cough. Precursor lesions can be either sharply circumscribed and grow exophytically, or be predominantly flat and diffuse, related in part to the amount of keratin present.

Macroscopy

Precursor lesions have a clinically diverse appearance, variously described as leukoplakia (white patch), chronic hyperplastic laryngitis or rarely erythroplasia/erythroplakia (red patch). A circumscribed thickening of the mucosa covered by whitish patches, or an irregularly growing, well-defined warty plaque may be seen. A speckled appearance of lesions can also be present, caused by unequal thickness of the keratin layer. However, the lesions are commonly more diffuse, with a thickened appearance, occupying a large part of one or both vocal cords. Their surface is rough, may be muddy brown to red (erythroplasia),

Table 3.6 Criteria used for diagnosing dysplasia

Architecture	Cytology
Irregular epithelial stratification	Abnormal variation in nuclear size (anisonucleosis)
Loss of polarity of basal cells	Abnormal variation in nuclear shape (nuclear pleomorphism)
Drop-shaped rete ridges	Abnormal variation in cell size (anisocytosis)
Increased number of mitotic figures	Abnormal variation in cell shape (cellular pleomorphism)
Abnormal superficial mitoses	Increased nuclear-cytoplasmic ratio
Premature keratinization in single cells (dyskeratosis)	Increased nuclear size
Keratin pearls within rete pegs	Atypical mitotic figures
	Increased number and size of nucleoli
	Hyperchromasia

perhaps with increased visible vascularity, or coated with diffuse or dispersed circumscribed whitish plaques (speckled leukoplakia) {1253,1332}. Few white patches are ulcerated (6.5%) or combined with erythroplasia (15%) {243}. Leukoplakia, in contrast to erythroplasia, tends to be well demarcated. In general, leukoplakia has a lower risk of malignant transformation than mixed white and red lesions, or speckled leukoplakia, which has an intermediate risk, and pure erythroplasia which has the highest risk of cancer development {2759}. However, no one clinical appearance is reliably diagnostic of any histologic grade of precursor lesion. Occasionally precursor lesions may appear clinically normal.

Histopathology

The epithelium of all precursor lesions is

generally thickened. However, in a minority of cases patchy atrophy, thinning of the viable cellular layers, may be present. By definition there is no evidence of invasion. The magnitude of surface keratinization is of no importance.

Allocation to categories within each of the classifications requires consideration firstly of architectural features and then of cytology.

1. Hyperplasia

Definition: Hyperplasia describes increased cell numbers. This may be in the spinous layer (acanthosis) and/or in the basal/parabasal cell layers (progenitor compartment), termed basal cell hyperplasia.

The architecture shows regular stratification and there is no cellular atypia.

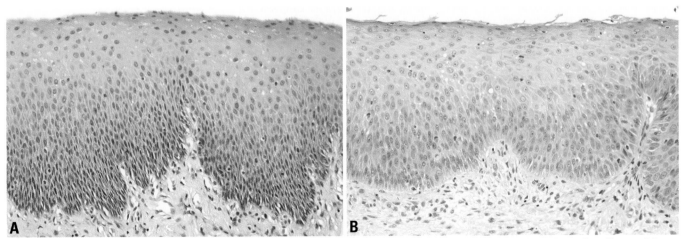

Fig. 3.40 Mild dysplasia (basal-parabasal cell hyperplasia, SIN1). **A** Note the increased number of basal-parabasal cells with hyperchromatic, uniform nuclei, perpendicularly oriented to the basement membrane. The upper part of the epithelium shows a regular spinous layer and thin parakeratotic layer on the surface. **B** Increased number of uniform, slightly enlarged basal and parabasal cells, perpendicularly oriented to the basement membrane. Increased number of regular mitoses are evident. At the right corner (lower half) the epithelial cells show minimal cytologic atypia. The upper half of the epithelium is composed of regular spinous cells, which become flattened toward the surface. A thin parakeratotic layer is present on the surface.

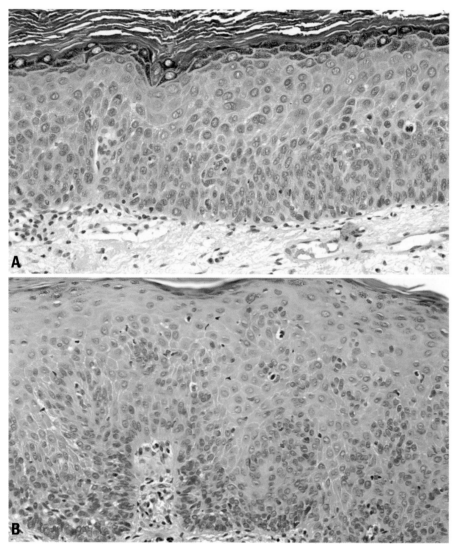

Fig. 3.41 Moderate dysplasia (atypical hyperplasia, SIN 2). **A** The epithelium is slightly thickened. More than half of the epithelium is occupied by increased number of slightly to moderately polymorphic epithelial cells with hyperchromatic nuclei and increased mitotic activity. The upper third shows spinous cell differentiation; prominent granular and keratotic layer is evident on the surface. **B** Hyperplastic epithelium with increased number of slightly to moderately polymorphic epithelial cells extending up to two thirds of the epithelium. A thin parakeratotic and keratotic layer is present on the surface.

2. Dysplasia (intraepithelial neoplasia, atypical epithelial hyperplasia potentially malignant lesions)

Definition: When architectural disturbance is accompanied by cytologic atypia the term dysplasia applies.

There is a challenge in the recognition of the earliest manifestations of dysplasia, and no single combination of the above features allows for consistent distinction between hyperplasia and the earliest stages of dysplasia as well as in attempting to rigidly divide the spectrum of dysplasias into mild, moderate and severe categories.

Mild dysplasia

In general architectural disturbance limited to the lower third of the epithelium accompanied by cytological atypia define the minimum criteria of dysplasia.

Moderate dysplasia

Architectural disturbance extending into the middle third of the epithelium is the initial criterion for recognizing this category. However, consideration of the degree of cytologic atypia may require upgrading.

Severe dysplasia

Recognition of severe dysplasia starts with greater than two thirds of the epithelium showing architectural disturbance with associated cytologic atypia. However, as noted in the previous paragraph, architectural disturbance extending into the middle third of the epithelium with sufficient cytologic atypia may be upgraded from moderate to severe dysplasia.

Carcinoma in-situ

The theoretical concept of carcinoma in-situ is that malignant transformation has occurred but invasion is not present. It is not always possible to recognize this morphologically. The following is recommended for the diagnosis of carcinoma in-situ: full thickness or almost full thickness architectural abnormalities in the viable cellular layers accompanied by pronounced cytologic atypia. Atypical mitotic figures and abnormal superficial mitoses are commonly seen in carcinoma in-situ.

Differential diagnosis

Reactive, regenerative or reparative squamous epithelium (for example in response to trauma, inflammation, irradiation or ulceration) may manifest atypical cytology or architectural disturbance. Nutritional deficiencies such as iron, folate, and vitamin B12, can also simulate dysplasia. Such lesions are not considered precursor lesions and should be distinguished from them. Clinical history is helpful, and morphologic changes suggestive of the inciting event (e.g. ulceration, inflammation, haemorrhage, radiation-induced mesenchymal and/or endothelial nuclear enlargement and hyperchromasia) may be present. The epithelial changes in these cases are generally less pronounced than in severe dysplasia/atypical hyperplasia or CIS, atypical mitoses are almost never present, and the epithelium may be thinned, or, if thickened, stratification and maturation often develop as the regenerative/reparative process matures.

Somatic genetics

In studies addressing the genetic changes underlying pre-malignant lesions of the head and neck, the larynx and hypopharynx are often dealt with in a broader anatomic context including the oral cavity. True to current models of carcinogenesis, malignant transformation of the mucosa lining the larynx and other

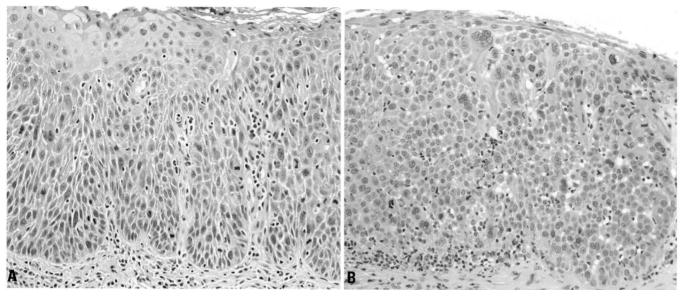

Fig. 3.42 Severe dysplasia (SIN 3, atypical hyperplasia). **A** The atypical epithelial cells occupy two thirds of the epithelial thickness. Note partially preserved epithelial stratification, expressed cytologic atypia and increased mitotic activity. Keratin layer is present on the surface. **B** Carcinoma in-situ (SIN 3). Prominent architectural disarray, marked cytologic atypia and increased mitotic figures with pathologic forms.

regions of the head and neck is fundamentally a genetic process that involves activation of key oncogenes and inactivation of critical tumour suppressor genes. These genetic alterations generally occur in order of progression, however, it is fundamentally the net accumulation of multiple genetic alterations that dictates the frequency and pace of progression to invasive carcinoma {318, 319}. Genetic progression does not imply a uniform orderly progression through various stages of histologic progression. By some estimates, progression from normal mucosa to invasive squamous cell carcinoma requires as many as ten independent genetic events {2156}.

Loss of heterozygosity studies indicate that the earliest alterations appear to target specific genes located on chromosomes 3p, 9p21, and 17p13 {318}. These alterations, particularly LOH at 9p21, may precede histopathologic evidence of dysplasia {317,2667}. Hyperplasia without any histologic evidence of dysplasia has been found to represent clonal populations of cells sharing the same genetic alterations found in SCC. Alterations that tend to occur in association with higher grades of dysplasia and SCC can include cyclin D1 amplification, pTEN inactivation, and LOH at 13q21, 14q32, 6p, 8, 4q27 and 10q23 {318,787}. Advanced precursor lesions of the head and neck demonstrate a spectrum of genetic alterations that is qualitatively

and quantitatively similar to SCC {230, 294,2436}.

For some of the chromosomal regions commonly lost or amplified in precursor lesions of the head and neck, the targeted genes have been identified. Two tumour suppressor genes residing at 9p21: p16 (CDKN2/MTS1) inhibit cell cycling via the Rb pathway, and p14(ARF) inhibits cell cycling via the p53 pathway {1022}. The p53 tumour suppressor gene resides at chromosome 17p13. p53 is involved in several cellular regulatory pathways including DNA repair, cell cycle control, and apoptosis {1115}. The cyclin D1 oncogene resides on chromosome 11q13 and is amplified in about a third of SCC {321,811}. However, for most regions of common chromosomal loss such as loss at chromosome 3p, the targeted gene(s) have not yet been well characterized.

Retrospective studies examining the prognostic value of molecular markers, including LOH of chromosomes 3p, 9p21, and 17q13 as well as general aneuploidy, have demonstrated that genetic alterations confer significant risk of malignant progression of precursor lesions. These precursor lesions included clinically defined leukoplakia, with corresponding histologic diagnoses varying along the spectrum of benign to precursor lesions mentioned above. In some cases, retrospective genetic analysis was able to define risk of malignant

progression in hyperplastic lesions {1627,2201,2492}.

Prognosis and predictive factors
Some precursor lesions are self-limiting and reversible, others persist and some progress to SCC {503}. The histopathologic degree of severity of these lesions can be a predictive factor {222,846, 1054,1689}. Simple and basal/parabasal cell hyperplasias have a minimal likelihood of malignant progression (0.9%). These patients do not require close clinical follow-up. Lesions classified as atypical hyperplasia (moderate to severe dysplasia) have a 11% rate of malignant transformation {1054}. Diagnosis of precursor lesions implies a need for close follow-up and complete excision depending on the clinical situation {846,1054}. Patients with carcinoma in-situ require more extensive management, depending on the clinical circumstance {504,1253, 1808,2151,2432}.

Papilloma / papillomatosis

N. Gale

Definition
Squamous cell papillomas are the most common benign epithelial tumours of the larynx, caused by HPV infection. The tumours can be multiple and often recur.

ICD-O codes
Papilloma	8050/0
Papillomatosis	8060/0

Synonyms
Recurrent respiratory papillomatosis (RRP), laryngeal papillomatosis, juvenile papillomatosis, adult papillomatosis.

Epidemiology
They rarely appear as solitary lesions, more frequently, especially in children, as recurrent respiratory papillomatosis (RRP). It is characterized by multiple contiguous lesions with great propensity for local recurrences. There is a bimodal age of distribution; the first peak is before the age of 5 (juvenile form), with no gender predominance. The second peak occurs between the ages of 20-40 years (adult form) with a 3:2 male predominance {178,586,618,1282,1519}. Its true incidence and prevalence are uncertain. A wide range in incidence, 0.4-4.3 /100,000, has been recorded for various regions worldwide {73,585,1253,1520}.

Etiology
HPV-6 and 11 are the most frequent genotypes associated with RRP as well as solitary papillomas {10,848,1484, 1788,2074,2101,2411}. Rarely, HPV 16,

18, 31, 33, 35 and 39 have been identified in RRP {389,2004,2074,2173,2461}. The mode of HPV infection in children is perinatal vertical transmission related to maternal genital infection {178,586, 2311}. An epidemiological triad has been identified: the first-born child, vaginal delivery and teen-aged mother correlating with juvenile RRP {1282}. Caesarean delivery has not been found to be entirely protective against the disease {2357}. Factors that influence the conversion of HPV exposure to active HPV infection resulting in epithelial proliferation are not known {944}. The mode of HPV infection in adults remains unclear. The reactivation of a latent infection acquired perinatally or adult acquired infection with orogenital contacts have been suggested {10,1281}.

Localization
The disease almost invariably involves the larynx, especially true and false vocal cords, subglottic areas and ventricles {10,126}. Papillomas may spread to other laryngeal sites; the most frequent sites of extralaryngeal spread are the oral cavity, followed by trachea and bronchi. Extralaryngeal extension of RRP has been identified in 30% of children and in 16% of adult patients {240}. Endobronchial and pulmonary dissemination occurs in 5% of patients with RPP {585}. Rare cases of isolated tracheal lesions without laryngeal involvement have been reported {2662}. The distribution of RRP follows a predictable pattern,

occurring mainly at anatomic sites in which ciliated and squamous epithelia are juxtaposed. An injury of ciliated mucosa after surgical procedures may result in squamous metaplasia creating an iatrogenic squamous-ciliary junction, thereby inducing a new background for additional tumours {1280}.

Clinical features
Squamous papillomas have been traditionally divided into juvenile and adult groups {586,1282,1519,2579} and additionally into multiple or solitary groups {1519,1524}. Although caused by the same viruses, they follow distinctly diverse and variable clinical courses. For children, extensive growth with rapid recurrences is characteristic. In some patients, RRP becomes indolent as the patient reaches adulthood. Disease progression is more frequent in the juvenile form, usually associated with subglottic papillomas and prior tracheotomy {2743}. Tracheobronchial extension of RRP is associated with morbidities such as pneumatocoeles, lung abscesses, tracheal stenosis and rarely malignant transformation {219}. The relatively small airway in children predisposes to airway obstruction. The clinical course in adults is usually not so dramatic, the development of respiratory distress and other complications are rare, although RRP can be aggressive with multiple recurrences {240,2074}.

Signs and symptoms
Adult laryngeal papillomas cause hoarseness {240,1253}. The disease is usually self-limiting.
Most children with laryngeal RRP present with dysphonia and stridor, less commonly with chronic cough, recurrent pneumonia, dyspnoea, and acute life-threatening events {178,240,587}. Delay, due to mistaken diagnoses, such as bronchitis, asthma, and other allergic manifestations, may lead to gradual respiratory distress and urgent tracheotomy, which is associated with more frequent extension into the tracheobronchial tree. The overall mortality rate of patients with

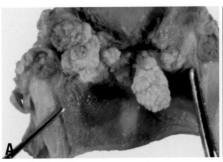
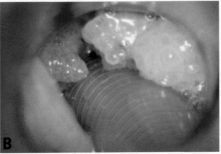

Fig. 3.43 Laryngeal papillomatosis. **A** Recurrent respiratory papillomatosis fills the endolaryngeal space. **B** Multilobulated grape like clusters of papillomas are located on the right side and anterior commissure of the larynx. (Endoscopic view)

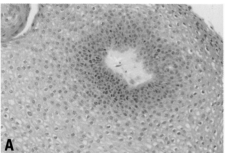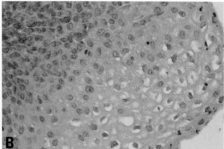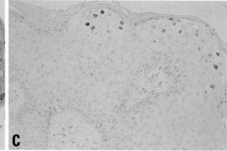

Fig. 3.44 Squamous papillomas of the larynx. **A** Higher magnification of a papillary branch. **B** Pronounced koilocytosis is evident in the upper part of the squamous epithelium. **C** Positive in-situ hybridization signal for HPV genotypes 6 and 11 in the upper part of the squamous epithelium.

RRP ranges from 4-14 % {126}, often due to asphyxia, infection, pulmonary complications, and malignant transformation {109,126,2437}.

Macroscopy
They are exophytic, branching, pedunculated or sessile masses, pink or red, with finely lobulated surface, disposed to bleeding with minor trauma, presenting either singly or in clusters.

Histopathology
Squamous papillomas are composed of finger-like or frond-like projections of squamous mucosa, containing thin fibrovascular cores. Secondary or tertiary branching of papillae may be present. Keratosis is minimal. Frequently, parabasal cell hyperplasia, usually extending up to the mid-portion with a perpendicular orientation of the cells to the basement membrane, is seen. Mitotic features may be prominent within this area. Koilocytosis is occasionally evident {2066}. Premature and abnormal keratinizing individual cells (dyskeratosis) if present, contributes to a disorganized appearance. Premalignant changes are not commonly observed, and should be reported when present {1253}.

Differential diagnosis
Adult papillary keratosis reveals keratotic, hyperplastic squamous epithelium with keratohyaline granules, occasionally atypia, and absence of koilocytes {126}. Verrucous carcinoma exhibits thicker squamous fronds with prominent keratosis, bulbous rete pegs, that infiltrate in a blunt, pushing manner. Papillary squamous carcinoma usually presents an architecture similar to RRP, but is cytologically malignant. Laryngeal verruca vulgaris is extremely rare, and shows the same features as in the skin {138}.

Histogenesis
RRP mainly originates from the squamous epithelium where ciliated and squamous epithelia are juxtaposed {1280}. HPV enters the basal cells through a microtraumatized squamous epithelium. Viral replication occurs in the spinous layer, causing a disturbance of epithelial maturation {2917}.

Prognosis and predictive factors
Clinical criteria
The clinical course of RRP is unpredictable, characterised by periods of active disease and remissions. The presence of HPV in apparently normal mucosa is thought to be a virus reservoir and the source of repeated recurrences {2171,2411}. RRP in the neonatal period is associated with poor prognosis, with a greater need for tracheotomy and likelihood of mortality {587}.

Histopathological criteria
Significant histological prognosticators of local recurrences and malignant transformation have not been identified {501, 908,2100}.

DNA ploidy, proliferation
DNA aneuploidy and Ki-67 proliferative

index, in contrast to histologic indices, have been found to predict disease recurrence and extension for children with RRP {2470,2471}.

HPV genotype
HPV 11 and 16 are associated with more aggressive disease, with frequent recurrence and progression in children and adults {2074,2110,2174}.

Malignant transformation
Malignant change is not common, but occurs in the setting of smoking, irradiation, or other promoters {2112}. It is an exceptional event in the absence of predisposing factors {196,959,2144,2356}. The overall incidence of cancer development for irradiated patients is 14% and 2% for the non-irradiated {126}. Malignancies occur preferentially in the tracheobronchial tree in children, and in the larynx in adults {944}. Prognosis in children is poor {2422}. HPV 11 is most frequently associated with malignant transformation of RRP {487,1465,1521, 2112}, followed by HPV 16 {619} and HPV 18 {2226}.

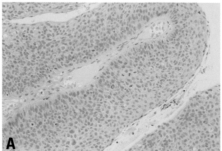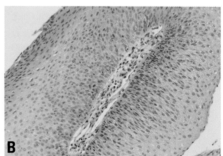

Fig. 3.45 Branch of a laryngeal squamous papilloma. **A** Note atypical hyperplasia of the covering epithelium. **B** Note basal and parabasal cell hyperplasia of the covering epithelium extending up to the half of the epithelial thickness.

Benign salivary gland-type tumours

J.W. Eveson

In the larynx, benign salivary gland-type tumours are rare and less frequent than the malignant varieties {1039}.

ICD-O codes
Pleomorphic adenoma   8940/0
Oncocytic papillary cystadenoma
                          8290/0

Pleomorphic adenoma
Most pleomorphic adenomas arise in the epiglottis or aryepiglottic folds and can reach several centimetres before producing symptoms. Microscopically, laryngeal pleomorphic adenomas are similar to those in other minor salivary glands.

Oncocytic papillary cystadenoma (OPC)
Synonyms: oncocytic cyst, oncocytic papillary cystadenomatosis of the larynx, oncocytic adenomatous hyperplasia, oxyphil adenoma, oncocytoma and adenolymphoma in laryngocele {1641,2845}.

Laryngeal oncocytic lesions usually consist of unilocular or multilocular cysts lined by cytologically bland oncocytic epithelium with or without intraluminal papillary ingrowths {748,1548}. These lesions probably represent duct hyperplasia and metaplasia rather than true neoplasia. Most patients are older than 50 years, and present with hoarseness or other symptoms. The most frequent locations are the false vocal cords and the laryngeal ventricular areas {850}. The lesions are not encapsulated, may be multicentric, and can have a Warthin-like lymphoid component {792}. Solid oncytomas of the larynx resembling those seen in major salivary glands are rare to absent. Recurrence is uncommon and they have no malignant potential.

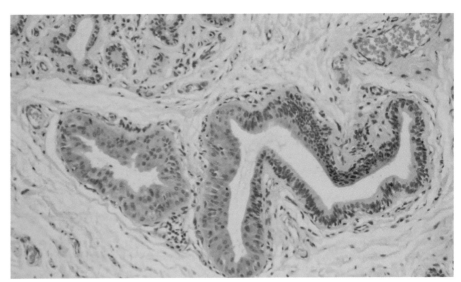

Fig. 3.46 Focal ductal oncocytic metaplasia and adjacent area of seromucous glands.

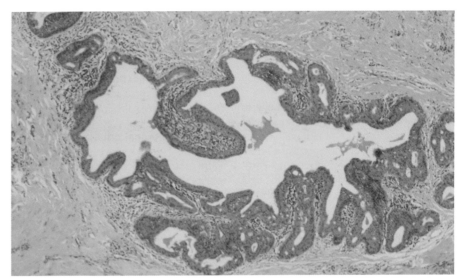

Fig. 3.47 Extensive ductal oncocytic metaplasia and hyperplasia with cystic dilatation.

Malignant soft tissue tumours

L.D.R. Thompson
J.C. Fanburg-Smith

Fibrosarcoma

ICD-O code   8810/3

In the past, the term "fibrosarcoma" was often applied indiscriminately to any malignant spindle cell tumour associated with collagen production. On critical review of these cases, supplemented with immunohistochemistry, it has become apparent that many alleged fibrosarcomas are examples of other entities {1636,2191}. With the possible exception of radiation-induced tumours, de novo fibrosarcoma is now recognized as a relatively uncommon tumour {1831}. The main differential diagnoses include spindle cell carcinoma and, occasionally, inflammatory myofibroblastic tumour, posttraumatic spindle cell nodule, and radiation-induced stromal atypia {2604, 2889}.

Malignant fibrous histiocytoma (MFH)

Definition
An aggressive, highly controversial malignant mesenchymal neoplasm composed of primitive round to spindle-shaped cells, often with admixed inflammatory and multinucleated giant cells, that grows either focally or diffusely in a storiform pattern.

ICD-O code   8830/3

Epidemiology
MFH of the larynx is an uncommon tumour. It occurs in all age groups (6-68 years) and is more common in males by a ratio of 3:1 {1985,2283}.

Etiology
Other than those related to prior radiation exposure, there are no known predisposing factors.

Localization
MFH is distinctly unusual in the hypopharynx and trachea. In the larynx,

the glottis is the site of predilection.

Clinical features
Symptoms vary according to location and include hoarseness, airway compromise, dysphagia or a sensation of a foreign body in the throat.

Macroscopy
The tumours are sessile to polypoid, firm, often ulcerated and have a yellow-tan to grey-white cut surface.

Histopathology
The histomorphology is highly variable but includes several of the following features: histiocyte-like cells, spindle-shaped cells, foam cells, pleomorphic multinucleated giant cells, typical and atypical mitoses, and necrosis. The tumour characteristically grows in a storiform pattern, either focally or diffusely.

Differential diagnosis
MFH must be distinguished from spindle cell carcinoma, which may be difficult on small biopsies. In spindle cell carcinoma, the tumour cells are typically positive for cytokeratin, as opposed to MFH. The presence of dysplasia or carcinoma in-situ in the overlying mucosa also indicates a carcinoma.

Prognosis and predictive factors
Surgery is the treatment of choice. The role of irradiation and chemotherapy is

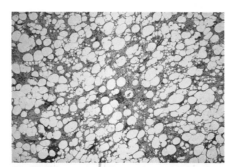

Fig. 3.48 Liposarcoma. The marked increase in cellularity with fibrous bands along with the increased nuclear to cytoplasm ratio even at this relatively low power is highly suggestive of a liposarcoma.

largely untested. In the absence of enlarged lymph nodes, a prophylactic neck dissection is not indicated {2283}. The tumour is unpredictable but certainly has the potential for local recurrence, haematogenous metastasis and death from disease.

Liposarcoma

ICD-O-code   8850/3

Primary liposarcomas of the larynx are rare, comprising less than 20% of all head and neck liposarcomas and fewer than 0.5% of all laryngeal neoplasms. Patients of all ages are affected, with a median of 64 years. There is a marked male to female predominance (nearly 10:1). The tumours, which occur almost exclusively in the supraglottic larynx or hypopharynx (pyriform sinus), most commonly cause airway obstruction. Imaging, especially with MR or CT, will document the lipomatous nature and extent of the mass. The tumours are firm, polypoid pedunculated, up to 10 cm in greatest dimension and demonstrate a lobulated, glistening, translucent cut surface often traversed by bands of fibrous tissue. The mucosa is usually intact. The majority of cases are well-differentiated lipoma-like liposarcomas (grade I), similar to their histologic counterparts in other anatomic sites, with infrequent reports of myxoid and pleomorphic types. Lipoblasts may be scanty necessitating multiple sections. Atypical cells, scattered lipoblasts, and infiltrative growth pattern differentiate liposarcomas from lipomas. In spite of surgical treatment, multiple recurrences are not uncommon (80% of patients). Metastasis has not been reported and the long-term prognosis is excellent (90% 5-year survival) {733,918,1155, 1371,2765,2772}.

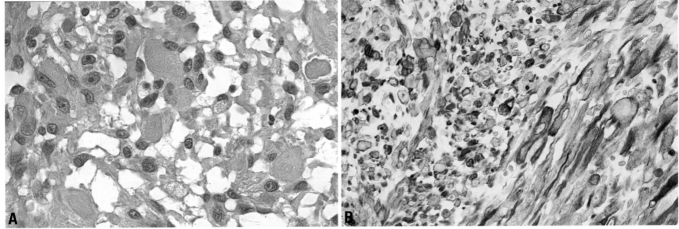

Fig. 3.49 Rhabdomyosarcoma. **A** Cells with eosinophilic and striated cytoplasm contain eccentrically placed nuclei with prominent eosinophilic nucleoli. Degeneration is noted. **B** The neoplastic cells are strongly immunoreactive with desmin, accentuated in both the "epithelioid" and spindled cells.

Leiomyosarcoma

ICD-O-code 8890/3

Leiomyosarcomas arising in the larynx are exceedingly rare accounting for less than 0.1% of all laryngeal malignancies. They present mainly in adults with no gender predilection. Symptoms are non-specific. Tumours can occur anywhere in the larynx but supraglottic lesions have been more frequently reported. They have a histology similar to leiomyosarcomas in soft tissues and demonstrate increased cellularity, nuclear and cellular pleomorphism, cytoplasmic vacuolization, necrosis, haemorrhage, and increased mitotic activity in addition to invasive growth. The diagnosis of leiomyosarcoma requires histologic, immunophenotypic (desmin, actins), and/or ultrastructural (parallel actin filaments, dense bodies and pinocytotic vesicles) confirmation as spindle cell carcinoma must always be excluded. Primary treatment is surgical. A variable prognosis is achieved {840,1247,1530, 1635,1686,1969,2208,2373,2706}.

Rhabdomyosarcoma

ICD-O code 8900/3

Rhabdomyosarcomas of the hypopharynx, larynx and trachea are poorly documented and exceedingly rare, comprising no more than 2% of all rhabdomyosarcomas {25,518,1084,1293, 1508,2215,2781}. They have been described in all age groups and, in the larynx, are centered around the glottic region. Possibly because of early presentation, prognosis has generally been good but death from disease has been recorded. The differential diagnosis includes a spindle cell carcinoma {915}.

Angiosarcoma

ICD-O-code 9120/3

Primary angiosarcomas of the larynx are exceedingly rare, with only a few well-documented reports. Despite the fact that nearly 50% of all angiosarcomas occur in the skin and superficial soft tissues of the head and neck, angiosarcoma accounts for less than 0.1 % of all head and neck malignancies. Laryngeal angiosarcoma is twice as frequent in men with a mean age at presentation in the 7th decade of life. Symptoms are non-specific; previous radiation exposure is frequently noted. The supraglottis is affected more frequently, specifically the epiglottis, where an increasing size is associated with a worse clinical outcome. Tumours demonstrate the typical histomorphologic features of angiosarcoma in other soft tissue sites. Tumour cells are consistently positive with Factor VIII-related antigen, CD34, and CD31. Contact ulcer, haemangioma, acantholytic squamous cell carcinoma and mucosal malignant melanoma are the principle differential diagnostic considerations. Surgical excision is the treatment

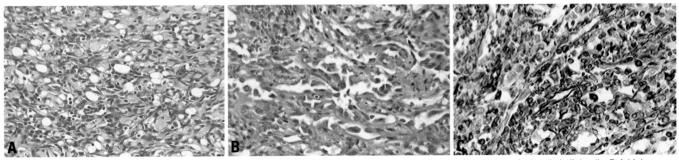

Fig. 3.50 Laryngeal angiosarcoma. **A** Intermediate power demonstrating the anastomosing vascular channels lined by atypical endothelial cells. **B** A high power showing nuclear atypia of the hobnailed endothelial cells in a laryngeal angiosarcoma. **C** Factor VIII R-Ag reacts strongly and diffusely with the neoplastic endothelial cells.

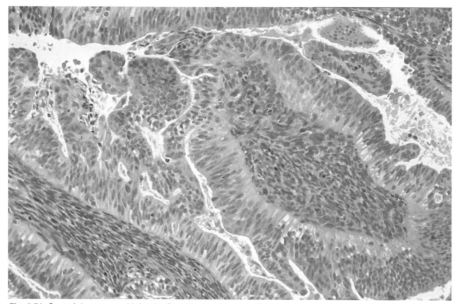

Fig. 3.51 Synovial sarcoma, biphasic. Stratified epithelial cells are surrounded by spindle cells.

fusiform submucosal masses, often demonstrating cystic or mucinous degeneration. The mucosa is usually intact, although larger tumours may ulcerate. Schwannoma is encapsulated and solitary with the nerve of origin attached peripherally. In contrast, neurofibroma is non-encapsulated, occasionally multiple or plexiform, especially when it is associated with NF1 and expands the nerve in a fusiform fashion rather than pushing it aside.

MPNST are infiltrative, mitotically active and often ulcerate the mucosa The tumour cells are immunoreactive, often patchy, with S-100 protein, vimentin, epithelial membrane antigen (EMA) and Leu-7. Distinguishing benign from malignant tumours on small biopsies may be difficult {385,659,1202,1235,1974,2508, 2591}.

of choice, with radiation therapy as necessary, yielding an overall patient survival of about 50% at 2 years. Large tumour size and previous radiation portends a worse prognosis {1556,1692, 2044,2055,2280,2591,2847}.

Kaposi sarcoma

ICD-O-code   9140/3

Kaposi sarcoma (KS) of the larynx is uncommon and only a few well-documented cases have been reported since 1983, coincident with the time frame during which HIV and AIDS were beginning to be recognized. This finding lends support to the strong association of KS of the larynx with the advanced HIV disease in epidemic AIDS rather than an association with the iatrogenic immunocompromised transplant, the endemic African, or the sporadic form. Men are almost exclusively affected, usually in the middle decades of life, presenting with upper airway obstruction. A flat to raised, violaceous, plaque-like mass is usually identified in the supraglottis, although glottic lesions are also frequent. Multifocal involvement is reported. The cut surface is fleshy and demonstrates recent and old haemorrhage. The histology is identical to the various stages of cutaneous KS, although the plaque-tumour stage with its sieve-like vasoformative pattern with eosinophilic, glassy-hyaline intra-

and extracellular globules (PAS positive) is most common. Human herpesvirus 8 (HHV-8) is usually positive, helping to confirm the diagnosis. Biopsy is contraindicated, as brisk haemorrhage will require emergent tracheostomy and possible death by exsanguination. Treatment is generally nonsurgical, encompassing radiotherapy or chemotherapy (systemic or intralesional). Laryngeal KS is usually non-lethal   {191,499,815,1487,1753, 2262,2552}.

Peripheral nerve sheath tumours (PNST)

ICD-O-codes
Schwannoma   9560/0
Neurofibroma   9540/0
Malignant peripheral nerve
sheath tumour (MPNST)   9540/3

Both benign (especially schwannoma and neurofibroma) and malignant peripheral nerve tumours (MPNST) can occur in the larynx, although vanishingly rare. Any age group can be affected and there is no gender predilection. Association of neurofibroma with neurofibromatosis-1 (NF1) has been reported in the larynx {385,2508}.
Macroscopically, benign and malignant PNST most often involve the supraglottis in relation to the superior laryngeal nerve. The tumours are of variable size and present as smooth, round or lobulated to

Synovial sarcoma

ICD-O-code   9040/3

Primary synovial sarcoma of the larynx and hypopharynx is rare, while secondary involvement by direct extension from the neck is slightly more common. Although all age groups may be affected, most patients are young and there is no gender bias. Symptoms are non-specific. The tumours are often exophytic or pedunculated, and infiltrative with surface ulceration. Both monophasic and biphasic synovial sarcomas have been described and are similar to the counterpart in the soft tissue. Immunohistochemically, both epithelial and spindle cells may be reactive with cytokeratin and epithelial membrane antigen (EMA), while only the spindle cells are positive for vimentin. Molecular studies reveal a characteristic translocation t(X;18)(p11.2;q11.2). The prognosis is variable but tends to be better than those arising in soft tissue {573,740, 1735,1780,2102}.

Inflammatory myofibroblastic tumour

B.M. Wenig

Definition
Inflammatory myofibroblastic tumour (IMT) is a distinct borderline lesion composed of myofibroblastic cells with a variable admixture of inflammatory cells, including mature lymphocytes, histiocytes, plasma cells and eosinophils, and collagen. It occurs predominantly in the soft tissue and viscera but also in the head and neck {2761}.

ICD-O code   8825/1

Synonyms
Inflammatory pseudotumour, plasma cell granuloma, plasma cell pseudotumour, pseudosarcomatous lesions/tumours.

Epidemiology
Head and neck IMTs are rare. There are very few comprehensive studies detailing their clinicopathologic features. In contrast to soft tissue and visceral IMTs, that occur predominantly in children and young adults, IMTs of the upper aerodigestive tract are more common in adults (median age of 59) and men {2761}.

Etiology
The etiology of IMT is unknown. Previous trauma, and immunosuppression have been implicated {858,2761}. Recently, human herpesvirus-8 DNA sequences and overexpression of interleukin 6 and cyclin D1 have been reported in IMTs {920}.

Localization
In the head and neck, nflammatory myofibroblastic tumours are most common in the larynx {396,686,1648, 2761} especially in the region of true vocal cord {2761}. Non-laryngeal sites include the oral cavity {632,677,1531}, tonsil {858,2736} parapharyngeal space {383,1165,2739}, sinonasal tract {1278, 1616,2165,2429,2739}, salivary glands {1178,2739,2794} and trachea {53}.

Clinical features
Laryngeal IMTs present with hoarseness, stridor, dysphonia, and/or a foreign body sensation in the throat {2761}. Constitutional and/or systemic signs and symptoms such as fever, weight loss, pain, malaise, anaemia, thrombocytosis, polyclonal hyperglobulinemia and elevated erythrocyte sedimentation rate seen in association with soft tissue and visceral IMTs are not usually a component of upper aerodigestive tract IMTs; however, they are occasionally reported {383, 2165}.

Macroscopy
The gross appearance of laryngeal IMT is a smooth, polypoid or nodular lesion with fleshy to firm consistency and varying dimensions.

Histopathology
IMTs are characterized by a submucosal, loose, cellular proliferation of spindled to stellate cells arranged in a storiform to fascicular pattern with a variable component of inflammatory cells. The surface epithelium may be intact, hyperplastic or ulcerated and show reactive epithelial atypia. The inflammatory infiltrate is comprised of mature lymphocytes, histiocytes, plasma cells, eosinophils and scattered neutrophils. The stroma is highly vascularized and ranges from oedematous to fibromyxoid to collagenous. The vascular component varies from widely dilated medium sized vascular channels to narrow, slit-like blood vessels that can be obsured by the myofibroblasts and inflammatory cells. Vascular thrombosis is not present.

This overall appearance is similar to a reactive process resembling granulation tissue or nodular fasciitis. The myofibroblasts are spindled to stellate with enlarged round to oblong nuclei, variable nucleoli and abundant, eosinophilic to basophilic appearing fibrillar cytoplasm. In some examples, the myofibroblasts have a more epithelioid or histiocytoid appearance, including round to oval nuclei, prominent nucleoli and ample cytoplasm. The myofibroblasts may also appear as slender axonal (spider-like) cells with elongated nuclei, inapparent nucleoli and long cytoplasmic extensions

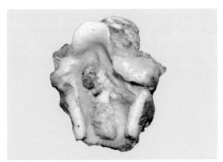

Fig. 3.52 Recurrrent inflammatory myofibroblastic tumour that necessitated laryngectomy appearing as an irregularly shaped polypoid lesion which initially originated in the glottic region but at recurrence extended to the supra- and subglottis.

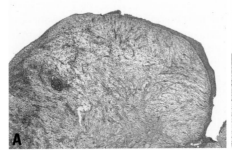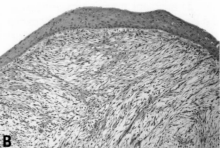

Fig. 3.53 Inflammatory myofibroblastic tumour. **A** Polypoid submucosal spindle cell proliferation with a myxoid and well-vascularized stroma, and an associated inflammatory cell infiltrate. Focally, storiform to fascicular growth. The surface epithelium varies from ulcerated to attenuated to intact squamous epithelium. **B** The submucosal spindle cell proliferation approximates the surface squamous epithelium, but there is usually no direct continuity or surface epithelial dysplasia.

creating a tadpole-like appearance. The myofibroblasts invariably maintain a low nuclear-to-cytoplasmic ratio. Focal nuclear pleomorphism may be present. Mitoses are common, sometimes even numerous, but never atypical. Necrosis and marked nuclear pleomorphism are not seen.

Immunoprofile

IMTs show strong diffuse cytoplasmic immunoreactivity for vimentin, and usually variable expression of smooth muscle actin and/or desmin. Cytokeratin staining may be seen but usually focal to absent.

Electron microscopy

The tumour cells show myofibroblastic and fibroblastic differentiation {707, 2761}.

Genetics

Recent evidence reveals the presence of anaplastic lymphoma kinase (ALK) gene rearrangements and expression in IMTs {486,949,1440,2865}. These rearrangements are common in IMTs of children and young adults {949,1440,2486} and are uncommon over the age of 40 {367,486,1440}. Both the gene rearrangements and protein activation are restricted to the myofibroblastic component, while the inflammatory cell component is normal {270,466,466,486,486, 949,1440}. Fusion of ALK to Ran-binding protein 2 gene in IMTs expand the spectrum of ALK abnormalities seen in IMT further confirming the clonal, neoplastic nature of IMTs {1593}.

Prognosis and predictive factors

Laryngeal IMT is usually cured by conservative resection {2761}. Corticosteroid and nonsteroidal anti-inflammatory agents have been used for treatment resulting in regression in some patients {795,2487}. A recurrence rate of approximately 25% has been reported for extrapulmonary IMTs {467}. IMT was originally believed to be a reactive non-neoplastic lesion. This has been refuted by the above genetic studies. An occasional

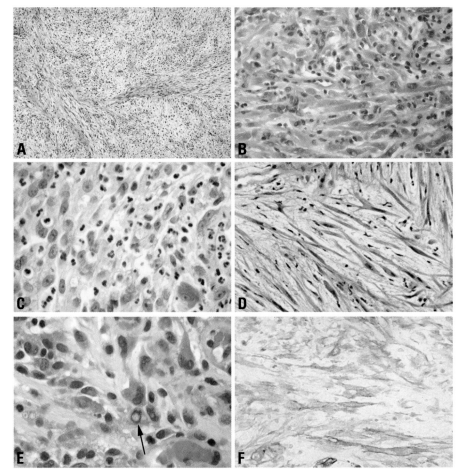

Fig. 3.54 Inflammatory myofibroblastic tumour. **A** Laryngeal IMTs show varied growth patterns including fascicular patterns. **B** The myofibroblasts appear spindle-shaped with enlarged round to oblong nuclei, inapparent to prominent eosinophilic nucleoli and abundant eosinophilic to basophilic appearing fibrillar cytoplasm. **C** In some examples, the myofibroblasts have a more epithelioid or histiocytoid appearance, including round to oval nuclei, prominent nucleoli and ample amount of cytoplasm. **D** The myofibroblasts may also appear as slender axonal (spider-like) cells with elongated nuclei, inapparent nucleoli and long cytoplasmic extensions, creating cells with a bipolar-to-multipolar (tadpole-like) appearance. **E** Scattered myofibroblasts show the presence of eosinophilic intranuclear inclusions (arrow). **F** The myofibroblasts in IMT show immunoreactivity for muscle specific actin.

IMT may follow an aggressive clinical course. Rarely non-head and neck visceral IMTs have metastasized {466}. It is difficult to predict on the basis of histology which IMTs will be more aggressive {1156,1363,2842}.

Benign soft tissue tumours

L.D.R. Thompson
J.C. Fanburg-Smith
L. Barnes

Lipoma

ICD-O code 8850/0

Lipomas of the larynx and hypopharynx comprise less than 0.5% of benign neoplasms at these sites, occur in all ages and affect both genders equally. The symptoms are non-specific but often include airway obstruction. In the larynx, supraglottic lesions predominate. Computed tomography and magnetic resonance document the lipomatous (low attenuation values and negative densitometry) nature and the extent of the mass. A lipoma is usually solitary, soft and sessile to polypoid. Tumours are composed of mature adipose cells, occasionally with foci of myxoid stroma. Distinction from well-differentiated liposarcoma is important. Association with systemic lipomatosis has been reported {1770}. Simple but complete excision is curative {329,409,1528,2756,2765}.

Leiomyoma

ICD-O- code 8890/0

Leiomyomas (angioleiomyoma) of the larynx comprise less than 0.2% of all laryngeal neoplasms. The tumour has been reported in all age groups, but primarily in adults, and is somewhat more common in males. The ventricle and false vocal cord are sites of predilection.

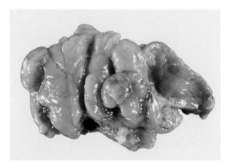

Fig. 3.55 Rhabdomyoma of the hypopharynx in an adult. Note the characteristic tan colour and multinodularity.

In addition to the usual type, vascular and rare epithelioid variants have also been described {1057,1179,1290,1686, 1913,2334}.

Rhabdomyoma

Definition
A benign mesenchymal tumour with skeletal muscle differentiation and a propensity for occurrence in the head and neck.

ICD-O code 8900/0

Epidemiology
Based on histology rather than age, rhabdomyomas are divided into three types: fetal, juvenile (intermediate), and adult.
Fetal rhabdomyoma (FRM) are 2-3 times more common in males and have been described in patients from birth to 65 years of age; about half of all patients are

15 years old or older at the time of diagnosis {597,1271}.
Juvenile rhabdomyomas (JRM) are 2 times more common in males and have been observed in patients from 5 months to 58 years of age (average 18 years) {508,1271}.
Adult rhabdomyomas (ARM) are 3-5 times more common in males and occur in an older population. About 80-90% of patients are over the age of 40 years (median 55-60 years, range 15 months to 82 years) {597,1272}.

Etiology
Whether RMs are hamartomas or true neoplasms is controversial. Cytogenetics examination of an ARM has demonstrated clonal chromosomal abnormalities which supports a neoplastic origin {886}. Extracardiac RMs should be distinguished from those in the heart. Cardiac RMs are hamartomas and often associated with tuberous sclerosis. Extracardiac RMs, with the rare exception of a FRM

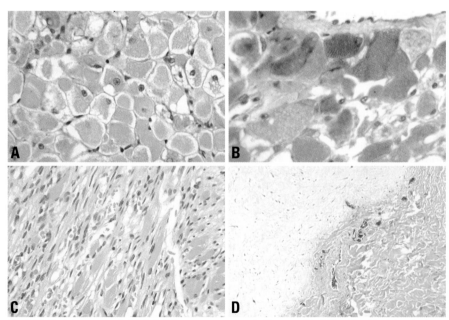

Fig. 3.56 Rhabdomyoma. **A** Adult rhabdomyoma composed of large epithelioid cells with pink cytoplasm and eccentric nuclei with prominent nucleoli. The cytoplasmic vacuoles represent glycogen. **B** Diffuse desmin staining of cells and cross-strations in the cell in the upper middle portion of the illustration. **C** Juvenile (intermediate) rhabdomyoma showing spindle-shaped rhabdomyoblasts. **D** Fetal myxoid rhabdomyoma. Note the sharp border.

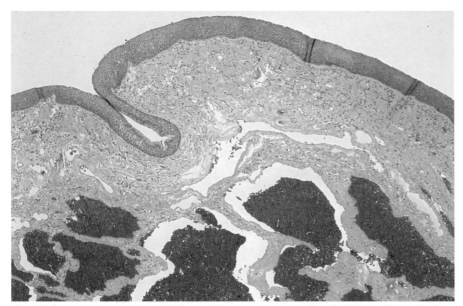

Fig. 3.57 Cavernous haemangioma with large, dilated vascular spaces. Note the intact surface epithelium.

ARMs are usually easily recognized. Infrequently, it may be confused with a pleomorphic rhabdomyosarcoma, granular cell tumour, hibernoma, oncocytoma, alveolar soft parts sarcoma, or crystal-storing histiocytosis {1268}.

Prognosis and predictive factors
In contrast to FRMs, which are generally solitary lesions, 3-10% of ARMs may be multifocal, either synchronous or asynchronous. Conservative but complete excision is the treatment of choice. Ten to 40% of ARMs may recur, either within a few months or 10-15 years later. FRMs, in contrast, demonstrate less tendency for recurrence. Some of the "recurrent" ARMs may represent additional primary tumours in a patient with multifocal disease. RMs have no malignant potential.

Haemangioma and Lymphangioma

ICD-O-codes
Haemangioma	9120/0
Lymphangioma	9170/0

Haemangiomas of the larynx are divided into juvenile (congenital) and adult types based on age of presentation, histologic appearance, and possibly patient outcome. Pediatric patients present at or within several months of birth with subglottic lesions that may result in potentially life-threatening airway obstruction and haemorrhage. In addition, about half of all pediatric patients with subglottic haemangiomas may have haemangiomas in other locations, most of which are cutaneous, rarely visceral. Adult haemangiomas are more often found in the supraglottic larynx. Grossly, haemangiomas are soft and compressible and range from red to blue, depending on the degree of vascularity. They may be either flat and diffuse or bulging and polypoid. The term 'haemangiomatosis' is sometimes used when the lesion is widespread and involves contiguous or noncontiguous sites. Microscopically, haemangiomas are categorized into capillary and cavernous types, and often demonstrate a lobular pattern of growth. Juvenile haemangiomas are usually cellular and of the capillary type while in adults, they are are more often cavernous.
Haemangiomas should be distinguished

occurring in a few patients with the nevoid basal cell carcinoma syndrome, are virtually never associated with a phakomatosis {929}.

Localization
RMs of the larynx and hypopharynx are uncommon {1225}. In the larynx, they tend to centre around the true and false vocal cords and ventricles.

Clinical features
The tumours generally present as hoarseness, airway obstruction, dysphagia, or sensation of a foreign body in the throat.

Macroscopy
FRMs are usually 1-5 cm, circumscribed and grey-white to tan-pink with a mucoid cut surface.
ARMs are circumscribed, tan to red-brown and multinodular. Most are less than 5 cm, but may be larger.

Histopathology
FRMs vary from sparse to moderately cellular and are composed of immature cells with little cytoplasm and small, round to spindled nuclei, with or without nucleoli. Strap cells with eosinophilic cytoplasm, occasionally with cross striations, may be seen, but are few in number. Mitoses, necrosis and nuclear pleomorphism are typically absent.
ARMs contain large, closely packed polygonal cells with light pink to bright eosinophilic cytoplasm and one or more

round to oval nuclei, sometimes with prominent nucleoli. The cytoplasm contains abundant glycogen, often appearing as vacuoles and producing a characteristic "spider cell". Rod-shaped cytoplasmic crystals ("jackstraws") may also be apparent. Cross striations are infrequent and, mitoses and necrosis are absent.
JRMs contain a large number of strap-shaped muscle cells with abundant eosinophilic cytoplasm with centrally located nuclei. Cytoplasmic vacuoles are common. The tumour often co-exists with typical areas of FRM.

Immunoprofile
RMs are positive for muscle specific actin, smooth muscle actin, desmin, and myoglobin. ARMs are also variably weakly positive for vimentin (35% of cases) and even S-100 protein (67% of cases), but negative for glial fibrillary acidic protein (GFAP), cytokeratin, and epithelial membrane antigen. FRMs are also variably positive for vimentin (75% of cases), S-100 protein (50% of cases), and GFAP (50% of cases).

Differential diagnosis
The FRM must be distinguished from embryonal rhabdomyosarcoma. The lack of significant infiltration of adjacent tissues; absence of cellular pleomorphism, mitoses, and necrosis; and the presence of muscle maturation at the periphery of the lesion are features indicative of a rhabdomyoma.

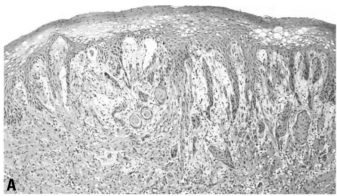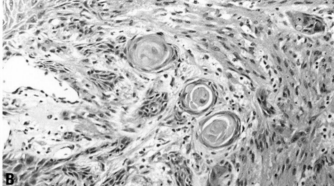

Fig. 3.58 Granular cell tumour. **A** Prominent pseudoepitheliomatous hyperplasia. The granular cells are spindle-shaped and may be confused with a desmoplastic stromal reaction. **B** Higher magnification of the pseudoepitheliomatous hyperplasia.

from telangiectasia, vascular stage of vocal cord polyps and granulation tissue. The distinction between haemangioma and telangiectasia may be difficult. But in the correct clinical setting of a positive family history of hereditary haemorrhagic telangiectasia (Rendu-Osler-Weber syndrome), typical lesions (in any location) and episodic bleeding can help to define the syndrome. Vascular vocal cord polyps occur exclusively on the true vocal cord and are separated from haemangiomas by a large amount of extravascular fibrin. Fibrin, if seen in haemangiomas, is always intravascular. The lobular growth of haemangioma distinguishes it from granulation tissue. If the lesion is biopsied rather than excised, unusually excessive bleeding may give a clue as to the type of lesion encountered. Although the preferred treatment is laser excision, therapy has included expectant management, systemic steroids, intralesional sclerosing agents and surgical excision {277,439, 1235,1680,2227,2305,2591}.

Lymphangiomas can occur in the larynx, but are extraordinarily rare. The distinction between a cystic hygroma with involvement of the larynx versus a pri-

mary lymphangioma underscores a semantic and clinical dilemma. The exact anatomic location and neck examination are needed to exclude a primary lymphangioma {659,1194,1235,1487}.

Granular cell tumour

Definition
A neural tumour composed of round and/or spindle cells with pink, granular cytoplasm due to abundant intracytoplasmic lysosomes.

ICD-O code   9580/0

Synonyms
Granular cell myoblastoma, granular cell schwannoma, Abrikossoff tumour.

Epidemiology
Granular cell tumours (GCT) of the larynx affect both sexes equally and occur over a broad age range (4-70 years), with a mean of 34 years {2247}. They are uncommon in children. Only 20 cases were identified in 1998 in patients less than 17 years of age {1114}.

GCTs of the trachea are even more

unusual. Of 30 cases, 84% occurred in women and the peak incidence was the fourth decade (range 6-56 years) {315}.

Localization
GCTs may occur anywhere in the larynx. In adults, the most common site is the posterior half of the true vocal cord, while in children the subglottis is the site of predilection. Tracheal tumours, in turn, arise most often in the cervical trachea.

Clinical features
GCTs are especially common in the Black population. Most patients have only a single tumour, but in 2-10% of individuals, multiple tumours may be found {924}. Hoarseness is the usual presenting symptom of laryngeal tumours while stridor or airway obstruction (often mistaken for asthma) is characteristic of those in the trachea.

Macroscopy
The majority of tumours are firm, polypoid or sessile, and less than two centimetres. They are covered by an intact (rarely ulcerated) mucosa, and on cross section are grey-white or yellow.

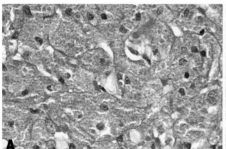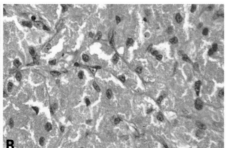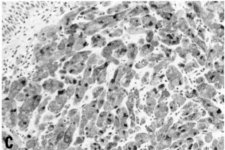

Fig. 3.59 Granular cell tumour. **A** Periodic acid-Schiff (PAS) stain with diastase accentuates the cytoplasmic granularity. **B** The granularity of the cytoplasm is due to lysosomes. **C** Strong immunoreactivity for S-100 protein.

Histopathology

GCTs are poorly circumscribed and composed of round or spindle cells, often in a syncytial pattern. The nuclei are small, hyperchromatic, and centrally located. The cytoplasm is eosinophilic and contains numerous periodic acid-Schiff-positive, diastase-resistant granules. The granules are also S100 protein and CD 68 positive, and ultrastructurally represent lysosomes.

Malignant granular cell tumour

Approximately 1-2% of all GCTs are malignant and exhibit either aggressive local behaviour or distant metastasis (lung, bone) {253,713}. Criteria for malignancy include: 1) necrosis, 2) spindling of cells, 3) vesicular nuclei with large nucleoli, 4) greater than 2 mitoses per 10 high power fields at 200X magnification, 5) high nuclear to cytoplasmic ratio, and 6) pleomorphism. Neoplasms that meet 3 or more of these criteria are classified as malignant. Those that meet only one or two criteria are regarded as atypical while those that show only focal pleomorphism but none of the other features are classified as benign.

Differential diagnosis

Small biopsies with sparse granular cells associated with pseudoepitheliomatous hyperplasia can easily be mistaken for squamous cell carcinoma. In the larynx, GCTs are typically non-ulcerated and occur on the posterior half of the true vocal cord in patients less than 50 years of age. In contrast, squamous cell carcinomas of the larynx are often ulcerated and arise on the anterior half of the true vocal cord in patients over the age of 50 years.

Prognosis and predictive factors

GCTs are radioresistent. Most can be removed endoscopically. Larger lesions may require an open excision. Although initial therapy is usually curative, 2-8% of patients may develop local recurrences. Some "recurrences", however, may represent new primary lesions in a patient with multifocal disease.

Haematolymphoid tumours

A.C.L. Chan
J.K.C. Chan
S.B. Kapadia

Non-Hodgkin lymphoma

Primary non-Hodgkin lymphomas (NHL) of the hypopharynx, larynx or trachea are very rare. They account for 1% of all primary extranodal NHL {809}. By contrast, secondary laryngeal lymphomas are more common and represent spread from cervical and mediastinal lymph nodes, and thyroid gland. Patients present with hoarseness, foreign body sensation, or mild airway obstruction. Supraglottic tumours are more frequent, but all regions of the larynx can be involved.

Most primary laryngeal NHL are B-cell lymphomas, especially diffuse large B-cell lymphoma (DLBCL) and extranodal marginal zone B-cell lymphoma of MALT type {63,601,1285,1771}. Rare cases of extranodal NK/T cell lymphoma of nasal-type {371,1761} and peripheral T-cell lymphoma {1285,1632,1761} have also been reported. Most patients (>90%) present with low clinical stage (Stage IE/IIE) {63,1285,1771}, but occasional patients can succumb to acute laryngeal obstruction {1771}. NK/T cell lymphomas and peripheral T-cell lymphomas have a poorer outcome as compared to B-cell lymphomas {63,1285,1761,1771}.

Patients with primary tracheal NHL may present with airway obstruction, dyspnoea, wheezing or cough. Most reported cases are extranodal marginal zone B-cell lymphoma of MALT type {762,1275}. Primary hypopharyngeal NHL is extremely rare {809}. Both extranodal NK/T cell lymphoma of nasal type {2455,2605} and extranodal marginal zone B-cell lymphoma of MALT type have been reported {2773}.

Plasmacytoma

Definition

Plasmacytoma is a monoclonal plasmacytic proliferation. A soft tissue plasmacytoma without bone marrow involvement is referred to as extramedullary plasmacytoma (EMP).

ICD-O code   9734/3

Localization

The larynx and pharynx are the most common head and neck sites for extramedullary plasmacytoma. For details see Chapter 1 on sinonasal tumours (pp. 61-63).

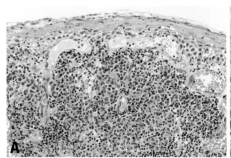
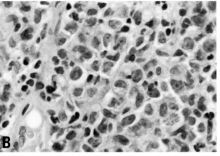

Fig. 3.60 Large B-cell lymphoma of larynx. **A** There is diffuse and dense infiltrate of large lymphoid cells beneath the surface stratified squamous epithelium. **B** The infiltrate comprises large lymphoid cells with irregularly folded nuclei and distinct nucleoli.

Tumours of bone and cartilage

J.E. Lewis
L. Barnes
L.Y. Tse
J.L. Hunt

Chondrosarcoma

Definition
Chondrosarcoma is a malignant tumour of the laryngeal framework characterized by the formation of neoplastic hyaline cartilage.

ICD-O code   9220/3

Epidemiology
Laryngeal chondrosarcoma (LCS) is the most common non-epithelial malignancy of the larynx, and comprises 75% of laryngeal sarcomas {1489}. Cartilaginous neoplasms are estimated to represent 0.07-0.2% of all laryngeal tumours {255}. Approximately 300 cases of cartilaginous laryngeal tumours have been reported; the majority are represented by chondrosarcomas. They affect adults in the 6-9th decades, with a mean age at diagnosis of 60-65 years. The male to female ratio is approximately 3:1.

Localization
LCS arise predominantly in the ossified hyaline cartilages. The cricoid ring is the most frequently involved, especially its posterior or posterolateral aspect, followed by the thyroid cartilage. Bulky tumours may encompass both structures, obscuring the exact site of origin. Chondrosarcoma of the epiglottis has only been rarely reported.

Clinical features
Patients with LCS typically present with hoarseness, and/or airway obstruction and dyspnoea. An external neck mass may be noted when it arises in the thyroid lamina. These tumours grow slowly and can be asymptomatic until they reach considerable size. On examination, the usual appearance is that of a subglottic swelling with intact mucosa. Vocal cord paralysis is a common finding at presentation. LCS have characteristic features on CT examination, with expansion of the affected cartilage by a relatively circumscribed, hypodense mass containing stippled to coarse calcifications. MR imaging may show better definition of the tumour boundaries but is less likely to detect internal calcifications {255,1888, 2598}. LCS are notoriously difficult to biopsy. Their characteristic imaging appearance precludes the necessity for preoperative biopsy.

Macroscopy
LCS are bulky, lobulated neoplasms that expand and distort the involved site. The cut surface is firm to hard, translucent, pale grey-blue, with gritty calcifications. Myxoid change, if present, is characterized by soft, cystic, or gelatinous areas. Dedifferentiated chondrosarcoma reveals fleshy areas resembling high-grade sarcoma.

Histopathology
The diagnosis and grading of LCS is based on general criteria for chondrosarcoma {1509}. The low power architecture of LCS is that of a lobulated neoplasm

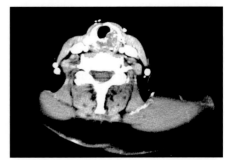

Fig. 3.62 Chondrosarcoma. CT scan of laryngeal chondrosarcoma demonstrating expansion of the posterior and left lateral aspect of the cricoid cartilage, narrowing the airway. Coarse internal calcifications are present.

with pushing borders. The tumour periphery shows invasive growth of neoplastic lobules into adjacent soft tissue or the marrow spaces of ossified cartilage. The overwhelming majority of LCS are low or intermediate grade, with variability from area to area {28,255,1152,1888}.

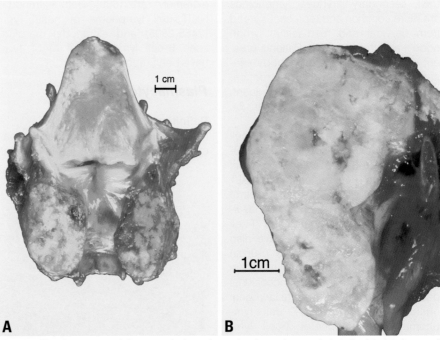

A **B**

Fig. 3.61 Chondrosarcoma. **A** Gross surgical specimen showing a characteristic bulky, lobulated mass of the posterior cricoid. **B** Cut section of cricoid chondrosarcoma with a solid, partly translucent, grey-white surface, with focal calcification.

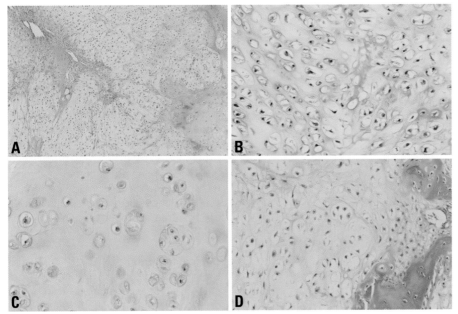

Fig. 3.63 Laryngeal chondrosarcoma. **A** Low power view demonstrating the characteristic lobulated growth pattern. **B** Moderately differentiated (grade 2) chondrosarcoma with greater degree of cellularity and nuclear pleomorphism. **C** Well differentiated (grade 1) chondrosarcoma with mild nuclear atypia and hyperchromasia. **D** Focal metaplastic bone formation in a laryngeal chondrosarcoma.

High-grade LCS are generally considered rare; although in the largest reported series they comprised 5% {2598}. Metaplastic bone formation and calcification are also common to LCS. Myxoid change is infrequent. Dedifferentiated and clear cell variants of LCS have been reported, albeit rarely {28,255,1888, 2598}. Dedifferentiated chondrosarcoma is characterized by the presence of two distinct components: well-differentiated chondrosarcoma and a high-grade, non-cartilaginous sarcoma. Clear cell chondrosarcoma is composed of chondro-

cytes with abundant clear cytoplasm and prominent cell membranes. LCS, similar to chondrosarcoma found elsewhere, expresses S-100 protein (strongly) and vimentin (focally) in immunohistochemical studies {255, 1888}.

Differential diagnosis

Low-grade LCS may be difficult to distinguish from chondroma. Grade 1 LCS show subtle increases in cellularity, with nuclear hyperchromasia and occasional binucleate forms. Irregular clustering of cell groups, or "cluster disarray" is found

in all grades of LCS {1152} and may be a useful feature in the distinction of low-grade chondrosarcoma from chondroma. The diagnosis of laryngeal chondroma should be reserved for small (less than 1-2 cm), clinically insignificant lesions, without discernible atypia. Any recurrent cartilaginous tumour of the larynx should be considered a chondrosarcoma {255}. Chondrometaplasia is characterized by small (less than 1 cm) nodules of bland, fibroelastic cartilage which are found in the submucosal soft tissue of the glottic region {747,1161}.

Precursor lesions

Understanding of the biologic potential of laryngeal cartilaginous neoplasms has evolved in recent years such that many reported laryngeal chondromas would now be interpreted as low-grade LCS {1888,2178,2598}. (See section on Chondromas).

Histogenesis

LCS usually develop in ossified cartilage. A pluripotential mesenchymal stem cell, which may be recruited in the process of ossification, is postulated to be the cell of origin {255}. Several authors have proposed that LCS may develop in a benign chondroma {2598}; this hypothesis remains highly controversial.

Prognosis and predictive factors

LCS are more indolent than chondrosarcomas arising elsewhere {2598}. This may be due to the fact that LCS are symptomatic at a smaller size when compared to their skeletal counterparts. LCS are managed with conservative surgery {255,1489,2598}. Incomplete resection (shelling out) is associated with local recurrence {2178}. Metastases from LCS, usually pulmonary, are distinctly unusual (<10%), and related to higher grade or dedifferentiation {2598}. LCS related mortality is very low {1489}. Myxoid change involving greater than 10% of the neoplasm correlates adversely with outcome {2598}.

Osteosarcoma

Definition

Osteosarcoma is a malignant tumour characterized by the direct formation of osteoid by neoplastic cells.

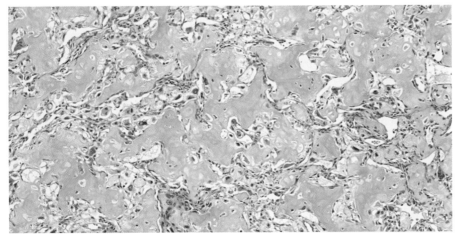

Fig. 3.64 Osteosarcoma of the larynx, characterized by large, pleomorphic osteoblasts and osteoid production.

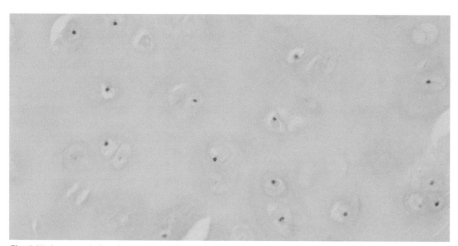

Fig. 3.65 Laryngeal chondroma presenting as hypocellular proliferation of chondrocytes, lacking nuclear atypia, which produce hyaline cartilage.

ICD-O code   9180/3

Epidemiology
Laryngeal osteosarcoma (LOS) is extremely rare, with fewer than 20 documented cases {198, 526,926,1604,1807, 2054,2154,2203,2327,2675}. LOS affects an older age group than osteosarcoma arising in long bone {2054}. They manifest in patients from about 50-80 years of age, nearly exclusively in males.

Localization
These sarcomas usually arise from the endolaryngeal soft tissue, vocal cords and/or anterior commissure, rather than the laryngeal framework.

Clinical features
LOS is typically a polypoid mass that impinges on the airway. Symptoms depend on the tumour site; hoarseness, dyspnoea, and airway obstruction are the most frequent complaints. Imaging studies reveal an invasive, mineralized mass, either situated primarily in the soft tissue of the glottis or expanding one of the laryngeal cartilages {1807,2203}. Biopsy may be difficult when the tumour is heavily mineralized.

Macroscopy
LOS of the vocal cord soft tissue is usually polypoid, and may show an intact or ulcerated mucosa. In the laryngeal framework, it forms a poorly defined, infiltrative mass. The cut surface is hard and gritty, with variable colouration.

Histopathology
Similar to other primary mesenchymal neoplasms, LOS typically retains a "Grenz zone" of tumour-free, superficial submucosa just beneath the non-dysplastic epithelium. LOS is uniformly high-grade {1604,2054}, composed of pleomorphic spindle cells. The amount of osteoid produced by the malignant cells can vary, but characteristic lace-like osteoid is present at least focally {926,1604}. Tumour giant cells may also be identified {198,526,1807}. Laryngeal osteosarcoma may also represent the high-grade sarcomatous component of dedifferentiated chondrosarcoma of the larynx {2675}.

Differential diagnosis
LOS must be distinguished from spindle cell carcinoma (SPCC) with heterologous osteoid production, since the spindle cell component of the latter tumour may be highly pleomorphic and focally produce osteoid {1604}. In contrast to LOS, SPCC is characterized by either 1) a concomitant squamous abnormality (dysplasia, carcinoma in-situ, or invasive SCC) or 2) evidence of epithelial differentiation in spindle cells. In addition, the malignant spindle cells of SPCC usually abut the overlying mucosa or merge with its basal layer in a feathering pattern, without the presence of a Grenz zone.

Prognosis and predictive factors
Reported cases of LOS have demonstrated aggressive clinical behaviour. Local recurrence is frequent, as are distant metastases, typically involving the lung. At least half of the reported patients have died of disease, most within a year of diagnosis {198,1604}.

Chondroma

Definition
A benign tumour composed of mature hyaline cartilage

ICD-O code   9220/0

Epidemiology
True chondromas of the larynx are extremely unusual and are greatly outnumbered by laryngeal chondrosarcoma (LCS) {2593}. The age incidence is difficult to estimate as many previous reports of chondroma probably represent LCS {465,591}.

Clinical features
Chondromas of the larynx primarily affect the cricoid and thyroid cartilages. Chondroma may be an incidental finding, or cause minor symptoms such as hoarseness. A clinically significant cartilaginous tumour is more likely to be LCS than a chondroma.

Macroscopy
Chondromas are well-circumscribed tumours. The cut surface is uniform, with a translucent, pale grey-blue appearance. A cartilaginous neoplasm greater than 2 cm in dimension more likely represents LCS.

Histopathology
Chondromas are composed of benign chondrocytes producing hyaline cartilage. They may show a lobular growth pattern. The appearance is uniform and monotonous with overall low cellularity. The chondrocytes are relatively evenly distributed, lack nuclear pleomorphism and mitotic activity and contain a single nucleus per lacuna {591,1489}. In LCS, the neoplastic chondrocytes are distributed in cell groups of varying size and cellularity (cluster disarray). However, because the histopathology of LCS is variable within a tumour, thorough sampling of any cartilaginous tumour is recommended. The diagnosis of chondroma should be reserved for small lesions that have been completely excised and entirely examined {591}.

Prognosis and predictive factors
Laryngeal chondroma does not recur after conservative excision. Any recurrent cartilaginous neoplasm of the larynx should be interpreted as LCS {591, 2593}.

Giant cell tumour

Definition
A benign but locally destructive neoplasm composed of sheets of ovoid to spindle-shaped mononuclear cells with uniformly dispersed osteoclast-like giant cells.

ICD-O code   9250/1

Synonym
Osteoclastoma

Epidemiology
Giant cell tumours of the larynx are very rare {590,982,1092,1642,2163}. They represented only 0.09% of almost 9000 benign and malignant laryngeal tumours {2785}. In total 28 cases have been reported comprised of 25 men and 3 women, aged 23-62 years (mean about 40-45 years).

Localization
The thyroid cartilage is most commonly involved, followed by cricoid cartilage and epiglottis {2785}.

Clinical features
The tumours enlarge slowly and manifest as palpable neck masses, hoarseness, airway obstruction, dysphagia or sore throat. On imaging, it often appears as a tumour exploding from within the cartilage, destroying it and extending into soft tissue of the neck or endolarynx.

Macroscopy
Most tumours have ranged from 2.4-7cm (mean about 4-4.5cm) and have been centred in the thyroid or cricoid cartilages, especially in the normally ossified

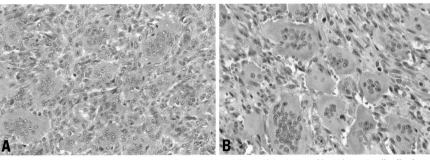

Fig. 3.67 A Giant cell tumour arising from the thyroid cartilage of the larynx. Note the even distribution of multinucleated giant cells. **B** The nuclei of the giant cells are similar to those of the mononuclear cells.

portions of these cartilages {2785}. On cut section, they are soft, red to grey-pink and frequently extend beyond the cartilage into the adjacent soft tissue. Haemorrhage and cystic degeneration are common.

Histopathology
The tumours are similar histologically to the giant cell tumour of bone and, as such, consist of a dual population of cells: mononuclear cells and osteoclast-like giant cells. The mononuclear cells appear as broad sheets of cells reminiscent of histiocytes. They are round, ovoid or spindled and have pink to amphophilic cytoplasm and round, vesicular nuclei with occasional prominent nucleoli. The giant cells are evenly distributed throughout the tumour and contain up to 20 or more nuclei per cell. The nuclei of the giant cells are identical to those of the mononuclear cells.

The stroma is vascular and contains many thin-walled vessels with small areas of haemorrhage and haemosiderin-laden macrophages. Mitoses are usually seen, averaging 4 per 10 high power fields (range 1-12 per 10 high power fields) {2785}. Atypical mitoses are not seen.

Differential diagnosis
This includes giant cell (reparative) granuloma, brown tumour of hyperparathyroidism, fibrous histiocytoma and a pleomorphic carcinoma. Giant cell granuloma of the cricoid cartilage is exceptionally rare {2587}. The giant cells in this tumour are not evenly distributed, but rather concentrate around areas of recent and/or old haemorrhage. A giant cell granuloma also exhibits more stromal fibrosis. A brown tumour is identical histologically to the giant cell granuloma, but is associated with elevated serum

calcium. A benign fibrous histiocytoma contains a more uniform storiform arrangement of fibroblasts and does not show a symmetrical distribution of giant cells. A malignant fibrous histiocytoma (giant cell type) exhibits significant nuclear pleomorphism and abnormal mitoses, none of which are seen in a giant cell tumour. A pleomorphic carcinoma will not only show abnormal mitoses and pleomorphism, but will also be positive for cytokeratin.

Prognosis and predictive factors
Complete, but conservative surgical excision is the treatment of choice. Large tumours may require a partial or total laryngectomy. Adjuvant therapy is unnecessary.

There have been no convincing records of local recurrence or malignant behaviour secondary to giant cell tumour of the laryngeal framework {1138,1181}.

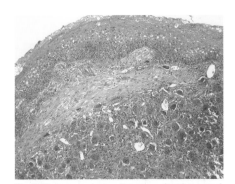

Fig. 3.66 Larynx giant cell tumour. A submucosal polypoid nodule without surface involvement or point of origin demonstrates many osteoclast-like giant cells.

Mucosal malignant melanoma

B.M. Wenig

Definition

Primary laryngeal mucosal malignant melanomas (PLMMM) are neural crest-derived neoplasms originating from melanocytes and demonstrating melanocytic differentiation.

ICD-O code   8720/3

Epidemiology

Approximately 15-20% of all malignant melanomas arise in head and neck sites, and of these over 80% are of cutaneous origin. Of the approximate remaining 20%, the majority are of ocular origin; mucosal malignant melanomas (MMM) of the upper aerodigestive tract represent from 0.5-3% of melanomas of all sites {735}. In the upper aerodigestive tract, the most common site of occurrence is the sinonasal tract. PLMMM are extremely rare, with less than 60 cases reported in the literature {51,77,631, 1277,1516,1668,1843,2754,2755}. PLMMM are much more common in men than in women with over 80% of cases occurring in men {2754}. PLMMM occur over a wide age range from 35-86 years with an average age of 58 years, and are most frequent in the 6th and 7th decades of life. Most cases of PLMMM occur in Caucasians but Blacks are also affected.

Etiology

There are no known etiologic factors for PLMMM. Melanosis {912,2022}, intralaryngeal naevi {2263,2287} and lentigo

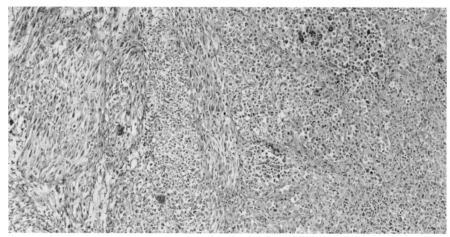

Fig. 3.69 Primary laryngeal mucosal malignant melanoma. This hypercellular proliferation shows an admixture of epithelioid and spindle-shaped cells. The epithelioid cells have a solid and nested growth, while the spindle-shaped component has a fascicular growth pattern.

{2630} of the larynx have been reported. It has been suggested that PLMMM may arise from malignant degeneration of intralaryngeal melanocytes or melanocytic lesions {2754}.

Localization

The majority (more than 60%) of PLMMM occur in the supraglottic larynx {2754, 2755}, including the epiglottis, arytenoids, aryepiglottic folds, ventricle, false vocal cord, and pyriform sinus {2755}. Other less common sites of occurrence include the glottic region along the true vocal cord and the posterior commissure. To date, there are no documented reports of PLMMM involving

the subglottic region.

Clinical features

The clinical presentation of PLMMM includes hoarseness, dysphagia, sore throat, intermittent haemoptysis, neck or jaw pain and a cervical neck mass. Symptoms generally occur over short periods of time, ranging from 3-6 months {2755}. Multicentric (synchronous, metachronous) MMM of other upper aerodigestive tract sites are not typically present.

Macroscopy

The macroscopic appearance of PLMMM vary and include nodular, mul-

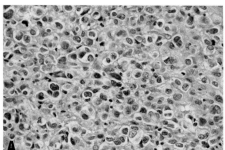 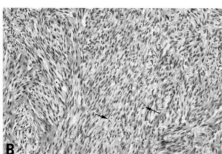 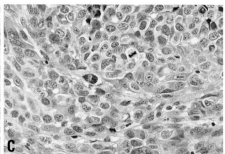

Fig. 3.68 Primary laryngeal mucosal malignant melanoma. **A** Features that can be seen in melanomas include clear appearing cytoplasm. **B** Spindle cell PLMMM comprised of a hypercellular spindle-shaped proliferation with storiform growth pattern; scattered mitotic figures are present (arrows). **C** More often, tumours are devoid of readily apparent melanin (amelanotic melanomas) or the melanin deposition is limited to isolated cells.

berry-like, sessile, polypoid, exophytic or pedunculated lesions with equally variable colour, including black, brown, red-pink, tan-grey and white {2754}. The size of the tumours range from 3-4 mm up to 8.0 cm in greatest dimension {2754}.

Histopathology

PLMMM are identical to melanomas at other sites.

In the presence of an intact laryngeal mucosa, continuity of the tumour with the surface epithelium (i.e., junctional or pagetoid changes) can be identified; however, even in the presence of intact surface epithelium, junctional changes may not be seen. Given the fact that normal melanocytes may localize to the sub-mucosal compartment within minor mucoserous glands or within the stroma {2754,2755}, junctional change is not required to render a diagnosis of PLMMM.

Prognosis and predictive factors

PLMMM has a poor prognosis. The average survival rate is usually less than 3.5 years {2159,2754} with a 5-year survival rate of less than 20% {2754}. Radical surgical excision is the treatment of choice. Adjuvant radiotherapy and chemotherapy are of questionable value in the management of PLMMM. Approximately 80% of patients with PLMMM have metastatic disease to the regional lymph nodes as well as to distant viscera (e.g., brain, lungs, bone). Pathologic criteria that are used to predict the biologic behaviour in association with cutaneous melanomas, including the depth of invasion, age and gender of the patient, and cytomorphology generally do not apply for PLMMM {2754,2755}. Further, prognostic significance has not been found for tumour thickness, level of invasion, ulceration, mitotic index or nerve/nerve sheath involvement for PLMMM {2080}.

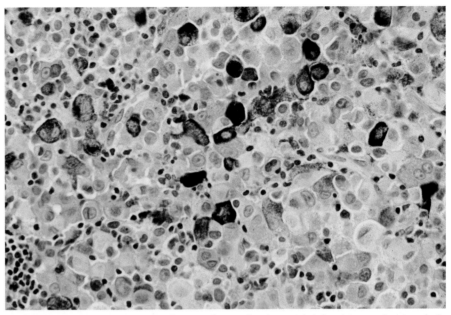

Fig. 3.70 Primary laryngeal mucosal malignant melanoma. Prominent and obvious intracytoplasmic melanin deposition is seen in this PLMMM; this extent of melanin deposition is unusual for MMM.

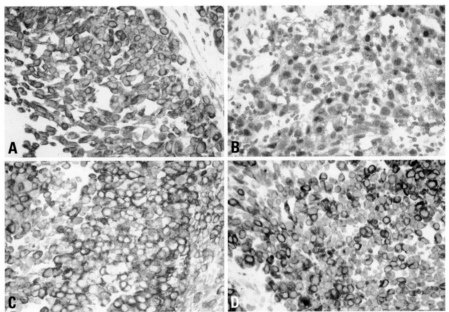

Fig. 3.71 Primary laryngeal mucosal malignant melanoma. Immunohistochemical reactivity in this epithelioid melanoma includes: **A** HMB-4 **B** S100 protein. **C** melan A and **D** vimentin.

Secondary tumours

L. Barnes
L.L.Y. Tse
J.L. Hunt

Definition

Tumours involving the hypopharynx, larynx and/or trachea that originate from, but are not in continuity with, other primary malignant neoplasms. Leukemias and lymphomas are excluded.

Epidemiology

Metastases to the larynx are uncommon. Only 11 cases over 20 years were identified in one series {160}. Eight additional cases were found in a review of more than 4000 laryngeal malignancies {7353}. In 1993, 134 cases were recorded in the world literature {735}. Metastases to the hypopharynx and trachea are even more unusual.

Age and sex distribution

Laryngeal metastases increase with age (median 58 years, range 24-83 years) and are more common in males by a ratio of 2:1 {160,741}.

Table 3.7 Site of origin of 120 tumours metastatic to larynx*

Site	Frequency (%)
Skin (melanoma)	39.1%
Kidney	13.3%
Breast	9.2%
Lung	7.5%
Prostate	6.7%
Colon	3.3%
Stomach	2.5%
Miscellaneous	18.4%

*Data based on reference {741}

Table 3.8 Site of origin of 12 tumours metastatic to trachea*

Site	Frequency (%)
Breast	33%
Colon	25%
Skin (melanoma)	17%
Uterine cervix	8%
Endometrium	8%
Ovary	8%

*Data based on references {179,485,1365,1599,1889,2775}

Etiology

The overwhelming majority of tumours that metastasize to the larynx are either malignant melanomas or carcinomas. Only 5% or fewer are from mesenchymal tumours (bone and soft tissue sarcomas).

The sites of origin of 12 tumours metastatic to the trachea are shown in Table 3.08.

Localization

Metastases to the larynx may be submu-cosal, cartilaginous or both. If cartilage is involved, it is usually only in the portion which has undergone ossification.

The most frequently affected site is the supraglottis (35-40% of all cases) followed by the subglottis (10-20%) and glottis (5-10%). Synchronous involvement of multiple laryngeal sites, however, is common and observed in about 35% of all cases {160,741}.

The pyriform sinus is the most frequent site of metastasis in the hypopharynx.

Clinical features

Generally, metastatic tumours to the larynx present with the usual supraglottic or glottic symptomatology. Richly vascular tumours, such as renal cell carcinomas and thyroid carcinomas, often result in haemoptysis. On rare occasions, the metastasis is the only evidence of an otherwise occult primary tumour.

Tracheal metastases result in cough, stridor, wheezing, dyspnoea and/or haemoptysis.

Tumour spread and staging

The majority of metastases to the larynx are haematogenous through the systemic circulation or the paravertebral venous plexus.

Prognosis and predictive factors

Metastases to the larynx, trachea or hypopharynx are usually associated with terminal, widespread disseminated disease. In some instances, the metastasis may be isolated or localized and, with appropriate therapy, a prolonged survival can be achieved.

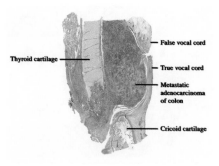

Fig. 3.72 Adenocarcinoma of the colon metastatic to the larynx. Note the involvement of both soft tissue and the inferior border of the thyroid cartilage.

CHAPTER 4

Tumours of the Oral Cavity and Oropharynx

Squamous cell carcinomas amount to more than 90% of malignant tumours of the oral cavity and oropharynx. As in other parts of the upper aerodigestive tract, there is a strong and synergistic association with tobacco smoking and alcohol abuse. In some regions, particularly the Indian subcontinent, oral cancer is among the most frequent malignancies, largely due to tobacco chewing.

The WHO Working Group has made an attempt to unify the terminology used to define the histological features of precursor lesions throughout the head and neck region. Although there has been considerable progress in the understanding of the genetic and molecular events underlying the progression of precancerous lesions to invasive carcinomas, this has yet to be translated into novel therapeutic strategies.

WHO classification of tumours of the oral cavity and oropharynx

Malignant epithelial tumours

Squamous cell carcinoma	8070/3
Verrucous carcinoma	8051/3
Basaloid squamous cell carcinoma	8083/3
Papillary squamous cell carcinoma	8052/3
Spindle cell carcinoma	8074/3
Acantholytic squamous cell carcinoma	8075/3
Adenosquamous carcinoma	8560/3
Carcinoma cuniculatum	8051/3
Lymphoepithelial carcinoma	8082/3

Epithelial precursor lesions

Benign epithelial tumours

Papillomas	8050/0
Squamous cell papilloma and verruca vulgaris	
Condyloma acuminatum	
Focal epithelial hyperplasia	
Granular cell tumour	9580/0
Keratoacanthoma	8071/1

Salivary gland tumours

Salivary gland carcinomas	
Acinic cell carcinoma	8550/3
Mucoepidermoid carcinoma	8430/3
Adenoid cystic carcinoma	8200/3
Polymorphous low-grade adenocarcinoma	8525/3
Basal cell adenocarcinoma	8147/3
Epithelial-myoepithelial carcinoma	8562/3
Clear cell carcinoma, not otherwise specified	8310/3
Cystadenocarcinoma	8450/3
Mucinous adenocarcinoma	8480/3
Oncocytic carcinoma	8290/3
Salivary duct carcinoma	8500/3
Myoepithelial carcinoma	8982/3
Carcinoma ex pleomorphic adenoma	8941/3
Salivary gland adenomas	
Pleomorphic adenoma	8940/0
Myoepithelioma	8982/0
Basal cell adenoma	8147/0
Canalicular adenoma	8149/0
Duct papilloma	8503/0
Cystadenoma	8440/0

Soft tissue tumours

Kaposi sarcoma	9140/3
Lymphangioma	9170/0
Ectomesenchymal chondromyxoid tumour	
Focal oral mucinosis	
Congenital granular cell epulis	

Haematolymphoid tumours

Diffuse large B-cell lymphoma (DLBCL)	9680/3
Mantle cell lymphoma	9673/3
Follicular lymphoma	9690/3
Extranodal marginal zone B-cell lymphoma of MALT type	9699/3
Burkitt lymphoma	9687/3
T-cell lymphoma (including anaplastic large cell lymphoma	9714/3
Extramedullary plasmacytoma	9734/3
Langerhans cell histiocytosis	9751/1
Extramedullary myeloid sarcoma	9930/3
Follicular dendritic cell sarcoma / tumour	9758/3

Mucosal malignant melanoma	8720/3

Secondary tumours

---

[1] Morphology code of the International Classification of Diseases for Oncology (ICD-O) {821} and the Systematized Nomenclature of Medicine (http://snomed.org). Behaviour is coded /0 for benign tumours, /3 for malignant tumours, and /1 for borderline or uncertain behaviour.

TNM classification of carcinomas of the oral cavity and oropharynx

TNM classification of carcinomas of the lip and oral cavity [1,2]

T – Primary tumour
TX   Primary tumour cannot be assessed
T0   No evidence of primary tumour
Tis   Carcinoma in situ
T1   Tumour 2 cm or less in greatest dimension
T2   Tumour more than 2 cm but not more than 4 cm in greatest dimension
T3   Tumour more than 4 cm in greatest dimension
T4a (lip)
      Tumour invades through cortical bone, inferior alveolar nerve, floor of mouth, or skin (chin or nose)
T4a (oral cavity)
      Tumour invades through cortical bone, into deep/extrinsic muscle of tongue (genioglossus, hyoglossus, palatoglossus, and styloglossus), maxillary sinus, or skin of face
T4b (lip and oral cavity)
      Tumour invades masticator space, pterygoid plates, or skull base; or encases internal carotid artery
Note: Superficial erosion alone of bone/tooth socket by gingival primary is not sufficient to classify a tumour as T4.

N – Regional lymph nodes##
NX   Regional lymph nodes cannot be assessed
N0   No regional lymph node metastasis
N1   Metastasis in a single ipsilateral lymph node, 3 cm or less in greatest dimension
N2   Metastasis as specified in N2a, 2b, 2c below
N2a   Metastasis in a single ipsilateral lymph node, more than 3 cm but not more than 6 cm in greatest dimension
N2b   Metastasis in multiple ipsilateral lymph nodes, none more than 6 cm in greatest dimension
N2c   Metastasis in bilateral or contralateral lymph nodes, none more than 6 cm in greatest dimension
N3   Metastasis in a lymph node more than 6 cm in greatest dimension

Note: Midline nodes are considered ipsilateral nodes.

M – Distant metastasis
MX   Distant metastasis cannot be assessed
M0   No distant metastasis
M1   Distant metastasis

Stage grouping

Stage 0	Tis	N0	M0
Stage I	T1	N0	M0
Stage II	T2	N0	M0
Stage III	T1, T2	N1	M0
	T3	N0, N1	M0
Stage IVA	T1, T2, T3	N2	M0
	T4a	N0, N1, N2	M0
Stage IVB	Any T	N3	M0
	T4b	Any N	M0
Stage IVC	Any T	Any N	M1

The regional lymph nodes are the cervical nodes.

TNM classification of carcinomas of the oropharynx [1,2]

T – Primary tumour
TX   Primary tumour cannot be assessed
T0   No evidence of primary tumour
Tis   Carcinoma in situ
T1   Tumour 2 cm or less in greatest dimension
T2   Tumour more than 2 cm but not more than 4 cm in greatest dimension
T3   Tumour more than 4 cm in greatest dimension
T4a   Tumour invades any of the following: larynx, deep/extrinsic muscle of tongue (genioglossus, hyoglossus, palatoglossus, and styloglossus), medial pterygoid, hard palate, and mandible
T4b   Tumour invades any of the following: lateral pterygoid muscle, pterygoid plates, lateral nasopharynx, skull base; or encases the carotid artery

N – Regional lymph nodes##
NX   Regional lymph nodes cannot be assessed
N0   No regional lymph node metastasis
N1   Metastasis in a single ipsilateral lymph node, 3 cm or less in greatest dimension
N2   Metastasis as specified in N2a, 2b, 2c below
N2a   Metastasis in a single ipsilateral lymph node, more than 3 cm but not more than 6 cm in greatest dimension
N2b   Metastasis in multiple ipsilateral lymph nodes, none more than 6 cm in greatest dimension
N2c   Metastasis in bilateral or contralateral lymph nodes, none more than 6 cm in greatest dimension
N3   Metastasis in a lymph node more than 6 cm in greatest dimension

Note: Midline nodes are considered ipsilateral nodes.

M – Distant metastasis
MX   Distant metastasis cannot be assessed
M0   No distant metastasis
M1   Distant metastasis

Stage grouping

Stage 0	Tis	N0	M0
Stage I	T1	N0	M0
Stage II	T2	N0	M0
Stage III	T1, T2	N1	M0
	T3	N0, N1	M0
Stage IVA	T1,T2,T3	N2	M0
	T4a	N0, N1, N2	M0
Stage IVB	T4b	Any N	M0
	Any T	N3	M0
Stage IVC	Any T	Any N	M1

The regional lymph nodes are the cervical nodes.

[1] {947,2418}.
[2] A help desk for specific questions about the TNM classification is available at www.uicc.org/index.php?id=508 .

Tumours of the oral cavity and oropharynx: Introduction

P.J. Slootweg
J.W. Eveson

Tumours of the oral cavity and oropharynx may be either epithelial, mesenchymal, or haematolymphoid. The epithelial tumours may be classified as those originating within the epithelium lining of the oral cavity and oropharynx and those derived from salivary gland tissue. Both will be included in this chapter, including precursor lesions where appropriate.

For the haematolymphoid diseases, the reader is referred to the WHO Classification of Tumours of Haematopoietic and Lymphoid Tissues {1197}, for mesenchymal ones to the WHO Classification of Tumours of Soft Tissue and Bone {775}.

Oral Cavity

The oral cavity extends from the lips to the palatoglossal folds. The outer vestibule is enclosed by the cheeks and lips and forms a slit-like space separating it from the gingivae and teeth. It is limited above and below by mucosal reflections from the lips and cheeks.

The space bordered by the teeth and gingivae is the oral cavity proper. It is bounded inferiorly by the floor of the mouth and tongue and superiorly by the hard palate. The buccal mucosa extends from the commissure of the lips anteriorly to the palatoglossal fold posteriorly. It is lined by thick, non-keratinized stratified squamous epithelium and contains variable numbers of sebaceous glands (Fordyce spots or granules) and minor salivary glands. The duct of the parotid gland (Stensen's duct) opens on a papilla or fold opposite the upper second permanent molar tooth.

The mucous membrane related to the teeth is the gingiva. The gingival mucosa surrounds the necks of the teeth and the alveolar mucosa overlies the alveolar bone and extends to the vestibular reflections. The junction between these two parts is marked by a faint scalloped line called the mucogingival junction. The gingival mucosa is pink and firmly attached to the underlying bone and necks of the teeth (attached gingiva) except for a free marginal area. It is usually non-keratinized or parakeratinized. The alveolar mucosa is reddish and covered by thin, non-keratinized stratified squamous epithelium. Minor salivary glands may be seen in the alveolar mucosa and occasionally the attached gingiva.

The hard palate is continuous anteriorly with the maxillary alveolar arches and posteriorly with the soft palate. A median raphe extends anteriorly from this junction to the incisive fossa into which the nasopalatine foramen opens. Most of the palatal mucosa is firmly bound to the underlying bone forming a mucoperiosteum. It is covered by orthokeratinized stratified squamous epithelium and posteriorly contains many minor mucous salivary glands.

The oral part of the tongue (anterior two thirds) lies in front of the V-shaped sulcus terminalis. It is mobile and attached to the floor of the mouth anteriorly by a median lingual fraenum. The dorsal part is covered by stratified squamous epithelium and contains several types of papillae. The most numerous are the hair-like filiform papillae which are heavily keratinized. There are less numerous and evenly scattered fungiform papillae which form pink nodules and contain taste buds. Taste buds here and in other oral sites are occasionally mistaken for junctional melanocytic proliferation or Pagetoid infiltration. In front of the sulcus terminalis there are 10-12 circumvallate papillae. These contain many taste buds on the surface and in a deep groove that surrounds each papilla. In addition, the ducts of minor serous salivary glands

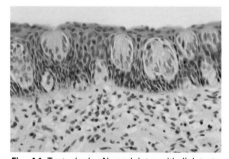

Fig. 4.1 Taste buds. Normal intraepithelial taste buds are sometimes confused with melanocytic lesions and pagetoid infiltration..

(von Ebner's glands) open into the base of the groove. At the postero-lateral aspect of the tongue where it meets the palatoglossal fold there are the leaf shaped foliate papillae. These also may contain taste buds on the surface and the core of the papillae often contains lymphoid aggregates similar to those in the rest of the Waldeyer ring. In addition, there are minor salivary glands in the underlying lingual musculature. The ventrum of the tongue is covered by thin, non-keratinized stratified squamous epithelium which is continuous with similar mucosa in the floor of the mouth. Minor salivary glands (glands of Blandin and Nuhn) are present, predominantly towards the midline and deep within the lingual musculature. They can extend to involve the tip of the tongue.

The floor of the mouth is a horseshoe-shaped area between the ventrum of the tongue medially and the gingivae of the lower teeth anteriorly and laterally. It extends to the palatoglossal folds distally and is in continuity with the retromolar pad behind the lower third molar tooth. The mucosa covers the major sublingual glands and the submandibular (Wharton's) ducts which open anteriorly onto the submandibular papillae on either side of the median sublingual fraenum. It is important to note that 75% of oral squamous cell carcinomas have been reported to arise in an area that comprises the floor of the mouth and adjacent lingual mucosa, sublingual sulcus and retromolar region {1767}. This region forms only about 20% of the total mucosal area. The zone of increased susceptibility has been called the 'drainage area' as it is thought that any carcinogens present in the mouth pool there before being swallowed. It is obvious, therefore, that any precursor lesions in these areas should be regarded as highly suspicious.

Oropharynx

The oropharynx lies behind the oral cavity. It is bounded superiorly by the soft palate and inferiorly by a hypothetical horizontal line level with the tip of the epiglottis. Anteriorly are the isthmus of the fauces and the posterior third of the tongue, and the lateral wall is formed by the palatopharyngeal arches and the palatine tonsils. The posterior wall contains the pharyngeal tonsils.

The palatine tonsils are two masses of lymphoid tissue situated in the triangular recess (tonsillar sulcus) between the anterior and posterior faucial pillars. They extend from the soft palate to the dorsum of the tongue. The surface is convoluted and deep clefts or crypts can penetrate almost its full thickness. The bulk of the tonsil consists of lymphoid tissue arranged in nodules or follicles. There are no afferent lymphatics and no subcapsular sinuses. Squamous cell carcinomas at this site can invade deeply into the underlying tissues, base of tongue and lateral pharyngeal wall. They also have a particular tendency to extend upwards into the nasopharynx.

The soft palate is a mobile, muscular flap attached to the posterior edge of the hard palate and extending to a free margin posteriorly. The uvula forms a small, conical, midline process. The oral surface of the soft palate is covered by non-keratinized stratified squamous epithelium and contains many minor mucous glands. The uvula contains mainly fat and a few muscle fibres but minor salivary glands may also be seen and occasionally salivary gland tumours develop at this site.

The pharyngeal part of the tongue is immobile and has a bossellated surface due to the presence of underlying lymphoid tissue forming the lingual tonsils. Minor salivary glands are also present.

Lymphatic drainage of mouth and oropharynx

The main sites of lymphatic drainage from the mouth and oropharynx are the jugulodigastric, submandibular and submental lymph nodes. Lymph vessels from the gingiva usually drain to the submandibular lymph nodes but those in the lower incisor region run to the submental nodes. Most of the vessels from the palate run to the jugulodigastric group but some involve the retropharyngeal nodes. There is a rich lymphatic plexus in the tongue and the main vessels can be subdivided into marginal and central. The marginal vessels drain the lateral third of the dorsum and contiguous later-

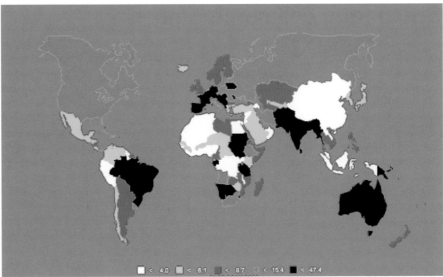

Fig. 4.2 Global incidence rates of tumours of the oral cavity and oropharynx (all ages) in males. Age-standardized rates (ASR, world standard population) per 100,000 population and year. From J. Ferlay et al., Globocan 2000 {730}.

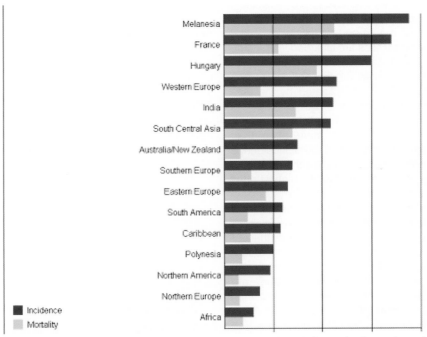

Fig. 4.3 Incidence and mortality rates for tumours of the oral cavity and pharynx (excl. nasopharynx), all ages, in males. Age-standardized rates (ASR, world standard population) per 100,000 population and year. From J. Ferlay et al., Globocan 2000 {730}.

al border and part of the ventrum of the tongue. They run to the ipsilateral submandibular nodes. Those towards the tip of the tongue drain to the submental nodes. Central lymph vessels drain to the submandibular nodes on both sides. Some marginal and central vessels run directly to the jugulodigastric group but some can pass direct to the jugulo-omohyoid nodes. Vessels from the area of the circumvallate papillae and posterior third

of the tongue drain to the jugulodigastric, jugulo-omohyoid or intermediate nodes, either unilaterally or bilaterally. Most of the lymphatics of the palatine tonsils drain to the jugulodigastric nodes.

Squamous cell carcinoma

N. Johnson
S. Franceschi
J. Ferlay
K. Ramadas
S. Schmid
D.G. MacDonald
J.E. Bouquot
P.J. Slootweg

Definition

An invasive epithelial neoplasm with varying degrees of squamous differentiation and a propensity to early and extensive lymph node metastases, occurring predominantly in alcohol and tobacco-using adults in the 5th and 6th decades of life.

ICD-O code   8070/3

Epidemiology

More than 90% of malignant neoplasms of the oral cavity and oropharynx are squamous cell carcinomas of the lining mucosae with relatively rare neoplasms arising in minor salivary glands and soft tissues. It is important to specify which anatomical sites are included in epidemiological data. Separate assessment of incidence rates for the oral cavity and oropharynx is complicated by the difficulty of assigning a site of origin to tumours that are often advanced.

Males are affected more often than females because of heavier indulgence in both tobacco and alcohol habits in most countries: in India the highest rates of intraoral cancer may be found in women who chew tobacco heavily. The male to female ratio is, however, globally lower for cancer of the oral cavity than for cancer of the oropharynx, perhaps suggesting that higher exposure to tobacco smoking and alcohol drinking are required to induce oropharyngeal than oral cancer {796}.

Globally some 389,650 cases occurred in the year 2000; 266,672 for the oral cavity (ICD-9 140-5) and 122,978 for the oropharynx (ICD-9 146,8-9) {1981}. This represents 5% of all cancers for men and 2% for women.

In males, the country with the highest rate in the western world is currently France, with extremely elevated rates also in French-speaking Switzerland, Northern Italy, Central and Eastern Europe (especially Hungary) and parts of Latin America. Rates are elevated amongst both men and women throughout South Asia. In the USA incidence rates are two-fold higher in Black men

than White men {1981}. Very high rates in the IARC database for Melanesia, presumably associated with areca nut and tobacco habits, are based on small numbers and need confirmation {730,1981}. The high incidence rates in Australasia are explained by lip cancer in fair-skinned races which has a comparatively low mortality rate.

Much of Europe and Japan is experiencing alarming rises in incidence, with a strong cohort effect, those born from approximately 1930 onwards showing significantly increased incidence and mortality. In North America there are statistically significant falls in Whites, but Blacks continue to show worse outcomes. Globally, with the exception of the most highly specialized treatment centres, survival rates have not improved for decades.

Significant increases in incidence in younger subjects, particularly males, have been reported from many western countries in recent decades {1534,2259}.

Etiology

Tobacco smoking and alcohol

The dominant risk factors are tobacco use and alcohol abuse, which are strongly synergistic {228}. Alcohol and tobacco account for 75% of the disease burden of oral and oropharyngeal malignancies in Europe, the Americas and Japan {227,1862}. For the highest levels of consumption compared to the lowest ones relative risks from 70 to over 100 have been shown {287,1811}. Relative risks in case-control studies showing a supermultiplicative effect in the oral cavity, between additive and multiplicative in the oesophagus, and multiplicative in the larynx, reflecting degree of contact with both these agents at these sites {797}.

Most of the rise in western countries in recent years has been attributed to rising alcohol consumption in northern Europe {1597 and rises in tobacco consumption in parts of southern Europe. Significant risk increases have also been reported amongst non-drinking smokers and, to a lesser extent, non-smoking heavy

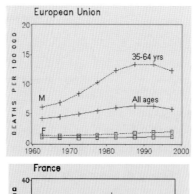
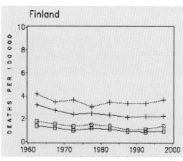
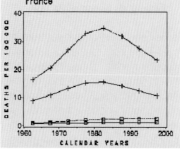
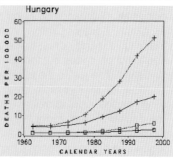

Fig. 4.4 Trends in mortality from cancer of the oral cavity and pharynx in some European countries. The large differences observed (currrently 10-fold in between Hungary and Finland) largely reflect past success and failure in tobacco and alcohol control. From F. Levi et al. {1483}.

drinkers {1406}. Studies that have attempted to estimate a difference between wine, beer and hard liquors generally indicate that heavy consumption of all types of alcoholic beverage confers risk, the differences in risk estimates being largely due to socio-cultural correlates of drinking patterns in various populations {142,1404}.

Ultraviolet light and contact with smoking appliances are important for lip vermillion.

Tobacco chewing

Oral smokeless tobacco is a major cause of oral {969} and oropharyngeal {2908} squamous cell carcinoma in the Indian subcontinent, parts of South-East Asia, China and Taiwan and in emigrant communities therefrom, especially when consumed in betel quids containing areca nut and calcium hydroxide (lime). Areca nut has been declared a known human carcinogen by an IARC Expert Group (2003). In India chewing accounts for nearly 50% of cancers of the oral cavity and oropharynx in men and over 90% in women {108}. Traditional tobacco products used in Sudan and the Middle East, which are powdered and fermented and mixed with sodium bicarbonate, contain very high levels of tobacco-specific nitrosamines and are highly carcinogenic {1171}. Those forms of non-flue cured smokeless tobacco used as oral snuff in Scandinavia and North America is less carcinogenic {1230} – though they cause nicotine addiction.

Human papillomavirus (HPV) infection

HPVs, especially those genotypes of known high oncogenic potential in uterine cervix and skin such as HPV 16 and 18, are found in a variable but small proportion of oral, and up to 50% of tonsillar and oropharyngeal SCCs, especially the tonsil. Recent studies suggest that HPV may be responsible for a small fraction of oral, and up to 40% of oropharyngeal, cancers {888,1077}. This has lead to speculation that HPV infection, perhaps arising from oral/genital contact, might be important in some cases {2284}. Of interest is the observation that HPV-containing cancers at these sites do not generally show TP53 mutations, contrary to HPV DNA-negative cancers {660,1077}. It is well known that HPV 16 E6 protein inactivates p53 protein, suggesting that HPV and smoking might operate, in part, on the same criti-

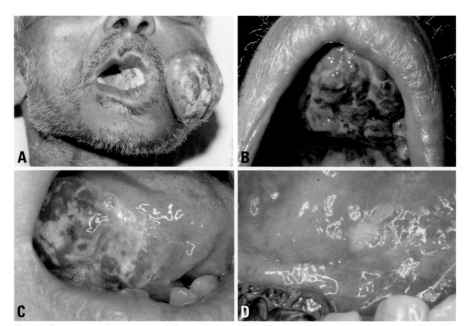

Fig. 4.5 Squamous cell carcinoma. **A** Exophytic growth involving the left buccal mucosa and overlying skin in a 65 year old male who chewed betel quid and smoked tobacco. **B** An exophytic growth arising from the left palate. **C** Squamous cell carcinoma of the tongue. **D** Early squamous cell carcinoma of lateral border of the tongue.

cal step in the multistage process of carcinogenesis at these sites.

Prevention

Recent work on risk factors in younger cases emphasises the importance of early and heavy tobacco and alcohol use, the protective effect of diets rich in fresh fruits and vegetables, but with a substantial minority without these established risk factors {1534}.

The protective effect of diets rich in trace elements and antioxidant vitamins is well demonstrated in many countries, especially in Italian studies {1628,2563}. Though more controversial, a contribution from poor oral hygiene is also suggested {108,2548}.

Second primary tumours

It has been recognised for a long time that patients with oral cancer are at risk of second tumours in the upper aerodigestive tract. This has been reported to occur in 10-35% of cases {2676}. These may be synchronous with the index tumour or, if occurring after an interval of longer than six months are described as metachronous. Recurrence of the index tumour after treatment can be diagnosed by the pathologist where the tumour is in deeper tissue and not associated with the epithelial surface. However, the most frequent situation of second tumours is when they

arise from surface epithelium adjacent to the treated index tumour. On morphological grounds these are diagnosed as second primary tumours. The increasing use of molecular biological techniques has allowed distinction to be made between molecularly distinct second primary tumours and second field tumours derived from the same genetically altered field as the index tumour {248}.

Localization

Tumours may arise in any part of the oral cavity. The most common sites vary geographically reflecting different risk factors. Lip SCC arise almost exclusively on the lower lip. Within the oral cavity, the subsites at which tumours may be located include: buccal mucosa, upper and lower gingiva, hard palate, anterior two-thirds of the tongue, including dorsal, ventral and lateral surfaces, and the floor of mouth. Many tumours are large at presentation and the tumour site is then recorded as essentially the centre of the tumour. Analysis of small symptomless tumours shows the highest frequency in floor of mouth, ventrolateral tongue and soft palate complex {1655}. This suggests that tumours arise at these sites, but spread preferentially to involve other sites such as tongue, being then recorded as lingual lesions. The clinical relevance of this observation is to emphasise the

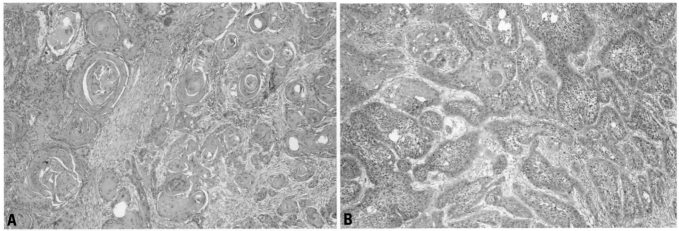

Fig. 4.6 A Well-differentiated squamous cell carcinoma (SCC), characterized by abundant formation of keratin pearls. **B** Moderately differentiated SCC. Cells form large anastomosing areas in which keratin pearls are formed. They are not very numerous and the main component consists of cells with pronounced cytonuclear atypia.

importance of close examination of high-risk sites. The oropharynx consists of the base of the tongue (posterior third), vallecula, tonsil with tonsillar fossae and pillars, glossotonsillar sulci, posterior wall and superior wall composed of the inferior surface of the soft palate and the uvula. The most common oropharyngeal site of involvement for SCC is the base of tongue.

Clinical features

Signs and symptoms

Patients with small oral and oropharyngeal SCC are often asymptomatic or may present with vague symptoms and minimal physical findings. Hence, a high index of clinical suspicion is needed to diagnose small lesions, especially if the patients have tobacco and alcohol habits. Patients may present with red lesions, mixed red and white lesions, or white plaques. Co-existing white plaques (leukoplakia) may be observed adjacent to carcinomas and this implies an origin in a pre-existing white lesion though the prevalence of this association varies considerably in different populations.

However, most patients present with signs and symptoms of locally advanced disease. The clinical features may vary according to the affected intraoral subsite. Mucosal growth and ulceration, pain, referred pain to the ear, malodour from the mouth, difficulty with speaking, opening the mouth, chewing, difficulty and pain with swallowing, bleeding, weight loss, and neck swelling are the common presenting symptoms of locally advanced oral and oropharyngeal cancers. Occasionally, patients present with enlarged neck nodes without any symp-toms from oral or oropharyngeal lesions. Extremely advanced cancers present as ulceroproliferative growths with areas of necrosis and extension to surrounding structures, such as bone, muscle and skin. In the terminal stages, patients may present with orocutaneous fistula, intractable bleeding, severe anaemia and cachexia.

Cancer of the buccal mucosa may present as an ulcer with indurated raised margin, exophytic or verrucous growth or with the site of origin depending upon the preferential side of chewing and placement of betel quid. In advanced stages, these lesions infiltrate into the adjacent bone and overlying skin. Cancer of the tongue may appear as a red area interspersed with nodules or as an ulcer infiltrating deeply, leading to reduced mobility of the tongue. These tumours are

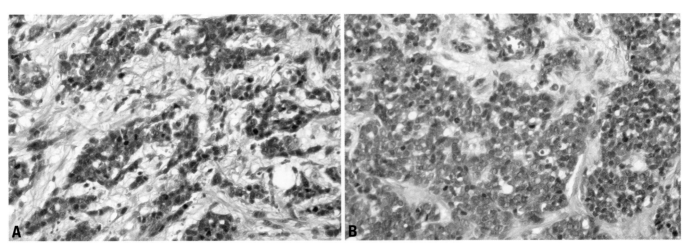

Fig. 4.7 Poorly differentiated SCC. **A** Cells with atypical nuclei and a small rim of eosinophilic cytoplasm form strands and small nests. **B** Cells in a poorly differentiated SCC tend to have more vesicular nuclei. The cells in this tumour are more cohesive, forming larger tumour areas than the lesion shown in A.

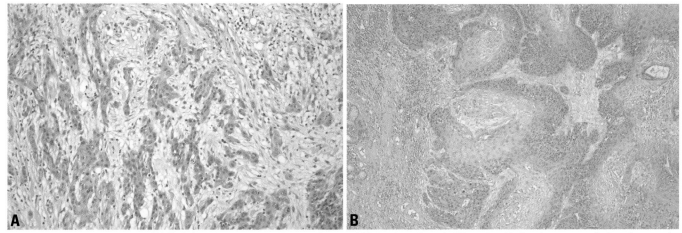

Fig. 4.8 Squamous cell carcinoma (SCC). **A** Growth pattern of a diffusely infiltrating SCC. In this moderately differentiated lesion, the tumour cells form tiny strands. This growth pattern is a prognostically unfavourable feature. **B** Moderately differentiated SCC growing in large cohesive fields. This pattern is prognostically more favourable than the diffuse growth shown in Figure A.

painful. Cancers of the floor of mouth may arise as a red area, a small ulcer or as a papillary lesion. Most patients present with discomfort or irritation at the site of the tumour. Advanced stages are associated with drooling. Cancers of the lower lip usually arise in the vermilion border and appear as a crusty indurated or ulcerated lesion. Cancers of the upper lip are rare, often originate on the skin and spread to the mucosa. Cancer of the gingiva usually presents as an ulceroproliferative growth. Tumours of the alveolar ridge may occasionally present as difficulty in wearing denture plates or as loosening of teeth associated with pain and bleeding during brushing of teeth. Tumours of the hard palate often present as papillary or exophytic growths, rather than a flat or ulcerated lesion.

Cancer of soft palate and uvula often appear as an ulcerative lesion with raised margins or as fungating masses. Tonsillar cancers generally appear as an exophytic or ulcerative lesion. Sometimes they can present as enlarged neck nodes without any other signs and symptoms. Cancer of the base of tongue presents late in the course of the disease as a grossly ulcerated, painful, indurated growth.

More than two-thirds of the patients with buccal mucosal and gingival cancers in South Asia present with submandibular lymph node enlargement. More than three fourths of patients with tongue, floor of mouth and oropharyngeal cancers in South Asia present with neck swellings implying clinically obvious lymph node metastasis. In the West lymph node involvement is common at presentation in oropharyngeal SCC.

Imaging

Intraoral and dental radiographs, in combination with orthopantomography, may help in identifying involvement of the underlying bone. Three-dimensional imaging with computed tomography (CT) and magnetic resonance imaging (MRI) is frequently used to supplement the clinical evaluation and staging of the primary tumour and regional lymph nodes. CT scan or MRI give more information about the local extent of the disease and also help to identify lymph node metastases. CT scanning is useful in evaluating involvement of cortical bone. MRI is more informative when evaluating the extent of soft tissue and neurovascular bundle involvement. The combination of soft tissue characterisation and anatomical localization afforded by CT and MRI make them valuable tools in the

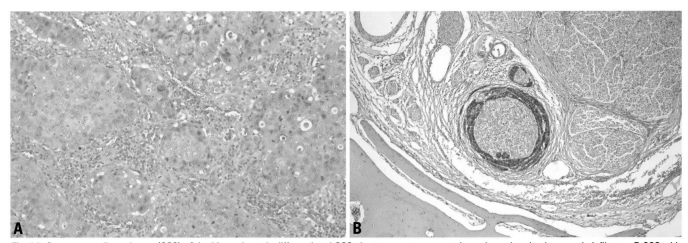

Fig. 4.9 Squamous cell carcinoma (SCC). **A** In this moderately differentiated SCC, the tumour stroma contains a dense lymphoplasmacytic infiltrate. **B** SCC with perineural growth, spreading alongside the inferior alveolar nerve.

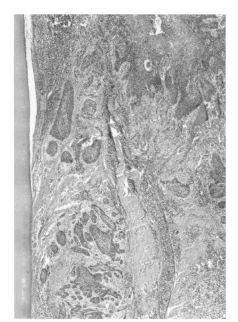

Fig. 4.10 Periodontal ligament involvement by a squamous cell carcinoma (SCC).

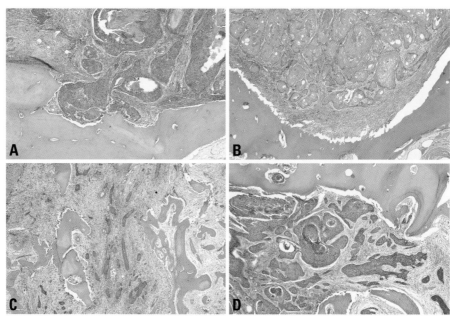

Fig. 4.11 Squamous cell carcinoma (SCC). **A** Superficial erosion of the mandibular bone has perforated the cortical bone. As there is no spread in the bone marrow, this case of SCC does not meet the requirements for classification as T4. **B** Saucerization by SCC. In this case of, there is substantial loss of bone due to endocortical tumour growth (meets the requirements T4). **C** Permeative infiltration of bone by SCC growing diffusely in the marrow cavities of the mandibular bone (T4). There is also heavy osteoclast-mediated bone resorption. **D** Bone invasion by SCC with diffuse growth in the mandibular bone.

preoperative assessment of patients with oral or oropharyngeal cancers. Distant metastasis from oral and oropharyngeal cancer is uncommon at presentation. At minimum, a routine radiograph of the chest is performed to rule out lung metastases.

Relevant diagnostic procedures
Optimal therapy and survival from oral cancer depend on adequate diagnosis and assessment of the primary tumour and its clinical extent. Physical examination should include visual inspection and palpation of all mucosal surfaces, bimanual palpation of the floor of the mouth, and clinical assessment of the neck for lymph node involvement.
The diagnosis is confirmed by biopsy. The specimen is taken from the clinically most suspicious area, avoiding necrotic or grossly ulcerated areas, and more than one biopsy site may need to be chosen.
In patients with enlarged cervical lymph nodes and an obvious primary in the oral cavity or oropharynx, the biopsy is always taken from the primary site and not from the lymph node. In such situations, fine needle aspiration cytology may be carried out to verify the involvement of the node.
If no obvious primary site is found in patients presenting with neck nodes, fine-needle aspiration of the lymph node can be performed to help establish the diag-

nosis. In patients for whom fine needle aspiration is non-diagnostic and SCC is strongly suspected, excisional lymph node biopsy is a last resort, as subsequent curative therapy may be compromised by this procedure. The search for an occult primary tumour may include direct pharyngolaryngoscopy with biopsy of high-risk sites like base of tongue, nasopharynx, and usually a diagnostic tonsillectomy, as well as other imaging modalities. Open lymph node biopsy is carried out only when the lesion cannot be identified by aspiration biopsy or in patients with suspected lymphoma.
Patients with SCC of the oral cavity or oropharynx have a risk of multiple primary tumours in the pharynx or larynx, as well as in the tracheobronchial region and oesophagus so routine panendoscopy is often performed to evaluate these sites.

Tumour spread and staging
Staging is carried out according to the TNM classification {947,2418}. Recent additions to the coding have been provided for micrometatses, isolated tumour cells, findings in sentinel nodes and tumour detection by molecular methods. Some of these are discussed in the following sections.
Local spread of oral SCC, in the early

stages, is relatively predictable in tissues that have not been previously irradiated. It is influenced by local anatomical features. Lip SCC spreads superficially and then into deeper tissues. Floor of mouth SCC spreads superficially rather than in depth, being unlikely to invade into the mylohyoid muscle or the sublingual gland until a late stage. Tumour involving the lateral margin of tongue, whether arising there directly or by superficial spread from the floor of mouth, tends to spread in depth. The intrinsic muscles of tongue run in small bundles in all directions such that invading tumour encounters some muscle running at right angles to the surface. The line of least resistance to tumour spread is therefore along these muscle bundles and into the tongue. Tumours of palate spread superficially rather than in depth and this is also true for more posterior tumours of the oropharynx.
For most oral SCC other than tongue, the extent of spread in an area can be predicted from the extent of surface involvement. Tongue and tonsil tumours can spread beneath intact normal appearing surface, giving a larger area of tumour involvement. Spread of oral SCC into bone is a frequent problem. The mandible is involved much more frequently than the

maxilla. In dentate jaws the usual route of entry into mandible is along the periodontal ligament. In edentulous areas of mandible the tumour spread is through the crest of the alveolus directly into the marrow spaces between trabeculae of cancellous bone {1682}. This occurs because of failure of formation of an intact cortex of alveolar bone as resorption of edentulous alveolus progresses. Tumours in the mandible can involve the inferior alveolar nerve {1683} with a particular likelihood of spread posteriorly along the nerve, sometimes extending well beyond the mandibular foramen. Cancers arising in gingiva or alveolus and those involving these sites by extension from adjacent sites are unlikely to invade into the mandible other than by periodontal ligament or the crest of edentulous alveolus. Extension into the mandible through foramina, for example the mental foramen from lip cancer, does occur, but is uncommon.

Spread in previously irradiated tissues

Tumour spread in previously irradiated soft tissues tends to be more extensive and less predictable than in normal tissues and as a consequence requires more extensive surgery if excision is attempted. Tumour invasion into irradiated mandible tends to occur wherever the tumour approaches bone, often at multiple sites {1682}.

Lymphatic spread

Spread to local lymph nodes worsens the prognosis in oral and oropharyngeal cancer. The mechanism of spread from the primary site to lymph nodes is almost always by embolism. Permeation in lymphatics adjacent to tumours is uncommon and it is debatable if this spread extends as far as lymph nodes. Once tumour is present in the neck, however, spread between nodes may be embolic or by permeation. The lymph nodes in the neck are divided into levels. The lymphatic draianage from different head and neck sites is realtively predictable {1789}. Levels at high risk for metastasis from oral cavity SCC are Levels I, II and III, and to a lesser extent Level IV. Although Level II is the most frequently involved, some tumours spread to Level III or IV, with or without involvement of Level I. This has given rise to the concept of skip metastsasis. In reality the lymphatic drainage is complex and does not follow a regular sequence of lev-

els of involvement in many patients {2817}. Bilateral spread to the neck is likely to occur from tumours involving the midline, especially tumours of posterior tongue or soft palate. Extracapsular spread of tumour involving lymph nodes is associated with a poor prognosis {2819}.

There have been many studies attempting to predict the presence of lymphatic spread from features of the primary tumour {872,2820}. Tumour size and site are relevant. Tumour differentiation is not a reliable predictor. The pattern of the invasive front is a useful predictor in that a non-cohesive front is associated with increased likelihood of metastasis. Other factors associated with increased risk of metastasis are perineural spread at the invasive front, lymphovascualr invasion and tumour thickness. The tumour thickness is measured from the deepest tumour invasion to the presumed original surface level, that is, ignoring exophytic growth or assessing the original surface level in ulcerated tumours. For diagnostic purposes a thickness of 5mm or greater is used as indicating increased risk of nodal spread {395}.

Haematogenous spread

Until relatively recently, haematogenous spread of oral and oropharyngeal cancer has been regarded as less important than local and lymphatic spread. However, its importance is increasing as loco-regional control improves. Blood borne spread most often involves lung {754,1958}. The best predictor of the likelihood of this spread is involvement of the neck at multiple levels. This suggests that the route of entry of tumours into the circulation is most often via the large veins in the neck and that haematogenous spread is in effect tertiary spread following extracapsular spread from neck nodes.

Sentinel node biopsy

This is currently an experimental technique {2057} that is under active evaluation by prospective clinical trials and it is not practised at all centres. It is a technique used primarily for staging a clinically N0 neck. in an effort to avoid a neck dissection. If a clinically N0 neck is followed untreated until tumour development occurs, the prognosis can be very poor {57,977}. Studies on the incidence of occult metastases in N0 necks {753} have shown tumour spread in only a small

minority of patients. Therefore, if neck dissection is undertaken either prophylactically or as a staging procedure, on patients with N0 necks, a large majority will have unnecessary surgery, as the neck will be found to be free from tumour. The sentinel node is the first draining lymph node from a tumour. It is assumed that if the sentinel node can be shown to be free from tumour, then the lymphatic basin is free from tumour and neck dissection is not required. By contrast, sentinel node positive patients can be selected for further therapy. Sentinel nodes are identified by a combination of lymphoscintigraphy and injection of blue dye in the tumour bed and then sampling draining nodes identified. In reality, more than one sentinel node is found in many cases {2345} indicating that tumours drain to more than a single first echelon node, presumably from different parts of the tumour.

Sampled sentinel nodes should be fully examined by the pathologist. This usually involves bisecting the node in the largest diameter and then undertaking extensive sampling. Some pathologists undertake frozen sections on bisected fresh nodes. If this is done it is important to use a technique whereby the cut surface is frozen on a flat surface and only early sections are examined. This is to ensure that as little node as possible is examined at this stage in order not to compromise full examination of the node. Paraffin processed blocks are then examined with H and E sections of the early sections of the blocks. If these show no tumour, more detailed sampling with immunocytochemistry for cytokeratins and sampling through the block is required. True serial sectioning is impracticable for routine use. A compromise is step sectioning at intervals of 150μm with examination of H and E sections and AE1/3 reacted sections {2202}. The importance of these sections is that suspicious areas on immunocytochemistry can be identified in the H and E sections. These may be viable tumour cells, but other possible causes of cytokeratin positivity, such as inclusion of normal salivary gland epithelium or thyroid follicles, either occult metastases or lateral aberrant thyroid, need to be identified. Another not infrequent finding is areas of cytokeratin positivity which on H and E appear as densely eosinophilic apparently non-viable tumour cells.

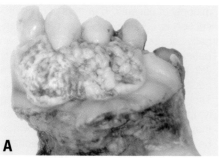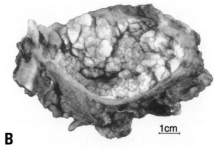

Fig. 4.12 A Verrucous carcinoma (VC) of the gingiva. **B** VC of the ginigva, spreading laterally to involve the cheek mucosa.

Interpretation of sentinel nodes can demand considerable pathological expertise. The outcome of the pathological assessment may be the presence of metastasis; micrometastasis, less than 2mm diameter tumour deposits, or isolated tumour cells {2477}. Micrometastasis has been defined {1073} as cells which have arrested and implanted. These may be in contact with a vessel or lymph sinus wall or may be extravascular. Single or small clusters of cells within lymph or blood vessels, but not in contact with the wall are defined as isolated tumour cells.

Histopathology

The histological features of SCC have been discussed in Chapter 3 on tumours of the hypopharynx, larynx and trachea. The findings in the oral cavity and oropharynx do not differ significantly from those of the larynx and hypopharynx. A minority of oral and oropharyngeal cancers show different histological subtypes that can be associated with differences in prognosis. These are discussed below. It is clearly important that pseudo epitheliomatous hyperplasia (PEH) is distinguished from SCC. PEH can occur in mucosa overlying a granular cell tumour, in necrotising sialometaplasia and in papillary hyperplasia of palate. PEH occurring with mucositis, particulary after irradiation, may be difficult to distinguish from squamous cell carcinoma.

The majority of cases of SCC present no difficulty in diagnosis for the experienced pathologist. However, the recognition of the earliest stages of invasion can be problematic. No consistent guidelines for this exist. The deepest layers of the epithelium and the interface between the epithelium and the lamina propria need to be examined in detail. This is frequently made more difficult where there is a prominent inflammatory infiltration.

Relevant features include the loss of a histologically well-defined interface, described previously as loss of basement membrane and disturbed architecture of the basal layers of the epithelium, particularly the replacement of basal cells by larger irregular cells with cytoplasmic processes extending into connective tissue. In some cases the degree of cytological atypia and mitotic feature may suggest malignancy, but these are not always present. To an extent the judgement about early invasion is subjective and it can be important for the pathologist to communicate the difficulty in interpretation to the clinician. Some pathologists will indicate that while no unequivocal evidence of invasion is demonstrated, they nevertheless feel that the lesion should be regarded as early invasive carcioma.

Somatic genetics

There is some variation in the genetic profile of oral and oropharyngeal SCC that reflects the site-specific impact of various casual agents and differences in clinical presentation. The carcinogens in tobacco smoke, for example, increase the prevalence and spectrum of TP53 mutations {268}. Compared to carcinomas that arise in patients who smoke, carcinomas in patients who have never smoked harbour fewer p53 mutations, disproportionately involve women, typically arise from the oral tongue, and affect very young or very old patients {1351,2258}. For carcinomas of the oropharynx, oncogenic human papillomavirus (HPV), particularly the HPV-16 subtype, is an important causative agent: More than 50% of oropharyngeal carcinomas harbour integrated HPV DNA {60,888,1999}. The E6 and E7 viral oncoproteins bind and inactivate the TP53 and retinoblastoma gene products respectively, disengaging two of the more critical pathways involved in

cell cycle regulation {2788}. These HPV-positive oropharyngeal tumours compose a distinct pathological entity with its own clinical spectrum and basaloid morphology {888,1012,2072}, illustrating the emerging role of genetic characterization as a potential means of determining prognosis and influencing management {1691}.

Genetic evidence has clarified the vague concept of "field cancerization". Most, if not all, multiple primary carcinomas of the upper aerodigestive tract derive from a common clonal progenitor cell that undergoes a common early genetic alterations {187,2271}. Genetic evidence has helped account for the perplexing problem of local tumour recurrence following seemingly complete tumour resection. In many instances, local tumour recurrence reflects extension of genetically damaged cells beyond the clinical and microscopic boundaries of carcinoma to the margins of surgical resection {268,1626, 1983,2777}.

Microsatellite analysis of exfoliated cells swabbed or rinsed from the oral cavity of patients with head and neck squamous carcinomas consistently harbour genetic changes that are identical to those in the primary tumours, suggesting a non-invasive test for specific DNA-sequence variants in saliva as a means of identifying patients with pre-invasive or invasive neoplasms {2430}. Clonal genetic changes identical to those found in primary head and neck SCC have been identified in circulating plasma or serum, suggesting a mechanism for early cancer detection and tumour surveillance {1853}. The use of highly sensitive genetic assays for detecting rare cancer cells at the margin of tumour resection shows promise for predicting the likelihood of tumour recurrence {268,1983}.

Prognosis and predictive factors

Tumour size and nodal status are the most significant prognostic factors {2060}. Histological grade correlates poorly with patient outcome {1292,2195}. The value of grading improves when only the deeply invasive margins of the tumour are evaluated {291,292,1927, 2818}. Tumours invading with pushing borders are less aggressive than tumours showing a noncohesive front showing diffuse spread with tiny strands or single cells. {1325,2132,2342,2653, 2841} Major risk factors that adversely influence prognosis are two or more positive regional nodes, extracapsular extension of nodal disease, or positive margins of resection {1429}. Other important histologic features associated with poor prognosis are tumour thickness and vascular invasion.

Molecular markers with unequivocal prognostic and/or predictive significance have not been identified {428,1052,1561, 2106}.

Verrucous carcinoma

ICD-O code   8051/3

Although uncommon, 75% of all cases of VC occur in the oral cavity. It is an exophytic, warty, slowly growing variant of SCC with pushing margins. It typically involves older males {950,1251,1677, 1695,2621}. Chronic smokeless tobacco use is accepted as the primary etiological factor for oral VC. Human papillomavirus subtypes 16 and 18 have been identified in up to 40% of oral VC {1927,2349}. Oral VC begins as a well-demarcated, thin white keratotic plaque which quickly thickens and develops papillary (blunted tips) or verruciform (pointed tips) surface projections. Occasional lesions present as erythaematous or pink papular masses. The colour depends on the amount of keratin produced and the degree of host inflammatory response to the tumour. This cancer almost always remains broad-based or sessile and can become quite extensive from lateral growth by the time of diagnosis. Rare fungating examples, however, may appear to be somewhat pedunculated. Smokeless tobacco keratosis (tobacco pouch) is often seen on adjacent mucosal surfaces in patients who chew tobacco or use snuff. Unless the tumour is infected or is encroaching on alveolar nerves in the jawbones, VC is an asymptomatic lesion. Surface ulceration and haemorrhage are not seen, unless a focus of SCC is present in the mass.

VC consists of thickened club-shaped papillae and blunt stromal invaginations of well-differentiated squamous epithelium with marked keratinization. The squamous epithelium lacks the usual cytologic criteria of malignancy, and by morphometry, the cells are larger than those seen in SCC {489}. Mitoses are rare, and observed in the basal layers; DNA synthesis (S-phase) is also limited primarily to the basal layers {737}. VC invades the stroma with a pushing, rather than infiltrating border. Dense lymphoplasmacytic host response is common. Intraepithelial microabscesses are seen, and the abundant keratin may evoke a foreign body reaction.

The surrounding mucosa shows progressive transition from hyperplasia to VC. A downward dipping of epithelium often "cups" the VC periphery, and is the ideal site for deep biopsy {174,1192}. With extensive surgical removal, and without neck dissection, the 5-year disease-free survival rate is 80-90%, although 8% of patients require at least one additional surgical procedure during that time {1870,1927}. Treatment failures usually occur in patients with the most extensive involvement or in those unable to tolerate extensive surgery because of unrelated systemic diseases. No molecular or other markers have yet shown prognostic significance for oral VC. However, one-fifth of these tumours contain a co-existing SCC which may not be identified without extensive histologic sectioning {1927}. Such hybrid tumours have a greater tendency to recur locally and a slight tendency to metastasize to the ipsilateral neck.

Basaloid squamous cell carcinoma

ICD-O code   8083/3

This is uncommon in the oral cavity, slightly more common in the oropharynx. It is described in the chapter on tumours of the hypopharynx, larynx and trachea.

Papillary squamous cell carcinoma
ICD-O code   8052/3

This is rarely recognized in the oral cavity and oropharynx other than as a component of a large SCC. It is described in the chapter on tumours of the hypopharynx, larynx and trachea.

Spindle cell carcinoma

ICD-O code   8074/3

This unusual variant is more common in the larynx than in the oral cavity and oropharynx, and is described in detail in the chapter on tumours of the hypopharynx, larynx and trachea.

Acantholytic squamous cell carcinoma

ICD-O code   8075/3

The lip is the most frequent oral site. There are no distinguishing clinical signs and the microscopical features are considered in the chapter on tumours of the hypopharynx, larynx and trachea. A variant of this tumour has been referred to as pseudovascular SCC.

Adenosquamous carcinoma

ICD-O code   8560/3

In the oral cavity this is a SCC with clear-cut areas of adenocarcinoma, most frequently seen as a component of a large SCC. It is described in the chapter on tumours of the hypopharynx, larynx and trachea.

Carcinoma cuniculatum (epithelioma cuniculatum)

ICD-O code   8051/3

This rare variant of oral cancer has similarities to the lesion more commonly described in the foot in which tumour infitrates deeply into bone. The oral tumours show proliferation of stratified squamous epithelium in broad processes with keratin cores and keratin filled crypts which seem to burrow into bone, but lack obvious cytological features of malignancy {40}. Diagnosis on biopsy specimens can be very difficult and correlation with the clinical and radiographic features is required.

Lymphoepithelial carcinoma

W.Y.W. Tsang
J.K.C. Chan
W. Westra

Definition

Lymphoepithelial carcinoma (LEC) is a poorly differentiated squamous cell carcinoma (SCC) or undifferentiated carcinoma, accompanied by a prominent reactive lymphoplasmacytic infiltrate. The morphological features are indistinguishable from those examples of nasopharyngeal nonkeratinizing carcinoma with a rich lymphoplasmacytic infiltrate.

ICD-O code   8082/3

Epidemiology

LEC is rare at these sites, and accounts for 0.8-2% of all oral or oropharyngeal cancers {1339,2741}. See Chapter 2.

Etiology

Epstein-Barr virus (EBV) has been tested in only a limited number of cases {819, 856,1802,1875,2405}, but it appears that tumours occurring in Chinese are usually positive for EBV, while those occurring in Caucasians are usually negative. The racial difference in the association with EBV is similar to LEC occurring in the major salivary glands (see Chapter 5).

Clinical features

The patients present with an intra-oral mass, which may be ulcerated. Some tumours can be bilateral {801,2038}. A proportion of patients present with neck mass due to regional lymph node involvement {119}.

Location and metastatic spread

More than 90% of all oral and oropharyngeal LEC occur in the tonsil and tongue base areas. The remaining cases are found in the palate and buccal mucosa {444,694,2822}. The tumour has a high propensity for regional cervical lymph node involvement (approximately 70% of cases at presentation) {119,444,1339}. Distant metastasis tends to occur in the liver and lung {119}.

Histopathology

LEC of the oral cavity and oropharynx shows morphologic features indistinguishable from its nasopharyngeal and sinonasal counterparts. The surface epithelium is often intact. The tumour is invasive, and comprises syncytial sheets and clusters of carcinoma cells with vesicular nuclei, prominent nucleoli and ill-defined cell borders. A rich lymphoplasmacytic infiltrate is present within the tumour islands and the surrounding stroma, which may appear desmoplastic.

The tumour cells are immunoreactive for pan-cytokeratin and epithelial membrane antigen. EBV encoded RNA (EBER) has been demonstrated by in-situ hybridization in oral / oropharyngeal LEC occurring in Chinese patients.

Prognosis and predictive factors

LEC of the oral cavity and oropharynx are radiosensitive, and in a high percentage of cases local control can be achieved even in the presence of regional lymph node metastasis {1339}. Local, regional and distant failures occur in 3%, 5% and 19% of cases respectively {444}. Distant metastasis is associated with a poor prognosis.

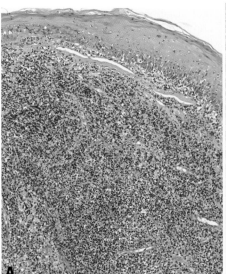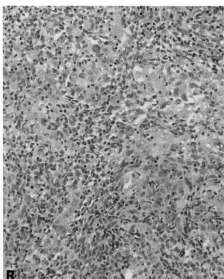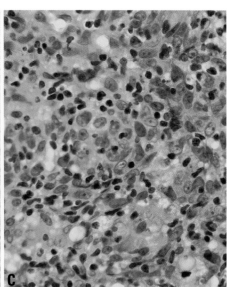

Fig. 4.13 A Lymphoepithelial carcinoma of the tonsil. The tumour infiltrates beneath an intact surface epithelium. In this example, the tumour islands are obscured by the heavy lymphoplasmacytic infiltrate. **B** Sheets and islands of tumour cells intimately admixed with lymphocytes and plasma cells. **C** Lymphoepithelial carcinoma of the palate. Carcinoma cells exhibit indistinct cell borders, pale chromatin and distinct nucleoli. Many lymphocytes are found among the carcinoma cells.

Epithelial precursor lesions

N. Gale
B.Z. Pilch
D. Sidransky
A. El Naggar

W. Westra
J. Califano
N. Johnson
D.G. MacDonald

The pathologic assessment of precursor lesions is similar throughout the upper aerodigestive tract. It is described in detail in the Chapter 3 on tumours of the hypopharynx, larynx and trachea (page 140).

Clinical features

The principal oral and oropharyngeal lesions which may be precursor lesions are white patches (leukoplakia) and red patches (erythroplasia/erythroplakia) or mixed red and white lesions. The majority of leukoplakias will not show dysplasia and correspond to the hyperplasia category. Red and mixed lesions (speckled leukoplakia) show a higher frequency of dysplasia, often of higher grade. The majority of leukoplakias will not undergo malignant change and may even regress particularly if apparent aetiologic factors are removed.

Histopathology

The epithelium of precursor lesions may be thick, but in the oral cavity it can also be atrophic. By definition, there is no evidence of invasion. The magnitude of surface keratinisation is of no importance. Allocation to categories within each of the classifications requires consideration firstly of architectural features and then of cytology.

Hyperplasia

Hyperplasia describes increased cell numbers. This may be in the spinous layer (acanthosis) and/or in the basal/parabasal cell layers (progenitor compartment), termed basal cell hyperplasia. The architecture shows regular stratification without cellular atypia.

Dysplasia, / squamous intraepithelial neoplasia / atypical hyperplasia

When architectural disturbance is accompanied by cytologic atypia, the term dysplasia applies. The terms squamous intraepithelial neoplasia (SIN) and atypical epithelial hyperplasia are used synonymously.

There is a challenge in the recognition of

the earliest manifestations of dysplasia and no single combination of the above features allows for consistent distinction between hyperplasia and the earliest stages of dysplasia. Dysplasia is a spectrum and no criteria exist to precisely divide this spectrum into mild, moderate and severe categories.

Mild dysplasia

In general architectural disturbance limited to the lower third of the epithelium accompanied by cytological atypia define the minimum criteria of dysplasia.

Moderate dysplasia

Architectural disturbance extending into the middle third of the epithelium is the initial criterion for recognizing this category. However, consideration of the degree of cytologic atypia may require upgrading.

Severe dysplasia

Recognition of severe dysplasia starts with greater than two thirds of the epithelium showing architectural disturbance with associated cytologic atypia. However, as noted in the previous para-

Table 4.01 Classification schemas that histologically categorize precursor and related lesions

2005 WHO Classification	Squamous Intraepithelial Neoplasia (SIN)	Ljubljana Classification Squamous Intraepithelial Lesions (SIL)
Squamous cell hyperplasia		Squamous cell (Simple) hyperplasia
Mild dysplasia	SIN 1	Basal/parabasal cell hyperplasia*
Moderate dysplasia	SIN 2	Atypical hyperplasia**
Severe dysplasia	SIN 3***	Atypical hyperplasia**
Carcinoma in-situ	SIN 3***	Carcinoma in-situ

*	Basal/parabasal cell hyperplasia may histologically resemble mild dysplasia, but the former is conceptually benign lesion and the latter the lower grade of precursor lesions.
**	'Risky epithelium'. The analogy to moderate and severe dysplasia is approximate.
***	The advocates of SIN combine severe dysplasia and carcinoma in-situ.

Table 4.02 Criteria used for diagnosing dysplasia

Architecture	Cytology
Irregular epithelial stratification	Abnormal variation in nuclear size (anisonucleosis)
Loss of polarity of basal cells	Abnormal variation in nuclear shape (nuclear pleomorphism)
Drop-shaped rete ridges	Abnormal variation in cell size (anisocytosis)
Increased number of mitotic figures	Abnormal variation in cell shape (cellular pleomorphism)
Abnormally superficial mitoses	Increased nuclear-cytoplasmic ratio
Premature keratinization in single cells (dyskeratosis)	Increased nuclear size
Keratin pearls within rete pegs	Atypical mitotic figures
	Increased number and size of nucleoli

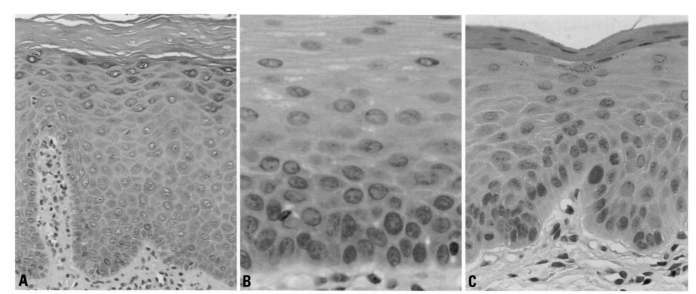

Fig. 4.14 A Acanthosis. Hyperplastic epithelium with thickened stratum spinosum. **B** Basal cell hyperplasia. Increase in progenitor compartment without dysplasia. **C** Mild dysplasia. Basal cell hyperplasia with relatively mild cytological change confined to lower third of epithelium.

graph architectural disturbance extending into the middle third of the epithelium with sufficient cytologic atypia is upgraded from moderate to severe dysplasia.

Carcinoma in-situ

The theoretical concept of carcinoma in-situ is that malignant transformation has occurred but invasion is not present. It is not possible to recognize this morphologically. The following is recommended for the diagnosis of carcinoma in-situ: full thickness or almost full thickness architectural abnormalities in the viable cellular layers accompanied by pronounced cytologic atypia. Atypical mitotic figures and abnormal superficial mitoses are commonly seen in carcinoma in-situ.

Differential diagnosis

Reactive, regenerative or reparative squamous epithelium, for example in response to trauma, inflammation, irradiation or ulceration, may manifest atypical cytology or architectural disturbance. Nutritional deficiencies such as iron, folate, and vitamin B12, can also simulate dysplasia. Such lesions are not considered precursor lesions and should be distinguished from them. Clinical history is helpful and morphological changes suggestive of the inciting event, such as ulceration, inflammation, haemorrhage, radiation-induced mesenchymal and/or endothelial nuclear enlargement and hyperchromatism, may be present. The epithelial changes in these cases are generally less pronounced than in dysplasia.

Relevance of dysplasia. It is reasonable to assume that the changes described in dysplasia are due to genetic changes in the epithelium occur, but it is unlikely that the mutations involved are the same ones as are associated with development of malignancy. More severe dysplasia has been traditionally believed to be associat-

ed with a greater likelihood of progression to malignancy. This might indicate that the greater the accumulation of mutations in tissue, the greater the chance that the critical mutations for malignancy will be present. The corollary is also true in that malignancy can arise from non-dysplastic epithelium {2493} presumably because these critical mutations can be present in the absence of the mutations causing dysplasia.

Genetics

There are no individual markers that reliably predict malignant transformation. The molecular biology techniques which show most promise as predictors of development of SCC are large scale genomic status (DNA ploidy) and loss of heterozygosity (LOH) at defined loci {2286}.

Dysplasia has been reported to be present in from 10-25% of leukoplakias

Table 4.03 Malignant transformation of oral leukoplakia (Reibel {2145})

Authors/Year	Country	Material (no. of cases)	Observation period (years)	Cases with malignant transformation (%)
Pindborg et al., 1968 {2049}	Denmark	248	3.9	4.4
Silverman and Rosen, 1968 {2362}	USA	117	1-11	6.0
Kramer et al., 1970 {1368}	UK	187	-	4.8
Mehta et al., 1972 {1699}	India	117	10	0.9
Silverman et al., 1976 {2358}	India	4762	2	0.13
Bánóczy, 1977 {118}	Hungary	670	9.8	6.0
Silverman et al., 1984 {2361}	USA	257	7.2	17.5
Lind, 1987 {1517}	Norway	157	9.3	8.9
Schepman et al., 1998 {2261}	Netherlands	166	2.5	12.0

{2286,2490}. Ploidy studies of dysplastic leukoplakias showed that the great majority of aneuploid lesions developed SCC in the follow-up period, by contrast with 60% of tetraploid lesions and only about 3% of diploid lesions {2490}. No correlation was found between the degree of dysplasia and DNA ploidy. Similar studies on erythroplasias {2491} confirmed the high predictive potential of aneuploidy in identifying cases which progressed to SCC. Nondysplastic white patches have also been studied {11} and although there was a much lower incidence of malignant transformation, 80% of such cases were aneuploid.

LOH studies have been undertaken contrasting oral lesions which progressed to SCC or carcinoma in-situ during follow-up with corresponding lesions which did not progress. LOH on two chromosome arms, 3p and 9p seemed to be particularly important in predicting progression {2201}.

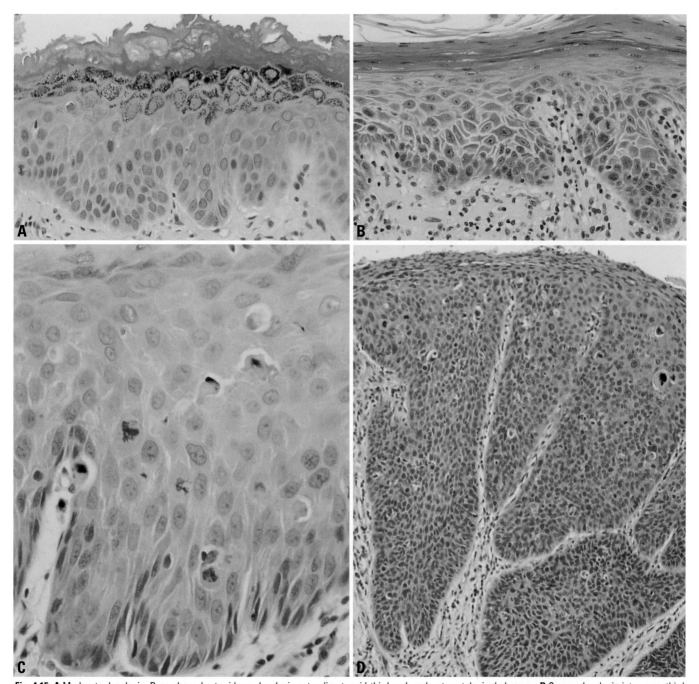

Fig. 4.15 A Moderate dysplasia. Drop shaped rete ridges, dysplasia extending to mid-third and moderate cytological changes **B** Severe dysplasia into upper third of epithelium with marked cytological change **C** Severe dysplasia into upper third of epithelium with prominent cytological change including abnormal mitoses. **D** Carcinoma in-situ. Abnormal cells seen throughout the full thickness of epithelium.

Proliferative verrucous leukoplakia and precancerous conditions

A.K. El Naggar
P.A. Reichart

Definition

Proliferative verrucous leukoplakia (PVL) is a rare but distinctive high-risk clinical form of oral precursor lesions. Because of the lack of specific histologic criteria, the diagnosis is based on combined clinical and histopathologic evidence of progression. Sequential biopsies show progressive dysplasia and the acquisition of aberrant TP53 protein.

Clinical features

PVL is an aggressive form of oral leukoplakia with considerable morbidity and strong predilection to malignant transformation {174,1005,1797,2360}. The etiology of this entity is unknown. The condition develops initially as focal clinical hyperkeratosis (leukoplakia) that progressively becomes a wide multifocal disease with gross exophytic features {174}. The aver-age age at diagnosis is 62 years; women are more commonly afflicted (ratio, 4:1). Typically, multiple oral sites are affected. The most common site in women is the buccal mucosa and the tongue in men. Carcinoma develops after a protracted period of time. The most common sites of the carcinoma are gingiva and tongue.

PVL is characterized by high recurrence rate and histological progression. Many cases are resistant to all forms of treatment, including laser microsurgery, surgical excision and radio-and chemotherapy. Conservative management of these lesions has been unsuccessful and wide surgical excision is the best hope for control.

Other precancerous conditions

Precancerous conditions (PCs) are generalized clinical states associated with a significantly increased risk for SCC. Epithelial atrophy, increased mitotic activity and impaired epithelial repair mechanisms are fundamental to PCs of different etiology.

Iron deficiency

Originally described in the context of sideropenic dysphagia, it is an important cause of epithelial atrophy. The association of iron deficiency with oropharyngeal squamous cell carcinomas has been observed since the mid-thirties of the 20th century {21}. However, a significant decrease of cases with hypopharyngeal cancers and iron deficiency was noted in Sweden in the seventies {1433}. Few cases of oral cancer and iron deficiency have been published in the last 20 years.

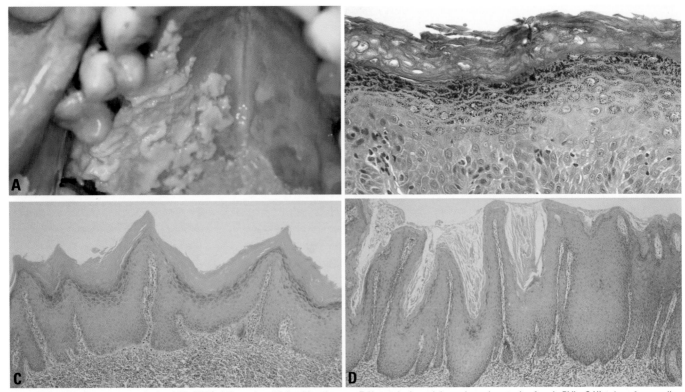

Fig. 4.16 Proliferative verrucous leukoplakia (PVL) **A** Extensive, thick, white plaques. **B** Hyperplasia and dense hyperkeratosis of early PVL. **C** Histology from a clinical case of PVL showing verrucous surface with hyperkeratosis, hypergranulosis and a dense inflammatory infiltrate in the corium. **D** Same case as shown on fig. C two years later showing more florid verrucous hyperplasia illustrating the progressive nature of the condition.

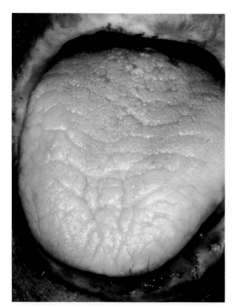

Fig. 4.17 Sideropenic dysphagia. Iron deficiency anaemia with depapillated tongue, depigmentation of the upper lip and epithelial erosion of the lower lip.

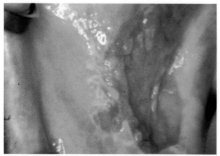

Fig. 4.18 Erythroplasia / erythroplakia associated with oral lichen planus (precancer).

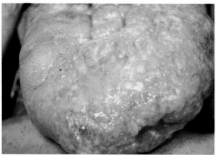

Fig. 4.19 Syphilis. Interstitial glossitis due to late stage syphilis with squamous cell carcinoma at the left tip of the tongue (Collection of J.J. Pindborg, M.D., Copenhagen).

Oral lichen planus

OLP is a chronic mucocutaneous immune inflammatory condition. Malignant transformation is still controversial {639,2359}; one review reporting malignant transformation rates between 0% and 5.6% {2116}.
The controversy is due to lack of uniform clinical and histological criteria for OLP and oral lichenoid lesions (OLL). The latter have also been termed interface mucositis or lichenoid mucositis. Oral lichenoid lesions have been considered by some to represent the lesion at risk if associated with dysplasia. In a recent study {2664} it was shown that all cases of malignant transformation (1.7%) involved cases of OLL and not OLP. Similarly, a study {2896} investigating whether OLP without dysplasia is premalignant by using microsatellite analysis for loss of heterozygosity (chromosomes 3p, 9p, 17p) did not support OLP as a lesion at risk.

However, until distinct clinical and histological criteria have been developed on how to differentiate OLP from OLL, both lesions have to be considered as 'at risk for malignant transformation'.

Oral submucous fibrosis (OSF)

This chronic, progressive condition of the oral mucosa {2115} is etiologically strongly associated with the chewing of areca nut which has recently been categorized by IARC as a human carcinogen {1}. It is almost exclusively seen in ethnic groups using areca nut alone or as a component of betel quid.

Clinically there is mucosal rigidity of varying intensity due to fibroelastic transformation of the juxtaepithelial connective tissue. Fibrous bands and mucosal pallor are characteristic {498}. Histologically, there is epithelial atrophy, keratosis and dysplasia in up to 25% of cases {498}. In a population-based prospective study, in India, SCC developed in 7% of patients with OSF over a period of 17 years {1798}.

Syphilis

Late stage (tertiary) syphilis associated with leukoplakia had a high risk of malignancy, but this is now largely of historical interest {1721}.

Xeroderma pigmentosum

This is a rare neurocutaneous disease with an autosomal-recessive mode of inheritance. The syndrome is caused by deficient nucleotide excision repair mechanisms {2090}. The skin, including the lips, is affected and shows epithelial atrophy and hyperpigmentation. Patients are extremely sensitive to light and show an increased predisposition to UV-associated malignancies of the skin. Carcinomas of the tongue have also

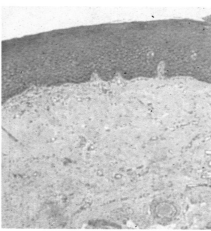

Fig. 4.20 Oral submucous fibrosis with a broad band of subepithelial collagenous tissue.

been described {1306,1994,2704}.

Lupus erythematosus

This is a chronic autoimmune disease of unknown etiology. Carcinomas, mainly of the lips, have been described in affected individuals {2264,2696}.

Epidermolysis bullosa dystrophicans (Hallopeau-Siemens type)

This disease of the skin and oral mucosa has an autosomal dominant pattern of inheritance. Oral leukoplakia and occasional cases of SCC have been observed in association with epidermolysis bullosa {226,2288}.

Papillomas

E.W. Odell

Definition

These form a range of localised hyperplastic exophytic and polypoid lesions of hyperplastic epithelium with a verrucous or cauliflower-like morphology. Lesions of fibroepithelial hyperplasia are not generally included. Not every papilloma can be allocated to one of the diagnostic categories described below.

ICD-O code   8050/0

Epidemiology

Papillomas are common, with a prevalence of approximately 0.1%-0.5% {94, 1342,2569}.

Etiology

HPV infection causes some papillomas {2076} and at least types 1,2,3,4,6,7,10, 11,13,16,18,30,31,32,33,35,38,45,52, 55,57,59,69,72,73 sequences have been detected in benign oral lesions. Clinically, latent HPV is common in oral mucosa and HPV DNA sequences can be detected in over 80% of individuals. There is no absolute association between the virus type and the type of papilloma {866} though focal epithelial hyperplasia is almost exclusively associated with types 13 and 32. HPV infection of oral tissue may be transmitted horizontally, including venereally, perinatally and possibly in utero {2518}.

Histopathology

Histological differential diagnosis for all types includes lesions of fibroepithelial hyperplasia: fibroepithelial polyps, fibrous epulis and papillary hyperplasia associated with candidal infection or dentures. These have a more prominent fibrous component and no viral change. Verruciform xanthoma is a solitary lesion with a very similar clinical and histological presentation.

Extensive multiple papillomas or diffuse papillomatous change raise the possibilities of HPV lesions in immunosuppression, acanthosis nigricans, naevus unius et lateris, focal dermal hypoplasia, Cowden syndrome, papillary and verru-

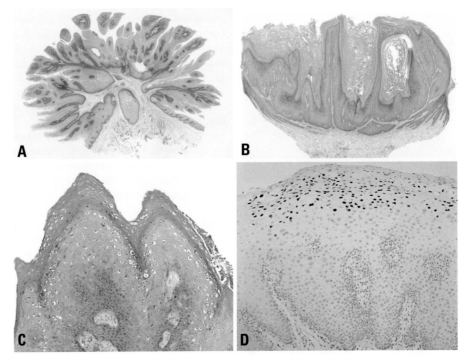

Fig. 4.21 Papilloma. **A** Typical papillary structure of squamous papilloma. This example is only lightly keratinised and negative for papilloma virus on immunocytochemistry. **B** Papilloma from the vermillion border showing extensive keratinisation. Note the inwardly facing rete ridges at the periphery. **C** Moderately keratinised papilloma of verruca vulgaris type showing koilocytic change in the upper prickle cell layers. **D** Strong and extensive staining for papilloma virus in a flat papilloma from an HIV infected individual. There is widespread infection in the upper prickle cell layer but the architecture of the epithelium is little changed. Note the sharp lesion margin on the left.

cous dysplastic lesions and papillary squamous {2488} or verrucous carcinoma. Florid oral papillomatosis is a clinical term for diffuse papillomatous change of the mucosa for which no specific cause can be identified and is not a defined clinico-pathological entity.

Squamous cell papilloma and verruca vulgaris

Definition

A benign, hyperplastic wart-like localised proliferation of the oral epithelium {2076}.

Epidemiology

Squamous papillomas are common in children and in adults in the 3rd to 5th decades but may be found at any age. There is an almost equal sex incidence with a slight male predominance.

Etiology

Evidence of causative HPV infection can be found in less than half of oral squamous papillomas {866,2516,2747}, and these lesions are the intraoral counterpart of verruca vulgaris. Many HPV subtypes have been detected including 2,4,6,7,10,40. The presence of HPV virion components ultrastructurally and immunocytochemically indicates active viral replication in the lesion. Virus transmission appears to be mostly horizontal or by autoinoculation. Lesions in children tend to arise at anterior oral sites and the source of infection is often verruca vulgaris on the skin, particularly on the fingers. Infectivity is low.

The remainder of squamous papillomas are of unknown etiology. HPV sequences may be detected by PCR but the significance of this is unclear.

Localization

Any oral site may be affected but the most common are the hard and soft palate, labial mucosa, tongue and gingiva.

Clinical features

Squamous papillomas are soft, pedunculated lesions formed by a cluster of finger-like fronds or a sessile, dome-shaped lesion with a nodular, papillary or verrucous surface. The surface may be white or of normal mucosal colour depending on the degree of keratinization {2076}. Lesions are usually single but fairly frequently multiple, particularly in children and for verruca vulgaris. Squamous papillomas grow rapidly over a period of a few months to a maximum of about 6mm diameter and then remain a constant size.

Histopathology

Lesions are exophytic and comprise folds of hyperplastic stratified epithelium that are usually thickly para- or orthokeratinized but may be non keratinised.
Squamous papillomas associated with HPV (oral verruca vulgaris) comprise a cluster of finger-like projections from a narrow base, each with a sharp keratinised tip, supported on ramifying cores of connective tissue containing dilated capillaries. Stratification of the epithelium is well ordered. Mitoses may be frequent and there may be mild anisonucleosis consistent with hyperplasia, but no atypia. The fronds are thickly keratinised, often with a prominent keratohyaline layer of large coarse granules. Small foci of HPV-infected cells (koilocytes) can usually be found in the upper prickle cell layer. These keratinocytes have crumpled, darkly stained nuclei with perinuclear haloes but appear very similar to vacuolated keratinocytes that are common in the normal oral mucosa. Koilocytes may be more frequent in early lesions. Less frequently, viral inclusions are found. Rete processes at the base often turn inwards and are symmetrical. Small foci of lymphocytic inflammation may lie in the fronds or at the base but inflammation is usually sparse unless the lesion is subject to trauma or other irritation {4,1929}. HPV may be identified by immunocytochemistry or in-situ hybridisation but this is not necessary for diagnosis {2076}.
Papillomas without detectable active HPV replication show more variation.

They may appear identical to verruca vulgaris but without koilocytes or prominent keratohyaline granules, or form rounded broad-based dome shaped lesions similar to condyloma. The hyperplastic epithelium may form papillary exophytic fronds or arborising rete processes. Some are flat zones of acanthotic hyperplastic epithelium with increased numbers of dermal papillae similar to plane warts of the skin.

Prognosis and predictive factors

Oral verruca vulgaris may regress spontaneously, particularly in children, but responds to simple excision or ablation by laser or cryosurgery. Recurrence is unusual provided all lesional tissue is removed and there is no malignant potential.

Condyloma acuminatum

Definition

Oral counterpart of anogenital condyloma acuminatum

Synonyms

Venereal wart; venereal condyloma

Epidemiology

Lesions are usually diagnosed between the mid 2nd and 5th decade with a peak in teenagers and young adults {2916}.

Etiology

Epithelial infection by HPV, most commonly types 6,11,16 and 18 though others have been detected {700,1380}. Transmission is usually venereal or by autoinnoculation from concomitant genital lesions {1975}.
Histological appearance is not an accurate indicator of a genital origin.

Localization

Most lesions arise on the labial mucosa, tongue and palate in anterior oral sites though any area may be affected {700, 2916}.

Clinical features

Condylomas are painless, rounded, dome-shaped exophytic nodules up to 15 mm in diameter, larger than squamous papillomas and verruca vulgaris. They have a broad base and a nodular or mulberry-like surface that is slightly red, pink or of normal mucosal colour. Lesions may be multiple and are then usually clustered {2076,2916}.

Histopathology

Condylomas are similar to squamous papillomas but with short blunt rounded fronds of hyperplastic epithelium of even length forming a smooth or nodular, flat or rounded surface. Keratin is usually absent or sparse, occasional examples show moderate keratin and are white clinically. Between the folds, crypts or clefts lined by epithelium extend close to the broad base and may be filled with keratin debris in keratinised lesions. Clusters of koilocytes identical to those described above are much commoner than in squamous papillomas and are usually a prominent feature. Unlike squamous papilloma, rete processes are bulbous and short, of even length and do not curve inwards {700,2076}.

Prognosis and predictive factors

Condyloma acuminatum often responds to simple excision or ablation by laser or cryosurgery but appears to carry a higher risk of recurrence than squamous papilloma. Unlike ano-genital condyloma, there is no documented risk of malignant transformation, regardless of the presence of high-risk HPV types.

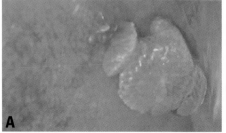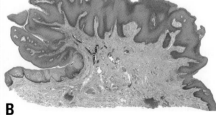

Fig. 4.22 Condyloma acuminatum. **A** Several sessile, cauliflower-like swellings forming a cluster. **B** Typical papilloma structure in condyloma showing the more rounded architecture in comparison with verruca vulgaris. Note a verrucous area on the left; many of these lesions have features of both types of papilloma.

Condyloma acuminatum in children raises the possibility of sexual abuse, but non-sexual transmission is possible {1380} and probably frequent.

Papillomas and papillomatosis in immunodeficiency

More florid presentations of HPV-induced lesions are found in immunosuppression, particularly in HIV infection. Lesions may be larger, multiple and coalesce to form extensive patches of affected mucosa. Occasionally the entire oral mucosa may become papillomatous and some of these presentations are not easily classified. Unusual HPV subtypes and multiple HPV subtypes are more frequent in immunosuppression. Occasional lesions in HIV infection are dysplastic and are of uncertain malignant potential.

Focal epithelial hyperplasia

Definition
Multiple oral papillomas induced by HPV 13 and 32

Synonym
Heck disease

Epidemiology
This is primarily a disease of children, adolescents and young adults. Originally described in Inuit and native Americans {69} but now recognised worldwide. The condition is endemic in some countries and prevalence may be as high as 40% of children in localised areas {94,332, 1014}.

Etiology
Infection by HPV types 13 and 32.

Localization
All areas of the oral cavity may be affected but the lesions are most common on the labial and buccal mucosa and the tongue {69,332,1014}.

Clinical features
Typically there are multiple asymptomatic lesions, each a soft rounded or flat plaque-like sessile swelling with a slightly nodular surface. They are usually pink in colour or sometimes white, and 2-10mm in diameter. Lesions develop in clusters or confluent patches {332}.

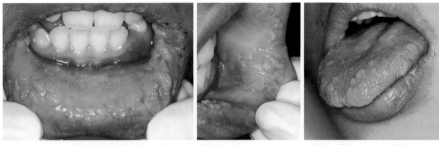

Fig. 4.23 Focal epithelial hyperplasia. Typical clinical appearance of multiple papillomatous nodules.

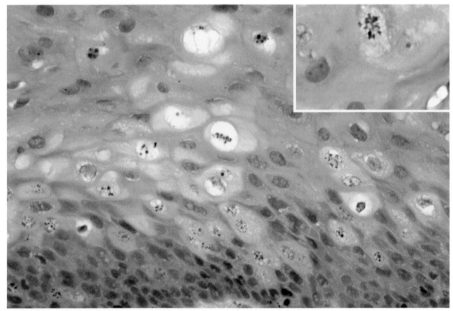

Fig. 4.24 Focal epithelial hyperplasia, viral change and mitosoid body (inset).

Individual lesions may appear and disappear during the course of the disease {1014}.

Histopathology
The histological features are more distinctive than squamous papilloma or condyloma. Each lesion is a slightly raised or rounded sessile swelling formed by a sharply demarcated zone of epithelial acanthosis, similar to condyloma acuminatum but with a less prominent papillomatous structure. The bulk of lesion is formed by exophytic acanthosis, without formation of well-defined projections of epithelium and the lesion contains minimal connective tissue papillae. Koilocytes similar to those of squamous papilloma are usually present and, in addition, there are usually characteristic "mitosoid bodies", which are nuclei with coarse clumped heterochromatin resembling a mitotic figure. Mitosoid bodies are characteristic but not specific for focal epithelial hyperplasia. The base of the lesion is flat and level with the adjacent epithelium without rete process enlargement {332,2076}. HPV may be detected on immunocytochemistry or by in-situ hybridisation but this is not necessary for diagnosis if the clinical presentation is typical {2076}.

Genetic susceptibility
Familial clustering and endemic areas may result from horizontal transmission.

Prognosis and predictive factors
The condition appears to resolve spontaneously after a period of years and is rarely found in adults. It has no malignant potential.

Granular cell tumour

P.M. Speight

Definition
A benign tumour of soft tissues which most often arises in the tongue and is thought to be of Schwann cell origin. It is composed of a poorly demarcated accumulation of plump granular cells which are often intimately associated with skeletal muscle.

ICD-O code   9580/0

Synonym
Granular cell myoblastoma

Epidemiology
Granular cell tumours are rare. Approximately 50% of all lesions arise in the head and neck and over half of these are found in the tongue. They arise in all age groups, with a peak between 40 and 60 years. In about 10-20% of patients the lesions are multiple. Females are affected more often than males with an M/F ratio of 2:1.

Etiology
No etiological factors are known. The lesion is thought to arise from Schwann cells. The granularity may be a senescent change associated with accumulation of lysosomes.

Localization
Granular cell tumours may arise in the skin, soft tissues, breast and lungs, but over 50% involve the head and neck and the tongue is the most common single site. Oral lesions may also be found in the buccal mucosa, floor of oral cavity or palate. Lesions may be multiple, affecting more than one intraoral site, or involving oral and extraoral sites {477}. Rare lesions have been reported in the salivary glands {331}.

Clinical features
The lesion typically presents as a smooth, sessile mucosal swelling 1-2 cm in diameter with a firm texture. The overlying epithelium is of normal colour or may be slightly pale. Occasionally there is candidal infestation of the superficial

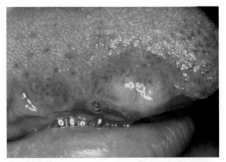

Fig. 4.25 Granular cell tumour. The typical presentation of granular cell tumour: a sessile swelling on the tongue covered by normal appearing epithelium.

epithelium and the lesion may then present as a discrete, white plaque.

Macroscopy
Tumours are usually 1-2 cm in diameter with a smooth surface. The cut surface shows a poorly demarcated lesion which is pale yellow or cream and firm on cutting.

Histopathology
The lesion is composed of plump eosinophilic cells with central small dark nuclei and abundant granular cytoplasm. The cells may be polygonal or elongated and have indistinct cell membranes, often giving the impression of a syncytium. The lesion is not encapsulated and the granular cells extend into adjacent tissues, typically skeletal muscle,

where they appear to merge with muscle cells {477,2791}. Granular cells extend up to the epithelium, often forming small islands in the connective tissue papillae. The granules stain positively with periodic acid Schiff (PAS).

A characteristic feature of granular cell tumour is that in up to 30% of cases the overlying epithelium shows pseudoepitheliomatous hyperplasia that may be misdiagnosed as carcinoma.

Immunoprofile
The lesion is strongly and uniformly positive for S-100 protein. Cells also express neurone-specific enolase, calretinin, inhibin-alpha and PGP 9.5, and show fine granular cytoplasmic positivity for the lysosome related antigen CD68 {764, 2791}.

Prognosis and predictive factors
Granular cell tumours are benign and rarely recur, even after conservative removal. Occasional lesions have behaved aggressively and malignant granular cell tumours have been described.

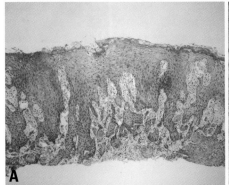
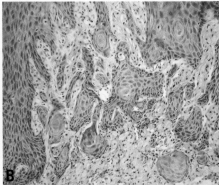

Fig. 4.26 Granular cell tumour. **A** Prominent pseudoepitheliomatous hyperplasia of the oral epithelium overlying a granular cell tumour. **B** The pseudoepitheliomatous hyperplasia can be mistaken for carcinoma, but careful examination shows eosinophilic granular cells in the connective tissues.

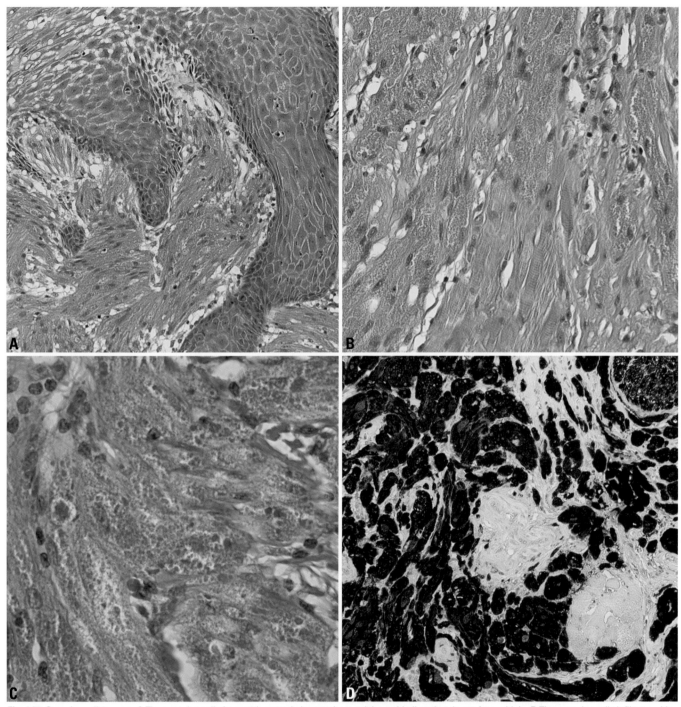

Fig. 4.27 Granular cell tumour. **A** The granular cells frequently extend close to the overlying epithelium, but do not fuse with it. **B** The granular cells infiltrate widely and often appear to merge with striated muscle cells. **C** The granules are PAS positive (Periodic acid Schiff stain). **D** The granular cells are strongly and uniformly positive for S-100 protein.

Keratoacanthoma

T. Löning
K.T. Jäkel

Definition

Keratoacanthoma is a benign tumour that is believed to arise from the epithelium of hair follicles.

ICD-O code   8071/1

Synonyms

Molluscum sebaceum, molluscum pseudocarcinomatosum, self-healing primary squamous carcinoma, tumour-like keratosis, idiopathic cutaneous pseudo-epitheliomatous hyperplasia.

Epidemiology

Keratoacanthoma occurs more often in whites, and is almost twice as frequent in men as in women. Although they have been seen in infants, keratoacanthomas are rare in persons under 20 years of age and the peak incidence is between the sixth and seventh decade {881}.

Etiology

Interestingly, the uptake of carcinogens (e.g. via particular smoking habits) may be relevant in human tumours {641}. No other risk factors are known. The concept of a common viral origin (papillomaviruses), popular for some years, has been abandoned.

In addition to the solitary type, clinical variants with multiple keratoacanthomas have been described, sometimes with a unilateral distribution {881}. Genetic factors may be involved in these cases, for familial clustering occurs, with multiple keratoacanthomas in affected individuals.

Localization

Keratoacanthomas preferentially occur on sun exposed hairy skin {881}. Thus, they are frequent on the skin of the face, including the lips (8% of cases), and extremely rare at hairless sites. Whether or not a "true keratoacanthoma" of the oral mucosa exists or not remains controversial {1929}. However, a small number of cases of the solitary form have been reported in intraoral sites {414,973}, and mucocutaneous linings may also be affected in the generalized forms (e.g. the Ferguson-Smith, Grzybowski and Witten and Zak types) {881}.

Clinical features

Keratoacanthoma is characterised by rapid growth followed by slow, spontaneous involution over several months {881}. Exact figures about regression time, however, are difficult to obtain, since the common mode of treatment is excision. The mature lesion is usually bud- or dome-shaped and is brownish or slightly reddish. Over time a central keratinous crater appears at the expense of the surrounding softer tumour tissue until finally a cup- or saucer-shape lesion develops that appears ulcerated, but is, in fact, lined by tumour epithelium and often covered with horn masses. An eruptive variant can be distinguished which is multifocal and often lacks the central keratin-filled crater. Following trauma and/or infection, true ulceration may occur, especially in areas like the lips, probably due to repeated scratching or biting. In the oral cavity, the above-described phenotypes rarely occur. Instead, the putative oral lesion mimics a broad spectrum of pseudoneoplastic and neoplastic lesions {1929}.

Macroscopy

The basic gross features of epidermal lesions have been already described. However, such prototypic lesions are rarely seen in the oral cavity. Instead, as in cases at the inner side of the vulva and within the anal canal, oral keratoacanthomas present as verrucous, speckled or even ulcerated lesions. Also, they may produce deep projections, which can extend through minor salivary glands and reach the surface of underlying bone.

Histopathology

Keratoacanthomas show a verrucous surface, and underneath keratinized clefts and penetrating squamous rete processes are found with deep keratin pearls. Atypia is minimal, and mitotic figures are rare or absent. Dense inflammatory infiltrates, including granulocytes typically are found in the adjacent stroma and within the deep parts of the tumour, so that the margins seem ill defined. The

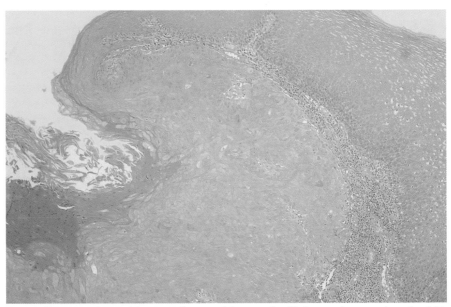

Fig. 4.28 Keratoacanthoma of the mucosal aspect of the upper lip with the cup-shape margin on the right, and the keratin-filled crater that is in the centre of the lesion on the left.

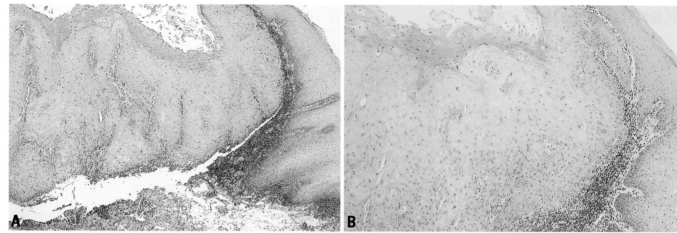

Fig. 4.29 Keratoacanthoma. **A** Intraoral keratoacanthoma with a marginal lip and a cup-shaped lesion, in this case with parakeratotic keratin, and the typical dense inflammatory infiltrate at the epithelial-stromal interface. **B** The higher magnification reveals the inflammatory infiltrate in detail, and the absence of cellular atypia in the lesional epithelium.

hallmark of keratoacanthoma is the overall architecture, with a cup-shaped appearance and a collar-like circumference.

A major diagnostic problem arises when destructive infiltration takes place as has been reported, including some cases in young individuals. When this kind of tumour growth occurs in the elderly, it is of course extremely difficult or even impossible to distinguish the lesion from carcinoma, particularly from carcinoma cuniculatum, which also shows minimal atypia despite its destructive growth pattern {1929}.

Histogenesis

A large body of evidence exists pertaining to the histogenesis of keratoacanthomas {881}. In fact, it is their origin from pilosebaceous follicles which has lead some authors to deny the existence of intraoral keratoacanthomas {1929}. This standpoint may be acceptable for sites of the oral cavity where pilo-sebaceous rudiments are rarely seen (e.g. gingiva). However, there are also cases reported in areas such as the buccal mucosa, which is a preferential site for the ectopic sebaceous glands (Fordyce spots). In addition, as also suggested for skin lesions, preprogrammed progenitor cells of the most superficial (intraepidermal) parts of the pilosebaceous unit may be sufficient as a source of (intraoral) keratoacanthoma.

Prognosis and predictive factors

Epidermal keratoacanthomas are clearly benign lesions {881}. However, for similar tumours of the external openings (oral cavity, vulva, anal canal) there are no reliable data, since these lesions are extremely rare, present diagnostic problems and therefore are usually completely excised. Recurrences after surgical excision do not occur.

Papillary hyperplasia

E.W. Odell

Papillary hyperplasia is an asymptomatic nodular or papillary mucosal lesion typically seen in the palate of patients who wear dentures. Most patients wear ill-fitting dentures, wear dentures continuously {2645} or have poor denture hygiene. Lesions also arise in non-denture wearers, in xerostomia or individuals with a high arched palate. Florid and extensive presentations occur in immunosuppression {937} and HIV infection {2150}. There is sessile nodular papillomatous hyperplasia of epithelium and supporting underlying fibrous tissue. There is usually parakeratinisation or less frequently orthokeratinisation. Rete processes are usually rounded or sharply defined at the base of the lesion but there may be pseudoepitheliomatous hyperplasia with keratin pearls and a poorly defined deep margin. Differential diagnosis includes diffuse HPV-induced papillomatosis, periorificial plasmacytosis {937} and verruciform xanthoma. Other multinodular lesions such as focal epithelial hyperplasia, acanthosis nigricans and Cowden syndrome appear similar histologically but have distinctive clinical presentations.

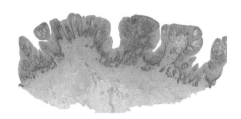

Fig. 4.30 Papillary hyperplasia. Low power view showing the overall architecture with nodular fibroepithelial hyperplasia and apparently detached islands of epithelium in the upper corium. Inflammation is slight in this example but depends on candidal infection and whether a denture overlies the lesion. It may be a very prominent feature.

Median rhomboid glossitis

E.W. Odell

Median rhomboid glossitis typically forms a patch of papillary atrophy near the midline of the dorsum of the tongue at the junction of the anterior two thirds and posterior third in the region of the embryological foramen caecum. It is no longer thought to be a developmental defect but the result of chronic candidal infection {719,2825}.

The epithelium lacks papillae, and shows psoriasiform hyperplasia and sometimes areas of pseudoepitheliomatous hyperplasia. A mild degree of atypia may be present. Fungal hyphae are present in the superficial epithelium but are usually sparse and revealed only in multiple sections. Scarring and nodularity persist after antifungal treatment. Differential diagnosis is aided by knowledge of the specific site and includes reactive fibroepithelial hyperplasia, granular cell tumour and other nodular lesions of the tongue. Occasionally the lesion can be difficult to differentiate from squamous cell carcinoma {931, 1932}, particularly when hyperplasia is extensive and epithelial processes reach or penetrate the underlying muscle.

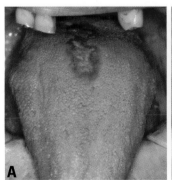
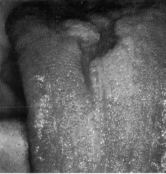
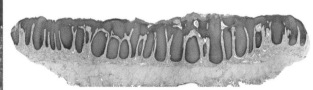

Fig. 4.31 Median rhomboid glossitis. A Two lesions of chronic candidiasis of the median rhomboid glossitis form. That on the left is flat and more typical, that on the right more nodular and irregular. B Typical median rhomboid glossitis with active candidal infection showing long bulbous rete hyperplasia and suprapapillary atrophy. Note the broad band of dense fibrosis separating the inflamed superficial corium from the underlying muscle.

Salivary gland tumours

J.W. Eveson

Epidemiology

Tumours of the oral cavity and oropharynx account for 9-23% of all salivary gland neoplasms in major series {669, 704,2301}. The most common sites are the palate (44-58%), lips (15-22%) and buccal mucosa (12-15%) {669,704,2301, 2711}. Variations in these series probably reflect patterns of referral in different institutions, together with geographical and ethnic differences.

Tumours of the oropharynx are relatively uncommon and form only 1.1-3.3% of all minor gland tumours {669,704,2448}. Most studies show a female to male ratio in the range of 1.2:1-1.5:1 {2711}.

Location

Nearly half of all oral and oropharyngeal salivary tumours are malignant, and in some sites, such as the lower lip, tongue and floor of the oral cavity, the large majority are carcinomas.. It is interesting to note that while 80-90% of labial salivary gland tumours involve the upper lip, there is a 3-5x greater risk of neoplasms in the lower lip being malignant {400,669, 704, 1871,1963}.

Most of the principle types of salivary gland tumour have been reported in the oral cavity. In some tumours such as canalicular adenoma, duct adenomas and polymorphous low-grade adenocarcinoma, the minor glands are by far the most frequent site of involvement. Whether there are genuine cases of intraoral Warthin tumour, or whether reported examples represent oncocytic hyperplasia and metaplasia with reactive lymphocytic infiltration, is contentious {2669}.

ICD-O codes

Acinic cell carcinoma   8550/3
Mucoepidermoid carcinoma
                                 8430/3
Adenoid cystic carcinoma
                                 8200/3
Polymorphous low-grade
adenocarcinoma   8525/3
Epithelial-myoepithelial
carcinoma   8562/3
Clear cell carcinoma,
NOS   8310/3
Basal cell
adenocarcinoma   8147/3
Cystadenocarcinoma   8450/3
Mucinous adenocarcinoma
                                 8480/3
Oncocytic carcinoma   8290/3
Salivary duct carcinoma 8500/3
Myoepithelial carcinoma 8982/3
Carcinoma ex pleomorphic
adenoma   8941/3

Acinic cell carcinoma

These are uncommon in minor glands {9, 280,340,410,734,864,2886} and form 2-6.5% of all intraoral salivary gland tumours {669,704,2711}. In one series, the age range was from 11-77 years, with a mean of 45 years, and a male to female ratio of 1.5:1 {2711}. The most common sites are the buccal mucosa, upper lip and palate where the tumours usually form non-descript swellings. The microscopical features are similar to those in major glands. However, in one series there appeared to be more areas consisting of solid sheets of epithelium with secretory material and fewer areas show-

the minor glands {2711}.

Mucoepidermoid carcinoma

This most common malignant salivary gland tumour involves minor glands, and accounts for 9.5-23% of all minor gland tumours {669,704,2711}. About half of the cases arise in the palate and other common sites include the buccal mucosa, lips, floor of oral cavity and retromolar pad. They appear to be much more frequent in the lower lip than the upper lip {1871}.

The tumour is often asymptomatic and detected during a routine dental examination. Many appear as bluish, domed swellings that resemble mucoceles or haemangiomas. Less commonly, the surface appears granular or papillary. Tumours of the base of tongue or oropharynx may cause dysphagia and sublingual tumours can lead to ankyloglossia and dysphonia. High-grade tumours are uncommon but can result in ulceration, loosening of teeth, paraesthesia or anaesthesia. Mucoepidermoid carcinoma is the most common salivary gland tumour to develop in a central location within the bone of the mandible or, less frequently, the maxilla {280}.

The microscopical features of minor gland mucoepidermoid carcinomas are the same as those seen in the major glands.

Adenoid cystic carcinoma

This lesion is relatively common in the minor glands. In the AFIP series 42.5% of all adenoid cystic carcinomas were in minor glands and 20.5% of the total was

Table 4.04 Percentage of malignant minor salivary gland tumours in different sites in published series.

	Upper Lip	Lower Lip	Lip NOS	Palate	Tongue	Cheek	Retro-molar	FOM*	Tonsil	Other
Auclair et al {669}	22.5	60.2	17.2	46.8	85.7	50.5	89.7	88.2	41.4	65.6
Waldron et al {2711}	14	86	-	42	-	46	91	80	-	69
Eveson & Cawson {704}	-	-	14.8	47	91.7	50	33.3	-	50	-
* Floor of the mouth										

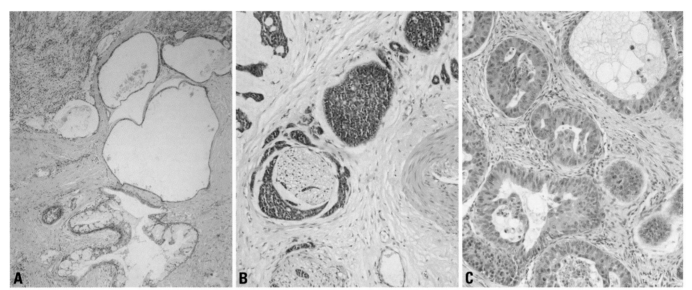

Fig. 4.32 A Mucoepidermoid carcinoma. Low power showing low-grade tumour with both cystic and solid areas and an inflamed, fibrous stroma. **B** Adenoid cystic carcinoma. This predominantly solid variant shows peri- and intraneural invasion. **C** Salivary duct carcinoma with large, somewhat oncocytic cells, cribriform areas, small papillae and comedo-type necrosis.

the tongue, tonsil and oropharynx, cheek, lips, retromolar pad and gingiva {899}. They are much more frequent in the upper lip than the lower lip {669,1871,2711}. Intraoral adenoid cystic carcinomas usually present as slow growing submucosal masses and ulceration may be seen, particularly in the palate. Pain, or evidence of nerve involvement, is usually only present in advanced tumours. Most tumours show the typical cylindromatous or cribriform variant microscopically, but some may have tubular areas and a few are predominantly solid {2711}.

Polymorphous low-grade adenocarcinoma
This tumour is seen almost exclusively in minor glands and is considered in detail in Chapter 5.

Epithelial-myoepithelial carcinoma
This tumour is rare in minor glands and the literature consists mainly of single cases or short series {154,436,493,784, 981,992,1177}. Tumours of the oral cavity and oropharynx formed only 10.3% of the AFIP series {669}. The palate is the most common site. The clinical presentation is non-specific and the microscopical features are the same as those in major glands.

Basal cell adenocarcinoma
This tumour is rare in minor glands. There were none in the AFIP series {669} but

there have been isolated case reports {563,785,1211,1540,2059,2703}. The most common sites are the palate, buccal mucosa and lip. They usually form asymptomatic, smooth or lobulated submucosal masses apart from one case that presented with dull pain and inflamed overlying mucosa {2703}. Microscopically they are similar to basal cell adenocarcinomas of the major glands.

Cystadenocarcinoma
These tumours are uncommon and about 32% developed in the minor glands where they are frequently papillary {411,790}. The most frequent sites are the palate, lips, buccal mucosa, tongue {1834} and retromolar regions. They are usually slow growing and painless but some palatal tumours have eroded the underlying bone and invaded the sinonasal complex. This tumour is considered in detail in Chapter 5.

Oncocytic carcinoma
This tuomur is rare and there were only two cases involving the oral cavity in the AFIP series of 26 cases {669}. One was in the palate and the other the buccal mucosa. Reported cases also include an additional case in the palate {274} and the AFIP case from the buccal mucosa {922}. The microscopical features are considered in Chapter 5.

Salivary duct carcinoma
This tumour is rare in minor salivary glands. A recent review documented 20 cases {1147} and a further 6 cases have been reported {1559,2673}. The most common location was the palate (65%). Other sites included the buccal mucosa and vestibule (19%), tongue (8%), retromolar pad (4%) and upper lip (4%). The age range was 23-80 years (mean 56 years). Some tumours formed painless swellings but many in the palate were painful and ulcerated or fungated. There were metastases to regional lymph nodes in 25% of cases and this was associated with a poor prognosis. The range of microscopical appearances was similar to that seen in the major glands.

Myoepithelial carcinoma
This is a rare salivary gland tumour and 26% of cases in a review of the literature (9 cases) involved the oral cavity or oropharynx {668} and only isolated cases have been published since this review {1827}. The most common location is the palate. The clinical signs and symptoms are non-specific and the microscopical features are considered in Chapter 5.

Carcinoma ex pleomorphic adenoma
Lesions involving the oral and oropharyngeal minor glands formed 17.5% of the AFIP series {669}. 63% of cases were in the palate and 10.5% were in the upper lip. There were no cases in the lower lip. Other sites included the tongue, buccal

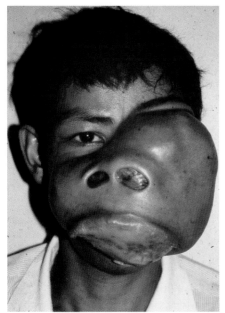

Fig. 4.33 Pleomorphic adenoma which started at palate involving the mid face and entire oral cavity.

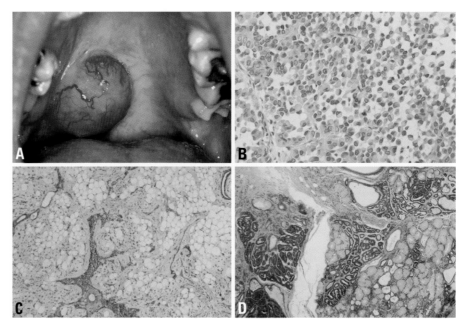

Fig. 4.34 A Pleomorphic adenoma. Tumour presenting as a firm swelling on the lateral aspect of the junction between the hard and soft palate. **B** Plasmacytoid, or hyaline myoepithelial cells are often a conspicuous feature of pleomorphic adenomas of minor glands. **C** Tumors may have an abundant lipomatous component that is occasionally misinterpreted as invasion. **D** Multifocal adenomatosis. Both basal cell adenoma and canalicular adenoma can show multifocal tumours and evidence of duct transformation within salivary gland lobules.

mucosa and tonsil/oropharynx. They usually form a painless mass of long duration and there may be a history of recent rapid growth, often with ulceration. The microscopical features are similar to those of major glands.

Mucinous adenocarcinoma is very rare while *clear cell carcinoma* is a controversial entity; both are discussed in Chapter 5.

Salivary gland adenomas

ICD-O codes

Pleomorphic adenoma	8940/0
Myoepithelioma	8982/0
Basal cell adenoma	8147/0
Canalicular adenoma	8149/0
Duct papilloma	8503/0
Cystadenoma	8440/0

Pleomorphic adenoma
These amount to 40-70% of minor gland tumours, the large majority of cases being located in the palate, lips and buccal mucosa {2711}. They usually present as painless, slow-growing, submucosal masses, but occasionally they are traumatised and bleed or ulcerate. They rarely exceed 3 sphere cm in diam-

eter. Oral pleomorphic adenomas are similar microscopically to tumours elsewhere but frequently lack encapsulation, especially in the palate. They tend to be cellular, and hyaline or plasmacytoid cell types are common. Squamous metaplasia is also frequently seen and may be extensive. Some tumours have a strikingly lipomatous stroma and this should not be misinterpreted as tumour invading fat. Cases of intraoral pleomorphic adenoma with florid pseudoepitheliomatous hyperplasia of the overlying mucosa have been reported following incisional biopsy {2541}.

Myoepithelioma
The minor glands are the common site for and myoepitheliomas account for about 42% of all of these tumours. Two thirds of the intraoral cases involve the palate {899}. They show the same range of morphological variation described in Chapter 5, but predominantly plasmacytoid tumours have a predilection for the palate of younger individuals {546}.

Basal cell adenoma
About 20% of basal cell adenomas involve the oral cavity and the upper lip and buccal mucosa are the most common sites {669}. They are histologically similar to those in major glands.

Cystadenoma
These lesions are uncommon and form 7% of benign minor gland tumours {668}. Of these, 30% arose in the lips, 23% in the cheek, 20% in the palate and 26% in other oral and oropharyngeal sites. Clinically they resemble mucoceles and rarely exceed 1cm in diameter. The pathology is discussed in Chapter 5.

Canalicular adenoma and duct papillomas arise almost exclusively in the minor salivary glands and are discussed in detail in Chapter 5.

Kaposi sarcoma

I. van der Waal
J. Lamovec
S. Knuutila

Definition

Kaposi sarcoma (KS) is a locally aggressive tumour that typically presents with cutaneous lesions in the form of multiple patches, plaques or nodules but may also involve mucosal sites, lymph nodes and visceral organs. The disease is uniformly associated with human herpes virus 8 (HHV-8) infection. KS rarely metastasizes and belongs to the group of intermediate type vascular tumours.

ICD-O code   9140/3

Epidemiology

Four different clinical and epidemiological forms of KS are recognized: 1. classic indolent form occurring predominantly in elderly men of Mediterranean/East European descent, 2. endemic African KS that occurs in middle-aged adults and children in Equatorial Africa who are not HIV infected, 3. iatrogenic KS appearing in solid organ transplant recipients treated with immunosuppressive therapy and also in patients treated by immunosuppressive agents, notably corticosteroids, for various diseases {2629}, 4. acquired immunodeficiency syndrome-associated KS (AIDS KS), the most aggressive form of the disease, found in HIV-1 infected individuals, that is particularly frequent in homo- and bisexual men. The relative risk of acquiring KS

in the latter patients is > 10,000 {909}; it has been reduced with the advent of highly active antiretroviral therapy (HAART) {212}, although this has not been proven yet for oral KS {1993,2120}.

Etiology

The disease is the result of a complex interplay of HHV-8 with immunologic, genetic, and environmental factors {392}. Oral exposure to infectious saliva seems to be a potential risk factor for the acquisition of HHV-8 {1995}. HHV-8 is found in KS cells of all epidemiological-clinical forms of the disease {2242} and is detected in the peripheral blood before the development of KS. Nevertheless, it has been observed that a declined incidence of KS did not appear to be caused by a decline in HHV-8 transmission {1959}.

Localization

The most typical site of involvement by KS is the skin, particularly of the face and lower extremities. During the course of the disease or initially, mucosal membranes such as oral mucosa, lymph nodes and visceral organs may be affected, sometimes without skin involvement. Oral KS most frequently occurs on the palate, followed by the gingiva and the tongue.

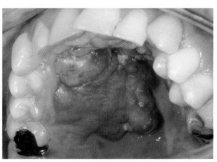

Fig. 4.35 Kaposi sarcoma of the palate.

Clinical features

Classic type of KS is characterized by the appearance of purplish, reddish blue or dark brown macules, plaques and nodules that may ulcerate. They are particularly frequent in distal extremities and may be accompanied by lymphoedema. The disease is usually indolent, lymph node and visceral involvement occurs infrequently. Classic KS may be associated with haematolymphoid malignancies.

In the endemic form of KS, the disease may be localized to skin and shows a protracted course. A variant of endemic disease, a lymphadenopathic form in African children is rapidly progressive and highly lethal.

Iatrogenic KS is relatively frequent. It develops in a few months to several years after the transplantation of solid organs or immunosuppressive treatment for a vari-

Table 4.05 Epidemiological-clinical types of Kaposi sarcoma

Type	Risk groups	Skin lesions -predilection sites	Visceral involvement	Course
Classic	Elderly men of Mediterranean/ East European descent	Lower legs	Rare	Indolent
Endemic	Middles-aged men and children in Equatorial Africa	Extremities	Fairly common - adults Frequent - children (lymph nodes)	Indolent - adults Aggressive - children
Iatrogenic	Immunosuppressed patients (post-transplant, other diseases)	Lower legs	Fairly common	Indolent or aggressive
AIDS-associated	Younger, mainly homo- and bisexual HIV-1 infected men	Face, genitalia, lower extremities	Frequent	Aggressive

From: WHO Classification of Tumours of Soft Tissue and Bone {775}.

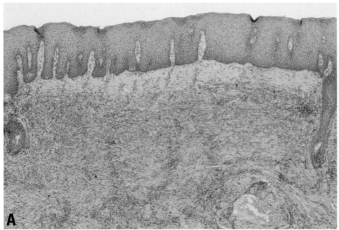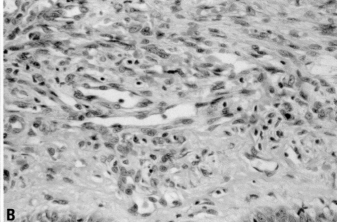

Fig. 4.36 Kaposi sarcoma. **A** Inflammatory-like aspect of palatal Kaposi sarcoma. **B** Vascular slits and sparsely distributed lymphocytes.

ety of conditions. The disease may resolve entirely upon withdrawal of immunosuppressive treatment although immunosuppressive treatment although its course is somewhat unpredictable.

AIDS-related KS is the most aggressive type of KS. Early oral KS is represented by solitary or multiple red or bluish flat lesions, while the later stage is characterized by a nodular, sometimes massive appearance with or without secondary ulceration.

Histopathology

Microscopic features of all four different epidemiological-clinical types of KS do not differ. Early lesions of the skin or the mucosa are uncharacteristic and present with subtle vascular proliferation {2216}.

In the patch stage, vascular spaces are increased in number, of irregular shape, and may dissect collagen fibres in the superficial corium. They often run parallel to the epithelium. The vascular proliferation is often perivascular and periadnexal. Endothelial cells lining the spaces are flattened or more oval, with little atypia. Pre-existing blood vessels may protrude into the lumen of new vessels. Admixed are sparse lymphocytes and plasma cells; frequently, extravasated erythrocytes and deposits of hemosiderin surround the vas-

cular structures. Slits lined by attenuated endothelial cells between collagen bundles are also seen. In some cases, there is a proliferation of spindle or oval endothelial cells around pre-existing blood vessels in the dermis or submucosa. Slit-like spaces, lymphocyte and plasma cell infiltration and extravasated erythrocytes are also observed.

In plaque stage, all characteristics of patch stage are exaggerated. There is more extensive angio-proliferation with vascular spaces showing jagged outlines. Inflammatory infiltrate is denser and extravascular red cells and siderophages are numerous. Hyaline globules (likely representing destroyed red blood cells) are frequently found.

Nodular stage is characterized by well-defined nodules of intersecting fascicles of spindle cells with only mild atypia and numerous slit-like spaces containing red cells. Peripherally, there are ectatic blood vessels. Many spindle cells show mitoses. Hyaline globules are present inside and outside the spindle cells. Some patients, usually with endemic nodular type KS, develop lesions that closely resemble lymphangioma.

The main differential diagnosis includes Kaposiform haemangioendothelioma {775}.

Immunoprofile

The lining cells of clearly developed vascular structures are usually positive for vascular markers, while the spindle cells consistently show positive reaction for CD34 and commonly for CD31 but are factor VIII negative. All cases, irrespective of epidemiologic subgroup, are HHV-8 positive. The new marker FLI1, a nuclear transcription factor, appears to be expressed in almost 100% of different vascular tumours, including KS {780}.

Prognosis and predictive factors

The evolution of disease depends on the epidemiological-clinical type of KS and on its clinical extent. It is also modified by treatment that includes surgery, radio- and chemotherapy. Patients with oral KS who did not receive triple antiretroviral therapy had a higher death rate than those having exclusively cutaneous manifestations of the disease {2192}.

Lymphangioma

I. van der Waal

Definition
A benign, cavernous/cystic vascular lesion composed of dilated lymphatic channels.

ICD-O code   9170/0

Epidemiology
Lymphangiomas are common paediatric lesions, which most often present at birth or during the first years of life. Lymphangiomas appear mostly in the head and neck area but may be found in any other part of the body.

Etiology
Early or even congenital appearance in life and lesional architecture are in favour of a developmental malformation, with genetic abnormalities playing an additional role in cystic lymphangioma of the neck in association with Turner syndrome {416}.

Clinical features
The lesion presents as a somewhat circumscribed painless swelling, which is soft and fluctuant on palpation. In oral involvement, the tongue is the site of predilection, the majority of lymphangiomas being located on the dorsal surface of the anterior part of the tongue. The size may vary from pinhead dimensions to massive lesions involving the entire tongue and surrounding structures. The typical lymphangioma of the

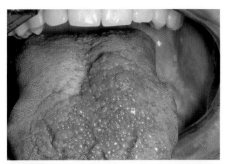
Fig. 4.37 Lymphangioma on the dorsum of the tongue.

tongue is characterized by irregular nodularity of the dorsum of the tongue with grey and pink, grapelike projections. Secondary haemorrhage in lymphangiomas is not a rare occurrence. CT scan reveals homogeneous non-enhancing areas {775}.
A staging system of lymphatic malformations of the head and neck based on the anatomic location has shown to be of relevance in predicting prognosis and outcome of surgical intervention {561,991}.

Macroscopy
Lymphangiomas form a multicystic or spongy mass, the cavities of which contain watery to milky fluid.

Histopathology
Lymphangiomas are characterized by thin-walled, dilated lymphatic vessels of different size, which are lined by a flat-

tened endothelium. There is no encapsulation. The lumina may be either empty or contain proteinaceous fluid, lymphocytes and sometimes a few erythrocytes. Longstanding lesions show interstitial fibrosis.

Immunoprofile
The endothelium demonstrates variable expression of FVIII-rAg, CD31 and CD34 {781}.

Electron microscopy
The endothelium of thin-walled vessels is not enveloped by a basement membrane and no pericytes are attached to it, thus directly contacting with the interstitium. With increasing calibre the vessels may acquire pericytes and smooth muscle, respectively.

Prognosis and predictive factors
Recurrences are due to incomplete removal. Current interest is centred on treating these lesions with sclerosing agents {2117}, interferon {1953} or bleomycin {2903A}. Malignant transformation does not occur. There is an exceedingly rare case report of a squamous cell carcinoma arising in a lymphangioma of the tongue {203}.

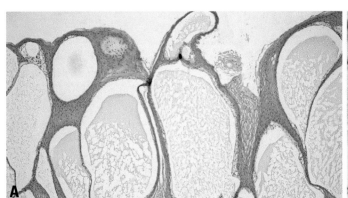
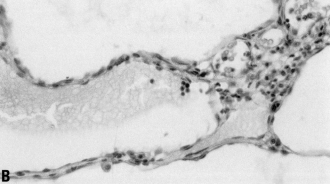
Fig. 4.38 Lymphangioma. **A** Cavernous lymphangioma. **B** Flattened endothelial lining in lymphangioma.

Ectomesenchymal chondromyxoid tumour of the anterior tongue

I. van der Waal

Definition

A benign ectomesenchymal chondromyxoid tumour that arises in the anterior tongue.

Epidemiology

In 1995, nineteen cases of the previously undescribed entity were reported. Ever since, a few additional case reports have been published {1169}. The reported age range varies from 9-78 years; there is no distinct sex predilection.

Clinical features

Most tumours presented as an otherwise asymptomatic, slow growing solitary nodule in the anterior dorsal tongue. The consistency may vary from firm to soft elastic.

Macroscopy

The cut surface has a gelatinous consistency with occasional foci of haemorrhage.

Histopathology

The tumour is usually well-circumscribed, but not encapsulated. Occasionally, muscle fibres and nerve branches may be entrapped within the tumour. It is composed of round, cup-shaped, fusiform, or polygonal cells with uniform small nuclei and moderate amounts of faintly basophilic cytoplasm; some tumours may show nuclear pleomorphism, hyperchro-

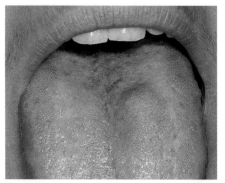

Fig. 4.39 Ectomesenchymal chondromyxoid tumour of the anterior tongue presenting as a small nodule.

matism, and multinucleation, while mitotic figures are scarce {2410}. In addition, the presence of myxoglobulosis-like changes has been reported {1169}. Alcian blue stains at pH 0.4 and 2.5 are positive, while mucicarmine is usually faintly positive in the extracellular matrix. The tumour cells do not stain with the periodic acid-Shiff (PAS). In the histological differential diagnosis other myxoid and chondroid lesions should be excluded, such as focal oral mucinosis, the mucous retention phenomenon, soft-tissue myxoma, nerve sheath myxoma, myxomatous changes in fibrous lesions, chondrosarcoma, chondroid choristoma, and variants of pleomorphic adenoma or myoepithelioma arising from minor salivary glands.

Immunoprofile

Reactivity with polyclonal and monoclonal anti glial fibrillary acidic protein (GFAP) is positive in almost all reported cases; reactivity with anti-cytokeratin monoclonal antibody has been positive in the majority of cases as well, while variable staining results were observed for S-100, CD57 and smooth muscle actin {2410}.

Histogenesis

The tumour cells are possibly derived from undifferentiated ectomesenchymal progenitor cells that have migrated from the neural crest {2410}.

Prognosis and predictive factors

Surgical excision is the treatment of choice. The recurrence rate is apparently low.

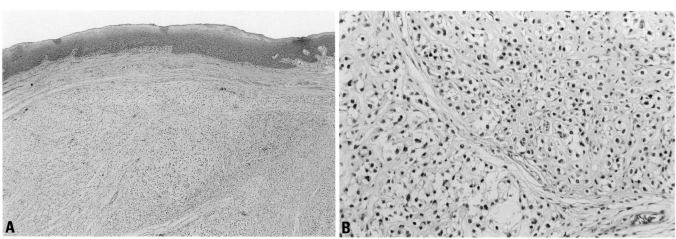

Fig. 4.40 A Rather well demarcated ectomesenchymal chondromyxoid tumour. **B** Net-like pattern of round or ovoid cells in a chondromyxoid background.

Focal oral mucinosis

I. van der Waal

Definition

Focal oral mucinosis (FOM) is the oral counterpart of focal cutaneous mucinosis and cutaneous myxoid cyst. It is postulated that FOM develops as the result of a fibroblastic overproduction of hyaluronic acid due to an unknown cause {2615}.

Epidemiology

Today, fewer than fifty cases have been reported. The lesion may occur at all ages, but it is rare in children {906}. There is no distinct sex predilection.

Clinical features

The clinical presentation is usually that of an otherwise asymptomatic fibrous or cystic-like lesion. The most common site is the gingiva; less common sites include the palate, cheek mucosa and tongue. The consistency may vary from soft elastic to firm.

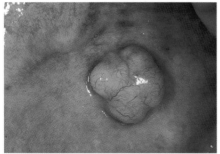

Fig. 4.41 Focal oral mucinosis. Fibroma-like swelling of the cheek mucosa based on focal oral mucinosis.

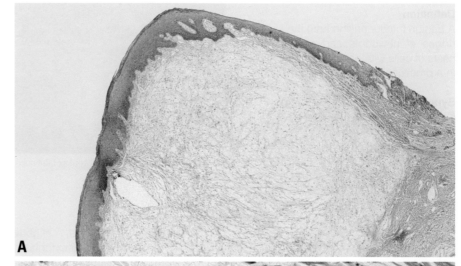

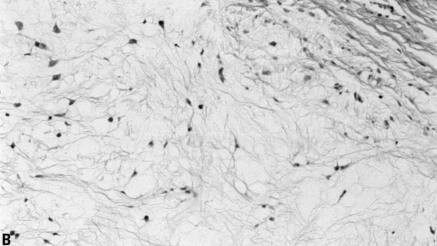

Fig. 4.42 Focal oral mucinosis. **A** Well-demarcated area of myxomatous connective tissue. **B** Delicate fibrillar processes extending from fibroblast cytoplasm.

Histopathology

The histopathology is characterized by a well-circumscribed area of myxomatous tissue in which fusiform or stellate fibroblasts are present {299}. Reticular fibres are sparse or absent. The mucinous material shows alcianophilia at pH 2.5. The histologic differential diagnosis includes soft-tissue myxoma, myxomatous change in fibrous lesions, nerve sheath myxoma, and mucous retention phenomenon. The lack of reticular fibres and the sharp delineation distinguishes FOM both from soft-tissue myxoma and from myxomatous changes in fibrous lesions {2615}. Nerve sheath myxoma usually shows a lobular architecture and, conspicuously, contains numerous mast cells. The mucous retention phenomenon is surrounded by a wall of granulation tissue or an epithelium-lined wall, while the mucoid material contains histiocytic cells; such features are lacking in FOM.

Prognosis and predictive factors

The lesion is treated by conservative surgical excision and has no tendency to recur.

Congenital granular cell epulis

I. van der Waal

Definition
A benign tumour arising from the alveolar ridges of newborns and composed of nests of cells with granular cytoplasm set in a prominent vasculature {2744}.

Synonym
Congenital epulis of the newborn

Epidemiology
In a review of the literature 216 cases have been collected since its first description in 1871. Females are affected ten times more often than males {2152}.

Clinical features
Congenital granular cell epulis (CGCE) occurs twice as often in the maxilla as in the mandible, usually presenting as a solitary, somewhat pedunculated fibroma-like lesion attached to the alveolar ridge near the midline. A few cases of simultaneous occurrence of a CGCE and a granular cell tumour of the tongue have been reported {1564,2848}. The size of a CGCE may vary from a few millimetres up to several centimetres.

Since the availability of ultrasound examination techniques, a number of cases have been diagnosed in the prenatal stage {1839,2000}.

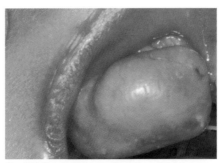

Fig. 4.43 Congenital granular cell epulis of the maxilla.

Histopathology
CGCE consists of large, slightly eosinophilic cells with granular cytoplasm set in a prominent vasculature. There is no cellular or nuclear pleomorphism, and mitotic activity is not usually observed. The presence of odontogenic epithelium scattered throughout the lesions has been reported. Immunohistochemically, the tumour cells are positive for vimentin and neuron specific enolase; there is no reactivity with cytokeratin, CEA, desmin, hormone receptors or S-100 {1968}. Pseudoepitheliomatous changes in the overlying epithelium, although common in the granular cell tumour, do not occur in CGCE. An extremely rare case of a congenital leiomyomatous epulis has been reported {2542}.

Histogenesis
The histogenesis is unknown. The lack of immunoreactivity with S-100 protein suggests that the tumour is derived from a cell line different from granular cell tumour. Furthermore, the hypothesis of a non-neoplastic lesion can be raised.

Prognosis and predictive factors
Spontaneous regression may occur, but surgical removal is usually indicated due to interference with feeding or respiration. The tumour has no tendency to recur after surgery.

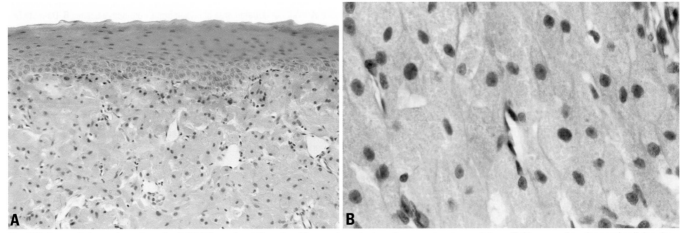

Fig. 4.44 Congenital granular cell epulis. **A** Slightly eosinophilic cells with granular cytoplasm in a prominent vasculature. **B** Absence of nuclear and cellular pleomorphism.

Haematolymphoid tumours

A.C.L. Chan
J.K.C. Chan

Non-Hodgkin lymphoma

Definition
Non-Hodgkin lymphomas (NHL) of the oral cavity and oropharynx are defined as lymphoid cell neoplasms in which the bulk of the disease occurs in the palate, tongue, floor of mouth, gingiva, buccal mucosa, lips, palatine tonsils, lingual tonsils or oropharynx.

ICD-O codes
Diffuse large B-cell lymphoma
(DLBCL)   9680/3
Mantle cell lymphoma   9673/3
Follicular lymphoma   9690/3
Extranodal marginal zone B-cell lymphoma of MALT type   9699/3
Burkitt lymphoma   9687/3
T-cell lymphoma (including anaplastic large cell lymphoma)   9714/3

Epidemiology
Although NHL is the second most com-mon cancer of the oral cavity, it only accounts for 3.5% of all oral malignancies {683}. NHL of the oral cavity and oropharynx account for 13% of all primary extranodal NHL, with approximately 70% of these occurring in the tonsils {809}. They affect patients over a wide age range (including children), but most patients are in the 6th and 7th decades. Burkitt lymphomas occur predominantly in children and young adults. Patients with an underlying immunodeficiency state (e.g. HIV Infection) are also usually younger.

Etiology
There is no known etiology in most patients. A minority of patients have an underlying immunodeficiency state (e.g. HIV infection, post-transplantation), which predisposes to the development of NHL. There is a strong association with Epstein-Barr virus (EBV) for lymphomas occurring in the setting of immunodeficiency as well as in extranodal NK/T cell lymphoma of nasal-type {371,962,1476, 2850}. Extranodal marginal zone B-cell lymphoma of MALT type may be associated with Sjögren syndrome {2476}.

Table 4.06 Frequency of the various types of primary lymphoma of the tonsil {1704}

Diffuse large B-cell lymphoma (DLBCL) ICD-O code 9680/3	64%
Mantle cell lymphoma ICD-O code 9673/3	10%
Follicular lymphoma ICD-O code 9690/3	8%
Extranodal marginal zone B-cell lymphoma of MALT type* ICD-O code 9699/3	6.5%
T-cell lymphoma (including anaplastic large cell lymphoma ICD-O code 9714/3)	6.5%
Burkitt lymphoma ICD-O code 9687/3	5%

* Reported as monocytoid B-cell lymphoma and immunocytoma in the original series.

Localization
The palatine tonsil is the most frequently involved site, followed by palate, gingiva and tongue {683,809,1476,2532}.

Clinical features
Patients with NHL of the lip, buccal mucosa, gingiva, floor of mouth, tongue or palate usually present with ulcer, swelling, discoloration, pain, paraesthesia, anaesthesia, or loose teeth. Those with NHL of the Waldeyer ring (tonsils) or oropharynx usually present with a sensation of fullness of the throat, sore throat, dysphagia, or snoring. The high-grade tumours often show rapid growth. Systemic symptoms such as fever and night sweat are uncommon {201}. Clinical examination reveals solitary or multiple lesions, in the form of an exophytic mass, ulcer or localized swelling. Some cases may mimic inflammatory

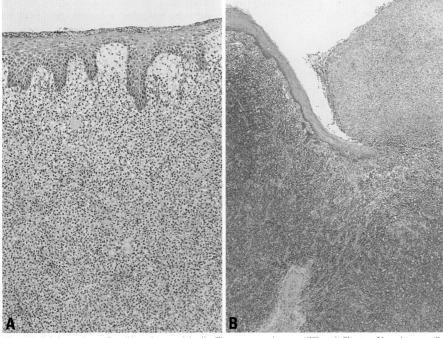

Fig. 4.45 A Primary large B cell lymphoma of the lip. The mucosa shows a diffuse infiltrate of lymphoma cells beneath an intact stratified squamous epithelium. **B** Primary large B cell lymphoma of the tongue. In this example, the mucosa is partly ulcerated.

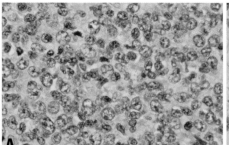
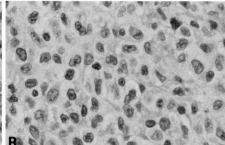
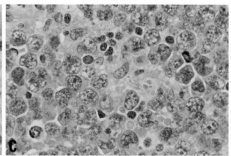

Fig. 4.46 Primary large B cell lymphoma of the oral cavity and oropharynx: cytological spectrum. **A** Large cells with predominantly round nuclei and membrane-bound nucleoli, consistent with centroblastic morphology. **B** Predominantly medium-sized cells with abundant pale cytoplasm. **C** Large cells with round or multilobated nuclei.

conditions, such as periodontitis. Tonsillar lymphoma usually manifests as asymmetric tonsil enlargement, although the disease can be bilateral in up to 9% of cases {2250}. The regional lymph nodes can be enlarged as a result of lymphoma involvement or reactive changes secondary to ulceration.

Tumour spread and staging
Three-quarters of patients have localized disease, with or without accompanying cervical lymph node involvement at presentation (Stage IE/IIE). Patients with lymphoma of the tonsil are prone to metachronous or synchronous gastrointestinal tract involvement, suggesting a homing mechanism among different mucosal sites {1998,2139,2250}.

Histopathology
Most NHL of the oral cavity and oropharynx are of B-cell lineage, with DLBCL being the commonest (>50%) {370,1476, 1704,2142,2530}. The surface stratified squamous epithelium is either intact or ulcerated. The stroma is densely infiltrated by lymphoma cells, which vary in appearance depending on the histologic type. In the tonsil, not uncommonly there are some residual lymphoid follicles due to incomplete involvement of the tissue.

Diffuse large B-cell lymphoma (DLBCL)
DLBCL is characterized by large to medium-sized cells which may resemble centroblasts. Nuclear multilobation is prominent in some cases. There can be areas of coagulative necrosis. In DLBCL of the tonsils, a focal follicular pattern may be present {2138}, and it has been argued that the follicles result from colonization of pre-existing follicles rather than de novo neoplastic follicle formation. In some cases, there may be an associated component of extranodal marginal zone B-cell lymphoma of MALT type or follicular lymphoma, indicating that the DLBCL represents high-grade transformation of the latter {1998}.

Mantle cell lymphoma
Lymphoma cells are usually monotonous, and frequently have small irregular nuclei, dense chromatin and scanty cytoplasm. They may show a mantle zone distribution around residual follicles. Rare cases can have a blastic appearance and are associated with a higher proliferation rate {19}.

Follicular lymphoma
Follicular lymphoma is characterized by follicles that frequently lack polarity and mantle zone. The neoplastic follicles consist of a mixture of centrocytes and centroblasts, often without accompanying tingible-body macrophages.

Extranodal marginal zone B-cell lymphomas of MALT type
These lymphomas most often involve the tonsil, and less commonly the palate, gingiva, buccal mucosa, tongue and lip {295,962,1476,1507,1629,1998,2225, 2531}. The surface epithelium is often intact. In a background of reactive lymphoid follicles, there is an interfollicular and perifollicular infiltrate of small to medium-sized cells with roundish or indented nuclei. Some cells have a moderate amount of clear cytoplasm, resembling monocytoid B-cells. There can be clusters of admixed plasma cells. Follicular colonization can be seen in some cases. A distinctive feature is invasion of the epithelial component (e.g. sur-

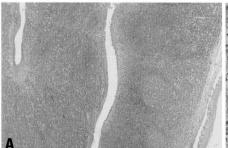
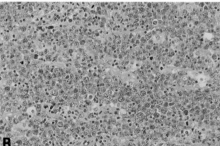
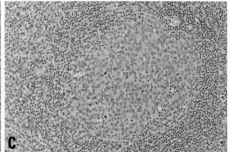

Fig. 4.47 Primary large B cell lymphoma of the tonsil with focal follicular features. **A** The left field shows the predominant component of diffuse large cell lymphoma. The minor component with follicles is shown in the right field. **B** The diffuse large B cell lymphoma component comprises large cells effacing the normal architecture of the tonsil. **C** Focally, there are follicles comprising a monotonous population of large cells. It is unclear whether this represents a grade 3 follicular lymphoma with diffuse large B cell lymphoma, or a diffuse large B-cell lymphoma with follicular colonization.

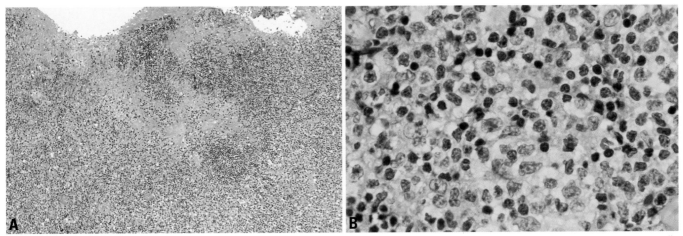

Fig. 4.48 Extranodal NK/T cell lymphoma of the palate. **A** The mucosa, which is densely infiltrated by lymphoma cells, shows ulceration. **B** The lymphoma cells comprise small, medium-sized and large cells with irregular nuclear foldings.

face or crypt epithelium, minor salivary glands), forming lymphoepithelial lesions.

Burkitt lymphoma
There is typically a starry sky pattern created by interspersed histiocytes. The lymphoma cells appear monotonous and medium-sized, with coarse chromatin, multiple small nucleoli and a small amount of basophilic cytoplasm. The cellular outline usually appears squared off. Frequent mitotic figures and apoptotic bodies are constant features.

Immunoprofile. B-cell lymphomas express pan-B markers such as CD19, CD20, CD22 and CD79a. Some DLBCLs can express CD10 and/or BCL6. Within the group of low-grade B-cell lymphomas, follicular lymphoma is characterized by CD10 and BCL6 expression,

mantle cell lymphoma CD5 and cyclin D1 expression, and extranodal marginal zone B-cell lymphoma none of these markers. Bcl-2 Immunoreactivity is helpful for distinction of follicular lymphoma from reactive follicular hyperplasia.

Extranodal NK/T cell lymphoma of nasal-type
Extranodal NK/T cell lymphoma of nasal-type can present primarily as an intraoral tumour in the palate, tonsil, oropharynx or lip {371,2639}. Please refer to the section of 'non-Hodgkin lymphoma' in 'Tumours of the nasal cavity and paranasal sinuses' for details.

T-cell lymphomas
Peripheral T-cell lymphomas, including anaplastic large cell lymphomas, can occasionally involve the oral cavity

{1476,2200,2530}. Some anaplastic large cell lymphomas (CD30+ T-cell lymphoproliferative disorder) of the oral cavity can regress spontaneously {760}. HTLV-1-associated adult T-cell lymphoma/leukaemia may also present as NHL of the Waldeyer ring {2616}.

Immunodeficiency-associated lymphomas
The lymphomas that develop in the oral cavity of patients with HIV infection are most commonly DLBCL with frequent EBV association (75%) {962,2141}, although EBV-associated T-cell lymphomas have also been reported in this setting {1476,2589}. A distinctive form of DLBCL, plasmablastic lymphoma, has recently been shown to exhibit a predilection for the oral cavity of HIV-positive subjects. It differs from the usual

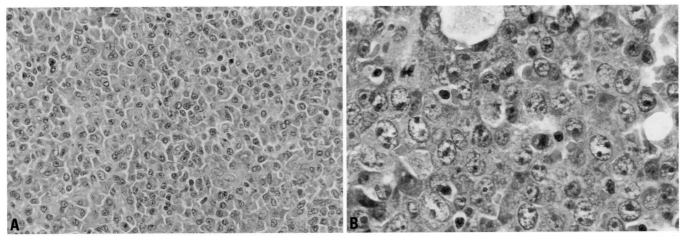

Fig. 4.49 Immunodeficiency-associated lymphoproliferative disorders. **A** Post-transplant lymphoproliferative disorder, plasmacytic hyperplasia, involving tonsil. **B** Plasmablastic lymphoma of the oral cavity in HIV-positive subject. The cells possess slightly eccentrically-located large vesicular nuclei, prominent nucleoli, and amphophilic cytoplasm.

DLBCL by the plasmablastic morphology, frequent lack of expression of CD45 and the pan-B marker CD20, and expression of plasma cell-associated markers (e.g. VS38c and CD138) {576}. EBV is identified in 60% of cases. Histologically, the tumour shows a starry-sky appearance and a high proliferation index. The large tumour cells have eccentric vesicular nuclei, central prominent nucleoli, abundant basophilic cytoplasm and paranuclear hof. There is no maturation into plasma cells.

Post-transplant lymphoproliferative disorder (PTLD) can also affect the oral cavity, and they are frequently associated with EBV (>80%). The 'early' lesions, including plasmacytic hyperplasia and infectious mononucleosis-like PTLD, commonly involve the tonsils of children or younger adults {355,356,2830}. The architecture of the tonsil is preserved, with expansion of the interfollicular areas by small lymphocytes, polyclonal plasma cells, plasmablasts and immunoblasts. Clonal immunoglobulin gene rearrangement is rare {355,2830}. Most lesions regress with reduction in immunosuppression, but rare cases may progress to polymorphic PTLD {2830}. Polymorphic and monomorphic PTLD can also present in the oral cavity (e.g. tonsil, gingiva, alveolus): the former shows architectural effacement, necrosis, cytologic atypia together with a full range of B-cell maturation, while the latter is indistinguishable from conventional DLBCL, and less commonly Burkitt lymphoma {1301,1926, 2131,2850}. Clonal immunoglobulin gene rearrangement is frequently demonstrated in polymorphic and monomorphic PTLD. Regression after reduction in immunosuppression may still be possible in some cases of polymorphic PTLD, but progression is usually the rule for monomorphic PTLD. (Please refer to 'Post-transplant lymphoproliferative disorders' in 'WHO classification of tumours: Tumours of haematopoietic and lymphoid tissues' for details).

Differential diagnoses

In *infectious mononucleosis*, the tonsils may appear histologically worrisome, with necrosis, partial effacement of architecture, and striking immunoblastic proliferation, mimicking DLBCL {431}. In contrast to the latter, there is usually a spectrum of lymphoid cells in different stages of differentiation and activation

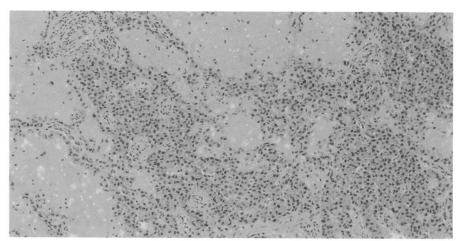
Fig. 4.50 Plasmacytoma of the tongue. The plasmacytoma is accompanied by blood lakes.

(immunoblasts, plasmablasts and plasma cells). On immunostaining, the large cells usually consist of a mixture of B- and T-cells, and there is no immunoglobulin light chain restriction. As a rule of thumb, infectious mononucleosis has to be seriously excluded before making a diagnosis of DLBCL in young patients.

Some cases of DLBCL (especially those in the tonsil) can exhibit deceptively cohesive growth and a sharp interface with the uninvolved mucosa, closely mimicking poorly differentiated carcinoma or malignant melanoma. Marked irregular nuclear foldings and amphophilic cytoplasm, if present, should point more towards a diagnosis of lymphoma. Appropriate immunostains can readily solve this diagnostic problem.

Anaplastic plasmacytoma can be difficult to distinguish from DLBCL, including the plasmablastic variant. An important clue to the diagnosis is the presence of coarsely clumped 'clock-face' chromatin in the few differentiated cells that are present. There are often intermingled atypical plasma cells. There is usually no association with EBV. A prior history of multiple myeloma, if present, would be a strong point to substantiate a diagnosis of plasmacytoma.

Extramedullary myeloid sarcoma (granulocytic sarcoma) is commonly misdiagnosed as large cell lymphoma. The clues to diagnosis are the fine chromatin, presence of cytoplasmic eosinophilic granules in some cells, and interspersed eosinophilic myelocytes. The diagnosis can be confirmed by immunoreactivity for myeloid or monocytic markers (e.g. myeloperoxidase, CD13, CD33, CD117, neutrophil elastase, lysozyme, CD68).

The differential diagnosis between extranodal marginal zone B-cell lymphoma of MALT type in the tonsil and *reactive lymphoid hyperplasia* can be extremely difficult, because of the presence of reactive lymphoid follicles, minimal atypia of the lymphoid cells in the former and presence of numerous plasma cells. Furthermore, lymphoepithelial lesions in the tonsil are difficult to assess since the tonsillar epithelium is normally extensively infiltrated by small lymphoid cells. The following features would favour a diagnosis of lymphoma: lymphoid cells infiltrating beyond the fibrous band at the base of the tonsil, presence of sheets of CD20+ B-cells between the lymphoid follicles, immunoglobulin light chain restriction, and molecular evidence of clonal immunoglobulin gene rearrangement.

Some *extranodal NK/T cell lymphomas of nasal-type* comprise predominantly small lymphoid cells with minimal atypia, rendering it difficult to distinguish from a reactive lymphoid infiltrate. Histologic clues to the diagnosis are the extensive necrosis and angiocentric growth. Demonstration of sheets of CD56+ or EBER+ cells would strongly support the diagnosis.

There is some morphologic overlap of anaplastic large cell lymphoma with *eosinophilic ulcer* (traumatic eosinophilic granuloma; atypical histiocytic granuloma) {645,674,701}, which is characterized by a rich inflammatory infiltrate (especially eosinophils) and occasional large cells {760}. Anaplastic large cell lymphoma can be distinguished from it by the presence of at least large aggregates of large atypical cells in areas and strong CD30 expression.

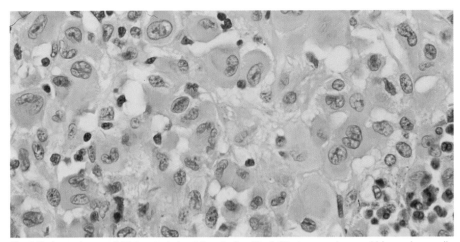

Fig. 4.51 Langerhans cell histiocytosis involving gingiva. The infiltrate comprises ovoid Langerhans cells with deeply grooved nuclei, thin nuclear membranes and abundant eosinophilic cytoplasm. There are typically many admixed eosinophils.

Prognosis and predictive factors

Patients with NHL of the oral cavity and oropharynx are treated by radiotherapy, chemotherapy or a combination of the two. Some studies have shown that adjuvant chemotherapy is associated with a better clinical outcome compared to radiotherapy alone {832,1009}. The five-year overall survival rate for localized disease ranges from 50% to more than 80% {146,832,1009,1614,2505}. High clinical stage, high histologic grade (large cell lymphoma), and T-cell or NK/T cell phenotype are poor prognostic indicators {146,1009,2250,2340,2809}.

Extramedullary plasmacytoma

ICD-O code   9734/3

Extramedullary plasmacytoma can occur in the oral cavity and oropharynx, see Chapter 1 for details.

Langerhans cell histiocytosis

ICD-O code   9751/1

Oral involvement occurs in 10% of patients with Langerhans cell histiocytosis (LCH). 78% of these patients have eosinophilic granulomas clinically, while the rest have multifocal multisystem disease {1021}. Common oral symptoms include swelling, pain, gingivitis, loose teeth and ulceration. The majority of patients with intraoral lesions have intraosseous lesions in the jaw bone, more commonly in the mandible. The intraoral soft tissues may be secondarily affected, especially the gingiva, but the palate, floor of mouth, buccal mucosa and tonsil can also be involved {1021, 2043}. In a minority of patients with intraoral soft tissue involvement, there is no

associated bony lesion {241,460,1731}. See chapter 7 for details.

Hodgkin lymphoma

Hodgkin lymphoma (HL) is predominantly a nodal-based disease, and primary extranodal presentation is very rare. When it presents in extranodal tissues, the Waldeyer ring, particularly the palatine tonsil, is a common site {1274,1756}. Most patients present with localized disease (stage I/II), with symptoms of chronic tonsillitis or tonsillar enlargement, with or without enlarged cervical lymph nodes. Other reported sites include the oropharynx {44,1756}, alveolar crest of mandible {1659}, and maxillary gingiva {2554}.

Most cases represent classical HL, as detailed in the WHO Classification of Tumours of Haematopoietic and Lymphoid Tissues {1197}, frequently of mixed cellularity subtype and showing strong association with Epstein-Barr virus (EBV) {1274}, although nodular lymphocyte predominant HL may also rarely present in the Waldeyer ring (palatine and lingual tonsils) {391,1274}.

Extramedullary myeloid sarcoma

ICD-O code   9930/3

Gingival infiltrates occur in 3.5% of patients with acute myeloid leukaemia, predominantly in the monocytic or myelomonocytic subtypes {622}. Clinically, there is diffuse enlargement of the interdental papillae, marginal gingiva and attached gingiva. The swollen gingiva has a spongy to firm consistency, bright red to purple in colour. There is no correlation between gingival leukaemic infiltrate and oral hygiene or peripheral white blood cell count {622}.

Rare cases of extramedullary myeloid sarcoma may present as an isolated tumour-forming intraoral mass. The most frequently involved sites are the palate and gingiva {52,761,2189,2614,2618}. While the tumour most often develops while the patient has active disease, it may precede the development of acute myeloid leukaemia, or arise as blastic transformation of an underlying chronic myeloproliferative disease or myelodys-

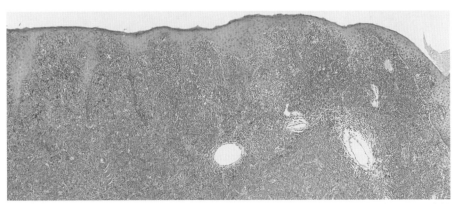

Fig. 4.52 Extramedullary myeloid sarcoma of the gingiva as the first sign of relapse of acute myeloid leukaemia. Beneath an intact stratified squamous epithelium, there is a diffuse and dense infiltrate of primitive myeloid cells.

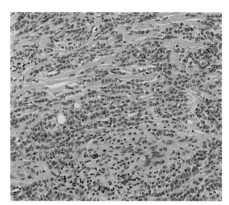

Fig. 4.53 Extramedullary myeloid sarcoma of the gingiva as the first sign of relapse of acute myeloid leukaemia. In areas, there is typically an Indian-file pattern of infitration.

zone or 'dysplasia' of FDC may represent the precursor lesion.

Histopathology

Histologically, the tumour usually grows beneath an intact stratified squamous epithelium. It usually exhibits pushing borders and comprises fascicles, whorls, nodules, storiform arrays or diffuse sheets of spindly to ovoid tumour cells sprinkled with small lymphocytes. The tumour cells usually show ill-defined cell borders, distinct nucleoli, and sometimes nuclear pseudoinclusions. There is a tendency for some nuclei to be haphazardly clustered, and scattered multincleated tumour cells are common. While nuclear pleomorphism is usually mild, some cases can show significant nuclear atypia and pleomorphism. The cytoplasm is eosinophilic, and often exhibits a fibrillary quality as a result of the presence of interdigitating cell processes. Very rarely, the tumour cells have distinct cell borders, and are polygonal or oval in shape. The mitotic count ranges from low to high, and some cases can show coagulative necrosis. Occasional cases may show irregular interspersed cystic spaces. Besides being intermingled among the tumour cells, the lymphocytes can show cuffing around the blood vessels.

The diagnosis has to be confirmed by demonstration of FDC markers (e.g. CD21, CD23 and CD35), although the staining can be patchy. Typically a mesh-

plastic syndrome. Histologically, there is a dense infiltrate of immature myeloid cells in the subepithelial soft tissue of the gingiva. Please refer to the section of 'Other uncommon haematolymphoid tumours' in 'Tumours of the nasal cavity and paranasal sinuses' for further details on extramedullary myeloid sarcoma.

Follicular dendritic cell sarcoma / tumour

Definition

Follicular dendritic cell (FDC) sarcoma/tumour is a rare neoplasm showing morphologic and phenotypic features of FDC.

ICD-O code   9758/3

Epidemiology, localization and clinical features

It is an uncommon tumour of adulthood, and can affect patients over a wide age range {368,2010,2043}. It can arise in nodal and extranodal tissues, and the oral cavity is among the more commonly involved extranodal sites {67,368,375, 2010,2043,2249}. The patients usually present with a painless mass involving the tonsil, palate or oropharynx.

Etiology

Occasional FDC sarcomas/tumours appear to evolve from an underlying hyaline-vascular Castleman disease; the two lesions can present simultaneously or the latter can precede the appearance of the former by several years {359,368,374}. Overgrowth of FDC in the interfollicular

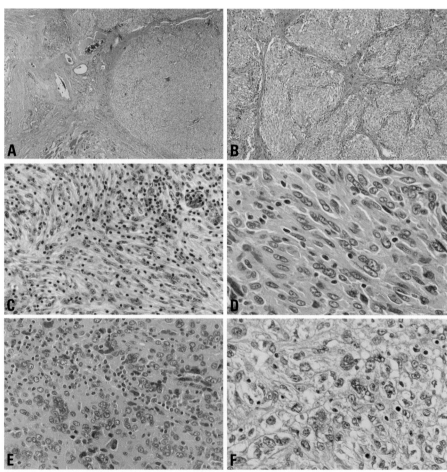

Fig. 4.54 Follicular dendritic cell sarcoma / tumour of oral cavity and oropharynx. **A** This palatal tumour invades in pushing fronts. The main tumour is seen in the right. Smooth-contoured nodules (upper field) invade the adjacent normal structures. **B** Uncommon nodular growth pattern, recapitulating the ability of follicular dendritic cells to form follicles. **C** Typical storiform pattern, accompanied by a sprinkling of lymphocytes. **D** This tumour consists of spindle cells with elongated nuclei, fine chromatin and small distinct nucleoli. Some cells have ill-defined cell borders, while others exhibit well-defined borders. **E** The tumour cell nuclei often appear haphazardly distributed, with some focal clustering. A few multinucleated tumour cells are also evident. The cytoplasm exhibits a fibrillary quality. **F** This example, composed of plump ovoid cells, shows a moderate degree of nuclear atypia and pleomorphism. Nucleoli are prominent.

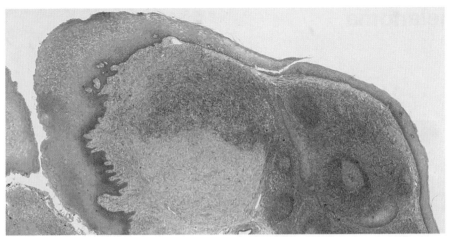

Fig. 4.55 Follicular dendritic cell sarcoma/tumour of the oral cavity. The surface epithelium is intact. This tumour shows partial involvement of the tonsil (left field).

work pattern is highlighted. Cytokeratin is negative. A proportion of cases express epithelial membrane antigen or muscle-specific actin. Occasional cases can weakly express the pan-B marker CD20 {2043}. Ultrastructurally, the tumour cells possess interdigitating long slender cytoplasmic processes and intercellular desmosome junctions. Differential diagnoses include soft tissue sarcoma, poorly differentiated carcinoma, meningioma, and malignant melanoma.

Prognosis and predictive factors
Most cases of FDC sarcomas/tumours have been treated by surgery, with or without adjuvant chemotherapy and radiotherapy, with variable success. FDC sarcomas/tumours are low to intermediate grade malignant tumours, with an overall local recurrence rate of at least 40% and a metastatic rate of at least 28% {368,2010,2043}. Since some patients can develop late metastasis (such as after more than 20 years) {438}, long-term follow up is essential. Poor prognostic factors include significant cytologic atypia, extensive coagulative necrosis, high proliferative index and large tumour size {368,2010}.

Mucosal malignant melanoma

P.M. Speight

Definition

Malignant melanoma is a malignant neoplasm of melanocytes or of melanocyte precursors. It is characterized by proliferation of atypical melanocytes at the epithelial-connective tissue interface associated with upward migration into the epithelium and by invasion of the underlying connective tissues. Although usually seen in the skin, melanomas may also arise from melanocytes in mucosae.

ICD-O code   8720/3

Epidemiology

Mucosal melanomas of the head and neck comprise just over 1% of all melanomas and of these about 50% arise in the oral cavity. Oral mucosal melanomas are therefore rare, representing about 0.5% of oral malignancies {1085} and less than 0.01% of all oral biopsies {122}. The annual incidence in the USA is about 0.02 per 100,000 {170}, but the lesion may be more common in other parts of the world including Japan where the oral cavity has been reported as the most common site for melanomas {2528}.

They arise in adults with an average age of about 55, but with a uniform age distribution from 20–80 years {122,617,1085, 2080,2127}. Very rare cases have been reported in children. In most large series there is a male predominance in a ratio of about 3:1 {122,617,2080} and some reports show males and females are almost equal {144,1843}.

Etiology

No etiological factors are known to be associated with oral melanoma.

Localization

Eighty percent of oral melanomas arise on the palate, maxillary alveolus or gingivae. Other sites include the mandibular gingivae, buccal mucosa, floor of mouth and tongue.

Clinical features

Oral melanomas are usually asymmetric

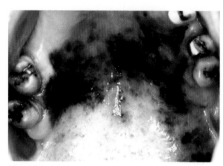

Fig. 4.56 Malignant melanoma. multiple or widespread areas of dark macular pigmentation affecting the palate. Irregular nodular areas are also seen.

with irregular outlines. They may be black, grey or purple to red, and rarely amelanotic. Typical lesions are composed of multiple or widespread areas of macular pigmentation with areas of nodular growth. Purely macular lesions may be seen but over 50% of lesions present as nodules or as a pigmented epulis. Ulceration is seen in about one third of cases and invasion of bone is common. Many reports document long-standing 'melanosis' before the onset of nodular lesions, with a history of up to 10 years. Oral lesions are usually advanced at presentation with up to 75% of patients having metastases to cervical lymph

nodes, and 50% with distant metastases, usually to lung or liver {144,617,1085}.

Macroscopy

Tumours are usually 1.5-4 cm in diameter with a black, macular or nodular surface. The cut surface is often homogeneously black or darkly pigmented.

Histopathology

Oral melanoma may have in-situ (radial) and invasive growth phases, but the histological classification is not analogous to cutaneous lesions. Mucosal lesions are similar to acral lentiginous melanoma of the skin {2652}, with junctional activity and upward migration but Pagetoid invasion is unusual. Atypical melanocytic lesions may progress to malignant melanoma but there is little evidence for progression of oral benign melanocytic naevi to invasive malignancy {1085, 2652}. Oral mucosal melanoma is, therefore, classified as in-situ oral mucosal melanoma, invasive oral mucosal melanoma, and mixed in-situ and invasive lesions. Borderline lesions may be termed atypical melanocytic proliferations {122,1085,2652}.

Most lesions at presentation are invasive or have mixed invasive and in-situ com-

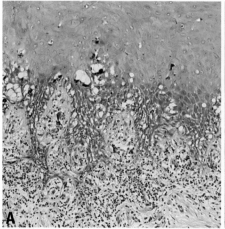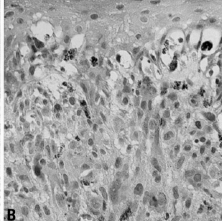

Fig. 4.57 A in-situ growth phase showing atypical and enlarged melanocytes at the epithelial-connective tissue interface. Melanocytes may show upward migration into the epithelium. **B** Invasive lesions showing considerable junctional activity, with atypical melanocytes invading into the underlying connective tissues.

ponents. Less than 20% are solely in-situ lesions. Typically, an oral melanoma is composed of sheets or islands of epithelioid melanocytes, which may be arranged in an organoid, or alveolar pattern. The cells have pale cytoplasm and large open nuclei with prominent nucleoli and occasionally they may be plasmacytoid. Sheets and fascicles of spindle cells may also be seen, but are usually a minor part of the lesion. Occasional lesions may be predominantly or wholly spindled. Over 90% of lesions contain melanin pigment that can easily be demonstrated with stains such as Masson-Fontana or Schmorl's.

When present, the in-situ component shows atypical naevoid cells arranged singly or in nests at the epithelial-connective tissue interface. Upward migration of the cells is common, but Pagetoid islands, similar to those of superficial spreading cutaneous melanomas, are not frequent. Invasion may be difficult to determine but the presence of obviously malignant cells in the lamina propria indicates invasion and islands of cells larger than those seen within the epithelium suggest an invasive growth phase.

Mitoses are surprisingly sparse but are seen more frequently in invasive lesions. The overlying epithelium is usually atrophic and just over half of lesions are ulcerated.

Immunoprofile

Over 95% of lesions are S100 positive and negative for cytokeratins {144}. Although sensitive, S100 is not specific. More specific markers include HMB45, Melan-A or anti-tyrosinase, which stain about 75% of lesions {2079}.

Genetics

Cutaneous melanomas may be associated with familial melanoma syndromes, and melanoma-prone kindreds show frequent loss of heterozygosity or mutations at several sites. Two tumour suppressor genes, CDKN2A (at 9p21, which codes for P16INK4A) and PTEN (at 10q23), and the oncogene CDK4 have been identified as important melanoma

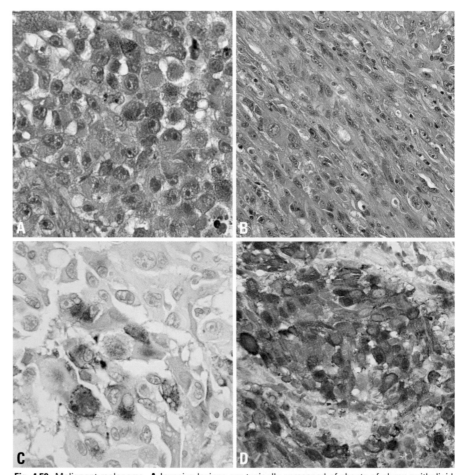

Fig. 4.58 Malignant melanoma **A** Invasive lesions are typically composed of sheets of plump epithelioid melanocytes. **B** Spindle cell areas are often seen. **C** HMB45 is one of the most specific markers for melanoma, but staining may be patchy. **D** S-100 antibodies are expressed strongly and uniformly in almost all lesions.

susceptibility genes {269,1252,2713}. However, associations with these genes have not yet been shown for oral melanomas, and expression of various tumour suppressor genes or oncogenes is variable and heterogeneous {1085,2555}.

Prognosis and predictive factors

The prognosis for oral melanoma is poor with an overall median survival of about 2 years and 5-year survival of less than 20% {122,170,1085}. Stage is a predictor of survival but even localized tumours (stage I) show a 5-year survival of less than 50%. Depth of invasion (Breslow

thickness and Clark's levels) is of limited value in oral lesions. This is due to lack of adequate studies and the fact that most oral melanomas are deeper than 4 mm at presentation {1085,1843,2080}. Nevertheless, lesions thicker than 5 mm may have a significantly worse prognosis. Other factors associated with poor prognosis include, vascular invasion, necrosis, a polymorphous tumour cell population, and increasing age {170,1085,1843,2080}.

Secondary tumours

E.W. Odell

Metastases to bone

Definition
Distant spread of malignant neoplasm to the head and neck from other parts of the body. This is almost exclusively via a haematogenous route.

Epidemiology
The most common malignant neoplasms within the jaws, apart from direct spread from mucosal carcinomas, are metastases and the most frequent primary sites are carcinomas of, in order of decreasing incidence, breast, kidney, lung, prostate and thyroid or colon {1098}. Maxillary and sinus metastases most frequently arise from renal carcinoma {202}.

Metastasis accounts for approximately 4% of all upper aerodigestive tract carcinoma {246}. The great majority of patients are elderly, with mean age at diagnosis of 55 years and the sex incidence varies from equal {2877} to a female preponderance accounted for by the prevalence of breast carcinoma. Asymptomatic mandibular metastases have been found in 16% of carcinoma patients at autopsy {1025} but only approximately 1% of carcinomas develop clinical metastasis to the jaws during the course of the disease. Sarcomatous metastases are extremely rare, usually Ewing sarcoma or osteosarcoma and arise in the second or third decade. Childhood malignant neoplasms also occasionally metastasise to the jaws.

Localization
The ratio of metastases in mandible to maxilla is 5:1 or greater. Most mandibular metastases develop in the angle of the mandible below the inferior dental nerve canal, a minority affect the alveolus.

Clinical features
Common signs and symptoms include loosening of teeth, swelling, failure to heal of a dental extraction socket {1101}, pathological fracture or nerve signs, particularly paraesthesia and anaesthesia in the mental region. Pain may be the only evidence of metastasis. After cortical perforation, a soft tissue mass may be present. Some metastases are asymptomatic chance radiographic findings.

The majority of jaw metastases are radiolucent and poorly defined but occasional lesions are circumscribed. A minority are osteosclerotic or mixed radiolucencies and these are usually breast or prostate carcinomas. Some show only subtle changes such as widening of the periodontal ligament or may be invisible on panoramic tomographic views and plain films. In such cases a bone scan may reveal the metastasis. Radiography has low diagnostic yield for metastases {1025}.

Tumour spread and staging
Jaw metastases are the presenting sign of malignancy in 20-30% of cases {1098,2877} but in most the primary lesion is known. Sometimes metastasis develops many years after treatment for the primary lesion, particularly with renal carcinoma. Metastatic spread to the jaws indicates UICC/AJCC Stage IV disease.

Histopathology
Histopathological appearances vary. Metastases are usually poorly-differentiated. If immunocyochemistry is required to aid clinical identification of sites of an occult primary lesion, prostate specific antigen and thyroglobulin are the most useful stains.

Prognosis and predictive factors
Metastasis to the jaws usually indicates widely disseminated disease and a poor prognosis with a 4-year survival of 10% {458}. Two thirds of patients die in less than 1 year {1101}. Depending on lesion type and dissemination, radiotherapy or hormone therapy may be provided. Surgery may occasionally be of value in palliative care.

Metastases to oral soft tissues

Metastasis to soft tissues is much more rare. It affects a similar age group, 40-70 years old, and the commonest sites for primary lesions in males are lung (one third of cases) followed by kidney and skin. The commonest primary site in females is breast {1100}. The commonest site for metastasis is gingiva (55%) because of its fine capillary bed, followed by tongue (30%), though any site may be affected. The predilection for gingiva is mostly lost after teeth are extracted {1100}. Lesions present as soft tissue masses, often ulcerated, resembling traumatic or reactive hyperplastic lesions.

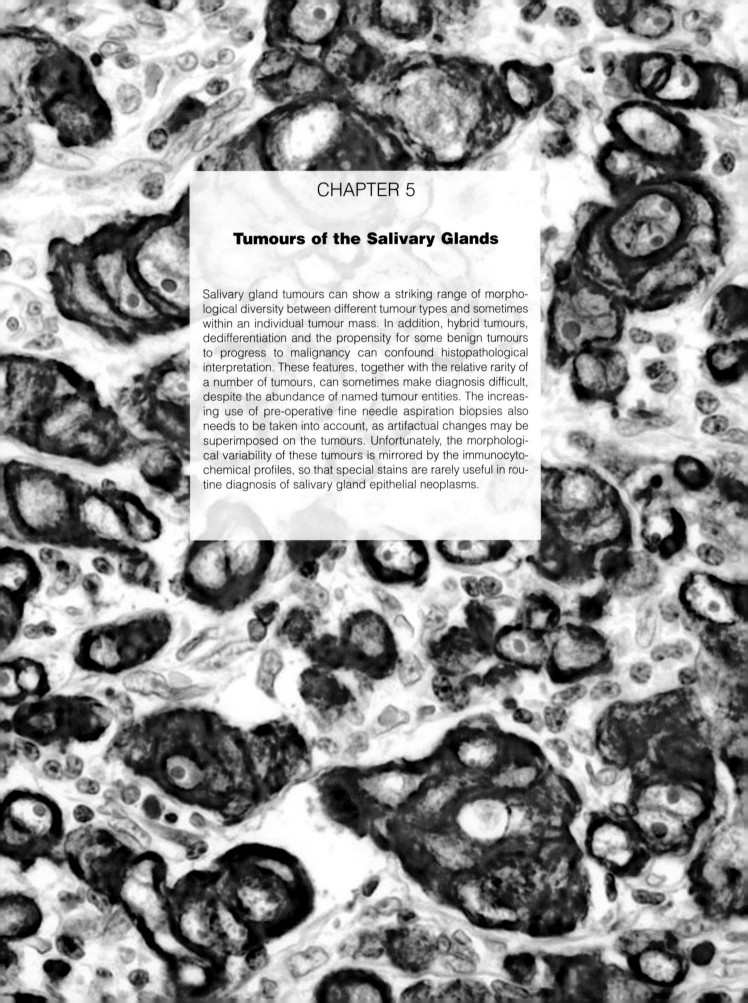

CHAPTER 5

Tumours of the Salivary Glands

Salivary gland tumours can show a striking range of morphological diversity between different tumour types and sometimes
within an individual tumour mass. In addition, hybrid tumours,
dedifferentiation and the propensity for some benign tumours
to progress to malignancy can confound histopathological
interpretation. These features, together with the relative rarity of
a number of tumours, can sometimes make diagnosis difficult,
despite the abundance of named tumour entities. The increasing use of pre-operative fine needle aspiration biopsies also
needs to be taken into account, as artifactual changes may be
superimposed on the tumours. Unfortunately, the morphological variability of these tumours is mirrored by the immunocytochemical profiles, so that special stains are rarely useful in routine diagnosis of salivary gland epithelial neoplasms.

WHO histological classification of tumours of the salivary glands

Malignant epithelial tumours

Acinic cell carcinoma	8550/3
Mucoepidermoid carcinoma	8430/3
Adenoid cystic carcinoma	8200/3
Polymorphous low-grade adenocarcinoma	8525/3
Epithelial-myoepithelial carcinoma	8562/3
Clear cell carcinoma, not otherwise specified	8310/3
Basal cell adenocarcinoma	8147/3
Sebaceous carcinoma	8410/3
Sebaceous lymphadenocarcinoma	8410/3
Cystadenocarcinoma	8440/3
Low-grade cribriform cystadenocarcinoma	
Mucinous adenocarcinoma	8480/3
Oncocytic carcinoma	8290/3
Salivary duct carcinoma	8500/3
Adenocarcinoma, not otherwise specified	8140/3
Myoepithelial carcinoma	8982/3
Carcinoma ex pleomorphic adenoma	8941/3
Carcinosarcoma	8980/3
Metastasizing pleomorphic adenoma	8940/1
Squamous cell carcinoma	8070/3
Small cell carcinoma	8041/3
Large cell carcinoma	8012/3
Lymphoepithelial carcinoma	8082/3
Sialoblastoma	8974/1

Benign epithelial tumours

Pleomorphic adenoma	8940/0
Myoepithelioma	8982/0

Basal cell adenoma	8147/0
Warthin tumour	8561/0
Oncocytoma	8290/0
Canalicular adenoma	8149/0
Sebaceous adenoma	8410/0
Lymphadenoma	
Sebaceous	8410/0
Non-sebaceous	8410/0
Ductal papillomas	
Inverted ductal papilloma	8503/0
Intraductal papilloma	8503/0
Sialadenoma papilliferum	8406/0
Cystadenoma	8440/0

Soft tissue tumours

Haemangioma	9120/0

Haematolymphoid tumours

Hodgkin lymphoma	
Diffuse large B-cell lymphoma	9680/3
Extranodal marginal zone B-cell lymphoma	9699/3

Secondary tumours

---

[1] Morphology code of the International Classification of Diseases for Oncology (ICD-O) {821} and the Systematized Nomenclature of Medicine (http://snomed.org). Behaviour is coded /0 for benign tumours, /3 for malignant tumours, and /1 for borderline or uncertain behaviour.

TNM classification of carcinomas of the salivary glands

TNM classification [1,2]

T – Primary tumour
TX   Primary tumour cannot be assessed
T0   No evidence of primary tumour
T1   Tumour 2 cm or less in greatest dimension without extraparenchymal extension*
T2   Tumour more than 2 cm but not more than 4 cm in greatest dimension without extraparenchymal extension*
T3   Tumour more than 4 cm and/or tumour with extraparenchymal extension*
T4a   Tumour invades skin, mandible, ear canal, or facial nerve
T4b   Tumour invades base of skull, pterygoid plates, or encases carotid artery

Note: *Extraparenchymal extension is clinical or macroscopic evidence of invasion of soft tissues or nerve, except those listed under T4a and 4b. Microscopic evidence alone does not constitute extraparenchymal extension for classification purposes.

N – Regional lymph nodes##
NX   Regional lymph nodes cannot be assessed
N0   No regional lymph node metastasis
N1   Metastasis in a single ipsilateral lymph node, 3 cm or less in greatest dimension
N2   Metastasis as specified in N2a, 2b, 2c below
N2a   Metastasis in a single ipsilateral lymph node, more than 3 cm but not more than 6 cm in greatest dimension
N2b   Metastasis in multiple ipsilateral lymph nodes, none more than 6 cm in greatest dimension
N2c   Metastasis in bilateral or contralateral lymph nodes, none more than 6 cm in greatest dimension
N3   Metastasis in a lymph node more than 6 cm in greatest dimension

Note: Midline nodes are considered ipsilateral nodes.

M – Distant metastasis
MX   Distant metastasis cannot be assessed
M0   No distant metastasis
M1   Distant metastasis

Stage Grouping

Stage I	T1	N0	M0
Stage II	T2	N0	M0
Stage III	T3	N0	M0
	T1, T2, T3	N1	M0
Stage IV A	T1, T2, T3	N2	M0
	T4a	N0, N1, N2	M0
Stage IV B	T4b	Any N	M0
	Any T	N3	M0
Stage IV C	Any T	Any N	M1

The regional lymph nodes are the cervical nodes.

---

[1] {947,2418}.
[2] A help desk for specific questions about the TNM classification is available at http://www.uicc.org/index.php?id=508.

Tumours of the salivary glands: Introduction

J.W. Eveson
P. Auclair
D.R. Gnepp
A.K. El-Naggar

Anatomy

Salivary glands are exocrine organs responsible for the production and secretion of saliva. They comprise the three paired major glands, the parotid, submandibular and sublingual, and the minor glands. The latter are numerous and are widely distributed throughout the mouth and oropharynx and similar glands are present in the upper respiratory and sinonasal tracts, and the paranasal sinuses.

Secretory acinus

The functional unit of salivary glands is the secretory acinus and related ducts, and myoepithelial cells. Acini may be serous, mucous or mixed. Serous acini form wedge-shaped secretory cells with basal nuclei. They surround a lumen that becomes the origin of the intercalated duct. The cytoplasm of serous cells contains densely basophilic, refractile zymogen granules that are periodic acid Schiff positive and diastase resistant. Their principle secretion is amylase. Mucous acinar cells also have basally placed nuclei and their cytoplasm is clear and contains vacuoles of sialomucin. The secretions of these cells pass through the intercalated ducts. These are often inconspicuous in routine histological sections. They are lined by what appears to be a single layer of cuboidal cells with relatively large, central nuclei. They are continuous with the much larger striated ducts. The intercalated ducts are lined by a single layer of cuboidal cells with relatively large, central nuclei and are linked to the much larger striated duct. The latter are lined by tall, columnar, eosinophilic cells that are rich in mitochondria. They have parallel infoldings of the basal cytoplasm and are responsible for modifying the salivary secretions. The striated ducts join the interlobular excretory ducts, which are lined by pseudostratified columnar epithelium that often contains few mucous cells.

Myoepthelial cells

Myoepithelial, or basket cells, are contractile and are located between the basement membrane and the basal plasma membrane of the acinar cells. They are variable in morphology and are inconspicuous in H&E sections. They contain smooth muscle actin, myosin and intermediate filaments including keratin 14. Immunohistochemical stains for the proteins highlights their stellate shape. They have long dendritic processes that embrace the secretory acini. Myoepithelial cells also surround the intercalated ducts but their presence in striated ducts is not firmly established. Ultrastructurally, the cytoplasm of myoepithelial cells contains actomyosin microfilaments running parallel with the outer surface of the cell, glycogen granules and lipofuscin, and pinocytotic vesicles may also be a conspicuous feature.

Parotid gland

The parotid gland is almost purely serous and the parenchyma is divided into lobules by fibrous septa. There is abundant intralobular and extralobular adipose tissue which increases in relative volume with age. The parotid gland contains randomly distributed lymphoid aggregates and lymph nodes that range from one to more than 20 in number. Not infrequently the lymph nodes contain salivary gland ducts or occasionally acini (Neisse Nicholson rests). Sebaceous glands, either individually or in small groups, are commonly seen if the tissue is widely sampled.

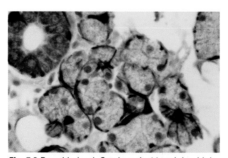

Fig. 5.0 Parotid gland. Cytokeratin 14 staining highlights dendritic myoepithelial cells.

Submandibular gland

The gland is mixed serous and mucous although the serous element predominates (~90%). In mixed acini the serous cells form caps, or demilunes, on the periphery of the mucous cells. The intercalated ducts are shorter and the striated ducts more conspicuous than those of the parotid gland.

Sublingual gland

The gland is also mixed but is predominantly mucous in type. The mucous acini form elongated tubules with peripheral serous demilunes.

Minor salivary glands

These are most numerous at the junction of the hard and soft palate, lips and buccal mucosa. The minor glands of the lateral aspects of the tongue, lips and buccal mucosa are seromucous whereas those in the ventral tongue, palate, glossopharyngeal area and retromolar pad are predominantly mucous. Salivary glands related to the circumvallate papillae (von Ebner's glands) are serous in type. The minor glands are not encapsulted, and those in the tongue and lip especially can be deeply located in the musculature.

Epidemiology

The epidemiology of salivary gland tumours is not well documented {2053}. In many studies the data are limited, as some are restricted to parotid gland neoplasms or tumours of major glands. In addition, most salivary gland tumours are benign and some cancer registries have only included malignant tumours. One study specifically excluded Warthin tumour, which is the second most common benign salivary neoplasm {698}. In addition, several investigators felt that their quoted incidence figures were an underestimate, particularly for benign tumours {963,1471,2053}.

The global annual incidence when all salivary gland tumours were considered varied from 0.4-13.5 cases per 100,000 population {669}. The frequency of malignant salivary neoplasms ranged from 0.4-2.6 cases per 100,000 population {1353,1960,2053,2503}. In the United States, salivary gland malignancies accounted for 6% of head and neck cancers, and 0.3% of all malignancies {2167}. There is also some geographic variation in the frequency of tumour types. In studies of patients from Denmark and parts of Pennsylvania, about 30% of all parotid tumours were Warthin tumours, a sevenfold increase of the expected frequency {1765,2075}. The reported frequency of mucoepidermoid carcinomas among British patients (2.1%) is much lower than the worldwide range of 5-15% {703,704, 1772,2580}. There was a very high reported incidence of salivary gland tumours in North American Inuits from 1950-1966 {1087,2255}. This was almost exclusively due to lymphoepithelial carcinomas that formed 25% of all malignancies in this population. Since then there has been a significant decline in the relative frequency of this tumour. A survey of different ethnic groups in Malaysia showed a higher frequency of salivary tumours in Malays than Chinese or Indians {1551}. Another study showed variations in the incidence of salivary tumours amongst different ethnic groups according to their city of residence {1705}. It should be noted that in some series malignant lymphoma and metastatic disease represent about 9% of major gland tumours, highlighting the need to include these neoplasms in differential diagnostic considerations {669,1916}.

Site, age and sex distribution

Between 64 and 80% of all primary epithelial salivary gland tumours occur in the parotid gland with most located in the superficial (lateral) lobe; 7-11% occur in the submandibular glands; fewer than 1% occur in the sublingual glands; and 9-23% occur in minor glands {669,679, 703,2301,2439}. Benign tumours represent 54-79%, and 21-46% are malignant. The proportion of malignant tumours, however, varies greatly by site. Malignant tumours comprise 15-32% of parotid tumours, 41-45% of submandibular tumours, 70-90% of sublingual tumours, and 50% of minor gland tumours. Eighty to 90% of tumours that occur in the tongue, floor of mouth, and retromolar areas are malignant. Females are more frequently affected, but there is some

gender variation according to the tumour type. The average ages of patients with benign and malignant tumours are 46 and 47 years, respectively, and the peak incidence of most of the specific types is in the sixth and seventh decades. However, the highest incidence of pleomorphic adenomas, mucoepidermoid carcinomas, and acinic cell carcinomas is in the third and fourth decades. In patients under 17 years of age, the frequency of mesenchymal tumours of the major glands is similar to that of epithelial tumours {1304,1413,2302,2337}. In this age group, pleomorphic adenomas, mucoepidermoid carcinomas and acinic cell carcinomas account for about 90% of epithelial tumours, and the frequency of benign and malignant tumours is essentially equal.

Among all patients, the most common tumour type is pleomorphic adenoma, which accounts for about 50% of all tumours. Warthin tumour is second in frequency among benign tumours and, in most large studies, mucoepidermoid carcinoma is the most common malignant tumour {669,679,703,2301,2439}. Most canalicular adenomas and polymorphous low-grade adenocarcinomas arise from minor glands whereas nearly all Warthin tumours occur in the parotid gland or periparotid lymph nodes.

Etiology

Viruses

A number of viruses have been implicated in the pathogenesis of salivary gland tumours. There is a strong association between Epstein Barr virus (EBV) and lymphoepithelial carcinomas {2253, 2636}, but this appears to be largely restricted to Asian patients {1173} and Greenlandic Inuits {986}. EBV has not been convincingly shown in other salivary gland carcinomas or neighbouring normal gland {2636}. A recent study did not support an etiological role for EBV or cytomegalovirus in benign parotid tumours {1407}. SV40 sequences have been demonstrated in human pleomorphic adenomas {1643} but there is no convincing association between human salivary gland tumours and other viruses, including polyoma virus and papilloma virus.

Radiation

There is compelling evidence implicating exposure to ionizing radiation and the

development of salivary gland tumours. Long-term follow-up studies of the survivors of the atomic bomb explosions in Hiroshima and Nagasaki show an increased relative risk of 3.5 for benign, and 11 for malignant salivary neoplasms {193,194,2543,2544}. The risk was directly related to the level of exposure to ionizing radiation. There was a high frequency of both mucoepidermoid carcinomas and Warthin tumours in these patients {2229}.

Therapeutic radiation, particularly of the head and neck region, has been linked with a significantly increased risk of developing salivary gland cancers {1725,1754,2197,2268}. There appears to be a risk from iodine131 used in the treatment of thyroid disease, as the isotope is also concentrated in the salivary glands {1111}.

There is evidence that exposure to routine dental radiographs is associated with an increased risk of salivary gland carcinoma {2088,2089}. Exposure to ultraviolet radiation has also been implicated {1832,2451,2452}. There appears to be no excess risk in those exposed to radon {1733}, or the microwaves of cellular telephones {92,1224}.

Occupation

It has been shown that workers in a variety of industries have an increased incidence of salivary gland carcinomas. These include rubber manufacturing {1127,1620}, exposure to metal in the plumbing industry {1730} and nickel compounds {1127}, woodworking in the automobile industry {2512} and employment in hairdressing and beauty shops {2513,2514}. An increased risk of salivary gland cancers was reported in people living in certain Quebec counties where asbestos was mined, and the risk was inversely proportional to the distance from the mines {935}.

Lifestyle and nutrition

No association was found between tobacco use and alcohol consumption and salivary gland cancers in a case/control study {1801}, confirming previous findings {1295,2792}. One study showed an elevated risk in men but not women {1127}. However, there is a strong association between smoking and Warthin tumour (Section on Warthin tumour). Exposure to silica dust and kerosene as a cooking fluid increased the risk of developing salivary malignancy in a Chinese population {2902}, and a higher level of risk of parotid carcinomas was associated with exposure to nickel, chromium, asbestos and cement dust in a European study {603}. An increased level of risk has been postulated in those with a high cholesterol intake {1128}.

Hormones

Endogenous hormones have been reported in normal and neoplastic salivary glands, but some of the results have been conflicting. Estrogen receptors were found in nearly 80% of normal glands in males and females and four out of eight salivary tumours in women had estrogen receptor levels similar to those of "hormonally dependent" breast carcinomas {606}. However, more recent studies have not confirmed this finding and questioned the methodology {616}. Estrogen receptors have been reported in a minority of cases of acinic cell carcinoma, mucoepidermoid carcinoma {1214} and salivary duct carcinoma {134}, but were not detected in adenoid cystic carcinoma {616,1214,1732,2335}. Estrogen or estrogen receptors have been reported in pleomorphic adenomas in some studies {1214,1764,1946}, but in others, estrogen receptors were absent {1851}.

Progesterone receptors have been reported in normal salivary glands {892,2335}. They have been detected in a minority of pleomorphic adenomas {892,1214} but high levels of expression were reported in recurrent pleomorphic adenomas and this was thought to be a prognostic factor {892}. However, a recent study failed to show progesterone receptors in all the benign salivary tumours examined {1851}. Progesterone receptors were seen in 2/10 acinic cell carcinomas and 3/10 mucoepidermoid carcinomas {1214} but were not detected in salivary duct carcinoma {134}. They have been reported in adenoid cystic carcinomas in some studies {1214,1965} but in others they were absent, or present in only a few tumours {616,1214}.

Androgen receptors are present in over 90% of salivary duct carcinomas {711, 712,1265}. A recent study showed immunoreactivity for androgen receptors in all their cases of salivary duct carcinoma, carcinoma ex pleomorphic adenoma and basal cell adenocarcinoma {1851}. There was also staining for the receptors

in a fifth of their cases of acinic cell carcinoma, mucoepidermoid carcinoma and adenoid cystic carcinoma.

Diagnostic imaging

Plain radiography and sialography are useful for ductal inflammatory disease, but computed tomography (CT), ultrasonography, CT sialography, and magnetic resonance imaging (MRI) are usually better for evaluation of suspected neoplastic disease. MRI is particularly useful when inflammatory disease is not suspected. It does not have the risks of radiation exposure nor complications with intraductal injection of contrast media, and it is often superior in demonstrating the interface of tumour and surrounding tissues. T1-weighted images of normal parotid have an image signal intermediate between fat and muscle whereas submandibular tissue is closer to muscle in intensity. With advanced age and fatty infiltration, the signal intensity of parotid tissue approaches fat. Most salivary gland tumours are brighter on T2 than T1 images but this difference is minimal in prominently cellular tumours. Lesions with higher water content, such as human immunodeficiency virus related parotid cysts, Warthin tumours, cystadenomas and cystadenocarcinomas, and cystic mucoepidermoid carcinomas, have a bright T2 signal.

Fine needle aspiration biopsy

Fine needle aspiration biopsy (FNA) can provide clinicians with rapid, non-surgical diagnoses. It can be performed at the time of initial consultation. Correlation of the clinical impression, cytologic diagnosis and radiographic imaging studies can then guide along different treatment pathways. FNA can be used both as a diagnostic test and as a screening tool to triage patients into different treatment groups i.e. surgical vs. medical management vs. to follow without intervention {2109}. FNA biopsy is useful in establishing whether a given lesion is inflammatory or neoplastic, is a lymphoma or an epithelial malignancy, or represents a metastasis or a primary tumour {424, 1585,2892}. Unnecessary surgery can be avoided in approximately one third of cases {668} especially in: (1) patients whose salivary gland lesion is part of a more generalized disease process, (2) inflammatory lesions where a clinical suspicion of malignancy is low, (3)

patients in poor health who are not good operative candidates, (4) patients with metastasis to a salivary gland or adjacent lymph node, (5) some examples of lymphoproliferative disease {763} or (6) in a primary soft tissue or skin appendage lesion arising in the area of a major salivary gland.

A number of series have examined the diagnostic accuracy of salivary FNA {26, 495,2474,2887} with false positive and false negative rates ranging from 1-14%. The rate of correctly establishing a diagnosis as benign or malignant ranges from 81-98% in most recent reports. However, a specific diagnosis can only be made in approximately 60-75% of cases {668}. False negative diagnoses due to inadequate sampling appear to be the most frequent error.

Frozen section examination

When considering all head and neck sites, the accuracy of frozen section diagnoses of the salivary gland is the most controversial. A review of 2460 frozen sections from 24 series revealed an overall accuracy rate for a benign or malignant diagnosis, excluding deferred diagnoses, of 96% {379,900,1697,2170, 2900}. False-positive rates (benign tumours initially diagnosed as malignant) were 1.1%, false-negative rates (malignant tumours initially diagnosed as benign) were 2.6%, and 2% of cases were deferred. If one subdivides the salivary gland lesions into benign and malignant groups, the accuracy rate (98.7%, excluding deferred diagnoses) is excellent for the benign lesions, which compose 80% of the frozen sections. However, in the malignant tumour group, the accuracy rate (85.9%) is suboptimal {900}.

The most common benign tumour overdiagnosed as malignant was pleomorphic adenoma. This was frequently called mucoepidermoid carcinoma or adenoid cystic carcinoma {904}.

Mucoepidermoid carcinoma is the malignancy most frequently associated with a false negative benign frozen section diagnosis, while acinic cell carcinoma, adenoid cystic carcinoma, carcinoma ex pleomorphic adenoma and an occasional lymphoma have also caused difficulty.

Staging

Staging of carcinomas of the major salivary glands is based on tumour size, local extension of tumour, metastasis to regional nodes, and distant metastases (see TNM classification). Recent changes in the staging system include a revision in the definition of T3 and the division of T4 into tumours that are resectable (T4a) and unresectable (T4b) {947,2418}. According to TNM rules, tumours arising in minor salivary glands are classified according to the criteria for other carcinomas at their anatomic site of origin, e.g., oral cavity. Spiro and co-workers have successfully applied the criteria used for squamous cell carcinoma of the oral cavity, pharynx, larynx, and sinus to mucoepidermoid carcinoma {2305,2863}.

Genetics

The goal of the molecular biological studies of salivary gland tumours is to define objective markers that may supplant the subjective phenotypic evaluation in the diagnosis, biological assessment and therapeutic stratification of patients with these tumours. The following molecular genetic events tentatively characterize some of these tumours:

(1) Chromosomes 3p21, 8q12 and 12q13-15 rearrangements and the PLAG-1 and HMGI-C genes in pleomorphic adenomas
(2) Translocations of chromosomes 11q21 and 19p13 in both Warthin tumour and mucoepidermoid carcinoma.
(3) Structural and molecular alterations at 6q, 8q, 12q in adenoid cystic and carcinoma ex-pleomorphic adenoma.
(4) Elevated HER-2 gene expression and gene amplification in mucoepidermoid, salivary duct and adenocarcinomas.

EGFR

Several studies have shown high expression of EGFR/HER-2/neu family members in mucoepidermoid and adenoid cystic carcinoma. The data suggest a biological role for members of this pathway in these tumours and their potential use as a target for therapy {887}.

C-erbB-2/HER-2/neu

This is an oncogene that encodes for a transmembrane glycoprotein receptor involved in cell growth and differentiation. The gene is a member of the EGFR signal transduction family and has been shown to be overexpressed in aggressive breast cancer. Studies in salivary gland adenocarcinoma, including sali-

vary duct and mucoepidermoid carcinoma, point to a general consensus on the association of HER-2 overexpression and adverse clinicopathologic features {725, 884,1058,2086,2198,2465}.

C-Kit

This is a proto-oncogene that encodes a transmembrane receptor type tyrosine kinase that belongs to the colony-stimulating factor-1 (CSF-1) and platelet-derived growth factors (PDGF;4-6). Upon binding to its ligand, a signalling cascade is initiated to stimulate growth and differentiation of haematopoietic cells {835}. Studies of C-kit in salivary gland tumours have largely focused on adenoid cystic carcinoma and findings vary considerably. C-kit expression appears to be restricted to adenoid cystic carcinoma {1215,2006} and myoepithelial carcinomas {1215} but absent in polymorphous low-grade adenocarcinoma {2006} and other types of salivary gland tumours {1215}.

None of the highly expressed tumours manifested genetic mutations at exons 11 & 17. The results confirm a previous study and underscore that a mechanism for gene activation and other genetic alterations may play a role {1117}. A more recent study of this gene indicates high expression in other types of salivary gland neoplasms as well (adenoid cystic carcinoma, polymorphous low-grade adenocarcinoma and monomorphic types of adenoma) {636}.

TP53

TP53 is a tumour suppressor gene located at the short arm of chromosome 17. The protein product acts as a transcription factor for cell differentiation, proliferation and death {636,1117,1485}. The role of this gene in salivary gland tumorigenesis remains unknown. Studies of different tumours have yielded variable results {554,1327,2198}. The incidence of p53 expression in other benign, malignant and hybrid tumours is low and does not correlate with recurrence {1823}. At present there is insufficient information on the correlation between p53 and outcome. These unsettling results reflect the lack of technical and interpretative uniformity in assessing this marker {2421}.

Expression profiles

A study of nine benign (4 Warthin tumours and 5 pleomorphic adenomas)

and three carcinomas (2 mucoepidermoid and one clear cell carcinoma), using cDNA of 19,000 human expressed sequence tags, identified a small set of genes that separate mucoepidermoid and clear cell carcinomas from normal and benign counterparts. Genes identified in carcinomas were apoptosis related {802}.

A study of adenoid cystic carcinoma using oligonucleotide array platform for 8920 human genes was recently reported {818}. The study identified a set of genes that included basement membrane and extracellular matrix-related genes and genes encoding transcription factors SOX4 and AP-2a and members of the Wnt/β-catenin signalling pathway.

A recent study of the gene expression in a cohort of pleomorphic adenomas and in spectrum of malignant tumours has also delineated a potential genetic profile that may be used in the biological investigation of these tumours {1652}.

Genetic susceptibility

There is no evidence of familial clustering. An association has been reported with dermal cylindromatosis in the setting of Brooke-Spiegler syndrome {1248}.

Prognosis and predictive factors

Prognosis correlates most strongly with clinical stage, emphasizing the importance of early diagnosis. The microscopic grade and tumour type have been shown to be independent predictors of behaviour and often play an important role in optimizing treatment {1264,1918, 2440,2447,2449,2519}. Locoregional failure of some types of salivary carcinomas results in a greater likelihood of distant metastasis indicating a need for aggressive initial surgery {2441}. As might be expected, there is often a positive correlation between grade and clinical stage.

Acinic cell carcinoma

G. Ellis
R.H.W. Simpson

Definition

Acinic cell carcinoma is a malignant epithelial neoplasm of salivary glands in which at least some of the neoplastic cells demonstrate serous acinar cell differentiation, which is characterized by cytoplasmic zymogen secretory granules. Salivary ductal cells are also a component of this neoplasm.

ICD-O code   8550/3

Synonyms

Acinic cell adenocarcinoma, acinous cell carcinoma. Acinic cell tumour is an inappropriate synonym since the malignant biologic behaviour of this neoplasm is well-established {2304}.

Epidemiology

Slightly more women than men are affected. There is no predilection for any ethnic group. Affected patients range from young children to elderly adults with a fairly even distribution of patients from the second to the seventh decades of life. Four percent of the patients are under 20 years old {668,1304,1954}.

Localization

The overwhelming majority, almost 80%, of acinic cell carcinomas occur in the parotid gland, and about 17% involve the intraoral minor salivary glands. Only about 4% develop in the submandibular gland, and less than 1% arise in the sublingual gland {668,2711,2886}.

Clinical features

They typically manifest as slowly enlarging, solitary, unfixed masses in the parotid region, but a few are multinodular and/or fixed to skin or muscle. A third of patients also experience pain, which is often vague and intermittent, and 5-10% develop some facial paralysis. While the duration of symptoms in most patients is less than a year, it can be up to several decades in some cases {478,668,670, 1435,2445}.

Macroscopy

Most are 1-3 cm in largest dimension. They are usually circumscribed, solitary nodules, but some are ill-defined with irregular peripheries and/or multinodularity. The cut surface appears lobular and tan to red. They vary from firm to soft and solid to cystic.

Tumour spread

Usually, acinic cell carcinomas initially metastasize to cervical lymph nodes and subsequently to more distant sites, most commonly the lung {670,960}.

Histopathology

While serous acinar cell differentiation defines acinic cell carcinoma, several cell types and histomorphologic growth patterns are recognized. These are acinar, intercalated ductal, vacuolated, clear, and non-specific glandular and solid/lobular, microcystic, papillary-cystic, and follicular growth patterns {161, 478,668,1492,2290,2304}.

Acinar cells are large, polygonal cells with lightly basophilic, granular cytoplasm and round, eccentric nuclei. The cytoplasmic zymogen-like granules are PAS positive, resistant to diastase digestion, and weakly stained or non-stained with mucicarmine. However, the PAS positivity can sometimes be very patchy and not immediately obvious. Intercalated duct type cells are smaller, eosinophilic to amphophilic, cuboidal with central nuclei, and surround variably sized luminal spaces. Vacuolated cells contain clear, cytoplasmic vacuoles that vary in number and size. The vacuoles are PAS negative. Clear cells are similar in size and shape to acinar cells but have non-staining cytoplasm that is non-reactive with PAS staining. Non-specific glandular cells are round to polygonal, amphophilic to eosinophilic cells with round nuclei and poorly demarcated cell borders. They often develop in syncytial sheets.

Tumour cells are closely apposed to one another in sheets, nodules, or aggregates in the solid/lobular growth pattern. Numerous small spaces that vary from several microns to a millimetre or more in size characterize the microcystic pattern. Prominent cystic lumina, larger than the

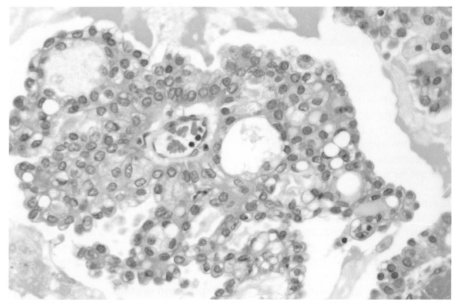

Fig. 5.1 Acinic cell carcinoma. Vacuolated cells in acinic cell carcinoma are similar in size to intercalated duct-type cells but have clear, cytoplasmic vacuoles, which sometimes distend the cellular membranes.

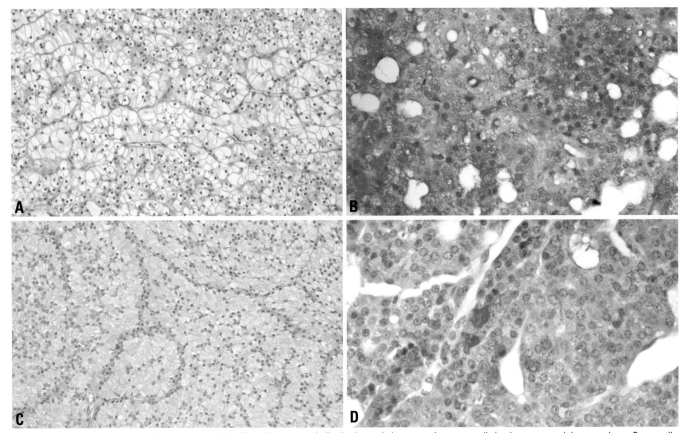

Fig. 5.2 Acinic cell carcinoma. **A** Clear cells in acinic cell carcinoma are similar in size and shape to acinar-type cells but have non-staining cytoplasm. Some cells have a variable amount of eosinophilic cytoplasm. **B** The cytoplasmic granules in serous acinar-type cells in acinic cell carcinoma stain with PAS and are resistant to diastase digestion. **C** Sheets of tumour cells, acinar-type cells in this case, with few or no cystic spaces characterizes a solid growth pattern in acinic cell carcinoma. **D** Often acinar type cells are scattered among nonspecific glandular cells. They are often inconspicuous with H&E-stain but highlighted with PAS stain (PAS stain).

microcystic spaces that are partially filled with papillary epithelial proliferations characterize the papillary-cystic pattern. This variant, in particular, may be very vascular and haemorrhagic and sometimes phagocytosis of haemosiderin by luminal tumour cells is a conspicuous feature. In the follicular pattern, multiple, epithelial-lined cystic spaces are filled with eosinophilic proteinaceous material, which produces a thyroid follicle-like appearance. Psammoma bodies are occasionally seen and are sometimes numerous. They are not restricted to the papillary-cystic variant and have been reported in FNA specimens.

Although a single cell type and growth pattern often dominate, many tumours have combinations of cell types and growth patterns. Acinar cells and intercalated duct-like cells often dominate while the other cell types seldom do. Clear cells are seen in only 6% of all acinic cell carcinomas {670}. They are usually focal and only rarely cause diagnostic confu-

sion. The solid/lobular and microcystic patterns are most frequent, followed by the papillary-cystic and follicular patterns.

A prominent lymphoid infiltrate of the stroma is associated with many acinic cell carcinomas {83,1717}. Whereas a heavy lymphoid infiltrate by itself has no prognostic significance, some tumours are well-circumscribed masses arranged in a microfollicular growth pattern and with a low proliferation index. They are completely surrounded by the lymphoid infiltrate (with germinal centre formation) and a thin fibrous pseudocapsule. These tumours appear to constitute a subgroup that behaves far less aggressively than other acinic cell carcinomas {1717}.

Immunoprofile

Although the immunoprofile is non-specific, acinic cell carcinomas are reactive for cytokeratin, transferrin, lactoferrin, alpha 1-antitrypsin, alpha 1-antichymotrypsin, IgA, carcinoembryonic anti-

gen, Leu M1 antigen, cyclooxygenase-2, vasoactive intestinal polypeptide, and amylase. The zymogen granules in the neoplastic acinar cells are often non-reactive with anti-α-amylase immunostain, an enzyme in zymogen granules of normal serous acinar cells. Reactivity for oestrogen receptor, progesterone receptor, and prostate-specific antigen has been described in some tumours {338, 429,995,1031,1049,1214,2230,2296, 2529,2571}. Approximately 10% of tumours are positive for S-100 protein {2529}.

Electron microscopy

Multiple, round, variably electron dense, cytoplasmic secretory granules characterize acinar type cells. The number and size of the granules varies. Rough endoplasmic reticulum, numerous mitochondria, and sparse microvilli are also typically. Some cells contain vacuoles of varying size and shape. Basal lamina separates groups of acinar and ductal

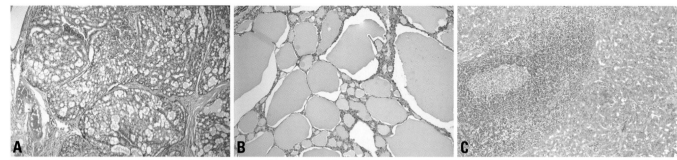

Fig. 5.3 Acinic cell carcinoma. **A** Variably sized luminal or cystic spaces, usually microscopic rather than macroscopic, identifies the microcystic pattern of acinic cell carcinoma. **B** Microcystic and macrocystic spaces, surrounded by tumour cells and filled with eosinophilic proteinaceous material, resemble thyroid follicles and characterize the follicular pattern, which is an infrequent variant of acinic cell carcinoma. **C** A prominent lymphocytic infiltrate of the stroma, usually with lymphoid follicles, is common and should not be misinterpreted as evidence of lymph node metastasis.

tumour cells from the stromal tissues. The light microscopically clear cells are the result of artefactual changes or dilatations of rough endoplasmic reticulum, lipid inclusions, enzymatic degradation of secretory granules, and intracytoplasmic pseudolumina {398,539,543, 971}.

Histogenesis

Most investigators consider that these tumours arise from neoplastic transformation of the terminal duct cells (intercalated duct cells) with histodifferentiation toward serous acinar cells. It has been shown {539,540}, however, that normal serous acinar cells undergo mitotic division, and some acinic cell carcinomas could arise from transformation of these cells.

Genetics

Cytogenetics

Multiple structural and numerical abnormalities of these tumours have been reported but no consistent or specific alterations can be defined. Deletions of chromosome 6q, loss of Y and trisomy 21 have been reported {2238}. A recent report of multiple analyses from one tumour showed various structural abnormalities, suggesting a polyclonal derivation {1218}.

Molecular genetics

In the largest molecular analysis of these tumours 21 (84%) of the 25 tumours studied showed LOH in at least one of the 20 loci on chromosomes 1,4,5,6 and 17 {647}. The most frequently altered regions were noted at chromosomes 4p, 5q, 6p and 17p regions. Chromosomes 4p15-16, 6p25-qter and 17p11 showed the highest incidence of alterations.

Another study of multiple spatially obtained samples from one tumour showed evidence for polyclonality suggesting different origins for this tumour {1218}.

Prognosis and predictive factors

The average among several studies is a recurrence rate of about 35% and a metastatic rate and disease-associated death incidence of about 16% {441,478, 670,960,994,1060,1112,1492,1845, 1938,2017,2515,2607}. Multiple recurrences and metastasis to cervical lymph nodes indicate a poor prognosis. Distant metastasis is associated with very poor survival. While tumours in the submandibular gland are more aggressive than those in the parotid gland, acinic cell carcinomas in minor salivary glands are less aggressive than those in the major salivary glands {340,864,1112, 2886}.

Attempts at histological grading have been controversial and inconsistent. Features that are often associated with more aggressive tumours include frequent mitoses, focal necrosis, neural invasion, pleomorphism, infiltration, and stromal hyalinisation {161,650,670,960, 2017,2445}. Occasional cases of dedifferentiation from a low-grade to a high-grade malignancy have been reported. These tumours are characterized by cytological pleomorphism, increased mitotic and proliferation indices and have a worse prognosis {594,1063,1911, 2459}.

Staging is often a better predictor of outcome than histomorphologic grading. Large size, involvement of the deep lobe of the parotid gland, and incomplete resection indicate a poor prognosis. The cell proliferation marker Ki-67 has shown the most promise as a predictor of biological behaviour. No recurrences of acinic cell carcinomas were seen when the percentage of positively immunostained tumour cells was below 5% whereas most patients with tumour indices above 10% had unfavourable outcomes {1060,2388}.

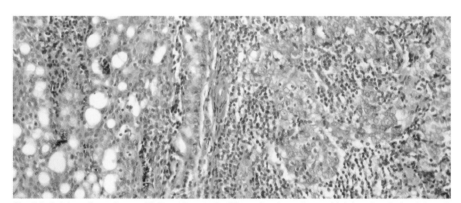

Fig. 5.4 Acinic cell carcinoma. High-grade, poorly differentiated carcinoma (right) and typical acinic cell carcinoma (left) in a single neoplasm has been designated as "dedifferentiated" acinic cell carcinoma.

Mucoepidermoid carcinoma

R.K. Goode
A.K. El-Naggar

Definition
Mucoepidermoid carcinoma is a malignant glandular epithelial neoplasm characterized by mucous, intermediate and epidermoid cells, with columnar, clear cell and oncocytoid features.

ICD code
8430/3

Synonyms
Mixed epidermoid and mucus secreting carcinoma. Mucoepidermoid tumour is an inappropriate synonym since the malignant biologic behaviour of this neoplasm is well established.

Epidemiology
Mucoepidermoid carcinoma (MEC) is the most common primary salivary gland malignancy in both adults and children {1560,2681,2711}.
MEC demonstrates a wide, nearly uniform age distribution, with diminution in paediatric and geriatric life {456,1850}. Mean patient age is approximately 45 years. Sixty percent of palate lesions are in patients under 40. Tongue neoplasms are reported at an older average age. There is a 3:2 female predilection, but higher female predominance for tongue and retromolar pad tumours {668}.

Localization
Approximately half of tumours (53%) occur in major glands. The parotid glands predominate, representing 45%, with 7% for submandibular glands and 1% in sublingual glands. The most frequent intra-oral sites are the palate and buccal mucosa.

Clinical features
Signs and symptoms
Most tumours present as firm, fixed and painless swellings. Sublingual gland lesions may demonstrate pain in spite of small size. Superficial intraoral neoplasms may exhibit a blue-red colour and mimic a mucocele or vascular lesion. The mucosa overlying palatal tumours can be papillary. Cortical bone is sometimes superficially eroded. Symptoms can include pain, otorrhoea, paraesthesia, facial nerve palsy, dysphagia, bleeding and trismus {703}.

Macroscopy
Tumours are firm, smooth, often cystic, tan, white or pink with well-defined or infiltrative edges.

Tumour spread and staging
Parotid gland tumours spread to adjacent pre-auricular lymph nodes, then to the submandibular region. Submandibular gland neoplasms spread to submandibular and the upper jugular lymphatic chain. Palatal lesions may extend

Table 5.1 Histopathologic features, point values and point scores used in grading mucoepidermoid carcinoma

Histopathologic feature	Point value
Cystic component < 20%	2
Neural invasion	2
Necrosis	3
4 or more mitoses / 10 hpf	3
Anaplasia	4
Tumour Grade	**Point Score**
Low	0 - 4
Intermediate	5 - 6
High	7 or more

into the upper respiratory tract and skull base. Lip lesions invade submental nodes and intraoral tumours metastasize to submandibular, post auricular and upper accessory nodes in neck level II. With advancing disease, levels III, IV and V may become involved. Distant metastases may be widespread to lung, liver, bone, and brain.

Histopathology
Mucoepidermoid carcinoma is characterized by squamoid (epidermoid), mucus producing and cells of intermediate type. The proportion of different cell types and their architectural configuration (including cyst formation) varies in and between tumours.

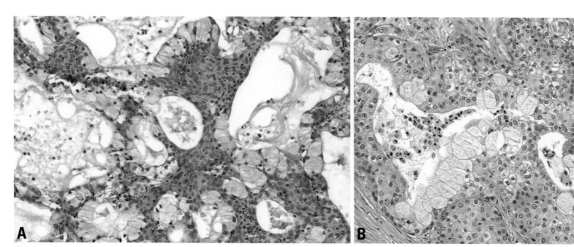

Fig. 5.5 Mucoepidermoid carcinoma. **A** Low-grade. **B** Intermediate grade.

They are usually multicystic with a solid component and sometimes the latter predominates. Some tumours have defined borders but infiltration of gland parenchyma is evident. Cystic spaces are lined by mucous cells with basaloid or cuboidal intermediate cells interspersed, and to a lesser degree, polygonal epidermoid cells, but keratinization is rare. Mucous cells are large, with pale cytoplasm and peripherally displaced nuclei. They typically constitute less than 10% of the tumour. Sialomucin content is demonstrated by mucicarmine or Alcian blue staining. Intermediate cells usually predominate. Clear, columnar and/or oncocytic cell populations may be present and occasionally are prominent {985, 1198,1996}. Clear cells demonstrate minimal sialomucin, but are diastase-sensitive periodic acid-Schiff positive, indicating glycogen content {666}. Focal sclerosis and/or mucus extravasation with inflammation is common. A sclerosing variant has been described {2657}. Neural invasion, necrosis, increased mitoses or cellular anaplasia are uncommon. At the tumour edge, a lymphocytic infiltrate with possible germinal centre formation can mimic nodal invasion {83}.

Grading

Several systems have been proposed to grade this neoplasm, but none has been universally accepted {86,258,695,1850, 2443}. However, one recent system using five histopathologic features has been shown to be reproducible in defining low, intermediate and high-grade tumours {86,972,1766}. In the submandibular gland low-grade tumours tend to behave more aggressively {921}.

Immunoprofile

Squamoid cells may be sparse in mucoepidermoid carcinoma and high molecular weight cytokeratins can help identify them.

Differential diagnosis

Differential diagnosis includes necrotizing sialometaplasia {263}, inverted ductal papilloma, cystadenoma {2292}, carcinomas composed of clear cells, adenosquamous carcinoma, squamous cell carcinoma and metastases.

Genetics

Cytogenetics

Several MECs have been reported to

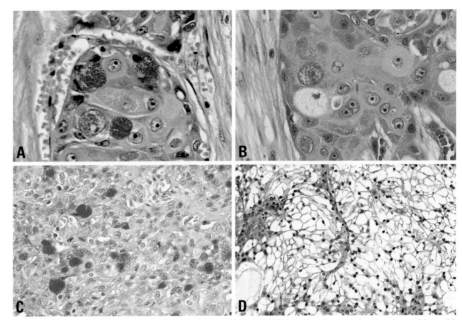

Fig. 5.6 Mucoepidermoid carcinoma (MEC). **A** Parotid gland MEC, intermediate grade, showing epidermoid cell anaplasia and mucous cells. Mucicarmine stain. **B** High grade parotid gland MEC exhibiting solid growth pattern of predominately epidermoid cells. **C** High grade. PAS stain showing scattered positive mucous cells. **D** Clear cell variant.

possess t(11:19) (q21;p13) translocation as the only abnormality (or with other structural and numerical alterations). This abnormality is also shared by acute leukaemia {655,1130,1904}.

Molecular genetics

Molecular studies of these tumours are few and limited in number of cases. They show infrequent genetic loss at chromosomes 9p21, 8q, 5p, 16q and 12p {351, 1228,2408}. Studies of the H-ras gene in these tumours have reported 18% mutations at codon 12 and/or 13 (one case) and no mutations at codon 61 {2858}. The mutations are mainly found in high-grade tumours {2859}. Recently molecular analysis of the t(11:19) (q21;p12) resulted in the identification of a fusion transcript resulting from the binding of exon-1 of a novel gene of unknown function, the mucoepidermoid carcinoma translocated gene-1 (MECT1), at 19p13 region with exons 2-5 of a novel member of the mastermind-like gene family (MAML2) at 11q21 region. This transcript activate the notch target genes.

Prognosis and predictive factors

Most patients have a favourable outcome. In one study, 8% of patients died of disease: 11% and 5% for major and minor gland tumours, respectively. Death correlated with high-grade histopatho-

logic features in minor gland and parotid gland tumours, but not in patients with submandibular gland tumours {921}. Death resulted from unresectable locoregional tumour, distant metastases or complications of adjunctive therapy {2609}.

The impact of grading on prognosis was described before and, additionally a MIB-1 index >10% correlates with high histopathologic grade, increased recurrence, metastasis and decreased patient survival {2387,2905}.

Currently, there are no prognostically useful genetic factors.

Adenoid cystic carcinoma

A.K. El-Naggar
A.G. Huvos

Definition

Adenoid cystic carcinoma is a basaloid tumour consisting of epithelial and myoepithelial cells in variable morphologic configurations, including tubular, cribriform and solid patterns. It has a relentless clinical course and usually a fatal outcome.

ICD code   8200/3

Epidemiology

Adenoid cystic carcinomas (AdCC) comprise approximately 10% of all epithelial salivary neoplasms and most frequently involve the parotid, submandibular and minor salivary glands. They comprise 30% of epithelial minor salivary gland tumours with the highest frequency in the palate, followed by the tongue, buccal mucosa, lip and floor of mouth. The tumour occurs in all age groups with a high frequency in middle-aged and older patients. There is no apparent sex predilection except for a high incidence in women with submandibular tumours {1663,1849,2016,2444}.

Clinical features

The most common symptom is a slow growing mass followed by pain due to the propensity of these tumours for perineural invasion. Facial nerve paralysis may also occur {1849,2016,2444,2519}.

Macroscopy

The carcinomas are solid, well-circumscribed but unencapsulated. They present as light-tan and firm masses of variable sizes. They are invariably infiltrative {161,1663,2439}.

Histopathology

Tumours consist of two main cell types: ductal and modified myoepithelial cells that typically have hyperchromatic, angular nuclei and frequently clear cytoplasm. There are three defined patterns: tubular, cribriform and solid. In the tubular form, well-formed ducts and tubules with central lumina are lined by inner epithelial and outer myoepithelial cells.

The cribriform pattern, the most frequent, is characterized by nests of cells with cylindromatous microcystic spaces. These are filled with hyaline or basophilic mucoid material. The solid or basaloid type is formed of sheets of uniform basaloid cells lacking tubular or microcystic formation. In the cribriform and solid variants small true ducts are invariably present but may not be immediately apparent. Each of these forms can be observed as the dominant component or more commonly as a part of a composite tumour {161,1663,1849,2016,2444, 2519}. The stroma within the tumour is generally hyalinized and may manifest mucinous or myxoid features. In some tumours there is extensive stromal hyalinization with attenuation of the epithelial component. Perineural and to a lesser extent, intraneural invasion is a common and frequently conspicuous feature of AdCC. Tumours can extend along nerves for a considerable distance beyond the clinically apparent boundaries of the tumour. In addition, the tumour may invade bone extensively before there is

Table 5.2 Differential diagnosis of adenoid cystic carcinoma

Tumour type	Pattern	Cellular features	Perineural invasion
Basal cell adenoma	Syncytial/ non-invasive	Uniform Basaloid	No
Epithelial-myoepithelial carcinoma	Tubular/biphasic	Uniform, with clear outer cells	Rare
Basaloid squamous cell carcinoma	Syncytial	Marked pleomorphism focal keratinization	Rare
Basal cell adenocarcinoma	Syncytial/invasive	Mild pleomorphism/ invasive	Yes
AdCC Solid	Syncytial	Mild pleomorphism	Yes
AdCC Tubular/cribriform	Ductal/ cylindromatous	Uniform biphasic Mild pleomorphism	Yes Yes
PLGA	Tubular papillary pattern variable	Mild pleomorphism	Yes
Cellular PA	Syncytial	Uniform	No

AdCC: Adenoid cystic carcinoma; PLGA: Polymorphous low-grade adenocarcinoma; PA: Pleomorphic adenoma

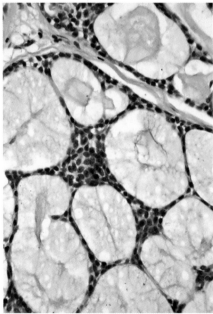

Fig. 5.7 Adenoid cystic carcinoma. Cribriform pattern with mucopolysaccharide filled spaces.

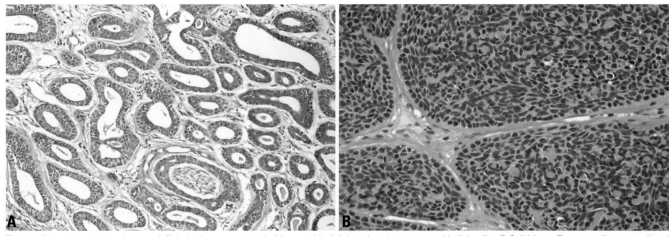

Fig. 5.8 Adenoid cystic carcinoma. **A** Tubular form, composed of inner epithelial ductal and outer myoepithelial cells. **B** Solid form. Tumour cells are small and basaloid with scanty cytoplasm.

radiographical evidence of osseous destruction.

Adenoid cystic carcinoma occasionally occurs with other different neoplasms (hybrid tumours) {505,1823,2297,2416}. Pleomorphic carcinomas and sarcomatoid transformation of adenoid cystic carcinoma have been reported, mostly in recurrent and metastatic disease {397, 418}.

Immunohistochemistry
In differentiating between polymorphous low-grade adenocarcinoma and adenoid cystic carcinoma, Ki-67 immunostaining may be helpful {2680}.
DNA content, C-kit and E-cadherin have been found to be associated with the biological behaviour of these tumours {636, 637,1215,1577}. Ki-67 and p53 have also been studied in these tumours {2844}, but no clear association with outcome have been reported. C-kit overexpression and its biological implication remains unknown. None of these markers, however, have been validated. Estrogen and progesterone receptor positivity has been reported in adenoid cystic carcinoma but the biological significance is currently unknown.

Differential diagnosis
Pleomorphic adenoma, polymorphous low-grade adenocarcinoma, epithelial-myoepithelial carcinoma, basal cell adenoma or adenocarcinoma and basaloid squamous carcinomas are the major entities to be differentiated from adenoid cystic carcinoma.

Genetics
Cytogenetics
The most consistent, although not exclu-sive, reported alterations have been at chromosomes 6q, 9p and 17p12-13 regions. The t(6;9) (q21-24;p13-23) has been reported in several tumours and is considered to be a primary event in at least a subset of these tumours {657, 1220,1906,2238}.

Molecular genetics
Frequent losses at 12q (33%) 6q23-qter, 13q21-q22 and 19q regions (40%) have been reported {657}. A study of the 9p21 regions and the p16 gene found only one tumour with LOH at this region and no mutations of the gene {351}. A recent study of 25 tumours found a high fre-quency of LOH at 6q 23-25 and this alter-ation correlated with histologic grade and clinical behaviour {2098,2458}. A recent genomic study identified new markers that may be helpful in future investigation of these tumours. Promoter methylation of the p16 was found in 20% of these tumours {1653}. Studies of other genes have been equally non-conclu-sive. Alterations of the p53 and Rb genes have been reported but no alter-ations in the K-ras have been found {2843}.

Prognosis and predictive factors
Factors that influence survival include histologic patterns, tumour site, clinical stage, bone involvement and status of surgical margins {1849,2016,2439,2444, 2519}. Generally, tumours composed of tubular and cribriform patterns pursue a less aggressive course than those with greater than 30% of solid component {2519}. Along with the histologic pattern, clinical stage greatly affects prognosis.

Other studies have failed to confirm the value of grading {2439,2444} and under-scored the significance of tumour size and clinical stage as the most consistent predictors of clinical outcome in patients with these tumours {2442,2449}. The 5-year survival rate is approximately 35% but the long-term survival is poorer. Eighty to 90% of patients die of disease in 10-15 years {993,2016}. The local recurrence rate ranges from 16-85% in several series of these tumours. Recurrence is a serious sign of incurabil-ity. Lymph node involvement is uncom-mon but has been reported to range from 5-25% and typically from tumours of the submandibular gland and is often due to contiguous spread rather than metasta-sis. The incidence of distant metastasis is estimated to range from 25-55%. The lung followed by bone, brain and liver are the common sites. Only 20% of patients with distant metastasis survive 5-years. The influence of perineural invasion on survival has been contradictory {860}. Wide local and radical surgical excisions with and without post-operative radiation is the treatment of choice {54,339, 1849,2439,2444,2519}. Radiation alone or with chemotherapy in the treatment of recurrent or metastatic disease has shown limited success. Radiotherapy, however, has been shown to improve local control in cases with microscopic residual disease {2670}. The value of chemotherapy in these tumours is limited and remains to be proven.

Polymorphous low-grade adenocarcinoma

M.A. Luna
B.M. Wenig

Definition

A malignant epithelial tumour characterized by cytologic uniformity, morphologic diversity, an infiltrative growth pattern, and low metastatic potential.

ICD-O code   8525/3

Synonyms

Terminal duct carcinoma, lobular carcinoma

Epidemiology

PLGA is the second most common intraoral malignant salivary gland tumour, accounting for 26% of all carcinomas {2711}. The female-to-male ratio is about 2:1. Patient age ranges from 16-94 years mean 59 years. Over 70% of the patients are between the ages of 50 and 70 years {342,697}. To date, only two tumours have been reported in the pediatric population {2641}.

Localization

Approximately 60% of the cases have involved the palate. Other intraoral locations are the buccal mucosa, retromolar region, upper lip, and the base of the tongue {342,697}. Uncommon locations include major salivary and lacrimal glands, nasopharynx and nasal cavity {1299,2763}.

Clinical features

A painless mass in the palate is the most common clinical sign. The duration of the lesion has varied from weeks to as much as 40 years {342}. Bleeding, telangiectasia, or ulceration of the overlying mucosa occurs occasionally.

Macroscopy

PLGA usually appears as a firm, circumscribed, but non-encapsulated, yellow-tan lobulated nodule up to several centimetres in greatest dimension (average 2.2 cm) {342}.

Histopathology

PLGA is characterized by cytologic uniformity, histologic diversity, and an infiltrative growth pattern. The tumour cells are small to medium size and uniform in shape with bland, minimally hyperchromatic, oval nuclei and only occasional nucleoli. Mitoses are uncommon and necrosis is not typical.

The striking feature of these carcinomas is the variety of morphologic configurations between tumours and within an individual tumour. The main microscopic patterns are: 1) lobular, 2) papillary or papillary-cystic (typically focal), 3) cribriform areas sometimes resembling those in adenoid cystic carcinoma, and 4) trabecular or small, duct-like structures lined by a single layer of cuboidal cells. The cells form concentric whorls or targetoid arrangements around blood vessels or nerves. Foci of oncocytic, clear, squamous or mucous cells may be found. Stroma may show areas of mucinosis or hyalinization. Despite the innocuous cytologic appearance, the neoplasm always invades adjacent soft tissues and is uncapsulated. Neurotropism is common in PLGA. Invasion of adjacent bone may be seen in tumours of the palate or mandible.

Immunohistochemistry

The neoplastic cells of PLGA are immunoreactive with antibodies to cytokeratin (100%), vimentin (100%), S-100 protein (97%), carcinoembryonic antigen (54%), glial fibrillary acidic protein (GFAP) (15%), muscle specific actin (13%), and epithelial membrane antigen (12%) {342,2011,2763}. Expression of galectin 3 has been reported to be significant in PLGA {2006}. Bcl-2 is over expressed in most cases of PLGA {342,2011}.

Differential diagnosis

The differential diagnosis includes pleomorphic adenoma (PA) and adenoid cystic carcinoma (AdCC), especially in small biopsy specimens. Unlike PLGA, PA is nearly always circumscribed and is composed of proliferating stromal, epithelial, and myoepithelial cells. It lacks the infiltrative, noncircumscribed character of PLGA. Although myxoid tissue is present in both tumours, the myxochondroid and chondroid areas present in PA are not evident in PLGA. Also, the typical benign plasmacytoid myoepithelial cells characteristic of palatal PA are seldom observed in PLGA. Staining with GFAP may be helpful in differentiating PA from PLGA.

The distinction between PLGA and AdCC is based primarily on cytologic features. Cells in PLGA are cuboidal or columnar. They have vesicular nuclei and often conspicuous eosinophilic cytoplasm without the basaloid features characteristic of AdCC. Papillary and fascicular growth patterns are extremely rare in AdCC. Furthermore, PLGA does not have large cribriform pseudocystic spaces that contain pools of haematoxyphilic glycosaminoglycans. The solid cellular areas of PLGA lack nuclear pleomorphism, necrosis, increased mitotic activity, and the numerous tubular structures characteristic of the solid variant of AdCC. The potential discriminating value of immunohistochemistry between cases of PLGA and AdCC remains controversial {547}, although some subtle differences may be apparent when series of these two neoplasms are studied {342,2006,2011,2391}.

Proliferative cell marker rates in PLGA are usually less than 6.4% (mean values 1.6% and 2.4%) {2391}. However, a higher proliferative rate (average 7%) has been reported by others investigators {2011}.

Genetics

Cytogenetic studies of this tumour are few. A total of 7 cases of which two were carcinoma ex-pleomorphic adenoma, have been reported. Alterations at 8q12 were found in two, 12q rearrangements in five, two showed a clonal t(6;9) (p21;p22) and one a monosomy 22 {1651}. Cytogenetic alterations in PLGA have frequently displayed chromosome 12 abnormalities affecting the q arm and the p arm {1651}.

Prognosis and predictive factors

The overall survival rate of patients with PLGA is excellent {164,342,696, 697,808}. A review of series with large numbers of cases and with long-term follow-up revealed a local recurrence rate between 9% and 17% and a regional metastases rate from 9-15% {342,697}. Distant metastases have seldom been reported {342,697}. Deaths attributed to tumour are unusual, and they occurred after prolonged periods {342,697}. In studies which accepted tumours with a predominant papillary configuration a higher incidence of cervical lymph node metastasis was reported {697}. The status of such tumours within the spectrum of PLGA is controversial. Dedifferentiation of PLGA has been reported and carries a less favourable prognosis. Such tumours should not be included under the rubric of typical PLGA {2368}.

Treatment consists of complete surgical excision. Neck dissection should be added for those patients with cervical adenopathy.

Cribriform adenocarcinoma of the tongue

A possible variant is cribriform adenocarcinoma of the tongue, but it is not yet clear whether this represents a genuine entity or just an unusual growth pattern in PLGA, with which there appears to be some overlap {1718}.

So far described only in one series, all cases presented with a mass in the tongue, usually the posterior part, and synchronous metastases in lateral neck lymph nodes, but no distant spread. There was an equal sex incidence and the mean age at presentation was 50.4 years (range 25-70).

The tumour grows beneath the surface epithelium and infiltrates soft tissue. It is divided by fibrous septa into lobules, which are solid or cribriform. A characteristic feature is that some nearly solid islands have a glomeruloid arrangement of broad microfollicular papillae separated from a layer of peripheral columnar cells by a narrow cleft. Small numbers of tubules are seen, and occasional spindling of tumour cells may occur. The nuclei are uniform, pale and often overlap, closely mimicking those of papillary carcinoma of the thyroid. Mitotic figures are sparse. No necrosis or significant

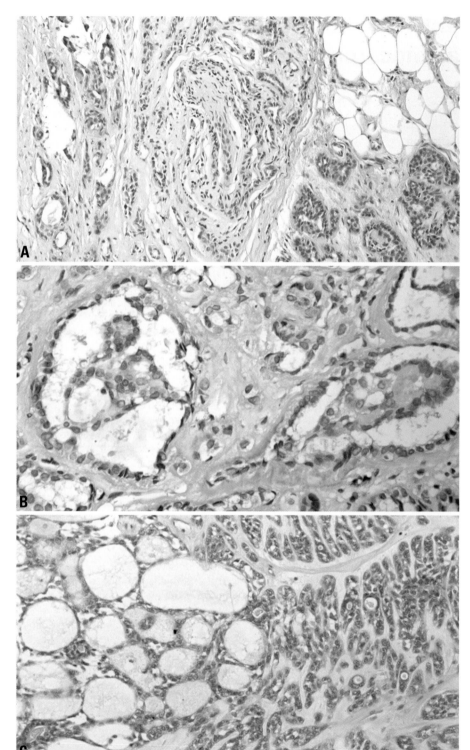

Fig. 5.9 Polymorphous low-grade adenocarcinoma (PLGA). **A** Destructive invasion of adjacent tissues. **B** PLGA with papillary cystic formations. **C** Cribriform growth pattern.

haemorrhage is seen, and the stroma includes hyalinized areas, and rarely psammoma bodies. The tumours are positive for cytokeratin, and more patchily for S-100 protein. Myoepithelial markers, such as actin are either negative or only focally positive. Thyroglobulin staining is consistently negative.

Epithelial-myoepithelial carcinoma

I. Fonseca
J. Soares

Definition
A malignant tumour composed of variable proportions of two cell types, which typically form duct-like structures. The biphasic morphology is represented by an inner layer of duct lining, epithelial-type cells and an outer layer of clear, myoepithelial-type cells.

ICD-O code
8562/3

Synonyms
Adenomyoepithelioma {176}, clear cell adenoma {494,2228}, glycogen-rich adenoma {913}, glycogen-rich adenocarcinoma {1758}, clear cell carcinoma {407}.

Epidemiology
Epithelial-myoepithelial carcinoma (EMC) represents around 1% of the salivary gland tumours. It is more prevalent in women (F: M=2:1). The patients range in age from 13 to 89 years, with the peak incidence in the 6th and 7th decades {436,493,614,784,1580}. Only two cases have been reported in the paediatric group {436,1775}.

Localization
EMC occurs mostly in major salivary glands, mainly in the parotid (60%), but also in the minor glands of oral mucosa and the upper {436,493,614,784,1580} and lower respiratory tract {610,1126, 1174,2002}.

Clinical features
EMC forms a painless, slow-growing mass. Tumours arising in minor glands frequently present as ulcerated, submucosal nodules and have less well-defined margins. Rapid growth, facial nerve palsy and/or associated pain are suggestive of concomitant high-grade areas.

Macroscopy
EMC is characteristically a multinodular mass, with expansive borders and lacking a true capsule. Cystic spaces may be present. Tumours of the minor glands are poorly circumscribed.

Histopathology
EMC has a lobulated growth pattern with a mixed tubular and solid architectural arrangement. Papillary and cystic areas can be identified in around 20% of the cases. Tumours from minor salivary and sero-mucinous glands show infiltration of surrounding tissues and there is ulceration of the overlying mucosa in about 40% of the cases.
The hallmark of EMC histology is the presence of bi-layered duct-like structures: the inner layer is formed by a single row of cuboidal cells, with dense, finely granular cytoplasm and central or basal, round nucleus. The outer layer may show single or multiple layers of polygonal cells, with well-defined borders; the cytoplasm is characteristically clear and the nucleus is vesicular and slightly eccentric. The double-layered pattern is preserved in papillary-cystic areas but solid tumour areas may be exclusively formed by clear cells. PAS positive, hyaline, eosinophilic strands of basement membrane-like material surround the duct-like structures and, in solid areas, divide the clear cells into theques. Coagulative necrosis at the centre of tumour nodules is uncommon. In rare cases, squamous differentiation and spindle cells are observed as well as an oncocytic appearance in the inner cell layer of neoplastic ducts.
Perineural and vascular invasion are frequent and bone invasion may occur.
None to 1-2 mitoses per 10 HPF can be identified in the clear cell population of EMC. Rare cases of dedifferentiation have been reported {42,783}.

Immunoprofile
Myoepithelial markers (smooth muscle actin, HHF35, p63 and/or calponin) stain the clear cell compartment. The luminal cells stain with cytokeratins.

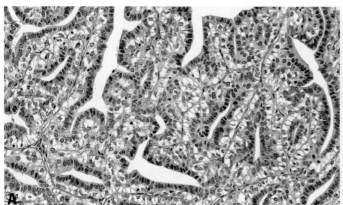
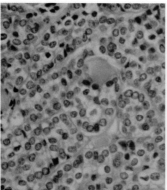
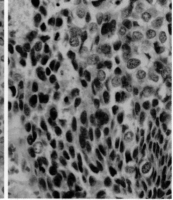

Fig. 5.10 Epithelial-myoepithelial carcinoma (EMC) of the parotid gland. **A** Double layered architecture formed by an inner layer of eosinophilic cuboidal cells and an outer layer of clear, myoepithelial-type cells. **B** Dedifferentiated EMC. There is co-existence of areas typical of EMC (left) with areas of undifferentiated carcinoma (right).

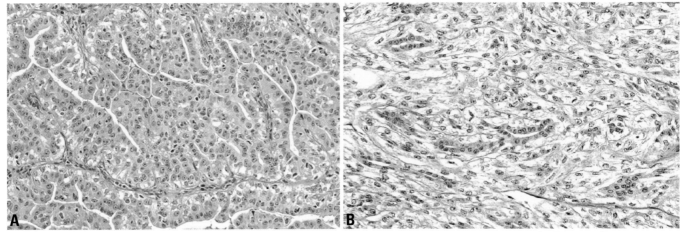

Fig. 5.11 Epithelial-myoepithelial carcinoma. **A** Ductal tumour cells of inner layer predominance. **B** Solid growth of clear, myoepithelial-type cells.

Differential diagnosis

The differential diagnosis of EMC includes all primary salivary gland tumours that are predominantly formed by clear cells: pleomorphic adenoma, myoepithelioma, oncocytoma and mucoepidermoid carcinoma. Differential diagnosis with clear cell carcinoma, NOS relies on the demonstration of the peculiar amyloid-like quality of the stroma and on the absence of myoepithelial markers. Metastatic kidney and thyroid carcinoma may be distinguished using immunohistochemistry; CD10 and high-molecular weight cytokeratin in the former and thyroglobulin in the latter.

EMC foci can be encountered within carcinoma ex pleomorphic adenoma as part of the carcinomatous component.

Genetics

A limited number of cases (6) have been karyotyped {656,1650,1751}, half of them showing non-distinctive chromosomal alterations and the remaining normal karyotypes.

Prognosis and predictive factors

Recurrence occurs in around 40% of cases and metastasis in 14%. The most common metastatic sites are cervical lymph nodes, lung, liver and kidney. Death from disease complications occurs in less than 10% of the patients {436,493,614,784,1580}. Five- and 10 year overall survival rates are 80% and 72%, respectively {784}.

Size and rapid tumour growth are associated with worse prognosis {42,783}.

Margin status is a major pathological prognostic factor. Incomplete surgical excision is associated with recurrence and metastasis. The poorer prognosis associated with tumours located in minor salivary glands may be due to the higher frequency of recurrences due to incomplete surgery. Atypia is associated with unfavourable outcome {784} whenever present in more than 20% of tumour area. EMC is usually diploid {784,992}. Aneuploidy and high mitotic counts have been reported in cases with unfavourable prognosis {784}. Areas of dedifferentiation also predict poor outcome, with recurrence and metastasis in 70% of patients {42,783}.

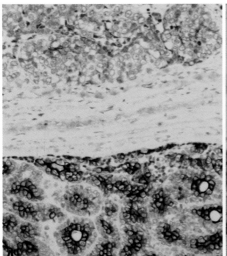
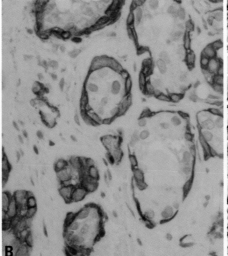
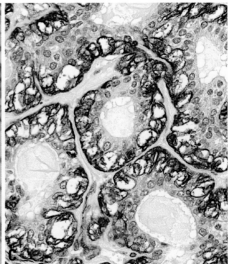

Fig. 5.12 Epithelial-myoepithelial carcinoma (EMC) of the parotid gland. **A** Dedifferentiated EMC. Low molecular weight cytokeratins emphasizes the loss of the biphasic pattern (lower). The differentiated component (upper) retains focal epithelial differentiation (CAM 5.2). **B** Immunostained for smooth muscle actin (SMA): the reverse image of that of the differentiated area is obtained, with intense staining of the outer layers. **C** Tumour cells of the outer layer are also strongly immunoreactive for calponin.

Clear cell carcinoma, not otherwise specified

G. Ellis

Definition

Clear cell carcinoma, not otherwise specified (NOS), is a malignant epithelial neoplasm composed of a monomorphous population of cells that have optically clear cytoplasm with standard haematoxylin and eosin stains. Because many types of salivary gland neoplasms commonly or consistently have a component of clear cells, clear cell carcinoma is distinguished by the absence of features characteristic of these other neoplasms and its monomorphous population of clear cells.

ICD-O code   8310/3

Synonyms

Clear cell adenocarcinoma; hyalinizing clear cell carcinoma.

Clear cell carcinoma has been confused with epithelial-myoepithelial carcinoma (EMC), and EMC have been reported as clear cell carcinoma {407}.

Epidemiology

The peak occurrence is in patients in the 40-70 year age range, and they are rare in children {668,2658}. There is no sex predilection.

Localization

Clear cell carcinomas are more frequent in the intraoral minor salivary glands than the major salivary glands {668,1728, 1931,2179,2369,2716}. The palate is most frequently involved, but buccal mucosa, tongue, floor of the mouth, lip, and retromolar and tonsillar areas are also affected.

Clinical features

The only sign in most cases is swelling, but mucosal ulceration and pain occur with some tumours. Patients have reported the durations of their tumours as 1 month to 15 years {2369}.

Macroscopy

Although the size of the primary tumour is usually 3.0 cm or less, the tumours usually are poorly circumscribed and infiltrate adjacent salivary gland, mucosa, soft tissues, bone, and nerves. The cut surface is greyish-white.

Histopathology

A monomorphous population of polygonal to round cells with clear cytoplasm characterizes clear cell carcinomas. In some cases, a minority of cells have pale eosinophilic cytoplasm. Nuclei are eccentric and round and frequently contain small nucleoli. PAS staining with and without prior diastase digestion of the tissue demonstrates cytoplasmic glycogen that varies from marked to not evident. The adjective glycogen-rich has been used by some to identify clear cell carcinomas with a prominent glycogen content {1028,2658}. With mucicarmine stain, intracytoplasmic mucins are usually absent. The tumour cells are arranged in sheets, nests, or cords, and ductal structures are absent. Mitotic figures are rare, but some tumours have a moderate degree of nuclear pleomorphism. In the hyalinizing type, the stroma is composed of thick bands of hyalinized collagen {727,1728}, but in other tumours it consists of interconnecting, thin fibrous septa that may be cellular or loosely collagenous. Clear cell carcinomas are unencapsulated and infiltrative.

Immunoprofile

While tumours are immunoreactive for cytokeratin, at least focally, immunohistochemical studies have given variable results for S100 protein, glial fibrillary acidic protein, actin, and vimentin {1028, 1728,1931,2348,2369,2658,2716}. Tumours that demonstrate histologic and immunohistochemical features of myoepithelial differentiation are best classified as clear cell variants of myoepithelioma or myoepithelial carcinoma {1719}.

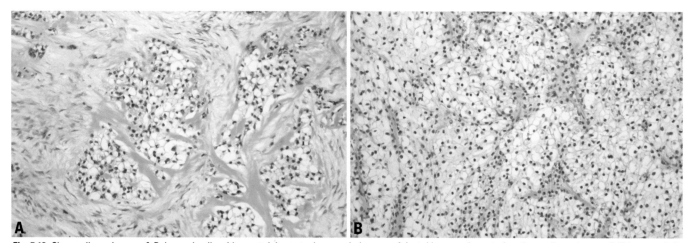

Fig. 5.13 Clear cell carcinoma. **A** Polygonal cells with nonstaining cytoplasm and absence of ductal lumens characterize clear cell carcinoma. **B** This example is composed of a mostly solid sheet of tumour cells with little stroma.

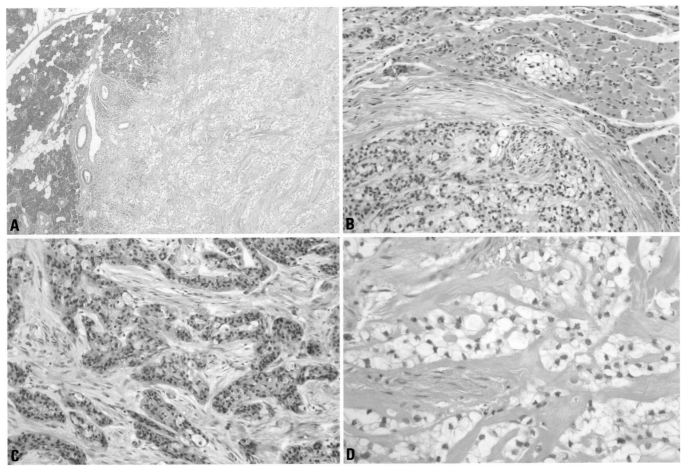

Fig. 5.14 Clear cell carcinoma. **A** Infiltration into adjacent lobules of normal parotid gland. **B** Clear cell carcinoma of the lip infiltrating skeletal muscle (top) and surrounding a peripheral nerve (lower centre). **C** PAS staining demonstrates a prominent cytoplasmic glycogen content. **D** Clear cell carcinoma of the parotid gland. Prominent hyalinized stroma separates nests of tumour cells.

Electron microscopy
Tight junctions, desmosomal attachments, tonofilaments, microvilli, and basal lamina are features of duct cell differentiation {399,1028,1728,1758,1931, 2369,2716}.

Histogenesis
Ultrastructural investigations have found features of ductal but not myoepithelial differentiation .

Prognosis and predictive factors
Prognosis is excellent. A few tumours have metastasized to cervical lymph nodes and, rarely, the lung, but no patients have succumbed to this neoplasm {155,948,1728,2716}.

Basal cell adenocarcinoma

G. Ellis

Definition
Dominated by basaloid epithelial cells, basal cell adenocarcinoma is cytologically and histomorphologically similar to basal cell adenoma but is an infiltrative epithelial neoplasm with potential for metastasis.

ICD-O code   8147/3

Synonyms
Basaloid salivary carcinoma, carcinoma ex monomorphic adenoma, malignant basal cell adenoma, malignant basal cell tumour, and basal cell carcinoma {159, 408,698,1163,1340,1576}. Tumours in infants reported as basal cell adenoma/carcinoma or hybrids are best classified as sialoblastomas.

Epidemiology
There is no sex predilection. The average age of patients is 60 years, and only adults have been affected {668,673, 1576,1792,2726}.

Localization
Over 90%, of these tumours occur in the parotid gland, and they are rare in the minor salivary glands of the oral cavity {668,673,2703}.

Clinical features
Rarely, patients complain of pain or tenderness; most tumours are asymptomatic except for swelling. The duration of tumours before excision ranges from weeks to years. Similar to some patients with basal cell adenomas, patients with basal cell adenocarcinomas may have a diathesis of multiple skin adnexal tumours and parotid basal cell adenocarcinomas {65,668,673,1163, 1576}.

Macroscopy
Basal cell adenocarcinomas most frequently occur in the superficial (lateral) lobe of the parotid gland. The cut surface has variable coloration of grey, tan-white, or brownish. The texture is homogeneous although some tumours are focally cystic. They are unencapsulated, but some tumours appear well-circumscribed while others are obviously infiltrative.

Histopathology
Basaloid epithelial cells, which vary from small, dark cells to larger, paler stained cells, form histomorphologic patterns that are described as solid, membranous, trabecular and tubular. A solid pattern, in which variable sized and shaped nests are separated by thin septa or thick bands of collagenous stroma, is most frequent. In the membranous type, tumours produce excessive amounts of eosinophilic, hyalinized basal lamina material that forms intercellular droplets and peripheral membranes. Interconnecting bands of basaloid cells characterizes the trabecular growth pattern. In the tubular type, there are luminal spaces among the basaloid cells. There are foci of squamous differentiation in some tumours. The nuclei of tumour cells along the interface with the collagenous stroma are often palisaded. The degree of cytologic atypia and the number of mitotic figures varies from one tumour to another but is often quite minimal. Infiltration of tumour cells into parotid parenchyma, dermis, skeletal muscle, or periglandular fat distinguishes basal cell adenocarcinoma from basal cell adenoma. Vessel or peripheral nerve invasion is evident in about a fourth of the tumours.

Immunoprofile
Immunohistochemical staining is variable among tumours. Tumour cells are reactive for cytokeratins and often focally reactive for S100 protein, epithelial membrane antigen, and carcinoembryonic antigen. Limited reactivity for smooth muscle actin and vimentin supports myoepithelial differentiation of some cells {2097,2793}.

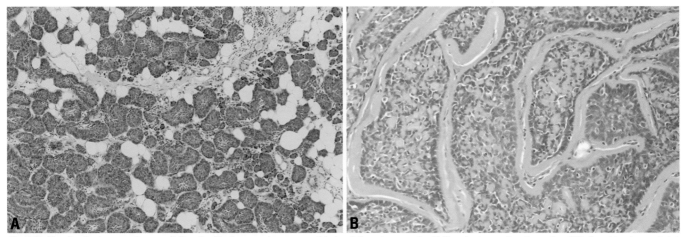

Fig. 5.15 Basal cell adenocarcinoma. **A** Basal cell adenocarcinoma, parotid gland. Invasive growth. **B** Abundant, prominently eosinophilic basal lamina material within and around nests of tumour is characteristic of the membranous pattern of basal cell adenocarcinoma.

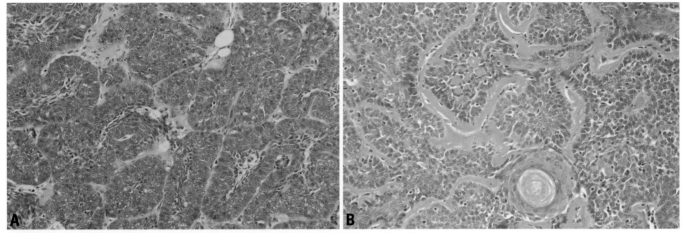

Fig. 5.16 Basal cell adenocarcinoma. **A** Basal cell adenocarcinoma of the parotid gland with solid pattern of growth. **B** Small, circular areas of squamous cells, sometimes with keratinization (bottom centre) occur in some basal cell adenocarcinomas.

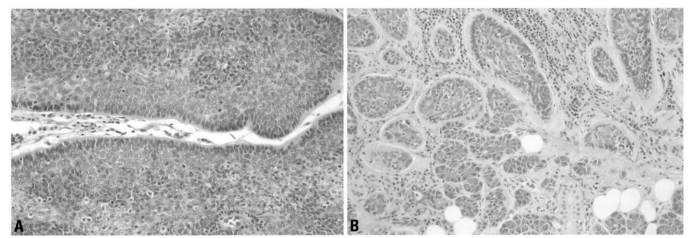

Fig. 5.17 Basal cell adenocarcinoma. **A** Alignment of the nuclei of the tumour cells along the stromal interface creates a palisaded appearance. **B** Nests of tumour cells infiltrate into adjacent parotid gland parenchyma.

Precursor lesions

Most basal cell adenocarcinomas probably develop de novo, but some arise by malignant transformation in basal cell adenomas {1576,1792}.

Genetics

Cytogenetics

Chromosomal gains at 9p21.1-pter, 18q21.1-q22.3, and 22q11.23-q13.31 as well as losses at 2q24.2 and 4q25-q27 have been described {2612}. The gain at 22q12.3-q13.1 is described as also common in adenoid cystic carcinoma.

Molecular genetics

A study of two familial cases and two sporadic basaloid tumours for alterations at the 16q12-13 regions showed high frequency (80%) of LOH in both sporadic and familial basaloid tumours and dermal cylindromas of the familial cases.

The minimally deleted region contained the *CYLD* gene. This study indicates that these tumours share the same alterations as dermal cylindromas and implicates the *CYLD* gene in their development {437}.

Prognosis and predictive factors

While they are locally destructive and often recur, basal cell adenocarcinomas only occasionally metastasize, and death of patients is rare {408,673,698,1163, 1340,1576,1792,1799}. Ki-67 and PCNA indices are low {782,2097}.

Malignant sebaceous tumours

D.R. Gnepp

Sebaceous carcinoma

Definition
Sebaceous carcinoma is a malignant tumour composed of sebaceous cells of varying maturity that are arranged in sheets and/or nests with different degrees of pleomorphism, nuclear atypia and invasiveness.

ICD-O code   8410/3

Epidemiology
There is a bimodal age distribution with a peak incidence in the third decade and the 7th and 8th decades of life (range 17-93 years) {669,896,901}. The male and female incidence is almost equal. Unlike sebaceous neoplasms of the skin {1132, 2214}, there is no increased risk of developing a visceral carcinoma in patients with a salivary gland sebaceous tumour.

Localization
Approximately 90% arise in the parotid area, with occasional tumours in the oral cavity, vallecula, sublingual gland, submandibular gland and epiglottis {107, 602,669,693,896}.

Clinical features
Patients typically present with a painful mass with varying degrees of facial nerve paralysis and occasional fixation to the skin.

Macroscopy
Tumours have ranged from 0.6-8.5 cm in greatest dimension and vary from yellow, tan-white, greyish-white, white, to pale pink {896}. They are well circumscribed or partially encapsulated, with pushing or locally infiltrating margins.

Histopathology
Tumours are composed of multiple large foci and nests or sheets of cells with hyperchromatic nuclei and abundant clear to eosinophilic cytoplasm. Cellular pleomorphism and cytologic atypia are present to varying degrees and are much more prevalent than in sebaceous adenomas. Squamous differentiation is common. There may be areas of basaloid differentiation, particularly at the periphery of cellular nests. Areas of necrosis and fibrosis are common. Perineural invasion is seen in greater than 20% of tumours; vascular invasion is infrequent. Rare oncocytes and foreign body giant cells with histiocytes may be observed, but lymphoid tissue with follicles or subcapsular sinuses is not seen.

Prognosis and predictive factors
The treatment of choice is wide surgical excision for low stage carcinomas. Adjunctive radiation therapy is recommended for higher-stage and grade tumours. The overall 5-year survival rate is 62% {669,896}. , slightly less than the survival for similar tumours arising in the skin and orbit (84.5%) {234}.

Sebaceous lymphadenocarcinoma

Definition
Sebaceous lymphadenocarcinoma is the malignant counterpart of sebaceous lymphadenoma. It is a carcinoma arising in a sebaceous lymphadenoma.

ICD-O code   8410/3
Synonym
Carcinoma ex sebaceous lymphadenoma.

Epidemiology
It is the rarest salivary gland sebaceous tumour. To date, only three have been reported {901,1525}. All three patients were in their seventh decade; two patients were male and one female.

Localization
The tumours arose within the parotid gland or in periparotid lymph nodes.

Clinical features
Patients had histories of a mass, two of which were present for more than 20 years.

Macroscopy
Tumour colour varies from yellow-tan to grey.

Histopathology
These carcinomas are partially encapsulated and locally invasive with foci of sebaceous lymphadenoma intermixed with or adjacent to regions of pleomorphic carcinoma cells exhibiting varying degrees of invasiveness. The malignant portion has ranged from sebaceous carcinoma to sheets of poorly differentiated carcinoma, with areas of ductal differentiation, adenoid cystic carcinoma-like areas or foci of epithelial-myoepithelial carcinoma. Perineural invasion, collections of histiocytes and a foreign body giant cell reaction may occur. Cellular atypia is not observed in the sebaceous lymphadenoma portion of the tumour.

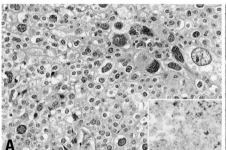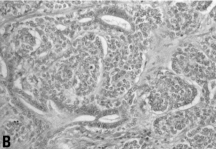

Fig. 5.18 A Sebaceous carcinoma. Solid growth of pleomorphic sebaceous tumour cells. Inset: Tumour cells are positive for fat stain (Sudan-III). **B** Sebaceous lymphadenocarcinoma composed of poorly differentiated carcinoma cells with areas of ductal differentiation.

Cystadenocarcinoma

P.L. Auclair

Definition
Cystadenocarcinoma is a rare malignant tumour characterized by predominantly cystic growth that often exhibits intraluminal papillary growth. It lacks any additional specific histopathologic features that characterize the other types of salivary carcinomas showing cystic growth. It is conceptually the malignant counterpart of the benign cystadenoma.

ICD-O code   8440/3

Synonyms
Papillary cystadenocarcinoma, mucus-producing adenopapillary (non-epidermoid) carcinoma {224,679,2463}, malignant papillary cystadenoma {2133}, and low-grade papillary adenocarcinoma of the palate {38,1742,2784}.

Epidemiology
There is no sex predilection. The average age of patients is 59 years; more than 70% are over 50 years of age {790}.

Localization
About 65% occur in the major salivary glands and most of these arise in the parotid. Involvement of the sublingual gland is proportionately greater than of other benign or malignant tumours {790}. The buccal mucosa, lips, and palate are the most frequently involved minor gland sites.

Clinical features
Cystadenocarcinomas usually manifest as a slowly growing, compressible asymptomatic mass. Tumours of the palate may erode bone.

Macroscopy
The tumours have multiple cystic spaces that are variable in size and often filled with mucin. They are grossly at least partially circumscribed and have ranged in size from 0.4-6 cm.

Histopathology
The tumours are usually well circumscribed but not encapsulated. Numerous haphazardly arranged cysts are evident that are partially filled with mucin, vary in shape and size, and have limited intervening fibrous connective tissue. Small solid neoplastic islands or duct-like structures may occur between the cysts or at the advancing front of the tumour. In about 75% of the cases the lumens of the cysts exhibit varying degrees of papillary proliferation. In either case, cell types that comprise the lining epithelium include, most often, small and large cuboidal, and columnar cells, but mucous, clear and oncocytic cells are occasionally noted. The columnar-rich tumours often predominate in the intraluminal papillary areas and account for their "gastrointestinal" appearance, but the cells usually fail to stain for neutral mucin. Although nucleoli are evident, the nuclei typically are uniformly bland and mitoses rare. However, a prerequisite for the diagnosis is that the cysts and smaller duct-like structures at least focally infiltrate the salivary parenchyma and surrounding connective tissue. The presence of ruptured cysts with haemorrhage and granulation tissue is common.

Differential diagnosis
Distinction from cystadenoma may be difficult and relies largely on identification of infiltrative growth into salivary parenchyma or surrounding tissues. Review of multiple sections is often helpful. Low-grade mucoepidermoid carcinoma is typically cystic but, unlike cystadenocarcinoma, usually has a wide variety of cell types and areas that are more solid than cystic. The papillary cystic variant of acinic cell carcinoma has focal acinar differentiation and a greater degree of epithelial proliferation. Epidermoid differentiation in cystadenocarcinomas is rare.

Prognosis and predictive factors
Cystadenocarcinoma is a low-grade adenocarcinoma treated by superficial parotidectomy, glandectomy of submandibular and sublingual tumours, and wide excision of minor gland tumours. Bone resection is performed only when it is directly involved by tumour {411,535, 790,2350}. In a study of 40 patients with follow-up data, all were alive or had died of other causes, four suffered metastasis to regional lymph nodes, one at the time of diagnosis and one after 55 months, and three experienced a recurrence at a mean interval of 76 months {790}.

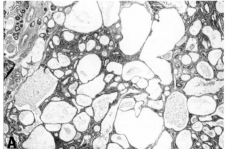 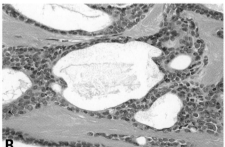 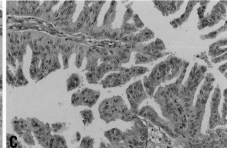

Fig. 5.19 Cystadenocarcinoma. **A** Focal collections of lymphoid tissue are present. No significant papillary luminal growth. **B** Cystic spaces are lined by morphologically bland low cuboidal epithelium, and are separated by loosely arranged fibrous stroma. **C** Papillary cystadenocarcinoma.

Low-grade cribriform cystadenocarcinoma

M.S. Brandwein-Gensler
D.R. Gnepp

Definition

A rare, cystic, proliferative carcinoma that resembles the spectrum of breast lesions from atypical ductal hyperplasia to micropapillary and cribriform low-grade ductal carcinoma in-situ.

Synonym

Low-grade salivary duct carcinoma

Epidemiology

To date, all but one tumour have been diagnosed in the parotid gland and one in the palate {259,578,899,2562}. There is a female predominance of 2:1.

Clinical features

Patients are usually elderly and all but one patient presented with cystic parotid tumours.

Histopathology

Low-grade cribriform cystadenocarcinomas (LGCCC) are unencapsulated, consisting of single or multiple cysts, accompanied by adjacent intraductal proliferation. The cysts are lined by small, multi-layered, proliferating, bland ductal cells with finely dispersed chromatin and small nucleoli. Within the cystic areas, they typically are arranged in a cribriform pattern and frequently have anastomosing, intracystic micropapillae lining the cavity, which may contain fibrovascular cores. Separate, smaller ductal structures are variably filled by proliferating ductal epithelium with cribriform, micropapillary and solid areas. The overall appearance is very similar to breast atypical ductal hyperplasia and low-grade ductal carcinoma in-situ. Many superficial cells contain cytoplasmic apocrine-type microvacuoles (PAS- positive/diastase-resistant) and/or fine yellow to brown pigment resembling lipofuscin. Focal invasion into the surrounding tissue can be seen, characterized by small solid islands and reactive inflammation and desmoplasia. Perineural or vascular invasion typically is not present. Cellular pleomorphism and mitotic figures are usually absent and necrosis is extremely uncommon. Occasional tumours may demonstrate transition from low to intermediate or high-grade cytology, with scattered mitotic figures and focal necrosis.

Immunoprofile

These tumours demonstrate strong, diffuse S100 positivity. Myoepithelial markers (calponin or smooth muscle actin) highlight cells rimming the cystic spaces, confirming the intraductal nature of most, or all, of each tumour. No myoepithelial cells are admixed within the proliferative cellular component. Those tumours studied for HER2-neu antigen are uniformly negative.

Variants

Originally, this tumour was reported as a low-grade variant of salivary duct carcinoma. However, as no data have accumulated definitely relating this entity to ductal carcinoma and since there frequently is a prominent cystic component, for the purposes of this WHO classification, the tumour is listed as a variant of cystadenocarcinoma.

Differential diagnosis

The following tumours require exclusion: papillary cystic variant of acinic cell carcinoma, (PCVACC) and other variants of cystadenocarcinoma. PCVACC contains vacuolated cells similar to the microvacuolated cells of LGCCC. However the vacuoles of the latter are smaller, refractile, and associated with a yellow to brown pigment, while areas with PAS positive diastase resistant fine cytoplasmic granules will be found in the former. Conventional cystadenocarcinoma differ from LGCCC by the lack of intraductal proliferation, golden brown pigment, solid cellular foci, and overall resemblance to atypical hyperplasia or carcinoma-in-situ of the breast. Cystadenocarcinoma tends to be an invasive tumour, whereas LGCCC is usually contained within cysts {790}.

Prognosis and predictive factors

Treatment is complete surgical excision. Although the number of cases with follow-up is small, none of the cases, to date, have recurred. Greater experience and longer follow-up periods are necessary to substantiate the excellent prognosis.

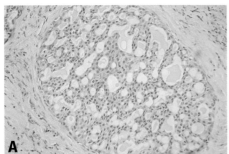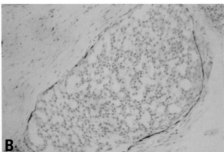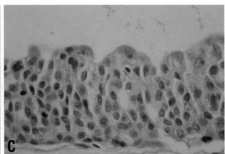

Fig. 5.20 Low-grade cribriform cystadenocarcinoma (LGCCC) **A** The intraductal proliferations of LGCCC resemble benign breast ductal hyperplasia. The fenestrations formed are "floppy", not rigid. **B** Calponin, a myoepithelial marker, highlights the largely intraductal nature of this neoplasm. LGCCC strongly expresses S100, in distinction to the papillocystic variant of acinic cell carcinoma. **C** Golden-brown pigment can be see within the relatively bland tumour cells of LGCCC.

Mucinous adenocarcinoma

K.H. Sun
Y. Gao
T.J. Li

Definition

Mucinous adenocarcinoma is a rare malignant tumour composed of epithelial clusters within large pools of extracellular mucin. The mucin component usually occupies the bulk of the tumour mass.

ICD-O code   8480/3

Epidemiology

It usually arises in patients over 50 years of age. Males are affected more frequently than females {859,1374,1909, 1957,2551}.

Localization

The most frequently affected sites are the palate and the sublingual gland, followed by the submandibular gland and the upper lip. Occurrence in the parotid gland is rare {859}.

Clinical features

The patients usually present with a slow-growing, painless swelling. However, local dull pain may be encountered in some cases. The tumour is firm and usually elevated.

Macroscopy

The tumour is nodular and ill defined. The cut surface is greyish-white, containing many cystic cavities with gelatinous contents.

Histopathology

The tumour is composed of round and irregular-shaped neoplastic epithelial cell nests or clusters floating in mucus-filled cystic cavities separated by connective fibrous strands. The tumour cells are cuboidal, columnar or irregular in shape, usually possess clear cytoplasm and darkly-stained, centrically placed nuclei. The tumour cells may have atypical nuclei, but mitotic figures are sparse. The tumour cells are arranged in solid clusters and tend to form secondary lumens or incomplete duct-like structures. Mucus-producing cells may arrange in a papillary pattern projecting into the mucous pools. Mucous acinus-like

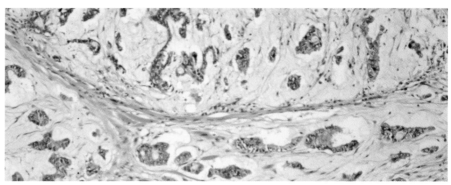

Fig. 5.21 Mucinous adenocarcinoma. Tumour cell clusters floating in mucus-filled cystic cavities separated by connective fibrous strands.

tumour islands may also be present. Both intracellular and extracellular mucin components show positive staining for periodic acid Schiff, Alcian blue and mucicarmine.

Immunoprofile

Immunocytochemically, the tumour cells express pankeratin AE1/AE3 as well as cytokeratins 7, 8, 18 and 19 that are usually found in simple epithelia {859,1374}. Expression of cytokeratins 4 and 13 is seen in about 10-20%. Negative staining is noted for cytokeratins 5/6, 10, 14, 17 and for smooth muscle actin (SMA).

Electron microscopy

The cytoplasm of the tumour cells is densely packed with numerous low-electron-density mucous droplets, and seromucous droplets containing electron-dense dots are also seen. Tumour cells possessing mucous or seromucous

droplets form a luminal structure, and they have irregularly arranged microvilli on the luminal side.

Differential diagnosis

Mucoepidermoid carcinoma, mucin-rich variant of salivary duct carcinoma and cystadenocarcinoma should be differentiated from mucinous adenocarcinoma. Mucoepidermoid carcinoma also shows extravasated mucin, but it consists of intermediate and epidermoid cells. Cystadenocarcinoma shows cystic spaces lined by epithelium. Extracellular mucin pools are not evident in acinic cell carcinoma.

Prognosis and predictive factors

Mucinous adenocarcinoma is insensitive to radiotherapy and has a propensity for local recurrence and regional lymph node metastases.

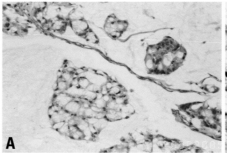
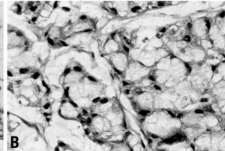

Fig. 5.22 Mucinous adenocarcinoma. **A** Clusters of mucin-producing cells and cuboidal cells floating in the mucous pools. **B** Mucous acinus-like tumour islands.

Oncocytic carcinoma

J.J. Sciubba
M. Shimono

Definition
Oncocytic carcinoma is a proliferation of cytomorphologically malignant oncocytes and adenocarcinomatous architectural phenotypes, including infiltrative qualities. These may arise de novo, but are usually seen in association with a pre-existing oncocytoma {1833}. Rarely, a benign appearing oncocytic tumour metastasizes following local recurrence {2498} and is designated carcinoma, despite the absence of malignant cellular morphology.

ICD-O code   8290/3

Epidemiology
Men are affected in two-thirds of cases. A wide age range from 25-91 years has been reported with a mean age of 62.5 years {71}. This neoplasm represents only 5% of oncocytic salivary gland tumours and less than 1% of all salivary gland tumours {922}.

Localization
Nearly 80% involve the parotid gland, 8% the submandibular gland, with all others in minor salivary glands.

Clinical features
Typically there is a painless, nondescript mass in the parotid or submandibular gland. In cases of malignant transformation of a benign oncocytoma a rapid increase in size is noted after a period of slow growth. Facial nerve involvement may cause pain, paresis or neuropathy {922}.

Macroscopy
They are firm, unencapsulated, tan to grey, unilocular or multilocular masses, occasionally with necrotic areas.

Histopathology
Sheets, islands and nests are composed of large, round to polyhedral cells with fine, granular, eosinophilic cytoplasm and central, round vesicular nuclei, often with prominent nucleoli {257}. Occasionally there are multinucleated cells. In some tumours there are duct-like structures of variable calibre. They are unencapsulated and often invade muscle, lymphatics and nerves. They are characterised cytologically by cellular atypia and pleomorphism.
Histochemically, phosphotungstic acid-haematoxylin (PTAH) staining reveals fine, blue, cytoplasmic granulues. Other methods to demonstrate mitochondria such as the Novelli technique, cresylecht violet V, Kluver-Barrera Luxol fast blue stains {2601} and antimitochondrial antibodies can also be used {2343}.

Immunoprofile
Ki-67 immunostaining has been suggested in separating benign from malignant oncocytoma {1188}. In addition, alpha-1-antitrypsin staining has been helpful {476}.

Electron microscopy
There are large numbers of mitochondria which are often abnormal in shape and size. Intracytoplasmic lumina lined with microvilli and lipid droplets have also been reported. A nearly continuous basal lamina, evenly spaced desmosomes and rearrangement of mitochondrial cristae have been demonstrated {218}.

Prognosis and predictive factors
These high-grade tumours are characterised by multiple local recurrences and regional or distant metastases {922,940}. In one series, 7 of 11 patients studied ultimately developed metastatic disease {1227}. It appears that the most important prognostic indicator is the presence or absence of distant metastases {1833}.

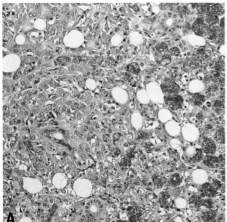
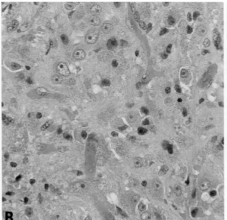
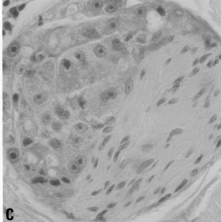

Fig. 5.23 Oncocytic carcinoma. **A** Invasion into the parotid gland. **B** Atypical tumour cells have prominent nucleoli and eosinophilic, granular cytoplasm. **C** Perineural invasion.

Salivary duct carcinoma

M.S. Brandwein-Gensler
A. Skálová
T. Nagao

Definition
An aggressive adenocarcinoma which resembles high-grade breast ductal carcinoma.

ICD-O code
8500/3

Synonyms
Cribriform salivary carcinoma of excretory ducts, high-grade salivary duct carcinoma

Epidemiology
Salivary duct carcinoma (SDC) is an uncommon, but not a rare form of salivary malignancy. De novo and/or ex-pleomorphic adenoma, SDC represents 9% of salivary malignancies.

The male:female ratio is at least 4:1. Most patients present after age 50 {135,259, 1488}. The parotid is most commonly involved, but submandibular, sublingual, minor salivary gland, maxillary and laryngeal tumours have been reported {682, 745,1383,2021,2583,2862,2909}.

Etiology
A unique case of SDC arising in a long-standing chronic obstructive sialadenitis has been reported {1113}.

Clinical features
Patients with SDC typically present with recent onset of a rapidly growing tumour that may fluctuate in size. Occasional patients have longer clinical histories. Pain and facial paresis may be present.

Macroscopy
SDC are usually firm, solid, tan, white or grey, with a cystic component. Infiltration of the adjacent parenchyma is usually obvious, but occasional tumours may appear to be circumscribed. SDC may also arise as the malignant component of a carcinoma ex pleomorphic adenoma, so that the macroscopic features of pleomorphic adenoma may also be present.

Tumour spread and staging
For SDC, perineural spread (60%) and intravascular tumour emboli (31%) are common. Most patients present with Stage III or IV disease, as lymph nodes are positive in 59% of patients {135}.

Histopathology
SDC resembles intraductal and infiltrating mammary duct carcinoma, both architecturally and cytologically. The diagnostic "ductal lesion" comprises pleomorphic, epithelioid tumour cells with a cribriform growth pattern, "Roman bridge" formation, and intraductal comedonecrosis. The tumour infiltrates and metastasizes with a cribriform pattern, or it totally recapitulates the intrasialodochal "ductal lesion". Solid and papillary areas may be seen, with psammoma bodies, as well as evidence of squamous differentiation. Cytologically, these cells have abundant, pink cytoplasm and large pleomorphic nuclei with prominent nucleoli and coarse chromatin. The cytoplasm may also be densely eosinophilic, granular, or oncocytic. Mitotic figures are usually abundant. Goblet cells are not seen. Rare tumours may have a prominent spindle cell or sarcomatoid growth pattern similar to the metaplastic ductal carcinomas of the breast {1064,1819,}. The mucin-rich SDC is a recently described variant of SDC {2371}. The tumour is composed of areas of typical SDC, but in addition, contains mucin lakes with islands of carcinoma cells. Another variant showing an invasive micropapillary component has also been reported {1820}.

Immunoprofile
SDC is immunoreactive for low- and high-molecular-weight cytokeratin, and markers such as carcinoembryonic antigen (CEA), LeuM1, and epithelial membrane antigen (EMA) {579,1488}. Strong nuclear reactivity for androgen receptors (AR) is reported in all SDC {1265,1488, 2371}. SDC cells are focally positive for

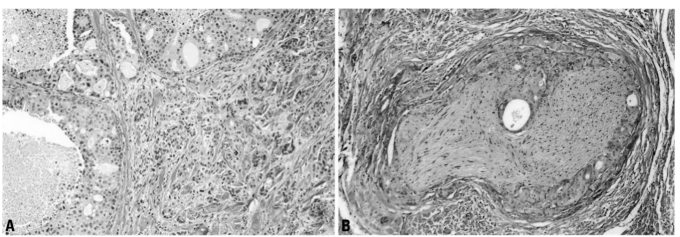

Fig. 5.24 Salivary duct carcinoma. **A** Note the cribriform ductal component with comedonecrosis and the invasive desmoplastic carcinoma on the right. **B** Perineural invasion.

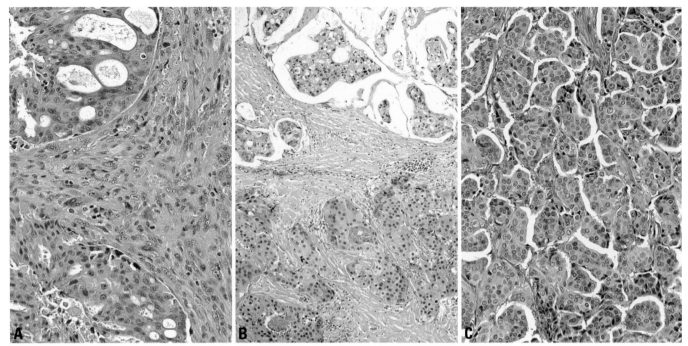

Fig. 5.25 Variants of salivary duct carcinoma. **A** Sarcomatoid variant. **B** Mucin-rich variant. **C** Invasive micropapillary variant.

apocrine marker GCDFP-15 and mitochondrial antigen (MIA), and typically negative for S-100 protein, myoepithelial markers, estrogen and progesterone receptors. Variable expression of prostatic markers (prostate specific antigen, prostatic acid phosphatase) is seen {555}. The MIB1 proliferative index is high, with an average value of 43% (range 25-80%). Most SDC show positive distinct membrane staining for HER-2/neu protein {1644,2392,2393}.

Differential diagnosis

Other diagnoses to consider for SDC include metastatic breast and squamous carcinomas, oncocytic carcinoma and mucoepidermoid carcinoma. Despite a superficial resemblance to squamous carcinoma, this diagnosis can be discarded as soon as the infiltrating cribriform pattern is recognized. Identification of sialodochodysplasia supports a primary parotid origin. Goblet cells are not seen with SDC (aside from intraductal goblet cell metaplasia), thus ruling out mucoepidermoid carcinoma.

Genetics

Only two studies of these tumours have been published. Seven of eight tumours had LOH in at least one marker on chromosome 9p21 {351} in one study. In the other study, a high incidence of LOH was

found at 6q,16q, 17p and 17q regions {1110}.

Amplification of HER-2/neu gene and gene product overexpression are reported in SDC {725,1644,1803,2392,2393}. Mutations and overexpression of the TP53 gene and protein are frequent {1110,1803,1823}. Loss of heterozygosity at microsatellite loci, TP53 point mutations and frequent alterations of certain loci on chromosome arm 6q have been reported {1110}. The chromosomal locus 9q21 contains the CDKN2A/p16 tumour suppressor gene that has been implicated in a variety of tumour types, including SDC {351}. More polymorphic genetic markers located at this particular region suggest that inactivation of CDKN2A/p16

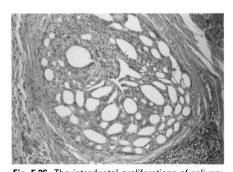

Fig. 5.26 The intraductal proliferations of salivary duct carcinoma resemble intraductal breast carcinoma. The tumour forms "rigid" intraductal fenestrations.

gene is associated with progression of SDC {351}.

Prognosis and predictive factors

SDC is one of the most aggressive salivary malignancies. A review of 104 cases concluded that 33% of patients developed local recurrence and 46% developed distant metastasis {135}. Sites for distant metastasis include lungs, bones, liver, brain and skin. Sixty-five percent of patients died of disease, between 5 months to 10 years, usually within 4 years of diagnosis. The clinical course is characterized by early distant metastases. Tumour size, distant metastasis, and HER-2/neu overexpression are putative prognostic parameters for SDC, while expression of p53 protein, DNA aneuploidy, and proliferative activity do not correlate with outcome {2393}. The clinical outcome for the mucin-rich variant of SDC is similar to that of conventional SDC {2371}. The invasive micropapillary variant appears to be particularly aggressive {1820}.

Adenocarcinoma, not otherwise specified

P. Auclair
J.E. van der Wal

Definition

Adenocarcinoma, not otherwise specified, is a malignant salivary gland tumour that exhibits ductal differentiation but lacks any of the histomorphologic features that characterize the other defined types of salivary carcinoma. The modifying term "not otherwise specified" should be included because most other epithelial salivary gland malignancies are also adenocarcinomas.

ICD-O code   8140/3

Synonyms

These tumours have often been reported as miscellaneous or unclassified adenocarcinomas or, simply, as adenocarcinoma {1662,1815,2447}. It appears that many reports include cases that should be classified as one of the more specific carcinoma types {668}. They should not be grouped together with tumours that arise from the seromucous glands of the nasal cavity, paranasal sinuses or larynx because in these sites they appear to have a more aggressive biologic behaviour {2447}.

Epidemiology

The inconsistent reporting of these tumours limits our understanding of them. In one report they are second in frequency only to mucoepidermoid carcinoma among malignant salivary gland tumours and account for about 17% of the carcinomas {668}. Women outnumber men slightly and the average patient age is 58 years. They are extremely rare in children.

Localization

About 60% and 40%, respectively, occur in the major and minor glands. The vast majority that involve the major glands occur in the parotid, and the minor gland tumours most often arise from the glands in the hard palate, buccal mucosa, and lips.

Clinical features

Most patients with tumours of major glands present with solitary, asymptomatic masses, but about 20% have pain or facial weakness {2447}. Pain is more often associated with tumours of the submandibular glands. Minor gland tumours may be ulcerated and about 25% of palatal tumours involve the underlying bone. Tumour duration ranges from one to 10 years {2447}.

Macroscopy

Adenocarcinoma, NOS, is often partially circumscribed but in many areas the periphery is irregular and ill defined. Areas of necrosis or haemorrhage may contrast with the white or yellowish cut surface.

Histopathology

Shared by all tumours in this group are the presence of glandular or duct-like structures, infiltrative growth into parenchyma or surrounding tissues, and lack of features that characterize other salivary adenocarcinomas. There is considerable variability in the architectural structure. Some have small confluent nests or cords of tumour cells, others large discrete islands with intervening trabeculae of fibrous connective tissue, and still others large solid, densely cellular sheets. This latter group reveals very limited stromal connective tissue.

Ductal differentiation is widespread in low and intermediate grade tumours but usually much more subtle in high-grade tumours. Small cysts are occasionally present in those with numerous ducts. Cuboidal or ovoid cells predominate in most tumours but scattered clear and oncocytic cells are occasionally evident. Small deposits of eosinophilic acellular material and extracellular mucin may be present.

Unlike most other salivary adenocarcinomas, the cytologic variability is useful for grading these tumours {2447}. Low-grade

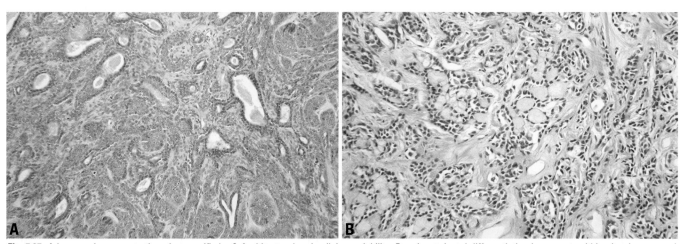

Fig. 5.27 Adenocarcinoma, not otherwise specified.. **A** Architectural and cellular variability. Prominent ductal differentiation is present, within closely arranged tumour islands. **B** Focal tubular structures with hyaline cores, reminiscent of adenoid cystic carcinoma.

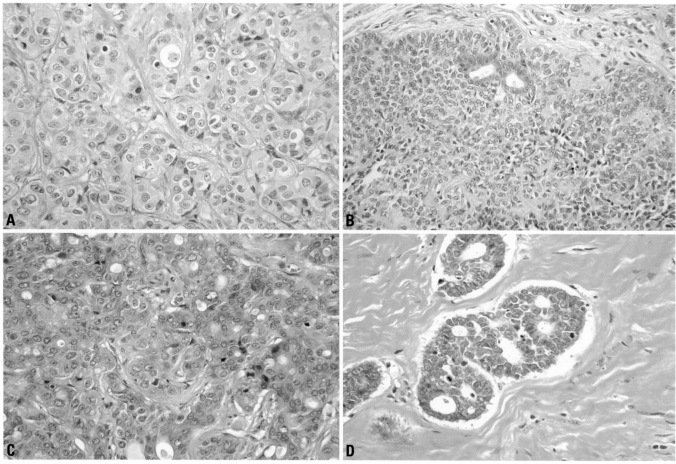

Fig. 5.28 Adenocarcinoma, not otherwise specified. **A** This example demonstrates an organoid arrangement of cells that have abundant eosinophilic and clear cytoplasm. **B** Low-grade tumours are characterized by distinct ductal differentiation, cells with limited nuclear variability and uniform nuclei that have small nucleoli, and rare mitoses. **C** Intermediate grade. Greater variability in the size, shape and staining of the nuclei is typically present. Nucleoli are often more prominent and scattered mitoses are often present. **D** Large, hyperchromatic, pleomorphic nuclei and frequent mitoses characterize high-grade tumours. Although ductal differentiation is present in these infiltrating tumour islands, other areas had large solid sheets of similar cells with rare to no ductal differentiation.

tumours demonstrate minimal variability of nuclear size, shape, or staining density, and rare mitoses. In some, the bland nuclear morphology suggests benignity and determination of their malignant nature is based largely on the identification of invasive growth. Intermediate grade tumours show nuclear variability and more frequent mitoses. High-grade tumours have enlarged, pleomorphic, hyperchromatic nuclei, focal necrosis, and frequent and atypical mitoses. The presence of ductal differentiation helps in the distinction from undifferentiated carcinoma.

Differential diagnosis
Because these tumours do not have pathognomonic histopathologic features, the possibility of metastatic adenocarcinoma should be considered. While immunohistochemical studies may be useful in this evaluation {2370} it should be remembered that immunoreactivity with prostate-specific antigen has been reported {2571,2574}.

Prognosis and predictive factors
Limited data suggest that the clinical stage, site of involvement and grade of tumour influence prognosis {1662,2447, 2708}. Minor gland tumours have a better prognosis than those of the major glands. Distant metastases may occur despite regional control and recurrence is more frequent with high-grade tumours {2447}. In one study, the 15-year survival for low, intermediate and high-grade tumours was 54, 31, and 3%, respectively, and the cure rate of the low-grade tumours was similar to that of acinic cell adenocarcinoma {2447}.

Myoepithelial carcinoma

A. Skálová
K.T. Jäkel

Definition

Myoepithelial carcinoma of the salivary glands is a neoplasm composed almost exclusively of tumour cells with myoepithelial differentiation, characterized by infiltrative growth and potential for metastasis. This tumour represents the malignant counterpart of benign myoepithelioma.

ICD-O code   8982/3

Synonym

Malignant myoepithelioma

Epidemiology

The mean age of patients at presentation is 55 years with a wide age distribution (range 14-86). Males and females are affected equally. In large series, myoepithelial carcinomas comprise less than two percent of all salivary gland carcinomas, but they may not be as rare as has been suggested before {2251,2304}. The very low historic incidence is probably due to their recent recognition as a separate tumour entity.

Etiology

No etiological factors are known.

Localization

Most cases (75%) arise in the parotid, but they also occur in the submandibular and minor glands.

Clinical features

The tumours are locally destructive. The majority of patients present with the complaint of a painless mass.

Macroscopy

Myoepithelial carcinomas are unencapsulated but may be well-defined with nodular surfaces. Tumour size varies considerably (2-10 cm). The cut surface is grey-white and can be glassy. Some tumours show areas of necrosis and cystic degeneration.

Tumour spread and staging

They can involve adjacent bone. Perineural and vascular invasion may occur. Regional and distant metastases are uncommon at presentation, but may occur late in the course of disease.

Histopathology

Myoepithelial carcinoma characteristically has a multilobulated architecture. The range of cell types in myoepithelial carcinoma reflects that seen in its benign counterpart. The tumour cells often are spindled, stellate, epithelioid, plasmacytoid (hyaline), or, occasionally, vacuolated with signet ring like appearance. Other tumours tend to be more cellular composed of spindle-shaped cells, and they can resemble sarcoma. Rarely, myoepithelial carcinoma is composed of a monomorphic population of clear cells

with myoepithelial features {1719}.
The tumour cells may form solid and sheet-like formations, trabecular or reticular patterns, but they can also be dissociated, often within plentiful myxoid or hyaline stroma. The neoplastic nodules frequently have necrotic centres. Pseudocystic or true cystic degeneration can occur. Sparse areas with squamous differentiation may be found. Rarely, myoepithelial carcinoma contains duct-like lumina usually with non-luminal cell differentiation of the lining cells. A tumour containing more than the occasional true luminal cell should not be included in the category of purely myoepithelial neoplasia.

Different cell types and architectural patterns may be found within the same tumour. In fact, most myoepithelial carcinoma s are less monomorphic than benign myoepithelioma. They also may demonstrate high mitotic activity with considerable variation {595,1154,1827, 2251}. Cellular pleomorphism can be marked, and necrosis may occur {1827, 2251}. However, unequivocal evidence of infiltrative, destructive growth is the major requirement for diagnosis, and it is this property that distinguishes myoepithelial carcinoma from benign myoepithelial tumours.

Immunoprofile

Reactivity for cytokeratin and at least one

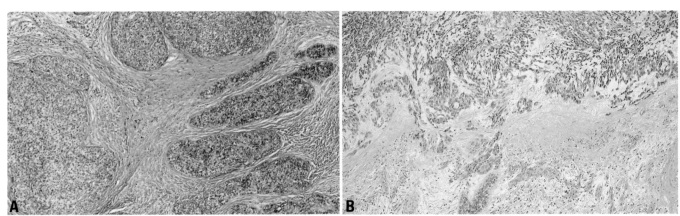

Fig. 5.29 Myoepithelial carcinoma. **A** Multinodular growth pattern. **B** Spindle cell malignant myoepithelioma invading soft tissues.

of the other myoepithelial markers, including smooth muscle actin, GFAP, CD10, calponin and smooth muscle myosin heavy chain, is required for diagnosis {595,1827}.

Electron microscopy

Ultrastructural criteria for the diagnosis of myoepithelial carcinoma include longitudinally oriented 6-8 nm fine cytoplasmic microfilaments with focal dense bodies, pinocytic vesicles, desmosomes and hemidesmosomes, basal lamina and intermediate filaments {41,640}.

Precursor lesions

Myoepithelial carcinomas may arise de novo, but it is important to note that about half of cases develop in pre-existing pleomorphic adenomas, or from benign myoepitheliomas, particularly in recurrences {595,1827,2251}.

Genetics

Comparative genomic hybridization has revealed infrequent abnormalities in these lesions with only three of 12 myoepitheliomas manifesting various chromosomal losses. Of myoepithelial carcinomas, five have manifested chromosome 8 alterations {1154}.

Prognosis and predictive factors

Myoepithelial carcinomas are locally aggressive salivary gland neoplasms that exhibit diverse clinical outcomes. Approximately one third of patients die of disease, another third have recurrences, mostly multiple, and the remaining third are disease free. Marked cellular pleomorphism and high proliferative activity correlate with a poor clinical outcome {1827,2251}. There is no difference in clinical behaviour of "de novo" myoepithelial carcinomas and of those arising in pleomorphic adenomas and benign myoepitheliomas {595,2251}.

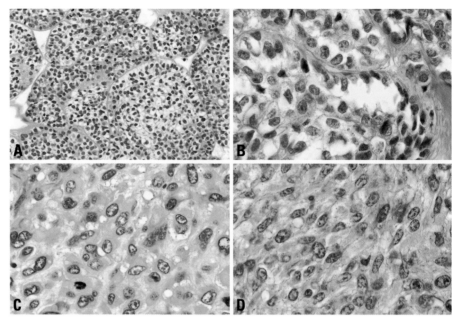

Fig. 5.30 Myoepithelial carcinoma. **A** Clear cell myoepithelial carcinoma composed of solid nodules separated by thin fibrous septa. **B** Epithelioid pleomorphic myoepithelial cells. **C** Hyaline (plasmacytoid) myoepithelial cells with prominent mitotic activity and abundant eosinophilic cytoplasm. **D** Spindle-shaped myoepithelial cells with abundant eosinophilic cytoplasm.

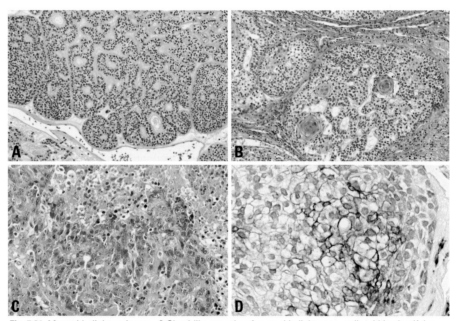

Fig. 5.31 Myoepithelial carcinoma. **A** Gland-like growths of myoepithelial tumour cells within plentiful myxoid or hyaline stroma. **B** Focal squamous metaplasia. **C** High mitotic activity and nuclear polymorphism. Focally, the tumour undergoes necrosis (right upper corner). **D** Positive staining for smooth muscle actin (SMA).

Carcinoma ex pleomorphic adenoma

D.R. Gnepp
M.S. Brandwein-Gensler
A.K. El-Naggar
T. Nagao

Definition

Carcinoma ex pleomorphic adenoma is defined as a pleomorphic adenoma from which an epithelial malignancy is derived.

ICD-O code   8941/3

Synonyms

Carcinoma arising in a benign mixed tumour, carcinoma ex benign mixed tumour, carcinoma arising in a pleomorphic adenoma, malignant mixed tumour.

Epidemiology

Many large series of carcinoma ex pleomorphic adenoma (Ca-ex-PA) have been reported and recently summarized: they comprise approximately 3.6% of all salivary tumours (range 0.9-14%), 12% of all salivary malignancies (range 2.8-42.4%), and 6.2% of all pleomorphic adenomas (range 1.9-23.3%) {898}. Ca-ex-PA usually presents in the 6th or 7th decades, approximately one decade later than patients with pleomorphic adenoma.

Etiology

Many Ca-ex-PA probably result from the accumulation of genetic instabilities in long-standing pleomorphic adenomas.

Localization

Ca-ex-PA most frequently arises in the parotid gland; but may also originate from the submandibular gland and minor salivary sites, most commonly the palate, occasionally with involvement of the nasopharynx {838}.

Clinical features

The typical history is that of a long-standing mass present much longer than 3 years with rapid growth over the previous few months; however, a significant proportion of patients present with a clinical history of less than three years {898,1533}. Patients frequently complain of a painless mass; but pain, facial nerve palsy, and skin fixation may also occur.

Macroscopy

The average size of Ca-ex-PA is more than twice that of its benign counterpart, ranging from 1.5-25 cm in greatest diameter {786,2624}. Grossly, Ca-ex-PAs are usually poorly circumscribed and many are extensively infiltrative. Occasionally, tumours are well circumscribed, scar-like or appear completely encapsulated {252,2624}.

Histopathology

The proportion of benign versus malignant components can be quite variable. Occasionally, extensive sampling is necessary to find the benign component and in rare cases, a benign remnant might not be found. But if there is clinicopathologic documentation of a previously excised pleomorphic adenoma in the same site, then the malignancy can also be classified as a Ca-ex-PA.

The malignant component is most frequently a poorly differentiated adenocarcinoma (salivary duct type or not otherwise specified) or an undifferentiated carcinoma; however, virtually any form of carcinoma may be found {898,1338, 1491}. An infiltrative, destructive growth pattern is the most reliable diagnostic criterion. Nuclear hyperchromasia and pleomorphism are frequent, although occasional tumours may demonstrate minimal atypia. This latter feature (tumour grade) directly correlates with prognosis. Necrosis is often present and mitoses are usually easy to find.

Ca-ex-PAs should be subclassified into non invasive, minimally invasive (≤1.5 mm penetration of the malignant component into extra capsular tissue) and invasive (>1.5 mm of invasion from the tumour capsule into adjacent tissues), as the first two groups usually have an excellent prognosis while the latter has a more guarded prognosis. The distinction between noninvasive and invasive tumours is based on destructive invasion through the capsule into peritumoral tissues.

Non-invasive Ca-ex-PAs are also referred to as carcinoma in-situ arising in a pleomorphic adenoma, intracapsular carcinoma ex pleomorphic adenoma or pleomorphic adenoma with severe dysplastic changes. Atypical changes within these tumours range from focal to diffuse often

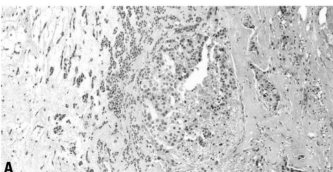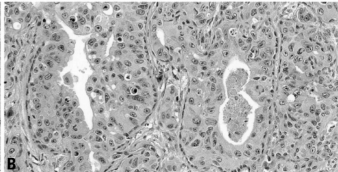

Fig. 5.32 Carcinoma ex pleomorphic adenoma. **A** Invasive type. Pleomorphic adenoma and carcinoma components are seen in the left and right, respectively. Carcinoma component is reminiscent of salivary duct carcinoma in this case. **B** Non-invasive type. Carcinoma cells replacing the inner ductal layer leaving outer benign myoepithelial layer.

with multifocal areas containing carcinoma, which frequently overgrows and replaces many of the benign elements. The earliest changes typically consist of tumour cells replacing the normal inner duct epithelial layer leaving the normal peripherally located myoepithelial layer intact.

Differential diagnosis
The most important differential diagnosis is between minimally invasive Ca-ex-PA and the more typical invasive Ca-ex-PA. This differential has prognostic significance, and affects decisions regarding the need for lymph node dissection and adjuvant radiotherapy. Also carcinomas may rarely arise in a histologically benign "adenoma" ("monomorphic" adenoma); they appear to have a more favourable prognosis {1576}.

Genetics
Cytogenetics
Deletions of chromosome 5(q22-23, q32-33) and t(10;12) (p15;q14-15) with 12q breakpoint at the 5' of the HMGIC and translocation of the entire gene to the 10 marker chromosome followed by deletion/amplification of the segment containing HMGIC and MDM2 genes have been reported {653,1220,2193}.
Rearrangements of 8q12 are a frequent finding. Alterations at 12q13-15 with amplification of HMGIC and MDM2 genes have also been reported {2125}. Cytogenetic evidence of amplification (homogeneously stained region and double minute) was found in 40% of these tumours. Both genes may contribute to the malignant transformation of pleomorphic adenoma. Alterations at chromosomes 6q deletion and 8q rearrangements have been reported.

Molecular genetics
Microsatellite analysis of these tumours has shown LOH at chromosome 8q and 17p. Concurrent analysis of the benign and malignant components of these tumours showed 8q and/or 12q in both components and additional alterations in 17p only in the carcinoma {651}. In another study homozygous deletion of the p16 gene on chromosome 9p21 was found in carcinoma of one case and microsatellite instability was noted in both the adenoma and carcinoma components in two tumours {2510}. A single case report of a carcinosarcoma, in

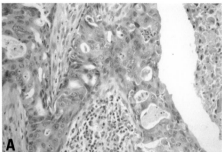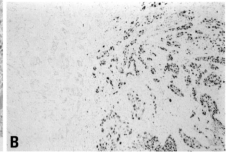

Fig. 5.33 Carcinoma ex pleomorphic adenoma. **A** Detail of adenocarcinoma with back-to-back glands composed of pleomorphic tumour cells with focal necrosis. **B** Many tumour cells are positive for MIB-1 in the carcinoma component (right), whereas only a few positive cells are observed in the pleomorphic adenoma component (left).

which the carcinoma and the sarcoma components were concurrently analyzed, showed lack of p53 alterations and concomitant LOH at different loci on chromosome 17 and 18 supporting monoclonality {932}.

Prognosis and predictive factors
In general, the recommended therapy is wide local excision with contiguous lymph node dissection. Adjuvant radiation therapy is recommended for widely invasive tumours. If the carcinomatous component is low-grade and/or minimally invasive and if the tumour is adequately excised, then adjuvant radiation therapy may not be necessary.
Patients with non-invasive or minimally invasive Ca-ex-PA typically have an excellent prognosis, similar to benign pleomorphic adenoma. Metastatic spread is exceptional {726}.
Invasive Ca-ex-PAs, as a group, are extremely aggressive malignancies with approximately 23-50% of patients developing one or more recurrences {786, 898,1491,1533}. The metastatic rate varies with each series; up to 70% of patients develop local or distant metastasis {877,898,1491}. Metastatic sites in order of frequency are lung, bone (especially spine), abdomen and central nervous system {786,2592}. Ca-ex-PA with capsular penetration of more than 1.5 mm is associated with a poor prognosis; survival rates at 5, 10, 15, and 20 years range from 25-65%, 18-50%, 10-35%, and 0-38%, respectively {786,877,1491, 1533,2592,2624}. Therefore, it is important to designate those Ca-ex-PA that are confined within the capsule and those invading through the capsule as non-invasive or invasive, respectively, and to differentiate within the latter group between widely invasive and minimally

invasive tumours.
One study showed that no patient with less than 8 mm invasion from the capsule died from the tumour, whereas all patients with invasion greater than 8 mm beyond the capsule ultimately died of disease {2624}. The local recurrence rate (LRR) in this latter series also correlated with extent of invasion; a LRR of 70.5% was found for tumours with invasion beyond 6 mm from the capsule, as compared to a LRR of 16.6% for tumours with invasion of less than 6 mm. In another study consisting of four patients with 5 mm of invasion beyond the tumour capsule, two died of disease and two were alive and well {1491}. The two patients with less than 5 mm of invasion (2 and 3 mm) were alive and well with no evidence of disease. Also, all four patients with intracapsular carcinoma were alive and well without evidence of disease progression.
The improved prognosis for minimally invasive tumours has been confirmed by Brandwein et al who observed recurrence free for periods ranging from 1-4 years (mean 2.5 years) {252}.
Tumour size and grade are also significant prognosticators in the more widely invasive Ca-ex-PAs. The five-year survival rates have been correlated with histologic subtype of the carcinoma component: there was a 30% survival rate for undifferentiated carcinomas, 50% for myoepithelial carcinomas, 62% for ductal carcinomas and 96% survival rate for terminal duct carcinomas {2624}. In addition, 63% of patients with high-grade carcinomatous components died of the disease, while patients with lower grade carcinomatous elements did not {1491}.

Carcinosarcoma

D.R. Gnepp

Definition
Carcinosarcoma is a malignant tumour composed of a mixture of both carcinomatous and sarcomatous elements.

ICD-O code 8980/3

Synonym
True malignant mixed tumour

Epidemiology
Carcinosarcoma is extremely rare; approximately 50-60 cases have been reported to date {47,898,911,932,1010, 1320,2377,2466}. The mean age at presentation was 58 years with a range of 14-87 years {899}. A number of patients have had a history of recurrent pleomorphic adenoma {2466} and several cases have arisen in a pleomorphic adenoma (carcinosarcoma ex pleomorphic adenoma) {899,1010,1320,1400}.

Localization
Two-thirds have arisen in the parotid gland, approximately 19% in the submandibular glands, and 14% in the palate {899}. One case has been reported in the tongue and one in the supraglottic region {691}.

Clinical features
Patients typically present with a mass, which may be painful.

Macroscopy
Tumours are well to poorly circumscribed.

Histopathology
The tumour is composed of mixtures of carcinomatous and sarcomatous elements in varying proportions {225}. Chondrosarcoma and osteosarcoma are the most common sarcomatous elements and moderate to poorly differentiated ductal carcinoma or undifferentiated carcinoma are the most common carcinomatous components. Local tissue infiltration and destruction are characteristic of this neoplasm.

Genetics
LOH at 17p13.1, 17q21.3 and 18q21.3 has been found in one carcinosarcoma. Sequencing studies excluded TP53 mutations, suggesting inactivation of another tumour suppressor gene at 17p13 {932}.

Prognosis and predictive factors
Treatment is wide surgical excision combined with radiotherapy. Almost 60% of patients die of local recurrence and/or metastatic disease (lungs, bones, central nervous system), usually within a thirty month period {47,899,2466}.

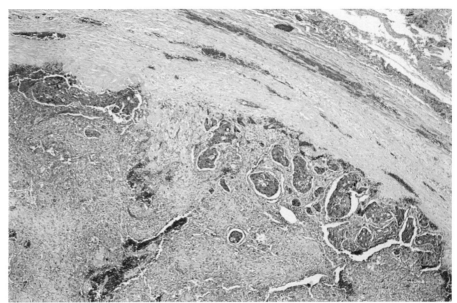

Fig. 5.34 Carcinosarcoma. Low power . The majority of this tumour is composed of poorly differentiated sarcoma with focal areas of poorly differentiated adenocarcinoma at the periphery.

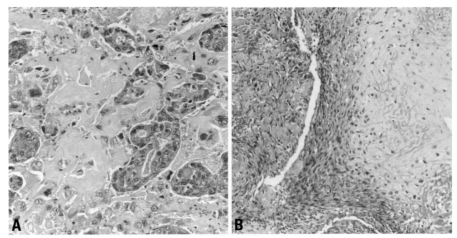

Fig. 5.35 Carcinosarcoma **A** Tumour composed of mixtures of adenocarcinomatous and osteosarcomatous components. **B** Midportion of tumour. Note areas with chondrosarcomatous differentiation (right side) and a small focus with osteosarcomatous differentiation (upper left)

Metastasizing pleomorphic adenoma

D.R. Gnepp

Definition
A histologically benign pleomorphic adenoma that inexplicably manifests local or distant metastasis.

ICD-O code   8940/1

Synonyms
Metastasizing benign mixed tumour, malignant mixed tumour.

Epidemiology
To date, approximately 40 cases have been described {406,2768}.

Etiology
It has been postulated that multiple recurrences and surgical procedures allow some tumours to gain venous access and metastasize.

Localization
Greater than three-quarters arise in the parotid gland, 13% in the submandibular gland and 9% in the palate.

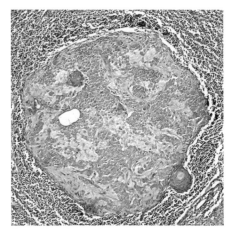

Fig. 5.36 Metastasizing pleomorphic adenoma. Note benign appearing tumour cells with numerous plasmacytoid myoepithelial cells, areas with a myxoid background and focal squamous and ductal differentiation; there are no atypical features.

Macroscopy
Tumours are well-circumscribed in primary and metastatic sites.

Histopathology
Characteristically, the primary salivary gland tumour and metastases are composed of the typical mixture of benign-appearing epithelial and mesenchymal components of a pleomorphic adenoma. The histology is not predictive regarding its ability to metastasize. Mitotic figures and nuclear pleomorphism may be seen, but the tumour is not overtly histologically malignant.

Prognosis and predictive factors
The treatment of choice is surgical excision. Metastasizing pleomorphic adenomas are characterized by multiple local recurrences and a long interval (1.5-55 years) between development of the primary tumour and its metastasis. Half of the tumours metastasize to bone, 30% to lung and 30% to lymph nodes; rarely tumours spread to other body sites. Forty percent of patients died with disease; 47% were alive and well, and 13% were alive with disease {899}.

Squamous cell carcinoma

J.E. Lewis
K.D. Olsen

Definition
A primary malignant epithelial tumour composed of epidermoid cells, which produce keratin and/or demonstrate intercellular bridges by light microscopy. It is essential to exclude the possibility of metastatic disease. By convention, the diagnosis of salivary squamous cell carcinoma is restricted to the major salivary glands, since minor salivary squamous carcinomas cannot be reliably distinguished from tumours of mucosal origin.

ICD-O code   8070/3

Synonym
Epidermoid carcinoma

Epidemiology
Primary squamous cell carcinoma (PSCC) probably represents less than 1% of salivary gland tumours. PSCC occurs in patents over a wide age range, but the majority present in the 6th through 8th decades, with a mean of 60-65 years. They are unusual in patients younger than 20 years, although several cases have been described in children {669}. There is a male to female ratio of approximately 2:1.

Etiology
In several studies, PSCC has been associated with a history of prior radiotherapy, with a latent period of 15-30 years {2329}.

Localization
Roughly 80% of PSCC arise in the parotid gland and 20% in the sub-mandibular gland. PSCC of the sublingual gland is quite unusual. Occasionally, cases arise from the mucosa lining Stensen's duct.

Clinical features
Patients with PSCC present with a rapidly enlarging mass, which is frequently painful. Tumours are firm and fixed and may be associated with facial nerve weakness. PSCC is typically high stage at the time of diagnosis {2329,2468}.

Macroscopy
PSCC is an invasive neoplasm with ill-defined margins. Most tumours are greater than 3 cm in size. The cut surface is typically solid, firm, and light grey or tan to white, sometimes with focal necrosis.

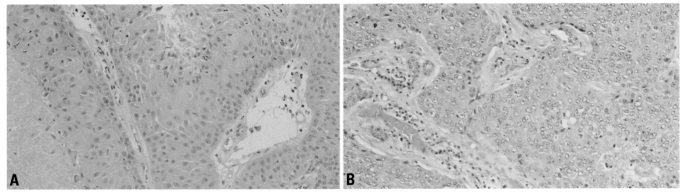

Fig. 5.37 A Squamous cell carcinoma. Moderately differentiated, keratinizing primary squamous cell carcinoma of the parotid gland. **B** Squamous cell carcinoma. Poorly differentiated, nonkeratinizing primary squamous cell carcinoma of the parotid gland.

Histopathology

The histology of PSCC of salivary origin is similar to that of well- to moderately-differentiated squamous cell carcinoma originating elsewhere in the head and neck. The tumour infiltrates the salivary parenchyma in irregular nests and trabeculae, accompanied by a fibrous to desmoplastic stromal response. Squamous metaplasia and dysplasia of salivary ducts are occasionally identified in association with PSCC. Perineural invasion and extension into adjacent soft tissue are common findings. There is a significant incidence of cervical nodal metastases (both clinically apparent and occult) at the time of initial surgery {779, 869,1456,2329}.

Differential diagnosis

The most critical distinction in the differential diagnosis of PSCC is ruling out the possibility of metastatic squamous cell carcinoma, whose incidence is greater than true PSCC. PSCC must also be distinguished from mucoepidermoid carcinoma (MEC). MEC is typically composed of a variable cell population, including mucocytes, basaloid, and intermediate

cells, in addition to epidermoid cells. However, prominent keratinization is not characteristic of MEC. MEC may exhibit cystic areas and focal clear cell differentiation, features not observed in PSCC. Histochemical stains for intracellular mucin to rule out high-grade MEC are recommended before making a definitive diagnosis of PSCC {669}. Squamous metaplasia in infarcted or surgically manipulated tumours can be misinterpreted as PSCC.

Keratocystoma is a recently described, rare lesion of salivary glands that may be confused with squamous cell carcinoma {1822}. It is characterized by multicytic spaces lined by stratified squamous cells containing keratotic lamellae and focal solid epithelial nests. The consistent absence of metastasis, necrosis or invasion, as well as the lack of cytological atypia and minimal cellular proliferative activity in keratocystoma is essential in distiguishing this lesion from PSCC.

Genetics

Cytogenetic studies in several cases of PSCC have yielded somewhat variable results, although it appears that various

6q deletions may be common, similar to the findings in other salivary carcinomas {1222}. Interestingly, this karyotype is unusual in squamous cell carcinoma of other head and neck sites {1222}.

Prognosis and predictive factors

PSCC is considered a relatively high-grade, aggressive salivary carcinoma. Five-year disease specific survival is approximately 25-30%. Local-regional recurrence develops in at least half of patients and distant metastases are found in 20-30% {2329}. Overall, 75% die of their disease, usually within 5 years {1456,2329}. In the largest published specific analysis of PSCC {2329}, tumour stage was the most important prognostic factor. Age greater than 60 years, ulceration, and fixation also had a significant negative impact on survival. Two additional series, which only considered parotid tumours, reported that age, facial nerve paralysis, deep fixation, and type of treatment were of statistical significance {869,1456}.

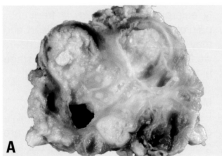
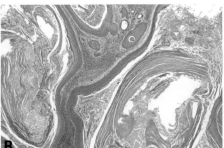
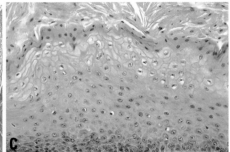

Fig. 5.38 Keratocystoma **A** Cut surface of the parotid tumour, showing multiple cystic formations filled with keratin material. **B** Low-power view showing multilocular cystic lesions filled with lamellar keratin material. **C** Portion of the cyst wall consists of stratified squamous epithelium with keratinization through parakeratotic cells. Note the lack of a granular cell layer. Tumour cells exhibit uniform, bland nuclei and abundant eosinophilic cytoplasm.

Small cell carcinoma

T. Nagao

Definition
Small cell carcinomas of the salivary glands are rare, malignant epithelial tumours characterized by a proliferation of small anaplastic cells with scant cytoplasm, fine nuclear chromatin, and inconspicuous nucleoli.

ICD-O code   8041/3

Synonyms
Small cell undifferentiated carcinoma, small cell anaplastic carcinoma, oat cell carcinoma, neuroendocrine carcinoma.

Epidemiology
They account for less than 1% of all salivary gland tumours and approximately 2% of salivary gland malignancies {668}. Most patients are older than 50 years at the time of initial diagnosis; however, these tumours have been described in younger patients {668,902}. The tumour has a slight predilection for males.

Localization
The tumours can involve major and intra-oral minor salivary glands, and are most common in the parotid gland.

Clinical features
Patients typically present with a painless, rapidly growing mass of several months duration. Cervical lymphadenopathy and facial nerve palsy are common findings. Paraneoplastic syndromes accompanied by the production of ectopic hormones are unusual {1746}.

Macroscopy
It is a firm, poorly circumscribed tumour that often infiltrates the surrounding salivary gland parenchyma and adjacent soft tissues. The tumour is usually grey to white and commonly accompanied by necrosis and haemorrhage.

Histopathology
Small cell carcinoma is characterized by sheets, cords, or irregular nests of anaplastic cells and a variable amount of fibrous stroma. The tumour cell nests may exhibit a peripheral palisading pattern. Rosette-like structures are occasionally seen. Tumour cells are usually 2-3 times larger than mature small lymphocytes and have round to oval nuclei with scant cytoplasm. Fusiform or polygonal cells as well as occasional larger cells are sometimes observed. Nuclear chromatin is finely granular, and nucleoli are absent or inconspicuous. Cell borders are ill defined, and nuclear moulding is common. Mitotic figures are numerous. A tumour may have small foci of ductal differentiation {902}. Focal areas of squamous differentiation also have been described {1030,2196}. Extensive necrosis and vascular and perineural invasion are common.

Immunoprofile
In most small cell carcinomas, the tumour cells express at least one neuroendocrine marker such as chromogranin A, synaptophysin, CD57 (Leu-7), CD56 (neural cell adhesion molecule) and neurofilament {907,1818}. However,

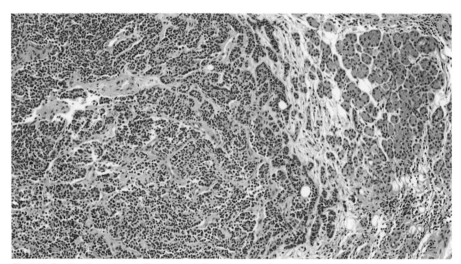
Fig. 5.39 Small cell carcinoma. The tumour infiltrates surrounding salivary gland tissue.

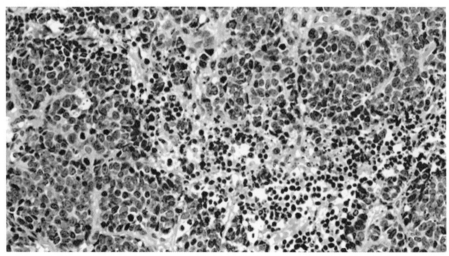
Fig. 5.40 Small cell carcinoma. Irregular nests of small tumour cells with marked necrosis.

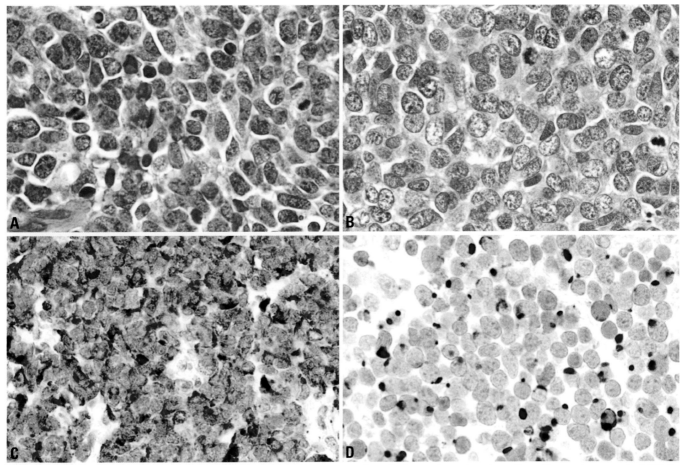

Fig. 5.41 Small cell carcinoma. High-power view showing tumour cells with scant cytoplasm, finely granular nuclear chromatin, and inconspicuous nucleoli. Mitotic figures are readily identified (A, B). **A** Tumour cell nuclei are oval to spindle, with dense chromatin. **B** The tumour cells are slightly larger than A and they have rather pale, dispersed chromatin and a little more abundant cytoplasm. **C** Tumour cells are diffusely immunopositive for chromogranin A. **D** Paranuclear dotlike pattern of immunoreactivity for cytokeratin 20.

immunoreactivity for neuron-specific enolase alone is insufficient evidence for confirming the neuroendocrine differentiation of the tumour. Most small cell carcinomas are positive for cytokeratins, which often have a characteristic paranuclear dotlike pattern of reactivity {372,1818}. The majority of the tumours are also positive for epithelial membrane antigen {907,1818}. Similar to Merkel cell carcinoma, but unlike pulmonary small cell carcinoma, three out of four salivary small cell carcinomas are cytokeratin 20 positive {1818}. Also, small cell carcinomas are negative for S-100 protein and HMB-45.

Electron microscopy
Electron microscopic examination shows membrane-bound neuroendocrine granules in about one-third of small cell carcinomas {907}. The tumour cells contain sparse cytoplasmic organelles, and either poorly or well-formed desmosomes interconnect the cells. Multidirectional differentiation with the presence of myofilament-like microfilaments and tonofilaments has been reported {1030,2628,2836}.

Prognosis and predictive factors
Local recurrence and distant metastases develop in more than 50% of patients

after the initial diagnosis. Cervical lymph node involvement is less common than haematogenous metastasis. The 5-year survival rate for patients with small cell carcinomas arising in the major salivary glands ranges from 13 to 46% {902, 1818,2042}. Overall survival is reduced for patients with a primary tumour larger than 3 cm, negative immunostaining for cytokeratin 20 and decreased immunoreactivity for neuroendocrine markers {1818}.

Large cell carcinoma

T. Nagao

Definition
Large cell carcinomas are rare, high-grade malignant salivary gland epithelial tumours composed of pleomorphic cells with abundant cytoplasm and absence of features of other specific tumour types.

ICD-O code   8012/3

Synonym
Large cell undifferentiated carcinoma.

Epidemiology
Large cell carcinomas are exceptionally rare {1151,1816}. In the majority of cases, the patients were older than 60 years. Males and females are affected equally.

Localization
The majority of large cell carcinomas arise in the major salivary glands, especially the parotid gland {1151,1432,1768, 1816,1828,2836}. A few tumours of minor salivary gland origin have been reported {1768}.

Clinical features
Many patients present with a rapidly growing firm mass that often is fixed to adjacent tissue. Facial nerve paralysis and cervical lymph node enlargement are common findings.

Macroscopy
A large cell carcinoma is usually a poorly circumscribed, solid tumour with greyish white or tan cut surface. Necrosis and haemorrhage are easily found. Invasion into the adipose and muscular tissue adjacent to the salivary gland is common.

Histopathology
The tumour is composed of large, pleomorphic cells (>30μm) with an abundance of eosinophilic or occasionally clear, cytoplasm. In some tumours there is striking dyscohesive architecture resembling lymphoma. The tumour cell nuclei have a polygonal or fusiform shape, prominent nucleoli, and coarse chromatin with a vesicular distribution. Cell borders are usually well-defined. Bizarre giant tumour cells may be present. Mitotic figures are readily identified. The tumour growth pattern consists of sheets and trabeculae, with a conspicuous tendency for necrosis. Organoid, rosette-like, and peripheral palisading patterns characterize some of the large cell carcinomas {1828}. Rare foci of ductal or squamous differentiation can be present in large cell carcinomas. Lymphoid cell infiltration is usually focal and patchy. Perineural and vascular involvement is prominent.

Immunoprofile
Some cases of large cell carcinoma may be positive for one of the neuroendocrine markers, including chromogranin A, synaptophysin, CD57 (Leu-7), PGP9.5, or CD56 (neural cell-adhesion molecule). No immunoreactivity for cytokeratin 20 was found. The Ki-67 (MIB-1) labeling index is high and often greater than 50%. In two reported cases, the tumour cells showed diffuse immunoexpression of bcl-2 protein, epidermal growth factor receptor, and cyclin D1 and reduced immunoexpression of p21/waf1 and p27/kip1 {1828}. Diffuse TP53 nuclear immunoexpression has been found in 4 of 5 cases {1803,1828, 2421}.

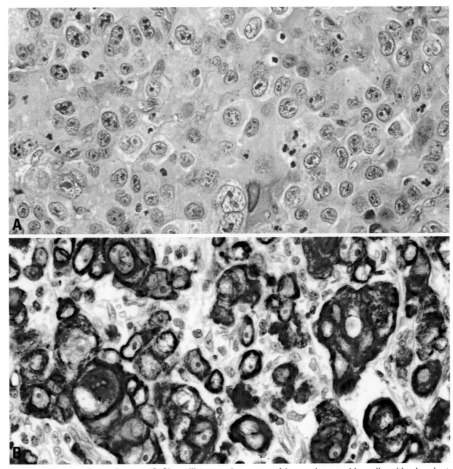

Fig. 5.42 Large cell carcinoma. A Sheet-like growth pattern of large pleomorphic cells with abundant eosinophilic cytoplasm and prominent nucleoli. **B** Strong immunoreactivity for cytokeratin.

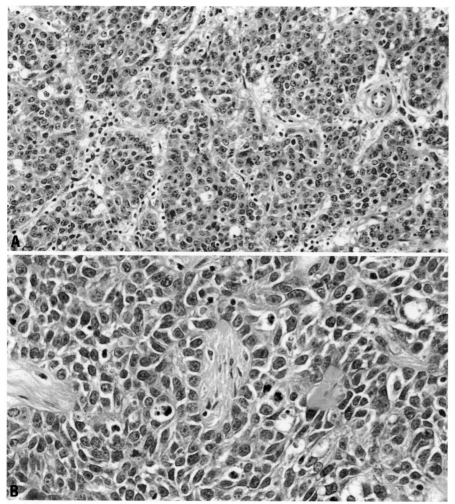

Fig. 5.43 Large cell carcinoma. **A** Organoid growth pattern. **B** Solid growth with peripheral palisading and rosette-like structures. Tumour cells have large and polygonal nuclei with vesicular chromatin and prominent nucleoli.

Electron microscopy

Ultrastructurally, tumour cells occasionally have a squamous or glandular differentiation not apparent on conventional light microscopic examination {1816, 2836}. Neuroendocrine differentiation is rare; neurosecretory granules have been described in 3 cases {1151,1432,1828}. Prominent desmosome-like junctions connect the tumour cells.

Genetics

Genetic studies of salivary gland large cell carcinoma are scant. TP53 mutation has been detected in two of three cases, and 1 case demonstrated loss of heterozygosity (LOH) at chromosome 17p {1803,1828}. Two cases of large cell neuroendocrine carcinoma exhibited LOH at chromosome 9p21 {1828}.

Prognosis and predictive factors

Large cell carcinoma is an aggressive tumour with a propensity for local recurrence, cervical lymph node metastases, and distant spread. However, one study has shown that cell size (small vs large type of carcinoma) has no influence on prognosis {1151}. Tumour size has been found to be a prognostic indicator; all patients with tumours larger than 4 cm died of disease with distant metastases {1151}.

Lymphoepithelial carcinoma

W.Y.W Tsang
T.T. Kuo
J.K.C. Chan

Definition

Lymphoepithelial carcinoma (LEC) is an undifferentiated carcinoma accompanied by a prominent non-neoplastic lymphoplasmacytic infiltrate.

ICD-O code   8082/3

Synonyms

Lymphoepithelioma-like carcinoma (LEC) {1173,1387}; malignant lymphoepithelial lesion {236,2253}; undifferentiated carcinoma with lymphoid stroma {459,2304}; undifferentiated carcinoma {986,1359}; carcinoma ex lymphoepithelial lesion {152}.

Epidemiology

LEC of the salivary gland is rare, accounting for less than 1% of all salivary gland tumours. It shows a striking racial predilection for Inuits (Eskimo) in the Arctic regions (Greenland, Canada, Alaska), South-eastern Chinese, and Japanese   {32,236, 986,1479,1821,2253,2326}. The Inuit populations have the highest worldwide incidence of malignant salivary gland tumours, with the majority represented by LEC {32,236,1708}. Slight female predominance, higher frequency of parotid gland involvement, more frequent high

stage disease and apparently more aggressive clinical course have been reported in Inuits {236,1428,1479,1708, 2253,2326,2636}. Patients affected by LEC span a wide age range from the first to the ninth decades, with most cases occurring in the fifth decade. There is a slight male predominance {236}.

Etiology

The near 100% association of Epstein-Barr virus (EBV) with salivary gland LEC from the endemic areas, and the presence of the virus in a clonal episomal form suggest an important role of EBV in tumourigenesis {31,236,986,1143,1387, 1428,1479,1821,2636}. Serologic studies show elevated titres of anti-EBV viral capsid antigen IgA or anti-EBV nuclear antigen IgG, though non-specific, in more than 50% of patients with salivary gland LEC from the endemic areas {31,236,1479,2253}. In patients from non-endemic areas, EBV is usually absent, although rare cases may harbour the virus {209,857,1173,1359}. These findings indicate complex interactions of ethnic, geographic and viral factors in the pathogenesis of salivary gland LEC.

Localization

The parotid gland is affected in approxi-

mately 80% of the cases, followed by the submandibular gland {1479,2253,2326, 2636}. LEC can also rarely occur in the minor salivary glands of the oral cavity, oropharynx and hypopharynx.

Clinical features

LEC presents as a parotid or submandibular swelling (which may be long-standing with recent rapid increase in size), with or without pain {236,857, 2253}. Advanced tumours may become fixed to the underlying tissues or the skin, although facial nerve palsy occurs in only about 20% of cases. Cervical lymph node involvement, which may be extensive, is seen in 10-40% of cases at presentation   {236,1000,1387,1479,2253, 2636}. There is no clinical or serologic evidence of an underlying Sjögren syndrome {1373,1479,2253}.

Since LEC of salivary gland is morphologically indistinguishable from nasopharyngeal carcinoma (which is much more common), it is important to examine and biopsy the nasopharynx thoroughly before accepting the salivary gland tumour as primary LEC {377,2252}.

Macroscopy

The tumours can be circumscribed or show frank invasion into the surrounding

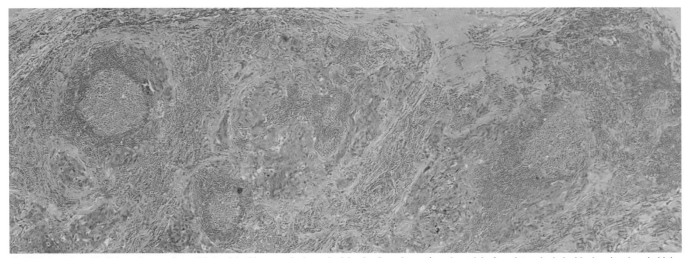

Fig. 5.44 Lymphoepithelial carcinoma of parotid gland. In this example, irregular islands of carcinoma (purple-staining) are intermingled with abundant lymphoid tissues which include lymphoid follicles (blue-staining).

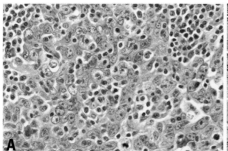
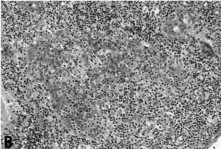
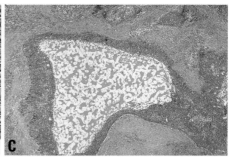

Fig. 5.45 Lymphoepithelial carcinoma of parotid gland. **A** Carcinoma cells are admixed with many small lymphocytes. Note indistinct cell borders, vesicular nuclei and prominent nucleoli. **B** Tumour islands are heavily infiltrated by lymphocytes. **C** Uncommon cystic change in the tumour islands.

gland and extraglandular soft tissues. They are fleshy and firm, and range from 1-10 cm in size (mean 2-3 cm) {2252}.

Tumour spread and staging
LEC has a propensity to spread to regional cervical lymph nodes {236, 1479,2636}. Distant metastasis, which can be found in up to 20% of cases at presentation, tends to occur in the lung, liver, bone and brain. In metastatic deposits, the prominent lymphoplasmacytic infiltrate characteristic of the primary lesion may or may not be present.

Histopathology
The tumour grows in infiltrative sheets, islands and cords separated by a lymphoid stroma. The tumour cells possess indistinct cell borders, lightly eosinophilic cytoplasm, oval vesicular nuclei with open chromatin, and conspicuous nucleoli. The nuclei usually show moderate variation in size, although rare cases exhibit fairly uniform-appearing nuclei. Necrosis and mitotic figures are usually easily found. Sometimes the tumour cells can be plump and spindly, with formation of fascicles {445}. Focal squamous differentiation in the form of increased amount of eosinophilic cytoplasm and vague intracellular bridges is occasionally present.

The tumour is by definition richly infiltrated by lymphocytes and plasma cells, often accompanied by reactive lymphoid follicles. The lymphoid component can sometimes be so heavy that the epithelial nature of the tumour may not evident. Histiocytes are abundant in the tumour islands in some cases, imparting a "starry sky" appearance {2253}. Other inconsistent findings are non-caseating granulomas with or without multinucleated giant cells, amyloid deposition {1387}, cyst formation in some tumour islands,

perineural and lymphovascular invasion. Tumour cells are immunoreactive for pan-cytokeratin and epithelial membrane antigen. The lymphoid cells include a mixture of B cells and T cells. Electron microscopy shows features of squamous differentiation, with desmosomes and tonofilaments.

In endemic cases, EBV-encoded RNA (EBER) and EBV-DNA can be detected in the tumour cells by in-situ hybridization. Immunohistochemical expression of EBV latent membrane protein 1 is more variable {377,857,986,1316,1479,2326}.

Differential diagnosis
Important differential diagnoses include metastatic undifferentiated carcinoma, malignant lymphoma, lymphoepithelial sialadenitis (no definite cytological atypia, presence of basement membrane-like material, no desmoplastic stroma, no EBV association), lymphadenoma (definite or subtle gland formation, no definite cytological atypia, no desmoplastic stroma, and no EBV association), and large cell undifferentiated carcinoma.

Precursor lesions
Most LEC arise de novo but rarely they may develop within lymphoepithelial sialadenitis (formerly myoepithelial sialadenitis) {938}.

Genetic susceptibility
Clustering of salivary gland LEC in family members has been reported {31,91, 1708}. One such family also showed dominantly inherited trichoepitheliomas, suggesting hereditary predisposition related to tumour suppressor genes {1708}.

Prognosis and predictive factors
Five-year survival rate of 75-86% has been reported in patients treated by

combined surgery (including neck dissection) and radiation therapy, although local recurrence can occur {236,1387, 1479,2252,2636}. The prognosis is significantly related to tumour stage. There have been attempts to grade LEC based on nuclear pleomorphism and mitotic activity {459,1373}, with suggestion that high-grade tumours are more aggressive, but there are currently no widely accepted or well-validated grading systems.

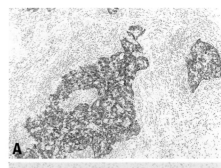
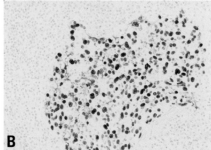

Fig. 5.46 Lymphoepithelial carcinoma of salivary gland. **A** Immunostaining for cytokeratin highlights the irregular tumour islands. **B** In-situ hybridization for EBV (EBER) selectively highlights the islands of carcinoma. The lymphoid cells in the background are negative.

Sialoblastoma

M.S. Brandwein-Gensler

Definition
This is a rare, potentially aggressive, parotid or submandibular tumour that is usually present at birth and recapitulates the primitive salivary anlage.

ICD-O code   8974/1

Synonyms
Congenital basal cell adenoma, basal cell adenoma, basaloid adenocarcinoma, congenital hybrid basal cell adenoma-adenoid cystic carcinoma, embryoma {2570,2685}.

Epidemiology
Most tumours are identified at birth or shortly thereafter; occasional children may be diagnosed after the age of two years. The male to female ratio is 2:1. Sialoblastomas are extremely rare; 23 such cases have been reported {48,156, 251,867,945,1016,1574,1688,1786, 1952,2353,2570,2685}.

Localization
The ratio of parotid to submandibular gland involvement is approximately 3:1.

Clinical features
Most babies present with a mass of the cheek or submandibular region. Occasional tumours may reach massive proportions and ulcerate skin. One baby presented with a concomitant hepatoblastoma {2353}, and two other children both had congenital nevi associated with their tumours {251,945}. Some babies have been diagnosed by prenatal sonography. Radiographically, these tumours appear as expansile, lobulated masses. True-cut preoperative biopsy can be diagnostic, and is useful in ruling out neoplasia that require neoadjuvant chemotherapy, such as rhabdomyosarcoma.

Histopathology
Sialoblastomas are composed of basaloid epithelial cells, with scanty cytoplasm, round to oval nuclei, single or few nucleoli, and relatively fine chromatin pattern. More mature cuboidal epithelial cells with pink cytoplasm can also be seen. These cells form ductules, bud-like structures and solid organoid nests, and may demonstrate peripheral palisading. The intervening stroma may appear loose and immature. Myoepithelial cells can be identified, and have been confirmed by ultrastructural study. More familiar salivary patterns such as adenoid cystic-like cribriform areas can be seen. The mitotic rate within sialoblastomas is highly variable, and may increase with subsequent recurrences {251}, as may necrosis, nuclear pleomorphism and MIB1 proliferative index.

It has been suggested that these tumours be separated into benign and malignant based on the absence or presence of invasion of nerves or vascular spaces, necrosis and cytologic anaplasia {251,1574}.

Immunoprofile
These tumours express S-100 and vimentin diffusely. Cytokeratin accentuates the ductal structures.

Histogenesis
It has been suggested that these tumours originate from retained blastemous cells rather than basal reserve cells {2570}. Dysembryogenic parotid changes have been described adjacent to the tumour, with proliferation of the terminal ductal epithelial bulbs {1952}.

Prognosis and predictive factors
Sialoblastomas have the potential to recur (22%), and can occasionally metastasize regionally (9%), and one fatality has been reported {251,1688}. Most of these children are cured by primary surgical resection.

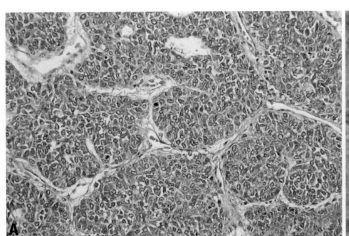
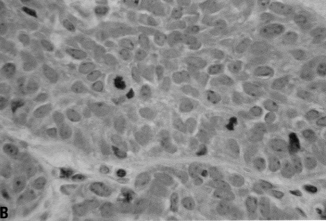

Fig. 5.47 Sialoblastoma. **A** Solid nests composed of basaloid cells. **B** Brisk mitotic rate within this sialoblastoma.

Pleomorphic adenoma

J.W. Eveson
K. Kusafuka
G. Stenman
T. Nagao

Definition

Pleomorphic adenoma is a tumour of variable capsulation characterized microscopically by architectural rather than cellular pleomorphism. Epithelial and modified myoepithelial elements intermingle most commonly with tissue of mucoid, myxoid or chondroid appearance.

Synonym

Mixed tumour

ICD-O code   8940/0

Epidemiology

Pleomorphic adenoma is the most common salivary gland tumour and accounts for about 60% of all salivary neoplasms {2439}. The reported annual incidence is 2.4-3.05 per 100,000 population {244, 2053}. The mean age at presentation is 46 years but the age ranges from the first to the tenth decades {703}. There is a slight female predominance {703,2711}.

Localization

About 80% of pleomorphic adenomas arise in the parotid, 10% in the submandibular gland and 10% in the minor salivary glands of the oral cavity, nasal cavity and paranasal sinuses and the upper respiratory and alimentary tracts {703}. The lower pole of the parotid gland is the most common location but deep lobe tumours can present as a parapharyngeal mass. The accessory parotid is occasionally involved.

Clinical features

Pleomorphic adenomas usually are slow growing painless masses. Small tumours typically form smooth, mobile, firm lumps but larger tumours tend to become bossellated and may attenuate the overlying skin or mucosa. Multifocal, recurrent tumours may form a fixed mass. Pleomorphic adenomas are usually solitary but they may show synchronous or metachronous association with other tumours, particularly Warthin tumour, in the same or other glands {2298}.
Pain or facial palsy are uncommon but

are occasionally seen, usually in relation to infarcted tumours. The size of most tumours varies from about 2-5 cm but some reported cases have been massive {388}. In the palate, tumours are usually seen at the junction of the hard and soft palate unilaterally. In the hard palate they feel fixed due to the proximity of the underlying mucoperiosteum.

Macroscopy

Pleomorphic adenomas tend to form well-defined, ovoid or round tumours. They are often encapsulated but the capsule varies in thickness and may be partially or completely absent, particularly in predominantly mucoid tumours. Those developing in the minor glands usually have a poorly developed or absent capsule. In major gland pleomorphic adenomas there is a distinct tendency for the tumour to separate from the capsule when handling the specimen.
The outer surface of larger tumours is frequently bossellated. The cut surface is typically homogeneous and white or tan. It may have a glistening appearance where there are cartilaginous or myxochondroid areas. There may be areas of haemorrhage or necrosis. Recurrent tumours are usually multifocal and may be widely dispersed.

Histopathology

Pleomorphic adenoma shows a remark-

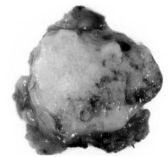

Fig. 5.48 Pleomorphic adenoma. Cut surface of the tumour showing a glistening appearance.

able degree of morphological diversity. The essential components are the capsule, epithelial and myoepithelial cells, and mesenchymal or stromal elements. The capsule varies in thickness and presence. A quantitative study showed the thickness ranged from 15-1750 mm {2732}. When tumours were serially sectioned areas of capsular deficiency were seen in all cases {1418}. In predominantly mucoid pleomorphic adenomas, the capsule may be virtually absent and the tumour abuts onto the adjacent salivary gland. Most tumours show areas where finger-like processes extend into the capsule. In addition, the tumour sometimes bulges through the capsule and forms what appear to be separate satellite nodules. These satellites are invariably attached to the main tumour by an isthmus {1418,1986}. There is a tenden-

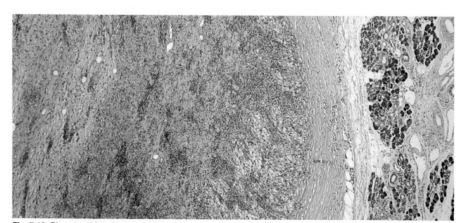

Fig. 5.49 Pleomorphic adenoma. Low-power view showing encapsulated tumour.

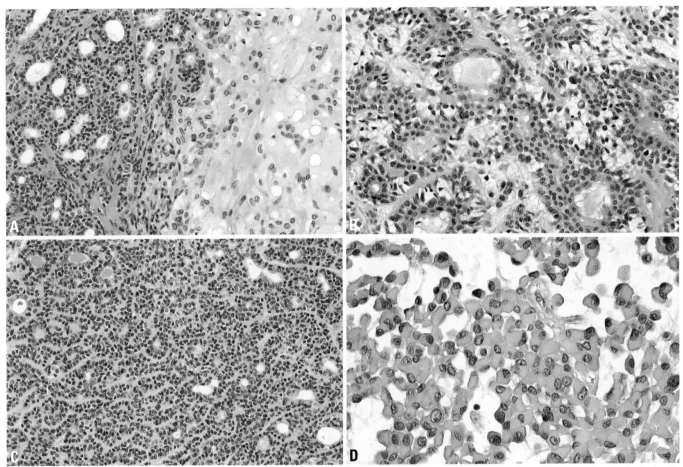

Fig. 5.50 Pleomorphic adenoma. **A** Epithelial component with ductal structures (left) and a mesenchymal myxoid component (right). **B** Ducts showing luminal cells and several layers of abluminal cells, the latter being merged into myxoid stroma. **C** Cellular type. **D** Plasmacytoid cells.

cy for clefts to form close to and parallel with the capsule. These clefts are within the tumour itself and leave tumour cells attached to the capsular wall.

The epithelial component shows a wide variety of cell types including cuboidal, basaloid, squamous, spindle cell, plasmacytoid and clear cells. Rarely, mucous, sebaceous and serous acinar cells are seen. These cells are cytologically bland and typically have vacuolated nuclei, without prominent nucleoli, and a low mitotic frequency. The epithelium usually forms sheets or duct-like structures. There is a wide range of epithelial cellularity; sometimes, the epithelial component forms the bulk of the tumour *(cellular pleomorphic adenoma)*. This phenomenon has no prognostic significance. The ducts show cuboidal luminal cells and there may be an abluminal layer of myoepithelial cells. These may be morphologically similar to the luminal cells or have clear cytoplasm and hyperchromatic and somewhat

angulated nuclei. In limited material tumours showing these features could easily be confused with adenoid cystic carcinoma and epithelial-myoepithelial carcinoma. The ducts often contain eosinophilic secretory material and are usually small but may be distended to form microcysts. Squamous metaplasia, sometimes with the formation of keratin pearls, can be seen in both ducts and sheets and occasionally there is mucous metaplasia or conspicuous clear cell change. These appearances can be confused with mucoepidermoid carcinoma. More rarely, sebaceous cells or serous cells with zymogen granules are seen. Another rare feature is the presence of multinucleated epithelial cells. Myoepithelial cells may form a fine reticular pattern or sheets of spindle-shaped cells. These may be palisaded forming a Schwannoma–like appearance. A very distinctive appearance is seen when the myoepithelial cells are plasmacytoid or hyaline {1552}. Focal oncocytic change

is not uncommon but occasionally the entire tumour is affected and may be mis-diagnosed as an oncocytoma {1973}. Crystalloid material in the form of collagenous crystalloids, tyrosine and oxalate crystals are occasionally present {324}.

The mesenchymal-like component is mucoid/myxoid, cartilaginous or hyalinised and sometimes this tissue forms the bulk of the tumour. Cells within the mucoid material are myoepithelial in origin and their cellular periphery tends to blend into the surrounding stroma. The cartilage-like material appears to be true cartilage and is positive for type II collagen and keratan sulphate. Occasionally it is the major component of the tumour. Bone may form within this cartilage or form directly by osseous metaplasia of the stroma. Deposition of homogeneous, eosinophilic, hyaline material between tumour cells and within the stroma can be a striking feature of some tumours.

It forms globular masses or sheets and

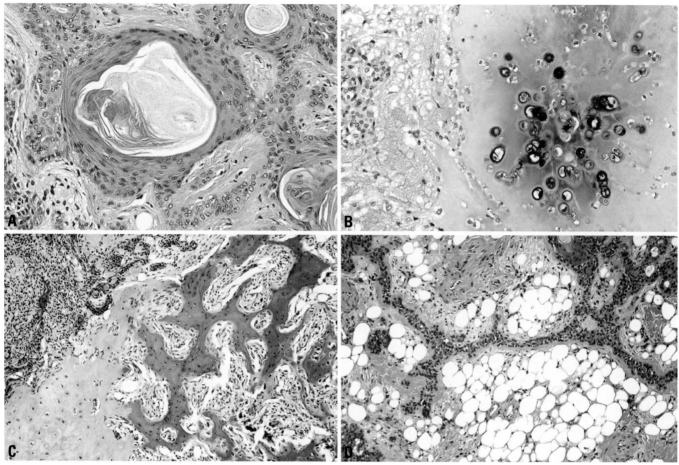

Fig. 5.51 Pleomorphic adenoma. **A** Squamous differentiation. **B** Chondroid differentiation. **C** Osseous differentiation. **D** Lipomatous differentiation.

typically is positive with stains for elastin. This material can push apart epithelial elements to give a cylindromatous or cribriform appearance that is readily mistaken for adenoid cystic carcinoma. Some longstanding tumours show increasing hyalinisation and the epithelial component is progressively effaced. It is important, however, to scrutinise the residual epithelial elements of such old, scarred pleomorphic adenomas as there is a significant risk of malignant progression in such tumours {85}. Tumours that have a lipomatous stromal component of 90% or more have been called lipomatous pleomorphic adenomas {1881, 2299}.

More extensive inflammation and necrosis can be seen following spontaneous infarction or fine needle aspiration. In such tumours there may be an increase in mitotic figures and some cellular atypia {361,1495}. In addition, squamous metaplasia may be present and these changes can be mistaken for malignancy. Some tumours show cystic degener-

ation with the neoplastic elements forming a rim around a central cavity.

Occasionally tumour cells can be seen within vascular spaces {475}. These are usually within the body of the tumour or at the periphery and this is assumed to be a peroperative phenomenon. Sometimes this is seen in vessels distant from the main tumour mass. However, this finding does not appear to have any significance in terms of tumour behaviour and, in particular, the risk of metastasis.

Immunoprofile

The inner ductal cells in the tubulo-glandular structures are positive for cytokeratin 3, 6, 10, 11, 13, and 16, whereas the neoplastic myoepithelial cells are irregularly positive for cytokeratin 13, 16, and 14 {311}. The neoplastic myoepithelial cells co-express vimentin and pan-cytokeratin and are variably positive for S-100 protein, a-smooth muscle actin, GFAP, calponin, CD10 and muscle-specific actin (HHF-35) {545}. Modified myoep-

ithelial cells in these tumours are also reactive for p63 {214}. The non-lacunar cells in the chondroid areas are positive for both vimentin and pan- cytokeratin, whereas the lacunar cells are positive only for vimentin {1776}.

The spindle-shaped neoplastic myoepithelial cells around the chondroid areas express bone morphogenetic protein (BMP) {1083} whereas the inner ductal cells in the tubulo-glandular structures and the lacuna cell in the chondroid areas express BMP-6 {1397}. Type II collagen and chondromodulin-I is present in the chondroid matrix {1396}. Aggrecan is present not only in the chondroid matrix but also in the myxoid stroma and in the inter-cellular spaces of the tubulo-glandular structures {2898}.

Genetics
Cytogenetics
Extensive cytogenetic studies of pleomorphic adenomas have shown that approximately 70% of the tumours are

karyotypically abnormal {306,1639, 2239}. Four major cytogenetic subgroups may be discerned:
> Tumours with rearrangements involving 8q12 (39%)
> Tumours with rearrangements of 12q13-15 (8%)
> Tumours with sporadic, clonal changes not involving 8q12 or 12q13-15 (23%)
> Tumours with an apparently normal karyotype (30%).
Whereas t(3;8)(p21;q12) and t(5;8)(p13;q12) are the most frequently observed translocations in the first subgroup, a t(9;12)(p24;q14-15) or an ins(9;12)(p24;q12q15) are the most frequent rearrangements seen in the second subgroup. In addition, many variant translocations have been identified in which a number of other chromosome segments are found as translocation partners of both 8q12 and 12q13-15. Secondary chromosome changes, including trisomies, dicentrics, rings and double minutes, are found in about one-third of the cases with abnormal karyotypes. Previous studies have also indicated that patients with karyotypically normal adenomas are significantly older than those with rearrangements of 8q12 (51.1 years versus 39.3 years, p < 0.001) and that adenomas with normal karyotypes are often more stroma rich than tumours with 8q12 abnormalities {306}.

Molecular genetics
The target gene in pleomorphic adenomas with 8q12 abnormalities is PLAG1, a developmentally regulated zinc finger gene {82,1279,2701}. Translocations involving 8q12 commonly result in promoter swapping/substitution between PLAG1 and a ubiquitously expressed translocation partner gene, leading to activation of PLAG1 expression. The breakpoints invariably occur in the 5´-noncoding regions of both the target gene and the promoter donor genes. The most commonly observed fusions are CTNNB1-PLAG1 and LIFR-PLAG1, resulting from t(3;8)(p21;q12) and t(5;8)(p13;q12) translocations, respectively {1279,2701}. Recently, cryptic gene fusions involving CTNNB1-PLAG1 and SII-PLAG1 were also found in karyotypically normal adenomas {82}. The PLAG1 protein is a nuclear oncoprotein that functions as a DNA-binding transcription factor. Deregulation of PLAG1 target genes, including IGF2, is likely to

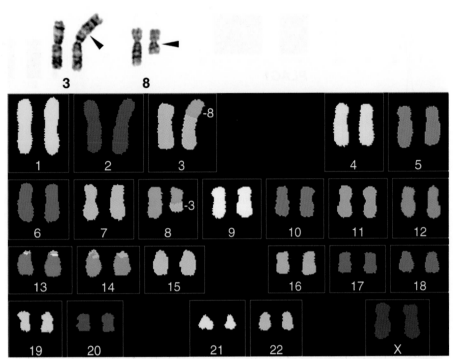

Fig. 5.52 Pleomorphic adenoma. Partial G-banded and complete SKY karyotypes of a pleomorphic adenoma showing the most common abnormality, a t(3;8)(p21;q12) translocation. Breakpoints on marker chromosomes are indicated by arrowheads.

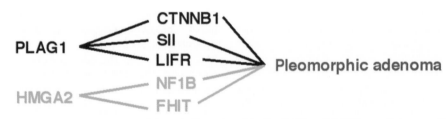

Fig. 5.53 Pleomorphic adenoma. Schematic illustration of the five PLAG1 and HMGA2 gene fusions specific and diagnostic for pleomorphic adenomas.

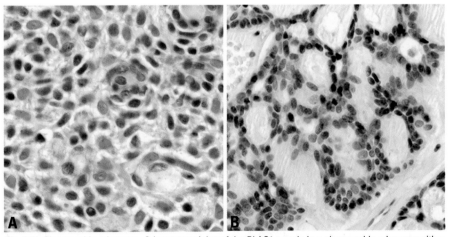

Fig. 5.54 Pleomorphic adenoma. **A** Immunostaining of the PLAG1 protein in a pleomorphic adenoma with a PLAG1-CTNNB1 fusion resulting from a t(3;8). **B** Strong immunoreactivity for HMGA2-NFIB fusion protein in a pleomorphic adenoma with ins(9;13).

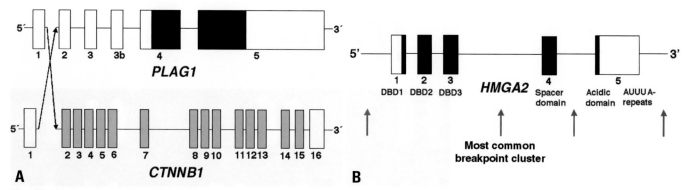

Fig. 5.55 Pleomorphic adenoma. **A** Schematic illustration of promoter swapping between *PLAG1* and *CTNNB1* in pleomorphic adenomas with t(3;8). Coding exons are indicated by filled boxes. Breakpoints are indicated by arrows. **B** Schematic illustration of the *HMGA2* gene. Coding exons are indicated by filled boxes. Breakpoints are indicated by arrows.

play a major role in the genesis of pleomorphic adenomas {2700}.

The target gene in adenomas with rearrangements of 12q14-15 is the high mobility group protein gene, HMGA2 (a.k.a. HMGIC) {878,879,2269}. HMGA2 encodes an architectural transcription factor that promotes activation of gene expression by modulating the conformation of DNA. The protein contains three DNA-binding domains that bind to the minor groove of AT-rich DNA. The majority of breakpoints in HMGA2 occur within the third large intron, resulting in separation of the DNA-binding domains from the highly acidic, carboxy-terminal domain. Two fusion genes, HMGA2-NFIB and HMGA2-FHIT, have been identified in adenomas with ins(9;12) and t(3;12), respectively {878,879}. Since no common functional domain has been found among the translocation partners, the critical event seems to be the separation of the DNA-binding domains from potential mRNA destabilizing motifs in the 3′-UTR, leading to deregulation of HMGA2 oncoprotein expression. High-level expression of HMGA2 resulting from gene amplification was recently suggested to be of importance for malignant transformation of pleomorphic adenomas {2194}.

The five PLAG1- and HMGA2-containing fusion genes so far identified are all tumour specific and may therefore be used as diagnostic markers for pleomorphic adenomas. The fusions may be detected either by RT-PCR or by interphase fluorescence in-situ hybridization {878,879,1279,2701}.

Molecular studies of the RAS and ERBB2 oncogenes have shown that mutation and activation of RAS frequently occur in pleomorphic adenomas, particularly in tumours with PLAG1 activation {1727, 2198,2464,2465}, whereas amplification and/or overexpression of ERBB2 seem to be rare {2198,2465}. Similarly, TP53 alterations are infrequent in adenomas {1907, 2198,2734}. In contrast, mutation and overexpression of TP53 are found in a relatively high proportion of carcinoma ex pleomorphic adenomas {1491,1907, 2169}. In addition, recent studies have shown that the TP53-related genes TP63 and TP73, which are novel myoepithelial markers, are overexpressed in basal and myoepithelial cells in pleomorphic adenomas {214,2734}. The pathogenetic relevance of the latter observations is uncertain. Studies using the human androgen receptor gene assay have demonstrated that the stromal and epithelial cells in pleomorphic adenomas are clonal and derived from the same progenitor cell {1455}.

Finally, it was recently demonstrated that pleomorphic adenomas contain Simian virus 40 (SV40) DNA sequences and express the SV40 large T antigen, suggesting that this oncogenic virus may be involved in the genesis and/or progression of this tumour {1643}.

Prognosis and predictive factors

Although pleomorphic adenoma is a benign tumour it can cause problems in clinical management due to its tendency to recur and the risk of malignant transformation. Recurrences are rare in the minor glands but in a meta-analysis of parotid tumours 3.4% of tumours recurred after 5 years and 6.8% after 10 years with a range of 1-50% {1083}. The variation of frequency of recurrence in this survey probably reflected the inclu-

sion of cases reported before superficial parotidectomy became a widely used treatment and the variability of long-term follow-up. Some single centre, long-term surveys however, have shown recurrence rates as low as 1.6% {2169}. Recurrences appear to be much more likely in younger patients {1436,1681}.

The possible reasons for recurrences or persistence in pleomorphic adenoma include:

- The diffluent nature of predominantly mucoid tumours {2157}.
- The variability of the thickness of the capsule, together with the tendency of the tumour to invade the capsule {1065}.
- Tumour nodules bulging through the capsule.
- Intratumoural splitting beneath the capsule.
- It is probable that the tumour cells have low biological requirements and this enables them to survive when spilt into the operative site.

Many recurrent pleomorphic adenomas are multifocal and some are so widely distributed that surgical control becomes impossible.

Myoepithelioma

A. Cardesa
L. Alos

Definition
Myoepithelioma is a benign salivary gland tumour composed almost exclusively of sheets, islands or cords of cells with myoepithelial differentiation that may exhibit spindle, plasmacytoid, epithelioid or clear cytoplasmic features.

ICD-O code   8982/0

Synonyms
Myoepithelial adenoma, benign myoepithelial tumour.

Epidemiology
Myoepitheliomas account for 1.5% of all tumours in the major and minor salivary glands and represent 2.2% and 5.7%, respectively of all benign major and minor salivary gland tumours {668}. Both sexes are affected with equal frequency {41,128,546,668,1647,2282,2367}. Most tumours occur in adults, but rare examples have been recorded in children {1527}. The age of patients with myoepithelioma ranges from 9-85, with an average of 44 years and the peak age of occurrence in the third decade {668}.

Localization
Myoepitheliomas develop preferentially in the parotid gland (40%) {668}. Minor salivary glands follow in frequency, especially in hard and soft palates {546,668, 2282,2367}. Other minor salivary gland sites can also be affected {41,1647}.

Clinical features
Myoepitheliomas usually present as slow growing painless masses {41,2282, 2367}.

Macroscopy
Myoepitheliomas are well-circumscribed, solid tumours that usually measure less than 3 cm in diameter {41,541,2367}. Myoepitheliomas have a solid, tan or yellow-tan, glistening cut surface {668}.

Histopathology
A variety of cell morphologies has been recognized, including spindle, plasma-

Table 5.03 Classification of clear cell tumours of the salivary glands.

Benign
Pleomorphic adenoma, myoepithelioma, sebaceous adenoma, oncocytoma and oncocytic hyperplasia

Malignant, primary
a). Carcinomas not usually characterized by clear cells, but with clear cell predominant areas;
      e.g. mucoepidermoid and acinic cell carcinomas.
b). Carcinomas usually characterized by clear cells;
      i. Dimorphic   epithelial-myoepithelial carcinoma.
      ii. Monomorphic   clear cell carcinoma.
                                  clear cell myoepithelial carcinoma.
      iii. Sebaceous carcinoma.

Malignant, metastatic
Carcinomas, especially kidney, thyroid, melanoma.

cytoid or hyaline, epithelioid, and clear {546}. Most are composed of a single cell type but combinations may occur. Spindle cells are arranged in interlacing fascicles with stroma-like appearance {1579}. Plasmacytoid cells are polygonal cells with eccentric nuclei and dense, nongranular or hyaline, abundant eosinophilic cytoplasm. Plasmacytoid cells are found more often in tumours arising in the minor salivary glands than in the parotid gland. These hyaline cells may simulate neoplastic plasma cells, skeletal muscle or "rhabdoid" cells {1575}. Epithelioid cells are arranged in nests or cords of round to polygonal cells, with centrally located nuclei and a variable amount of eosinophilic cytoplasm. The surrounding stroma may be either collagenous or mucoid. Some myoepitheliomas are composed predominantly of clear polygonal cells with abundant and optically clear cytoplasm, containing large amounts of glycogen but devoid of mucin or fat. These tumours may show intercellular microcystic spaces.

In other myoepitheliomas, occasional duct-like structures and intercellular microcystic spaces may be present.

An unusual reticular variant of myoepithelioma characterized by netlike arrangements of interconnected cell cords, extending through a loose, vascularized stroma, has been reported {546}.

Immunoprofile
The cells of myoepithelioma are usually positive for cytokeratins, especially for CK7 and 14. The reactivity of the spindle cells is variable for α-smooth muscle actin, muscle specific actin (MSA), calponin, S-100, GFAP and smooth muscle myosin heavy chain. There is considerable variation of tumour expression of MSA. The spindle cells react strongly for MSA, the epithelioid cells react sporadically, and the plasmacytoid and clear cells are often nonreactive {805}.

Electron microscopy
Ultrastructural studies confirmed the epithelial and myoepithelial differentiation of myoepithelioma {538,541}.

Differential diagnoses
Distinction from pleomorphic adenoma is based on the relative lack of ducts and the absence of myxochondroid or chondroid areas. Myoepitheliomas with clear cells, or mixed epithelioid and clear cells have to be separated from other salivary gland tumours with clear cells, such as: mucoepidermoid carcinoma, acinic cell carcinoma, epithelial-myoepithelial carcinoma, oncocytoma and clear cell carcinoma. All these tumours lack the characteristic immunoprofile of the myoepithelial cells. In contrast to carcinomas, myoepitheliomas have a non-infiltrative, well-circumscribed periphery.

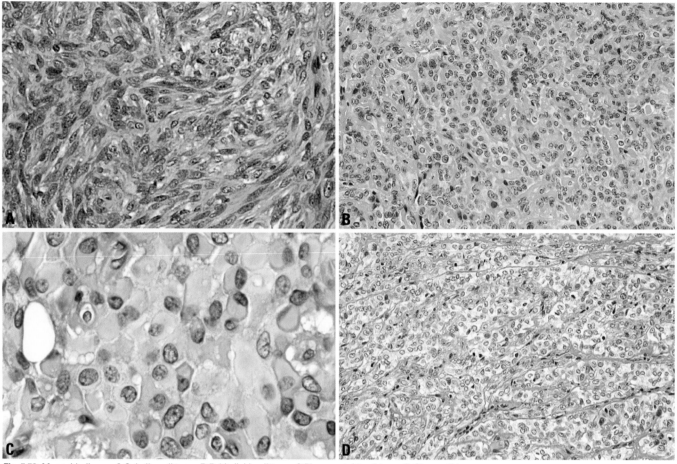

Fig. 5.56 Myoepithelioma. **A** Spindle cell type. **B** Epithelioid cell type. **C** Plasmacytoid cell type. **D** Clear cell type.

Predominantly spindle cell myoepitheliomas must be distinguished from benign and malignant mesenchymal tumours.

Genetics

Cytogenetic studies have demonstrated structural alterations of chromosomes 1, 9, 12, and 13: t(1;12)(q25;q12), del(9)(q22.1q22.3), del(13)(q12q22) in a parotid myoepithelioma {654}. Mutations of TP53 have been observed in 3 of 12 (25%) myoepitheliomas {2734}.

Prognosis and predictive factors

According to well-documented series myoepitheliomas are less prone to recur than pleomorphic adenomas {2282}. However, higher recurrence rates have been reported by others {41,646}. Recurrence is correlated with positive margins at the first excision {646}. The recommended treatment is complete surgical excision. Benign myoepitheliomas can undergo malignant transformation, especially in long standing tumours or in tumours with multiple recurrences {41}.

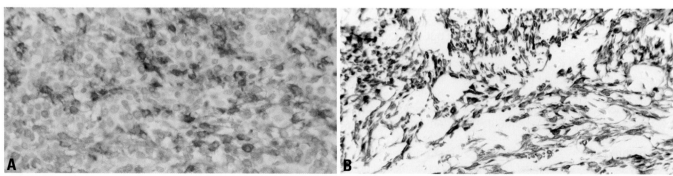

Fig. 5.57 Myoepithelioma. **A** α-SMA stain. **B** Spindle cell type: cytokeratin 7 stain.

Basal cell adenoma

V.C. de Araujo

Definition
Basal cell adenoma (BCA) is a rare benign neoplasm characterized by the basaloid appearance of the tumour cells and absence of the myxochondroid stromal component present in pleomorphic adenoma.

ICD-O code   8147/0

Epidemiology
Accurate epidemiological data are hard to obtain since in the past BCA was included within non-pleomorphic tumours. The BCAs are rare, accounting for 1-3% of all salivary gland tumours. They are typically seen in adults in the 7th decade with a 2:1 female predilection {2303}, except for the membranous type that has an equal female:male distribution {668}.

Localization
The majority arise in the major glands, and the parotid is the most frequent site of occurrence (~75%), followed by the submandibular gland (~5%) {162,2881}. It is extremely rare in minor salivary glands, the upper lip being the most common site, followed by the buccal mucosa {704,2711}.

Clinical features
Most tumours are solitary, well-defined, movable nodules. They are usually firm but occasionally cystic. The membranous type (dermal analogue tumour) {153} may be multiple and co-exist with dermal cylindromas or trichoepitheliomas {1033,1582,2867}.

Macroscopy
Most of the tumours present as small, well-circumscribed, encapsulated nodules measuring between 1-3 cm, except for the membranous type that may be multinodular or multifocal. On cut section they are solid and homogeneous or cystic, with a greyish-white to brown colour.

Histopathology
Microscopically, BCAs are composed of basaloid cells with eosinophilic cytoplasm, indistinct cell borders and round to oval nuclei, distributed in solid, trabecular, tubular, and membranous patterns. However, tumours may present with more than one of these patterns, usually with the predominance of one. The solid type is composed of sheets or islands of variable shapes and sizes, usually with peripheral palisading of cuboidal to columnar cells. The islands are separated by strands of dense collagenous tissue. The trabecular type is characterized by narrow strands, trabeculae or cords of basaloid cells separated by cellular and vascular stroma. A rare but distinctive feature is the presence of a richly cellular stroma composed of modified myoepithelial cells {542}. Ductal lumina are often observed among the basaloid cells and these cases are considered as tubulo-trabecular type. The membranous type of BCA has thick bands of hyaline material at the periphery of basaloid cells and as intercellular coalescing droplets. In the tubular type, ductal structures are a prominent feature. All variants may demonstrate cystic change, squamous differentiation in the form of whorls or 'eddies', or rare cribriform patterns. Occasional tumours, particularly of the tubular type, are largely oncocytic.

Immunoprofile
Immunopositivity for keratin, myogenic markers, vimentin and p63 indicate ductal and myoepithelial differentiation {214, 553,1598,2883}. Also the palisading cells of the solid type can stain for vimentin and myogenic markers. The pattern of expression reflects the different differentiation stages of the tumour cells, varying from the solid type, the less differentiated, to the tubular type, the most differentiated.

Genetics
Genetic aberration has been described in three cases of BCA. Two cases presented trisomy 8 and one case the 7;13 translocation and/or inv(13) {1136,2385}.

Prognostic and predictive factors
BCA is usually a non-recurrent tumour, except for the membranous type, that has a recurrence rate of approximately 25% {1582}. Although exceedingly rare, malignant transformation of BCA has been reported {1825}.

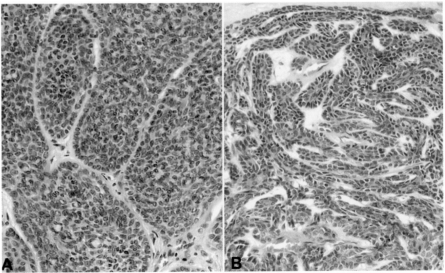

Fig. 5.58 Basal cell adenoma. **A** Solid type - Varied size nests of cuboidal cells. Note the palisading of nuclei in peripheral cells. **B** Trabecular type, with anastomosing cords of basaloid cells.

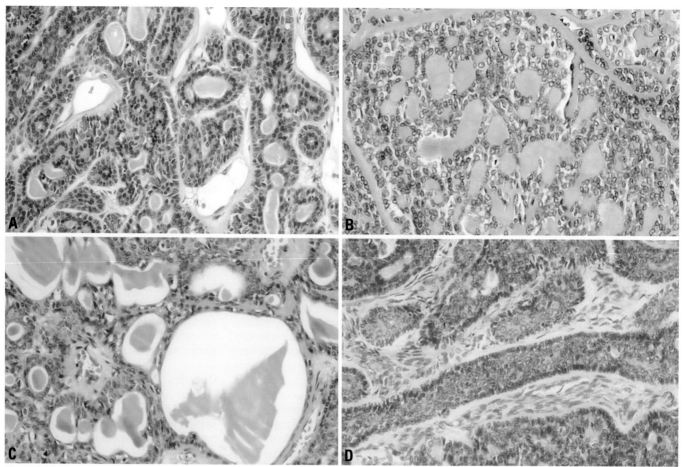

Fig. 5.59 Histological types of basal cell adenoma. **A** Tubular type, with small duct lumens lined by cuboidal eosinophilic cells. **B** Membranous type, with prominent hyaline material around and inside epithelial islands. **C** Occasional features found in basal cell adenoma include variable sized cystic spaces. **D** High cellularity of the stroma represented by spindle-shape cells.

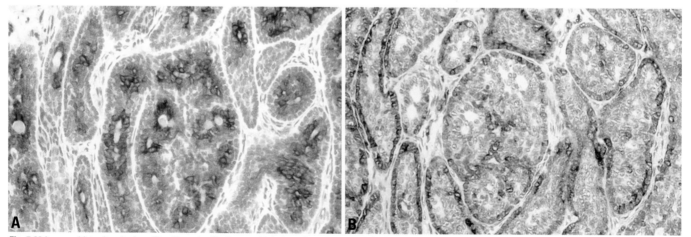

Fig. 5.60 Immunohistochemical profile of basal cell adenoma. Tubulo-trabecular type. **A** CK7 positivity in ductal cells. **B** Smooth muscle actin expression in myoepithelial cells.

Warthin tumour

R.H.W. Simpson
J.W. Eveson

Definition
A tumour composed of glandular and often cystic structures, sometimes with a papillary cystic arrangement, lined by characteristic bilayered epithelium, comprising inner columnar eosinophilic or oncocytic cells surrounded by smaller basal cells. The stroma contains a variable amount of lymphoid tissue with germinal centres.

ICD-O code   8561/0

Synonyms
Adenolymphoma, cystadenolymphoma, papillary cystadenoma lymphomatosum. Warthin tumour is preferred to avoid any possible confusion with a lymphoid malignancy, and with the separate entity, lymphadenoma {1591}.

Epidemiology
In most countries, Warthin tumour is the second commonest tumour of the salivary glands. In the United States (US) it comprised about 3.5% of all primary epithelial tumours (5.3% in the parotid) {668}. Other studies revealed higher percentages, such as 14.4% of primary epithelial tumours of the parotid gland in the United Kingdom (UK) {703}, 27% in Denmark {2075}, and 30% in Pennsylvania, USA {1765}. Warthin tumour occurs in Caucasians and Asians {451}, but has a lower incidence in African-Americans {668} (although this may now be increasing {2856}) and in Black Africans {2590}. The mean age at diagnosis is 62 years, (range 12-92) {668}, and it is rare before 40. The relative sex incidence has changed during the last half-century: In 1953 the male to female ratio was 10:1 {786}, whereas in 1996 it was 1.2:1 {668}, and in 1992 it was equal {1765}. In the UK in 1986 the ratio was 1.6:1 {705}.

Localization
Warthin tumour is almost exclusively restricted to the parotid glands and the periparotid lymph nodes. Most cases involve the lower pole although 10% are in the deep lobe. Occasional tumours (2.7% in one series) arise within adjacent lymph nodes {664}. Very rare examples have been reported in other glands {2669}, but some tumours thought initially to be within the submandibular gland have usually arisen from the anterior tail of the parotid or from lymph nodes {668}. Warthin tumour is clinically multicentric in 12-20% of patients (either synchronous or metachronous), and is bilateral in 5-14% {899,1610}. In addition, serial sectioning revealed additional sub-clinical lesions in 50% of cases {1417}.

Etiology
There is a strong link between Warthin tumour and cigarette smoking {633,2052} – the incidence is eight times that of non-smokers {1360}. In addition, the increased numbers of female smokers during the second half of the 20th century closely parallels the increase in Warthin tumour in women, and largely explains the change in sex incidence during this period {1421,2856}. The mechanisms are not clear but in has been speculated that irritants in tobacco smoke cause metaplasia in the parotid {2866}.

Radiation exposure may be relevant as there is an increase in Warthin tumour among atomic bomb survivors {2229}. There is also said to be a higher frequency of autoimmune disorders in patients with Warthin tumour than in those with pleomorphic adenomas or healthy subjects {899}.

At present, the balance of probabilities is that EBV does not play a significant role in the etiology of Warthin tumour {2733}. The metaplastic (infarcted) variant can follow trauma, particularly from FNA biopsy {596,706}.

Clinical features
Most patients present with a painless mass, on average, 2-4 cm, although

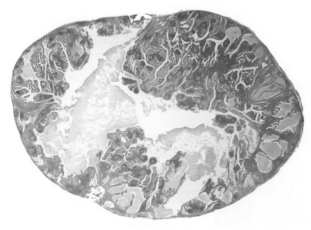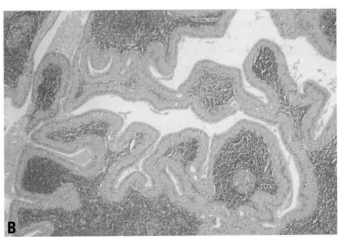

Fig. 5.61 A Warthin tumour. Low power showing lymphoid stroma, cystic change and intraluminal papillary epithelial projections. **B** Intermediate power showing oncocytic epithelium and characteristic lymphoid stroma with germinal centres.

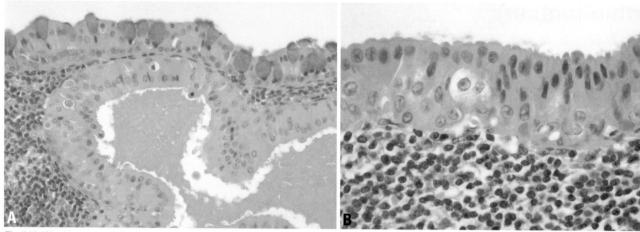

Fig. 5.62 Warthin tumour **A** Conspicuous mucous metaplasia. **B** Luminal layer of palisaded oncocytic cells with apocrine blebs, and less numerous abluminal cells.

occasional cases have reached 12 cm {2783}. The mean duration of symptoms is 21 months, but in 41% of patients it is less than six months {705 Many patients notice fluctuation in size of the tumour, especially when eating {1711}. Pain has been reported in 9% {705}, particularly those with the metaplastic variant {2866}. Facial paralysis is very rare, and is the result of secondary inflammation and fibrosis, and likewise can be seen in the metaplastic variant {706,1876}.

Warthin tumour is able to concentrate Technetium (99mTc), appearing as a "hot" lesion. It is usually well-circumscribed, but secondary inflammation can cause the edges to become indistinct.

Macroscopy

Most Warthin tumours are well-circumscribed, spherical to ovoid masses, and partly cystic. The cysts vary from small slits to spaces up to several centimetres, and contain clear, mucoid, creamy white or brown fluid. Solid areas are tan to white, and often firm and fibrous in the metaplastic variant. In all cases of Warthin tumour, the parotidectomy specimen should be examined for other lesions.

Histopathology

The tumour is sharply demarcated with a thin capsule. There are cystic and solid areas, composed of epithelial and lymphoid components. The cysts and slit-like spaces vary in size and shape, and papillary structures project into the lumina. The papillae have fibrovascular cores often with lymphoid stroma. The epithelium comprises two layers of cells: the

oncocytic luminal cells are tall and columnar, and show palisading of their bland single ovoid nuclei. The surface often shows apocrine blebbing and cilia are occasionally identified {705}. Deep to this layer lie smaller flattened or cuboidal basal cells. Their cytoplasm is similar, but less abundant. No significant nuclear atypia or mitotic activity is identified. Small foci of squamous metaplasia, scanty goblet cells and very occasional sebaceous cells are seen.

The stroma comprises lymphoid tissue displaying varying degrees of reactivity, and germinal centres are usual. Increased numbers of mast cells and plasma cells may also be seen. The cystic spaces contain eosinophilic secretions with occasional crystal formation and laminated bodies resembling corpora amylacea.

Some tumours, variously termed, infarcted, infected or metaplastic, account for 6-7% of Warthin tumours {706,2295}. They are likely to be encountered more frequently in the future with the increasing use of pre-operative FNA. There is

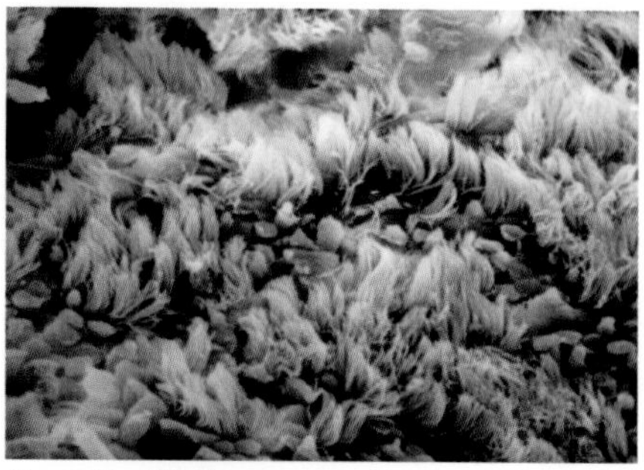

Fig. 5.63 Warthin tumour. Electron micrograph showing ciliated epithelium.

extensive necrosis, in which a ghost architecture of papillary structures is often identified – this can be highlighted with a reticulin stain. Non-keratinizing squamous metaplasia is prominent, consisting of tongues and cords of often spongiotic squamous cells extending into surrounding tissues in a pseudo-infiltrative pattern. Cytological atypia can be prominent, and mitotic figures numerous, but none is abnormal. Goblet cells can also be seen, but should not be numerous. At the periphery of the lesions, there is extensive fibrosis, with dense hypocellular collagen and myofibroblastic spindle cell proliferation. There is a heavy mixed inflammatory infiltrate, comprising neutrophils, chronic inflammatory cells, as well as sheets of macrophages, some with foamy cytoplasm. Lipogranulomas, with or without cholesterol crystals, are not uncommon. Areas of residual undamaged Warthin tumour can be found, but not in every case, and there may thus be few clues to the nature of the original lesion {596,706}.

Immunoprofile

Lymphoid marker studies have shown B (CD20), NK (CD56) and T (CD3) cells, including helper (CD4) and suppressor (CD8) subtypes. This profile of lymphocyte subsets is similar to that in normal or reactive lymph nodes {432}.

Special stains and immunohistochemistry have little to offer in the diagnosis of Warthin tumour, although there may be a role in diagnosing the metaplastic variant with epithelial markers, particularly when no residual viable Warthin tumour can be identified {596,2279}.

Cytopathology

The cytopathological findings reflect the histopathological appearance, except that mast cells are more noticeable. The other cellular elements are oncocytic epithelial cells and lymphocytes, with a background of cell debris and proteinaceous material {776}. Uncommon findings include ciliated cells {2899}, squamous cells, mucous cells, siderophages, giant cells, calcifications and crystalloids {776}. The diagnostic sensitivity of FNA cytology is moderately accurate {1984}, but the error rate is clinically significant, as for example, the findings in lymphocyte-rich acinic cell carcinoma are almost identical {2135}.

Differential diagnosis

Of all salivary gland tumours, the typical type of Warthin tumour is usually unmistakeable. Papillary cystadenoma is similar and possibly related, but any lymphoid tissue is scanty. There is some resemblance to other lymphoepithelial cystic lesions such as simple benign lymphoepithelial cyst (unrelated to AIDS), lymphoepithelial sialadenitis (LESA) with cystically dilated ducts, cystic lymphoid hyperplasia of AIDS and MALT lymphoma with cystically dilated ducts {2372}. An important differential is from cystic metastases in intra and peri-parotid lymph nodes – the malignant nature of most should be obvious, but a recently-reported variant of papillary thyroid carcinoma has been described as "Warthin-like" {113,1572}. It is characterised by a heavy lymphoid stroma and oncocytic metaplasia of the epithelium. The best guide to its true nature is that the nuclei display typical chromatin clearing, inclusions and groove-formation, and the epithelial cells show immunohistochemical expression of thyroglobulin.

If there is marked cytological atypia and mitotic activity, the metaplastic variant can be mistaken for squamous or mucoepidermoid carcinoma, either primary or metastatic {596}. The resemblance is particularly close if there has been total infarction of the original Warthin tumour. Clues to the true nature of the lesion include any ghost papillary architecture in the necrotic zones. Also, the squamous metaplasia lacks keratinization (seen in most squamous carcinomas), and mucinous goblet cells are usually much less numerous than in low-grade cystic mucoepidermoid carcinoma.

Histogenesis

There are two principal theories of the histogenesis {668}: one is an origin from intercalated and basal cells of heterotopic salivary ductal inclusions in intra- or peri-parotid lymph nodes. In particular, this explains the distribution of Warthin tumour and its absence from other salivary tissue lacking incorporated lymph nodes. The alternative theory is that Warthin tumour is a benign epithelial neoplasm or proliferation that attracts a heavy lymphoid reaction, similar to that seen in certain other salivary neoplasms {83,1717,2372}.

More recently, it has been suggested that Warthin tumour initially develops in a parotid lymph node as an adenomatous epithelial proliferation responding to as yet unidentified stimuli (probably including tobacco either as a direct stimulus or a promoter), followed by lymphocytic infiltration. The stage of this process seen at the time of surgery determines the proportions of epithelial and lymphoid elements {20}.

Genetics

Cytogenetic studies have shown Warthin tumour to have three main stemline groups, one with a normal karyotype, a second with numerical changes only (loss of Y chromosome or trisomy or monosomy 5) and a third group involving structural changes with one or two reciprocal translocations {1711}. Damage to the mitochondrial DNA may account for the ultrastructural changes seen in the mitochondria, as well as the oncocytic change seen morphologically {1494}.

Analysis of the X chromosome-linked human androgen receptor gene showed that Warthin tumour is non-clonal, and thus likely to be non-neoplastic {1118}. This finding supports morphological observations that suggested Warthin tumour (as well as various thymic and head and neck cysts) resulted from the induction of cystic changes in branchial cleft epithelium by an inflammatory infiltrate, accompanied by oncocytic change in the epithelium {2199,2509}.

A study of 13 cystadenolymphomas (Warthin tumours) showed minimal chromosomal alterations in these tumours {1905}. Interestingly, at least two tumours with cytogenetic analysis have been reported to have t(11;19) (q21;p13) translocation, suggesting a link to mucoepidermoid carcinoma {305,1638}. It is interesting, that the rearrangements on 8q and 12q have, so far, been found to be mutually exclusive {306,2239}.

Prognosis and predictive factors

Primary treatment is surgical, either superficial parotidectomy or enucleation. After this, most studies show low recurrence rates of about 2-5.5% {668,705}, presumably the result of multifocality.

Malignant change is rare, at about 1% {669,2295}, and may involve the epithelial or lymphoid components. Some patients give a history of radiation {1984,2229,2295}. Several types of carcinoma have been described, including squamous {2390}, adenocarcinoma {2295}, mucoepidermoid {1826,2294}, oncocytic {2585}, Merkel cell {788} and undifferentiated. The differential diagnosis includes squamous or mucous metaplasia, and metastases of extra-salivary malignancies to a pre-existing Warthin tumour. Lymphomas include nodal types {115,1694,2338}, and one report of lymphoepithelial lesions suggesting a MALT-type neoplasm {113}.

Warthin tumour is sometimes seen in association with other benign salivary tumours, particularly pleomorphic adenoma {664,905,1458,2338,2395}, although it is not clear if this is greater than would be expected by chance with what is after all not an uncommon tumour. Another study found an increased incidence of extra-salivary neoplasms. A common etiology of cigarette smoking explains the carcinomas of the lung, larynx and possibly the bladder, whilst the others (lymphoma, kidney and breast cancers) could just be a coincidence {1610}.

Oncocytoma

A.G. Huvos

Definition
Benign tumour of salivary gland origin composed exclusively of large epithelial cells with characteristic bright eosinophilic granular cytoplasm (oncocytic cells).

ICD-O code   8290/0

Synonym
Oncocytic adenoma, oxyphilic adenoma

Epidemiology
Oncocytoma accounts for about 1% of all salivary gland neoplasms and occurs most commonly in the 6-8th decades {257}. The mean age of the patients is 58 years. There is no sex predilection.

Etiology
Approximately 20% of all the patients will have a history of radiation therapy to the face or upper torso or long-term occupational radiation exposure five or more years prior to tumour discovery {257}. Patients with previous radiation exposure are on the average 20 years younger at tumour discovery than those without a documented history of irradiation.

Localization
Among oncocytic major salivary gland tumours, 84% occur in the parotid (male to female ratio of 1:1), and the remainder arise in the submandibular gland {2601}. Minor salivary gland sites include the lower lip, palate, pharynx, and buccal mucosa.

Clinical features
Symptoms vary according to the site of occurrence and most commonly present as a painless mass, less frequently nasal or airway obstruction.

Imaging
CT scan: Well-defined area of increased density in the host salivary gland. Radionucleotide imaging shows increased uptake of technetium-99m that does not disappear following sialogogue administration. This finding plays an important role in the diagnosis and is related to the presence of oncocytes and their increased mitochondrial content.

Macroscopy
On gross examination, oncocytomas are usually 3-4 cm in size and possess a well-defined capsule. The cut surface is light brown and lobular.

Histopathology
Histologically, the oncocytic cells are arranged in a solid or trabecular pattern. Microcyst formation can rarely be observed. The oncocytes display ample granular acidophilic cytoplasm. Typically the predominant cells have abundant oncocytic cytoplasm and an oval, vesicular nucleus (light cells). In addition, there are cells with very brightly eosinophilic cytoplasm and pyknotic nuclei (dark cells). The cells are arranged in uniform sheets and they may aggregate into clusters, and sometimes they form duct-like structures. Rarely, oncocytomas present with large polyhedral clear cells in an organoid distribution. A thin fibrovascular stroma is also present. An intimate mixture of typical eosinophilic and clear cell oncocytes may be encountered within the same tumour. Tumours with a predominantly clear cell component are referred to as clear cell oncocytoma {665}. The optically clear cell appearance is due to fixation artefact and/or intracytoplasmic glycogen deposition {551,2291}.
The tumour cells typically stain with phosphotungstic acid haematoxylin (PTAH). Electron microscopy shows elongated cristae and a partial lamellar internal structure {1227}. The nuclei of the oncocytes are irregular and contain inclusions and glycogen granules.

Differential diagnosis
The most important differential diagnosis of oncocytoma includes acinic cell carcinoma and clear cell carcinoma. Mucoepidermoid carcinoma with prominent clear cell alteration and metastatic renal cell carcinoma may also be practical considerations. Also, stroma-poor Warthin tumour, oncocytic carcinoma, and metastatic thyroid carcinoma should be included.
The clear-cut separation of an oncocytic adenomatous (nodular) hyperplasia of the parotid gland from a multinodular oncocytoma (a true neoplasm) is not always possible since the two entities overlap histologically {223,882,2427}.

Prognosis and predictive factors
Complete surgical excision is the treatment of choice. Radiotherapy is not indicated especially since oncocytes are radioresistant.
Local recurrence of an oncocytoma is extremely rare, but when it occurs, it may be multiple and bilateral. The incidence of bilateral oncocytomas is 7%. It seems there is an association between bilateral disease, tumour recurrence, and marked clear cell change (clear cell oncocytosis).

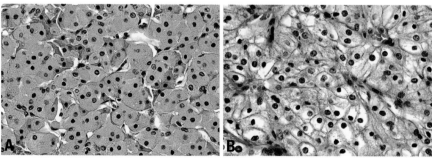

Fig. 5.64 Oncocytoma **A** Tumour cells having eosinophilic, granular cytoplasm and showing both light and dark cells. **B** Clear cell variant.

Canalicular adenoma

J.A. Ferreiro

Definition
The tumour is composed of columnar epithelial cells arranged in thin, anastomosing cords often with a beaded pattern. The stroma is characteristically paucicellular and highly vascular.

ICD-O code   8149/0

Synonyms
Basal cell adenoma, canalicular type, monomorphic adenoma, canalicular type, adenomatosis of minor salivary glands

Epidemiology
There is a peak incidence in the seventh decade (mean 65 years). The age range is 33-87 years. It is uncommon before the age of 50 {529,668,1864} and the female-to-male ratio is 1.8:1 {529,668}. It comprised 1% of all salivary gland neoplasms and 4% of minor salivary gland neoplasms in a major series {668}.

Localization
Canalicular adenoma has a peculiar predilection to involve the upper lip (about 80% of tumours) {529,1864}. The next most common location is the buccal mucosa (9.5% of tumours) {1864}. Rarely, canalicular adenoma can involve the major salivary glands {529}.

Clinical features
These tumours present as enlarging nodules with no accompanying symptoms such as pain or paralysis. The overlying mucosa shows typical coloration but in some cases may appear bluish.
A peculiar presentation of canalicular adenoma is that of multiple /multifocal canalicular adenomas {1308,1866,2206}. When this occurs, the upper lip and buccal mucosa are typically involved but other sites can be affected.

Macroscopy
Canalicular adenomas range in size from 0.5-2.0 cm in diameter and are grossly well circumscribed. The colour is light yellow to tan {668}.

Histopathology
The microscopic appearance at low magnification likewise shows circumscription. Some canalicular adenomas have a fibrous capsule while smaller tumours often do not. It is not uncommon to see multifocal microscopic canalicular adenomas adjacent to a larger canalicular adenoma. In addition, very small foci of adenomatous tissue can be seen which may represent the earliest recognizable microscopic manifestation of canalicular adenoma. Superimposed necrosis can occur in some cases {36}.
The epithelial component manifests as two rows of columnar cells which alternately are situated opposed to each other and alternately widely separated. This leads to the characteristic appearance of these tumours - canaliculi - where the epithelial cells are widely separated. The alternating arrangement of closely opposed and widely separated epithelial cells also leads to the characteristic beaded appearance of these tumours. The epithelial cells forming the cords are typically columnar but can be cuboidal. Nuclei are regular and show no pleomorphism. Nucleoli are inconspicuous and mitotic figures are rare. The stroma is characteristic and a useful clue to the diagnosis. It is paucicellular but shows a prominent vascular pattern. The capillaries often have an eosinophilic cuff of connective tissue.

Immunoprofile
Canalicular adenomas stain with anti-keratin, anti-vimentin and anti S-100 antibodies {758}. Rare focal GFAP positivity is seen {758}. Canalicular adenomas are devoid of staining when more sensitive markers of myogenous differentiation such as smooth muscle actin, smooth muscle myosin heavy chain and calponin are used {2883}.

Differential diagnosis
The most important are adenoid cystic carcinoma and basal cell adenoma. Multifocality and cribriform pattern should not be misinterpreted as carcinoma.
Hybrid tumours composed of canalicular adenoma and basal cell adenoma have been reported {2297}.

Prognosis and predictive factors
The prognosis is excellent and recurrences are rare even if the tumours are treated with just a local excision or lumpectomy. Whether new tumours are true recurrences or are a manifestation of the multicentric growth pattern is difficult to ascertain.

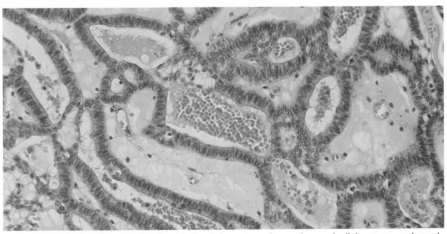

Fig. 5.65 Canalicular adenoma, showing thin, beaded anastomosing cords, paucicellular stroma and prominent vascularity.

Sebaceous adenoma

D.R. Gnepp

Definition
It is a rare, usually well-circumscribed tumour composed of irregularly sized and shaped nests of sebaceous cells without cytologic atypia, often with areas of squamous differentiation and cystic change.

ICD-O code   8410/0

Epidemiology
They account for 0.1% of all salivary gland neoplasms and slightly less than 0.5% of all salivary adenomas {2301}. The mean age is 58 years (22-90 years) and the male:female ratio is 1.6:1 {896, 901}. Unlike cutaneous sebaceous neoplasms {1132,2214}, there is no increased risk of developing a visceral carcinoma.

Localization
Approximately 50% of tumours arise in the parotid gland, 17% in the buccal mucosa, 13% in the retromolar region or area of the lower molars and 8% in the submandibular region {896}.

Clinical features
Patients typically present with a painless mass.

Macroscopy
These adenomas range in size from 0.4-3.0 cm in greatest dimension, are commonly well circumscribed to encapsulated and are greyish-white to yellow {896,901}.

Histopathology
They are composed of sebaceous cell nests often with areas of squamous differentiation with minimal atypia and pleomorphism with no tendency to invade local structures. Many tumours are microcystic or composed predominantly of ectatic ductal structures. The sebaceous glands frequently vary markedly in size and tortuosity and are often embedded in a fibrous stroma. Occasional tumours demonstrate marked oncocytic metaplasia. Histiocytes and/or foreign

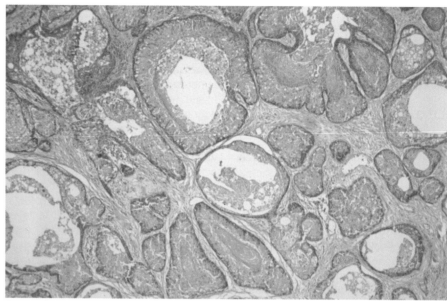
Fig. 5.66 Sebaceous adenoma. Multiple, variably sized nests of sebaceous cells in a slightly fibrotic stroma.

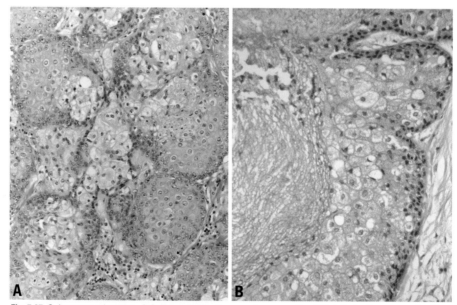
Fig. 5.67 Sebaceous adenoma. **A** Solid nests of sebaceous tumour cells. **B** Detail of sebaceous cells. Note bland tumour cells with lightly eosinophilic vacuolated cytoplasm and prominent holocrine secretion.

body giant cells can be seen focally. Lymphoid follicles, cytologic atypia, cellular necrosis, and mitoses are usually not observed. Infrequently, these tumours may be part of a hybrid neoplasm {2297}.

Treatment and prognosis
Treatment consists of complete surgical excision. They do not recur.

Lymphadenomas: sebaceous and non-sebaceous

D.R. Gnepp
W. Cheuk
J.K.C. Chan
T. Nagao

Definition

Sebaceous lymphadenoma is a rare, well-circumscribed to encapsulated tumour composed of variably sized and shaped nests of sebaceous glands without atypia often intermixed with different proportions of variably sized ducts, within a background of lymphocytes and lymphoid follicles. Lymphadenoma is a similar tumour lacking sebaceous differentiation.

ICD-O code

Sebaceous lymphadenoma
8410/0

Epidemiology

Approximately 75% of sebaceous lymphadenomas are first diagnosed in the 6-8th decades of life (25-89 years). There is no sex predominance.

Lymphadenoma is a rare tumour, with only 5 cases having been reported in the literature {83,1399,1591}. From the limited available data, all patients are male ranging in age from 17-57 years.

Localization

Well over 90% of sebaceous lymphadenomas occurred in or around the parotid gland with one tumour arising in the anterior midline of the neck {896}, and two tumours occurring in the oral region {1393,1654}. All cases of lymphadenomas reported so far have occurred in the parotid gland {83,1591}.

Clinical features

Patients typically present with a painless mass.

Macroscopy

Tumours have ranged from 1.3-6.0 cm in greatest dimension. They are usually encapsulated, solid, multicystic, or unicystic masses that range from yellow to grey. Sebum is commonly found in many of the cysts.

Histopathology

Sebaceous lymphadenoma.

The majority of sebaceous lymphadenomas are composed of variably sized sebaceous glands admixed with salivary ducts in a diffuse lymphoid background. Others consist mainly of lymphocytes and lymphoid follicles surrounding ductal structures with only occasional sebaceous glands. All tumours have a lymphoid background, and about one half have well-developed lymphoid follicles. In addition, tumours may contain small areas of identifiable residual lymph node and focal necrosis has rarely been observed. Occasional tumours may also contain or be intermixed with components of a Warthin tumour or membranous basal cell adenoma {896,901}. Histiocytes and foreign body giant cell inflammatory reactions secondary to extravasated sebum are commonly observed. This foreign body reaction can be helpful in differentiating these tumours from mucoepidermoid carcinoma (MEC). Unlike MEC, which contains a variety of cell types; mucin positivity is never found in the clear sebaceous cells. However, intracellular and extracellular mucin may be occasionally found within ducts adjacent to sebaceous cells.

Lymphadenoma

It can take the form of anastomosing trabeculae or solid tubules surrounded by basement membrane-like material, or cystically-dilated glands filled with proteinaceous materials. Papillary structures can be found in some cases. The lining cells are cuboidal to columnar and show no significant cytologic atypia or mitotic activity. Basal cells can be identified in some areas. However, the epithelial component can be obscured by abundant admixed and intraepithelial lymphocytes; the diastase-peroxidase acid Schiff stain can help in highlighting the basement membrane around the epithelial nests. The lymphoid stroma comprises dense populations of lymphoid cells with lymphoid follicle formation. The lymphoid component is generally considered to represent tumour-associated lymphoid proliferation {83,604}, hence conventional salivary gland adenomas occurring within intraparotid or cervical lymph node are excluded.

Differential diagnosis

The most important differential diagnosis of lymphadenoma is lymphoepithelial carcinoma; distinguishing features of lymphadenoma are lack of mitotic activity, lack of invasive growth with desmoplastic stroma, presence of subtle or overt ductal differentiation, and absence of EBV association. Metastatic adenocarcinoma in lymph node is characterized by recognizable nodal structures, definite nuclear atypia and invasive growth. Lymphadenoma can be distinguished from lymphoepithelial sialadenitis by the circumscribed borders as well as a more proliferative epithelial component.

Treatment and prognosis

Treatment consists of complete surgical excision. These tumours rarely recur.

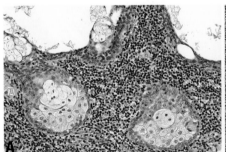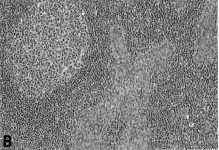

Fig. 5.68 A Sebaceous lymphadenoma. Sebaceous glands in a diffuse lymphoid background. **B** Lymphadenoma, non-sebaceous type. Epithelial tumour cell islands in lymphoid stroma with lymphoid follicle.

Ductal papillomas

R.B. Brannon
J.J. Sciubba

Ductal papillomas are a group of relatively rare, benign, papillary salivary gland tumours known as inverted ductal papilloma, intraductal papilloma, and sialadenoma papilliferum. They represent adenomas with unique papillary features with a common relationship to the excretory salivary duct system, a non-aggressive biologic behaviour, and a predilection for the minor salivary glands. They tend to occur in the middle-aged and elderly and rarely in children. The three types of ductal papillomas possess distinct clinical and histologic features allowing differentiation from each other and other adenomas with a papillary pattern.

Inverted ductal papilloma

Definition
Inverted ductal papilloma is a luminal papillary proliferation arising at the junction of a salivary gland duct and the oral mucosal surface epithelium and exhibits an endophytic growth pattern that forms a nodular mass.

ICD-O code   8503/0

Synonym
Epidermoid papillary adenoma

Epidemiology
The true incidence of inverted ductal papilloma (IDP) is unknown, but it is thought to be relatively rare based on the sparse number of reported cases. Lesions have arisen in adults with an age range of 28-77 years and a male predilection {264}.

Localization
All of the reported sites have been in the minor salivary glands—the most common location is the lower lip followed by the buccal mucosa/mandibular vestibule. Other reported sites have been the palate and the floor of mouth {264}.

Clinical features
IDP typically presents as a painless nodular submucosal swelling, often with a dilated pore or punctum surfacing the swelling {1046}. Lesions have been described as being present from months to several years.

Macroscopy
Lesions have ranged from 0.5-1.5 cm. They are nodular masses that are often papillary and occasionally cystic.

Histopathology
The neoplasms are unencapsulated. Well demarcated endophytic epithelial masses that are typically continuous with the mucosal epithelium. The mucosal epithelium has a central pore-like opening in the mucosal surface. The peripheral borders of the epithelial mass show a broad, smooth "pushing" interface juxtaposed to the connective tissue stroma. The epithelium proliferates in broad papillary projections that extend into the luminal cavity and are composed predominantly of epidermoid and basal cells that show columnar epithelium on the surface of the papillae. Acinar aggregates or individual mucocytes can be found in the columnar epithelial layer and/or in the subjacent epidermoid component. The epithelial cells are cytologically bland with little or no pleomorphism. Mitotic figures are rare.

Differential diagnosis
IDP must be differentiated from mucoepidermoid carcinoma since both have epidermoid and mucous cells. Inverted ductal papilloma does not have the multicystic, multinodular, and infiltrative growth pattern of mucoepidermoid carcinoma. Papillary features are rarely found in mucoepidermoid carcinomas.

Prognosis and predictive factors
There have been no reported recur-

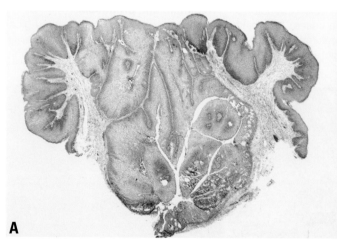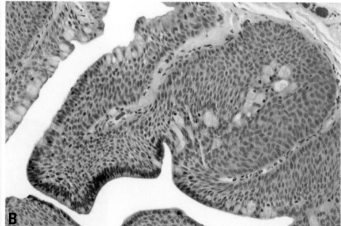

Fig. 5.69 Inverted ductal papilloma. **A** low power view demonstrates a centrally endophytic epithelial proliferation with bosselated deep and lateral margins. **B** Goblet cells and epithelium with columnar features line portions of the lumen.

rences following conservative surgical excision based on 12 cases with adequate follow-up time {264}.

Intraductal papilloma

Definition
Intraductal papilloma is a luminal papillary proliferation of duct epithelium that arises from a segment of the interlobular or excretory duct and causes unicystic dilatation.

ICD-O code   8503/0

Epidemiology
The intraductal papilloma is very rare. Age range is 8-77 years with most cases occurring in the 6th and 7th decade of life {264,1375}. Sex distribution is essentially even.

Localization
The minor salivary glands are more frequently involved than the major glands. Intraductal papillomas are most commonly found in the lips and buccal mucosa. Tumours have been reported in the palate and tongue as well. Of the major glands the parotid is most frequently involved, but cases in the submandibular and sublingual glands have also been cited {264,1008,1749}.

Clinical features
Intraductal papillomas of major and minor salivary glands present as painless, well-defined solitary masses or swellings. Duration can range from weeks to years.

Macroscopy
Grossly, intraductal papillomas are well-circumscribed, unicystic nodules that range in size from 0.5-2.0 cm. The lumina contain finely granular, often friable tissue and mucinous material.

Histopathology
The tumour is entirely confined within a circumscribed or encapsulated unicystic cavity. The lumen is partially or completely filled with many branching papillary elements consisting of fibrovascular cores surfaced by columnar to cuboidal cells of one to two layers that originate from a focal point in the wall. Mucocytes, often goblet-like, are interspersed throughout the epithelium lining the pap-

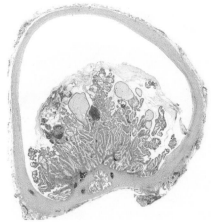

Fig. 5.70 Intraductal papilloma. A cystic cavity is bounded by a thin fibro-collagenous layer. Emerging from a narrow region along the inner aspect of the lumen is an exophytic and papillary growth.

illary elements. These mucous-containing cells can be few to many in number. The epithelium that lines the cyst-like cavity is composed of the same type of epithelium as the papillary fronds. In many instances, the cystic structure has a dense fibrous connective tissue wall surrounding it. Cytologic atypia and mitotic figures are virtually absent {264}.

Differential diagnosis
In contrast to intraductal papillomas, papillary cystadenomas are morphologically multicystic with numerous small to medium-sized cystic spaces. In the pap-

illary cystadenoma the intraluminal growth is often characterized by multiple papillary projections with a variety of epithelial cell types, but usually the papillary growth occupies the lumen to a limited degree.

Prognosis and predictive factors
Excision appears to be curative based on five cases with an adequate follow-up of 2-5 years {1186,1302,1375,1829, 2039}.

Sialadenoma papilliferum

Definition
Sialadenoma papilliferum is an exophytic papillary and endophytic proliferation of mucosal surface and salivary duct epithelium.

ICD-O code   8406/0

Epidemiology
Sialadenoma papilliferum is a rare neoplasm {2711}. The age range is 31-87 years (mean age 59) with a male to female ratio of 1.5:1 {264}.

Localization
The vast majority of cases have occurred in the minor salivary glands. Major salivary gland involvement is very rare with the parotid gland being the most frequently involved. Over 80% of the neo-

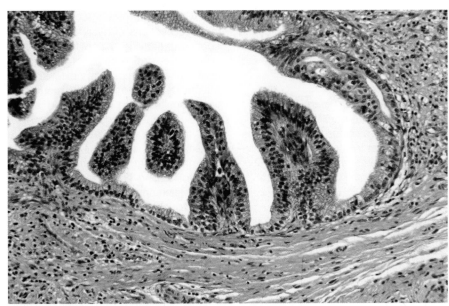

Fig. 5.71 Intraductal papilloma. Extending into the lumen of the cystic space are fronds of columnar epithelium supported by a central fibrovascular core.

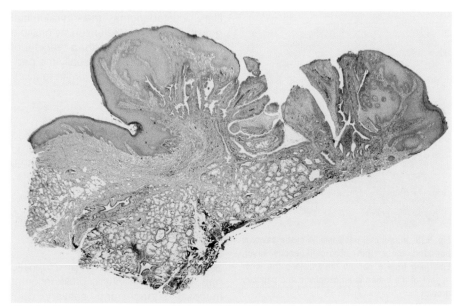

Fig. 5.72 Sialadenoma papilliferum. Surface growth is exophytic and papillary to verrucous in nature with clusters of underlying minor salivary gland tissue deep to the surface.

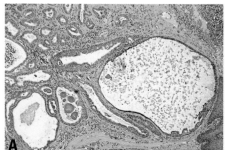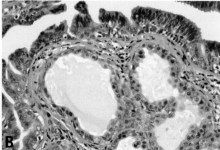

Fig. 5.73 Sialadenoma papilliferum. **A** Ductal ectasia of varying caliber with lining cells forming short luminal projections or nodular thickenings. **B** Ductal structures are lined by cuboidal cells with large, uniform and centrally placed nuclei as well as a tall columnar cell population.

be present {2344}. The lack of encapsulation of the ductal structures can at times give the false impression of an invasive growth pattern.

Differential diagnosis

The differential diagnosis typically centres around three lesions: squamous papilloma, inverted ductal papilloma, and mucoepidermoid carcinoma. Squamous papilloma is composed entirely of squamous epithelium and lacks the endophytic growth pattern and glandular differentiation of sialadenoma papilliferum. Inverted ductal papilloma in contrast to the sialadenoma papilliferum, lacks the glandular complexity, and is a well-circumscribed tumour with blunted, pushing non-infiltrative margins. The invasive pattern and variable mixture of epidermoid, intermediate, mucous, and clear cells found in mucoepidermoid carcinoma set it apart from sialadenoma papilliferum.

Prognosis and predictive factors

The recurrence rate for sialadenoma papilliferum is in the 10-15% range based on 20 reported cases with adequate follow-up {264}. Therefore, it is characterized by a higher risk of recurrence than the other types of ductal papillomas of the salivary gland. Complete surgical excision is the treatment of choice.

plasms occur on the hard and/or soft palate. Buccal mucosa is the second most common site. Other intraoral sites are the upper lip, the retromolar pad, and the faucial pillar {264}.

Clinical features

The sialadenoma papilliferum typically manifests as a painless, exophytic papillary growth that is often interpreted clinically as a squamous papilloma. Duration ranges from months to several years.

Macroscopy

Gross findings usually show a well-demarcated papillary or verrucoid, sessile to pedunculated surface morphology. Overall, the tumours generally range from 0.5-1.5 cm in size.

Histopathology

The neoplasm consists of a biphasic pattern with a glandular component consisting of collections of cysts and duct-like spaces underlying a papillary or verrucous type proliferation of squamous epithelium. These papillary extensions of squamous epithelium are supported by fibrovascular cores and extend above the level of the adjacent mucosa. At or near the base of the fronds there is a transition from squamous epithelium to columnar ductal epithelium, which lines the proliferating ductal elements. These ductal elements consist of small and ectatic ducts, some of which show cystic enlargement. The ducts and their papillary folds are lined by a double row of cells showing a basal layer composed of cuboidal cells and a luminal lining of low columnar cells. Mucocytes can be interspersed throughout the lining of ductal cells as well as in the squamous component. Columnar oncocytic cells may also

Cystadenoma

A. Skálová
M. Michal

Definition

Cystadenoma is a rare benign epithelial tumour characterized by predominantly multicystic growth in which the epithelium demonstrates adenomatous proliferation. The epithelial lining is frequently papillary and rarely mucinous.

ICD-O code   8440/0

Synonyms

Monomorphic adenoma, cystic duct adenoma {2301}, Warthin tumour without lymphoid stroma {668}, intraductal papillary hyperplasia {401}, oncocytic cystadenoma.

Epidemiology

The frequency of cystadenoma is between 4.2-4.7% of benign tumours {668,2711}. There is a female predominance and the average age of patients with cystadenoma is about 57 years (range 12-89).

Localization

About 45% of all cases of cystadenoma arise in the parotid; the majority of tumours are located in minor salivary glands, particularly in the lips and buccal mucosa {668,2711}.

Clinical features

Cystadenomas of the major glands typically present as slowly enlarging painless masses. In oral mucosa, these tumours produce smooth-surfaced nodules that resemble mucoceles.

Macroscopy

Cut section reveals multiple small cystic spaces or a single large cyst surrounded by lobules of salivary gland or by connective tissue.

Histopathology

Cystadenomas are often well circumscribed and surrounded by complete or incomplete fibrous capsules. The tumours are composed of cystic spaces, the number and size of which is variable. Twenty percent of cystadenomas are unilocular {2711}. Most cases are multilocular with individual cystic spaces separated by limited amounts of intervening stroma. The lumens often contain eosinophilic material with scattered epithelial, inflammatory or foamy cells. Rarely, psammoma bodies or crystalloids have been described within the luminal secretion {2389}. The lining epithelium of these cystic structures is mostly columnar and cuboidal. Oncocytic, mucous, epidermoid and apocrine cells are sometimes present focally or may even predominate. An oncocytic variant of cystadenoma is composed predominantly of oncocytes in unilayered or bilayered papillary structures thus resembling the epithelium of Warthin tumour without lymphoid stroma. Cystadenomas often show a mixture of cell types in the epithelial lining. An unusual case of oncocytic cystadenoma with apocrine, mucinous, sebaceous and signet ring cell appearance has been described {1715}. Squamous epithelium may be present focally but rarely predominates. Cystadenomas of the salivary glands are usually devoid of foci of solid growth, cytologic atypia, fibrosis and apposed lymphoid tissue {790}. Cystadenoma occurs in two major variants, as papillary and mucinous cystadenoma.

Papillary cystadenoma is composed of large multilocular or unilocular cysts with multiple papillary projections. The lining epithelium is, in some cases, composed of oncocytic cells.

Mucinous cystadenoma is composed of multiple cysts lined by mucous tall columnar epithelium with small basally situated nuclei and eosinophilic to clear cytoplasm. The lumens contain PAS and mucicarmine positive abundant mucus. The columnar epithelial lining has a uniform thickness with limited papillary growth.

Prognosis and predictive factors

Cystadenomas are benign tumours, and conservative but complete surgical removal is recommended. The tumours are unlikely to recur but rare cases of mucinous cystadenoma with malignant transformation have been described {1716}.

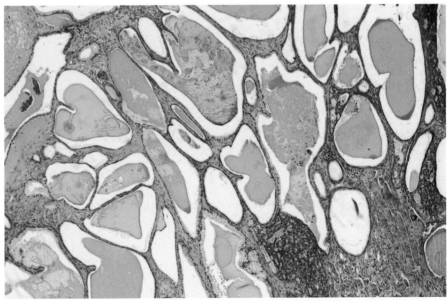

Fig. 5.74 Cystadenoma, composed of cystic spaces, the number and size of which is variable.

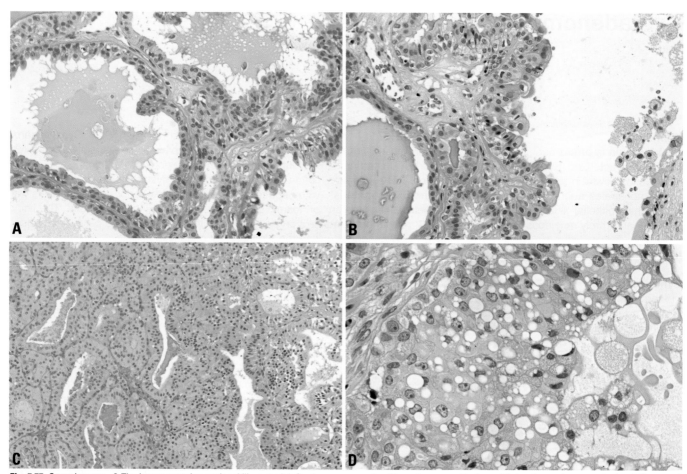

Fig. 5.75 Cystadenoma. **A** The lumen contains eosinophilic material. Cystic spaces are lined by columnar epithelium with focal apocrine metaplasia. **B** Scattered foamy cells within the secretion. **C** Oncocytic variant of cystadenoma is composed of prevailing oncocytes present in unilayered or bilayered papillary structures thus resembling Warthin tumour without lymphoid stroma. **D** Oncocytic cystadenoma with apocrine, mucinous, sebaceous and signet ring cell appearance.

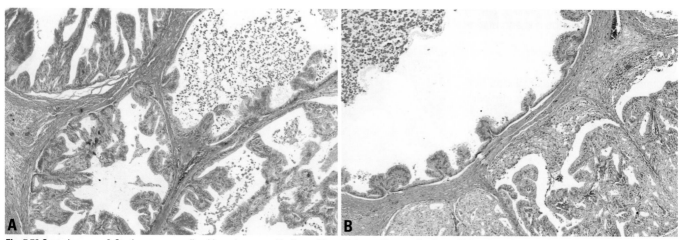

Fig. 5.76 Cystadenoma. **A** Cystic spaces are lined by columnar epithelium with multiple papillary projections. **B** Prominent intracystic papillary growth pattern.

Soft tissue tumours

D.R. Gnepp

Excluding haematopoietic neoplasms, pure mesenchymal tumours account for 1.9-4.7% of salivary gland tumours {347, 669,678,2301} with benign soft tissue lesions being more common than sarcomas. The ratio of benign to malignant mesenchymal tumours varies from series to series, ranging from 18:1-2.4:1 {669,2301}. Over 85% of soft tissue tumours arise in the parotid gland, over 10% involve the submandibular gland and, rarely, a tumour arises in the sublingual gland.

Vascular tumours are the most common benign mesenchymal neoplasm, accounting for almost 40% of the benign tumours {669,2301}. Seventy-five to 80% of the vascular neoplasms are haemangiomas, typically the juvenile or cellular variant, with the greatest incidence occurring in the first decade of life {430}. Most other vascular tumours are lymphangiomas. Other major salivary gland benign soft tissue neoplasms include neural tumours, most frequently neurofibroma or schwannoma {669} and fibroblastic/myofibroblastic tumours, most frequently nodular fasciitis, and fibromatosis with an infrequent myofibromatosis, fibroma, haemangiopericytoma, solitary fibrous tumour {953,2248} or inflammatory pseudotumour (inflammatory myofibroblastic tumour {775}) {2794} being reported. Lipomas, including the pleomorphic variety {934} and miscellaneous other tumours including granular cell tumour {2222}, angiomyoma, glomangioma, myxoma, fibrous histiocytoma, giant cell tumour, osteochondroma and rarely a metastatic sarcoma may be also seen. Several cases of lipomas entrapping salivary glandular tissue have been recently described and termed sialolipomas {810,1824}, including a congenital case {1129}.

Salivary gland sarcomas arise in an older population than their benign soft tissue counterparts. They are rare tumours, accounting for only 0.3% of salivary gland neoplasms {347}. Almost any type of sarcoma can arise primarily in the salivary gland {87,669,1583}. In the largest

Table 5.04 Salivary gland sarcomas*

Tumour type	Armed Forces Institute of Pathology Registry {87}	MD Anderson Medical Center {1583}	University of Hamburg Registry {2301}
Haemangiopericytoma	14		
Malignant schwannoma	13	2	2
Fibrosarcoma	12	2	
Malignant fibrous histiocytoma	9	3	4
Rhabdomyosarcoma	7	2	2
Angiosarcoma	5		
Synovial sarcoma	4		
Kaposi sarcoma	3	3**	
Leiomyosarcoma	3		
Liposarcoma	2		
Alveolar soft part sarcoma	2		
Epithelioid sarcoma	1		
Extraosseous chondrosarcoma	1		
Osteosarcoma		2	
Malignant haemangioendothelioma			1
Sarcoma, poorly differentiated	9		
TOTAL	**85**	**14**	**9**

*Excluding lymphomas
**Arose in intraparotid lymph nodes

published series, haemangiopericytoma, malignant schwannoma, fibrosarcoma and malignant fibrous histiocytoma were the most common neoplasms, accounting for 16, 15, 14, and 11% of reported sarcomas, respectively {87}. These are aggressive neoplasms; 40-64% of patients develop recurrences, 38-64% develop metastases (usually haematogenous), and the mortality rate ranges from 36-64% with death occurring frequently within 3 years of diagnosis {87,1583}. The most successful treatments are wide surgical excision or surgery combined with radiation. For more specific information about each type of tumour, refer to the other texts {775,2745}.

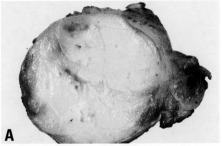 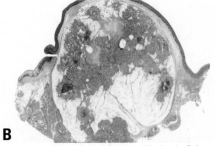

Fig. 5.77 Sialolipoma. **A** A well-circumscribed, encapsulated, yellow mass of the parotid gland. **B** Low-power view of a palatal tumour showing a mass clearly demarcated from the adjacent salivary gland tissue. The tumour consists of salivary gland tissue and adipose element, in approximately equal amounts in this case.

Haemangioma

E. Odell

Definition
This is characterized by a proliferation of endothelial cells and pericytes.

ICD-O code   9120/0

Synonyms
Benign or infantile haemangioendothelioma, infantile haemangioma, cellular haemangioma, immature capillary haemangioma, juvenile haemangioma

Epidemiology
Haemangiomas of the salivary glands account for approximately 0.4% of salivary tumours {668}. Lesions may present at any age but two thirds of cases are diagnosed in the first two decades {668,2301}. They are twice as common in females as males.

Localization
The haemangioma occurs almost exclusively in the parotid gland.

Clinical features
Lesions are asymptomatic soft swellings. They usually appear during the first 6 months of life and grow slowly. Most eventually involute by the age of 5-6 years {914,1413}. A bluish colour may be visible through skin but the overlying skin is not usually involved. Lesions are usually limited to the parotid gland but some are part of an angiomatosis that extends to involve the parapharyngeal space, infratemporal fossa or base of skull {1625}.
Diagnosis may be aided by imaging {312,624}.

Macroscopy
Lesions cause diffuse enlargement of the gland.

Histopathology
The lesion is composed of varying sized and shaped vascular spaces. The juvenile variant comprises small round densely packed endothelial cells and pericytes clustered within sheets that extend diffusely through the gland but divided into lobules by the gland septa. Lesional cells replace acinar cells, enlarging the lobules but leaving ducts scattered through the lesion. Mitoses are sparse or moderate in the juvenile form. In the early stages no vascular lumens are present but these develop with time to be the dominant feature {668,2301, 2745}. Mature lesions are typical capillary haemangiomas with thin endothelial cell linings and no atypia. Thrombi and phleboliths may be present and foci of normal salivary tissue may persist in the mature lesion {668,914,1814,1817,2301}.

Prognosis and predictive factors
Neonatal and infantile lesions grow rapidly initially but the majority involute before age 7 years and often much earlier {668,874,1413,1625,2301,2626,2632, 2745,2790}. No treatment may be required and any intervention should be delayed. Steroids reduce growth and are the main treatment; pressure therapy {2626} or embolisation {265} may be considered if large. Occasional cases show progressive growth {2185}.

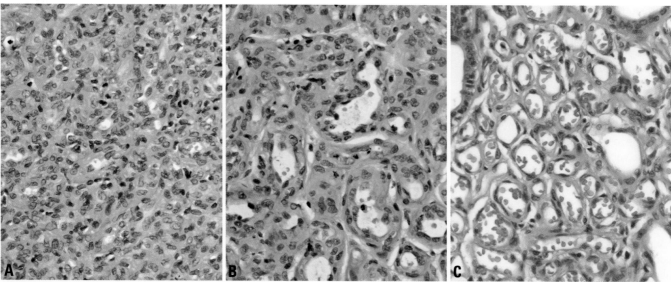

Fig. 5.78 Juvenile haemangioma. **A** Immature appearance with little lumen formation from a patient under 1 year in age. **B** More mature area with well-organised vessels. **C** Highly vascularized haemangioma.

Haematolymphoid tumours

A.C.L. Chan
J.K.C. Chan
S.L. Abbondanzo

Hodgkin lymphoma

Involvement of the salivary glands by Hodgkin lymphoma is very rare. Combining data from four large series on primary lymphomas of the salivary glands, Hodgkin lymphoma only accounts for 4% of all cases {473,893, 1164,2267}. Both classical Hodgkin lymphoma and nodular lymphocyte predominant Hodgkin lymphoma have been reported {101,391,893}, and all have involved the parotid gland only. Some of these tumours have originated from intraparotid lymph nodes, and thus are strictly-speaking not genuine primary extranodal lymphomas of the salivary glands. Rarely, Hodgkin lymphoma can arise within a Warthin tumour {1702}. Please refer to the WHO Classification of Tumours of Heamatopoietic and Lymphoid Tissues {1197}.

Non-Hodgkin lymphoma

Overview

Primary salivary gland non-Hodgkin lymphomas (NHL) are uncommon, accounting for only 5% of all primary extranodal NHL {809} and 2% of all salivary gland

tumours {893}. For a case to be considered as primary in the salivary gland, the bulk of disease should occur in this site, and the glandular parenchyma should be involved. A major problem in definition is caused by the normal presence of intraglandular lymph nodes in the parotid gland. Strictly speaking, cases of NHL limited to these lymph nodes without glandular parenchymal involvement should be considered as nodal NHL instead. However, the distinction is not always easy because cases with extensive parenchymal and nodal involvement can still have originated from intraglandular lymph nodes.

The most commonly affected gland is the parotid gland (75% of all cases), followed by the submandibular gland (20%) {473,893,1164}. Most patients are in the sixth decade, and multiple glands (especially bilateral) are involved in about 10% of cases {473}. The patients present with a palpable mass, and pain and tenderness are observed in a minority of cases.

Histologic types of NHL affecting the salivary glands

Most NHL occurring in salivary glands are B-cell lymphomas. In some older series, follicular lymphoma is the most common, accounting for about half of all

cases {473,893,1164}. However, many of these tumours are probably nodal lymphomas arising from intraglandular lymph nodes with subsequent infiltration of the glandular parenchyma, or represent extranodal marginal zone B-cell lymphoma of MALT type with prominent follicular colonization. In follicular lymphoma, lymphoepithelial lesions may be present in occasional cases {1017}. Extranodal marginal zone B-cell lymphoma of MALT type is probably the most common type of lymphoma truly of salivary gland origin. It is frequently associated with Sjögren syndrome. Mantle cell lymphoma can also present as salivary gland involvement, but staging often reveals additional sites of disease. It is important not to misdiagnose mantle cell lymphoma for extranodal marginal zone B-cell lymphoma, because of the worse prognosis of the former.

Diffuse large B-cell lymphoma accounts for about 15% of all NHL of the salivary glands {473,893,1164}. The tumour is infiltrative, with destruction of the salivary gland parenchyma and interstitial infiltration among residual salivary acini. The tumour comprises large lymphoid cells that may resemble centroblasts or immunoblasts, and express pan-B markers. Some cases represent transforma-

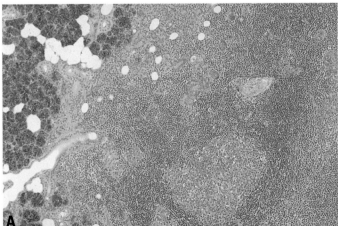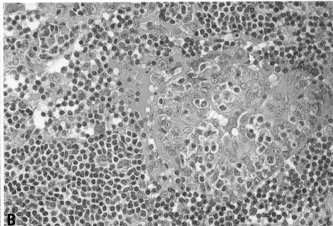

Fig. 5.79 Lymphoepithelial sialadenitis (LESA). **A** Reactive germinal centre in LESA associated with Sjögren syndrome. **B** Higher magnification of benign lymphoepithelial lesion (BLEL) without monocytoid B cell halo.

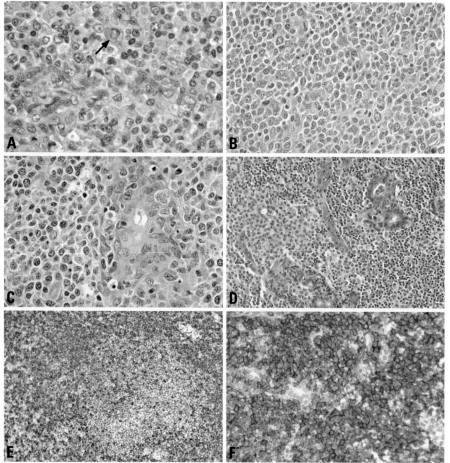

Fig. 5.80 Extranodal marginal-zone B-cell lymphoma. **A** Characteristic cellular heterogeneity of EMZBCL with monocytoid B, centrocyte-like and lymphoplasmacytoid cells with an occasional intranuclear inclusion (arrow). **B** Focal area of large cells in EMZBCL of salivary gland. **C** Ductal invasion by large cells in EMZB-CL. **D** Invasion of the epimyoepithelial (lymphoepithelial) islands by neoplastic cells. **E** Bcl-2 reactivity in the colonizing neoplastic cells in EMZBCL but not in the reactive germinal centre cells. **F** Diffuse reactivity for CD20 in EMZBCL.

tion from an underlying extranodal marginal zone B-cell lymphoma of MALT type {2103}.

Anaplastic large cell lymphoma (ALCL), peripheral T-cell lymphoma unspecified, and extranodal NK/T cell lymphoma of nasal-type can also rarely affect the salivary glands {373,1081,1203}. Please refer to the section of 'non-Hodgkin lymphoma' in 'Tumours of the nasal cavity and paranasal sinuses' for details.

Rare cases of NHL can arise in the lymphoid stroma of Warthin tumour, with follicular lymphoma being the most frequent type {307,1694}. The lymphoma discovered in the Warthin tumour may be the presenting feature of more generalized disease.

Differential diagnosis

Some benign conditions can mimic NHL histologically. Lymphoepithelial sialade-nitis (LESA), a condition associated with Sjögren syndrome, is a precursor lesion for extranodal marginal zone B-cell lymphoma of MALT type, and will be discussed in details in the next section.

Kimura disease is a benign lesion of unknown etiology, commonly affecting the soft tissues in the head and neck region of young adults. It shows a predilection for Asian populations. Involvement of the major salivary glands is frequent {369,1385,1497,2581}. It is characterized by reactive lymphoid follicles, vascularization of germinal centres, heavy eosinophilic infiltration, proliferation of high endothelial venules and prominent sclerosis. See Chapter 7 for details.

Chronic sclerosing sialadenitis (Küttner tumour) is a chronic inflammatory disorder affecting the submandibular gland {366}. It can be bilateral. Since the gland

is enlarged and hard, it usually imparts a clinical suspicion for malignancy. Histologically, there is a heavy lympho-plasmacytic infiltrate, accompanied by reactive lymphoid follicles, atrophy of salivary acini, periductal fibrosis and interlobular sclerosis. In the early phases, the striking lymphoid infiltrate can lead to a misdiagnosis of lymphoma. In contrast to lymphoma, the follicles are obviously reactive, the interfollicular lymphoid cells lack atypia, a permeative infiltrative pattern is lacking, there is a mixture of B and T cells, and the B cells are polytypic.

Rosai-Dorfman disease (sinus histiocytosis with massive lymphadenopathy) can also affect the major salivary glands {791,2760}.

Prognosis and predictive factors

The prognosis of salivary gland lymphomas depends on the histologic type and clinical stage. T cell lymphomas and extranodal NK/T cell lymphomas are generally associated with a poorer outcome. A study reports that cases of probable nodal origin have a worse prognosis compared to those of probable extranodal-parenchymal origin {1193}.

Extranodal marginal zone B-cell lymphoma (EMZBCL)

Definition

A low-grade B-cell lymphoma arising in mucosa-associated lymphoid tissue (MALT).

ICD-O code   9699/3

Epidemiology

Primary EMZBCL of the salivary gland is an uncommon neoplasm that usually develops in the setting of lymphoepithelial sialadenitis (LESA) in patients with Sjögren syndrome {59,98,710,2210, 2266,2915}. It occasionally occurs in the absence of an autoimmune disease or in association with another autoimmune process. EMZBCL occurs primarily in adults with an age range of 55-65 years and shows a slight female predominance. It may occasionally be seen in children and young adults {2524}.

Etiology

Since most cases of EMZBCL arise in the

setting of LESA in association with Sjögren syndrome, it is postulated that this low-grade B cell lymphoma develops subsequent to the accumulation of mucosa-associated lymphoid tissue (MALT) that is acquired as a result of the autoimmune process.

Localization

EMZBCL usually presents as a persistent unilateral or bilateral mass in the parotid gland region, although any major or minor salivary gland may be involved {1181}. The regional lymph nodes may also be enlarged due to involvement by the tumour.

Clinical features

EMZBCL may occur in the salivary gland as a manifestation of either primary or disseminated disease {473,813}. Presenting signs include persistent enlargement of the involved salivary gland(s), sometimes in association with regional lymphadenopathy or monoclonal gammopathy {56}. The patient may also show signs of other autoimmune diseases such as rheumatoid arthritis, systemic lupus erythematosus or Hashimoto thyroiditis {1181}. Occasionally, EMZBCL may present in a cervical lymph node with subsequent development in the salivary gland. There is a variable period of time between the documented occurrence of LESA and the development of malignant lymphoma, which has been reported to range from 6 months to 29 years {630,710,2266}. When EMZBCL of the parotid gland develops, there is a tendency for it to remain localized for long periods of time, as is the case with EMZBCL at other anatomic sites, including the stomach {468}.

Macroscopy

The cut surface of EMZBCL of salivary gland is yellowish- tan in colour and has a "fish-flesh" appearance. Microcysts may be present.

Tumour spread and staging

The majority of patients with EMZBCL of salivary gland present with Stage IE (extranodal) or IIE disease. Dissemination most often occurs to cervical lymph nodes and other mucosal sites such as lung, conjunctiva and stomach {710,1003}.

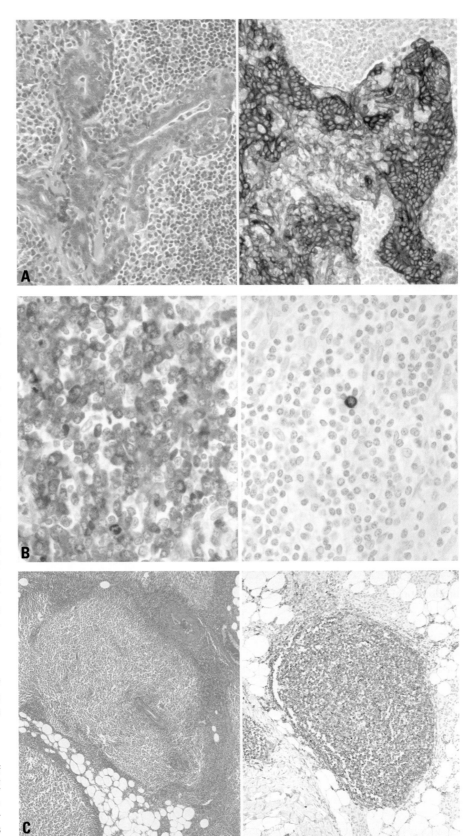

Fig. 5.81 Extranodal marginal-zone B-cell lymphoma (EMZBCL). **A** Lymphoepithelial lesion (left) highlighted by antibody to cytokeratin (right). **B** EMZBCL. Immunoglobulin light chain restriction for kappa (left) compared to lambda (right). **C** Follicular lymphoma of salivary gland with monotonous, neoplastic follicles extending into periglandular fat (left) and demonstrating reactivity for bcl-2 (right).

Histopathology

EMZBCL of the parotid gland occurs in a background of lymphoepithelial sialadenitis (LESA) in almost all cases. The histologic features include a vaguely nodular to diffuse heterogeneous B-cell infiltrate that totally or subtotally effaces the normal glandular architecture. It is variably comprised of atypical small lymphocytes, centrocyte-like (cleaved) cells, monocytoid B-cells, immunoblasts, lymphoplasmacytic cells and plasma cells. Plasma cell differentiation may be striking, causing confusion with a plasmacytoma. Intranuclear inclusions (Dutcher bodies) may be seen in the plasma or lymphoplasmacytic cells. Reactive germinal centres, often colonized by neoplastic B cells, are often present {1182}. Lymphoepithelial lesions, representing infiltration of the ductal and epithelial structures by neoplastic B cells, are seen in both LESA and EMZBCL. Ductal dilatation occasionally imparts a multicystic appearance to the gland. An important early change that occurs in EMZBCL of parotid gland, developing in the setting of LESA, is the formation of "halos", comprised of monocytoid and centrocyte-like B cells surrounding epimyoepithelial islands (lymphoepithelial lesion) {1162}. These cells may coalesce into broad, interconnecting sheets. Clusters of epithelioid histiocytes and prominent fibrosis may also be noted. There may be single or multifocal foci of large cell transformation adjacent to the low-grade component.

Immunoprofile

The B cell immunophenotype is confirmed by immunoreactivity for CD20 or CD79a. The lymphocytes and monocytoid B cells express surface immunoglobulin. The neoplastic B cells are negative for CD5, CD10, CD23 and bcl-1 (Cyclin D1). Bcl-2 reactivity in the neoplastic, colonizing B cells (but not in the residual, reactive germinal centre cells) is also characteristic. An antibody to cytokeratin may be useful to highlight the epithelial remnants in the lymphoepithelial lesions.

Differential diagnosis

The distinction between EMZBCL and LESA may be extremely difficult. Although histologic evaluation remains the gold standard for diagnosis, immunohistochemical, flow cytometric or molecular genetic analyses may be required. In both reactive follicular hyperplasia and EMZBCL, benign germinal centres are present but in the latter entity, the follicles may be colonized by neoplastic B-cells that express bcl-2. A dense diffuse B cell infiltrate, intranuclear inclusions (Dutcher bodies) and cytologic atypia are characteristically seen in EMZBCL. Lymphoepithelial lesions may be seen in both LESA and EMZBCL. The demonstration of light chain restriction by immunohistochemistry or flow cytometry supports the monoclonality of the B cell lymphoma. Extranodal marginal zone lymphoma with prominent nodularity may simulate a follicular lymphoma (FL). It is necessary, therefore, to distinguish the reactive, colonized germinal centres in EMZBCL from the neoplastic germinal centres in FL. The majority of cases of FL will show immunoreactivity for bcl-2 and will express the germinal centre cell markers CD10 and bcl-6.

Somatic genetics

There are clonal rearrangements of the immunoglobulin genes {2,104,608,630, 2103,2524}. The significance of this finding, however, is somewhat unclear and controversial since gene rearrangements have also been found in histologically benign cases of LESA {105,770,2103} and in the salivary gland lesions of Sjögren syndrome patients who subsequently developed overt lymphoma {1238}. The cell of origin of EMZBCL lymphoma has not been definitively identified and has been postulated to be of post germinal centre origin. In some cases, however, the variable regions of the immunoglobulin genes have been shown to undergo somatic hypermutation, suggesting that this tumour may arise from germinal centre B cells {104}. Although no specific oncogene has been described in association with MALT lymphoma, numerical chromosomal abnormalities, especially Trisomy 3 {293,2823, 2824}, and the chromosomal translocation, t (11;18) (q21;q21) {1961} have been reported in EMZBCL in various anatomic sites.

Prognosis and predictive factors

The prognosis of salivary gland EMZBCL lymphoma is usually very favourable. Tumours that are localized (Stage IE) at the time of presentation and demonstrate purely low-grade histology have an excellent prognosis. With lymph node involvement (Stage IIE), the prognosis is usually similar to primary nodal low-grade B cell lymphomas. Although EMZBCL of salivary gland may show histologic transformation to a higher grade, similar to what has been reported in the stomach, the clinical significance of this finding remains unclear. There is no conclusive evidence that treatment of EMZBCL prevents transformation to a higher grade. With or without treatment, EMZBCL of the salivary gland is usually an indolent neoplasm that does not result in significant morbidity or mortality. There are reports, however, of patients with EMZBCL associated with LESA subsequently developing extensive extra salivary gland lymphoma or nodal large B-cell lymphoma.

Salivary gland extramedullary plasmacytoma

Please refer to Chapter 1 for details.

Secondary tumours

T. Löning
K.T. Jäkel

Definition
A metastatic tumour involving salivary glands that originates in a distant site.

Epidemiology
Secondary tumours comprise about 5% of all malignant tumours of salivary glands {669,2293,2300}, but this incidence is considerably higher in some countries {199}. The peak incidence is in the 7-8th decade. Almost 70% of cases occur in males. The majority of cases are squamous cell carcinoma and melanoma is second in frequency.

Localization
The large majority of metastases are located in the parotid, while fewer are seen in the submandibular gland. Metastases occur within the interstitial tissue and the intra-/periglandular lymph nodes with a slight predominance of extranodal infiltrates {2300}.

Clinical features
Eighty percent of secondary tumours of the parotid are metastases from head and neck neoplasms. On the other hand, 85% of metastatic tumours in the sub-mandibular glands are from distant sites {899}. Primary sites frequently are the upper and middle parts of the facial region (including skin, mucous membranes, deep soft tissues as well as eyes and ears) {443,692,1917,1987}. A further 10% originate from distant tumours among which lung carcinoma (especially the small cell carcinoma type), kidney and breast carcinomas are the most common {669,806,1585,2219,2293, 2300}.
However, almost 10% of the secondary tumours remain undefined as to their origin.

Histopathology
Generally, metastases retain to some extent the histological pattern and cyto-logical characteristics of the respective primary tumour.

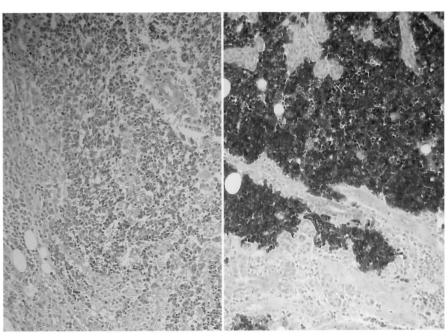

Fig. 5.82 Small cell carcinoma diffusely infiltrating the salivary gland tissue. Tumour cells are marked by immunoreactivity to synaptophysin (right).

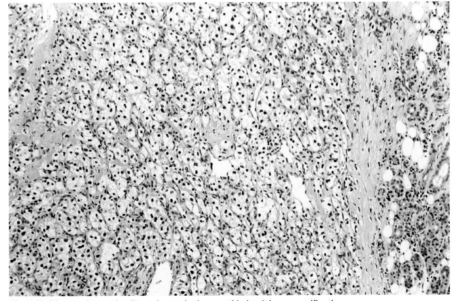

Fig. 5.83 Metastatic renal cell carcinoma in the parotid gland. Low magnification.

CHAPTER 6

Odontogenic Tumours

Odontogenic tumours and tumour-like lesions constitute a group of heterogeneous diseases that range from hamartomatous or non-neoplastic tissue proliferations to benign neoplasms to malignant tumours with metastatic potential. They are derived from epithelial, ectomesenchymal and/or mesenchymal elements of the tooth-forming apparatus. Odontogenic tumours are rare, some even extremely rare, but can pose a significant diagnostic and therapeutic challenge.

WHO histological classification of odontogenic tumours

MALIGNANT TUMOURS

Odontogenic carcinomas

Metastasizing (malignant) ameloblastoma[1]	9310/3
Ameloblastic carcinoma – primary type	9270/3
Ameloblastic carcinoma – secondary type (dedifferentiated), intraosseous	9270/3
Ameloblastic carcinoma – secondary type (dedifferentiated), peripheral	9270/3
Primary intraosseous squamous cell carcinoma – solid type	9270/3
Primary intraosseous squamous cell carcinoma derived from keratocystic odontogenic tumour	9270/3
Primary intraosseous squamous cell carcinoma derived from odontogenic cysts	9270/3
Clear cell odontogenic carcinoma	9341/3
Ghost cell odontogenic carcinoma	9302/3

Odontogenic sarcomas

Ameloblastic fibrosarcoma	9330/3
Ameloblastic fibrodentino–and fibro-odontosarcoma	9290/3

BENIGN TUMOURS

Odontogenic epithelium with mature, fibrous stroma without odontogenic ectomesenchyme

Ameloblastoma, solid / multicystic type	9310/0
Ameloblastoma, extraosseous / peripheral type	9310/0
Ameloblastoma, desmoplastic type	9310/0
Ameloblastoma, unicystic type	9310/0
Squamous odontogenic tumour	9312/0
Calcifying epithelial odontogenic tumour	9340/0
Adenomatoid odontogenic tumour	9300/0
Keratocystic odontogenic tumour	9270/0

Odontogenic epithelium with odontogenic ectomesenchyme, with or without hard tissue formation

Ameloblastic fibroma	9330/0
Ameloblastic fibrodentinoma	9271/0
Ameloblastic fibro-odontoma	9290/0
Odontoma	9280/0
Odontoma, complex type	9282/0
Odontoma, compound type	9281/0
Odontoameloblastoma	9311/0
Calcifying cystic odontogenic tumour	9301/0
Dentinogenic ghost cell tumour	9302/0

Mesenchyme and/or odontogenic ectomesenchyme with or without odontogenic epithelium

Odontogenic fibroma	9321/0
Odontogenic myxoma / myxofibroma	9320/0
Cementoblastoma	9273/0

Bone-related lesions

Ossifying fibroma	9262/0
Fibrous dysplasia	
Osseous dysplasias	
Central giant cell lesion (granuloma)	
Cherubism	
Aneurysmal bone cyst	
Simple bone cyst	

OTHER TUMOURS

Melanotic neuroectodermal tumour of infancy	9363/0
see Chapter 1, pp. 70-73	

---

[1] Morphology code of the International Classification of Diseases for Oncology (ICD-O) {821} and the Systematized Nomenclature of Medicine (http://snomed.org). Behaviour is coded /0 for benign tumours, /3 for malignant tumours, and /1 for borderline or uncertain behaviour.

Neoplasms and tumour-like lesions arising from the odontogenic apparatus and maxillofacial skeleton: Introduction

H.P. Philipsen
P.A.Reichart
P.J. Slootweg
L.J. Slater

Definition

Odontogenic tumours are lesions derived from epithelial, ectomesenchymal and/or mesenchymal elements that still are, or have been, part of the tooth-forming apparatus. These tumours, therefore, are found exclusively within the maxillofacial skeleton (intraosseous or centrally located), or in the soft tissue (gingiva) overlying tooth-bearing areas or alveolar mucosa in edentulous regions (extraosseous or peripherally located). The tumours may be generated at any stage in the life of an individual. Knowledge of basic clinical features such as age, gender, and location can be extremely valuable in developing differential diagnoses of odontogenic tumours.

Prior consensus conferences on taxonomy of odontogenic tumours, cysts and allied lesions {2048,2050,2051,2148, 2595} confirmed that the characteristic morphological and inductive relationship between the various parts of the normal tooth germ are reproduced, to a greater or lesser extent, in many of the tumours and tumour-like lesions of the odontogenic tissues. The observation of these features is important both in the identification of the lesions and in their classification. For example, normal dentin is easily identified because of its tubular structure, but if for some reason this tubular structure is absent it is difficult to distinguish between atypical poorly mineralized dentin (dentinoid) and atypical osteoid. However, if an osteoid-like tissue develops in direct juxtaposition to odontogenic epithelium, this relationship provides presumptive evidence that the material is dysplastic dentin.

The classification used here is based firstly on a lesion's behaviour, with a classification into benign, malignant and non-neoplastic. Subdivisions of "benign" lesions are then based on the types of odontogenic tissues involved: odontogenic epithelium with mature, fibrous stroma without odontogenic ectomesenchyme; odontogenic epithelium with odontogenic ectomesenchyme, with or without hard tissue formation; mesenchyme and / or odontogenic ectomesenchyme with or without the presence of odontogenic epithelium.

Epidemiology

Data from China, Hong Kong, Nigeria, Zimbabwe, Germany, Turkey, Japan, Canada, South Africa and the US show marked differences in relative frequencies between benign odontogenic tumours {1569,2110A}. According to the PRC study, the most frequent tumour was ameloblastoma, solid/multicystic type (A-S/M, 58.6%) comparable to that found in Hong Kong (59.4%), Japan (57%) and in two African countries (Zimbabwe and Nigeria), 79.1% and 58.5%, respectively. This contrasts with the rates in series involving populations in the US and Canada, where the most frequent tumour was odontoma (73.8% and 56.4%, respectively) with A-S/M accounting only for 12.2% and 14.8%, respectively. It seems that one reason for these discrepancies may be found in the source of the data. Odontogenic tumour patients from PRC, Hong Kong, Japan and several African countries are diagnosed and treated in Maxillofacial Units of Medical Hospitals, whereas patients from the US and Canada generally are monitored in Dental Schools or Hospitals. Odontomas frequently are diagnosed on routine panoramic images performed in a dentist's surgery or in a Dental School without previous biopsy. In several developing countries cases are not registered or

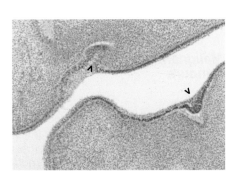

Fig. 6.1 Early stage of dental anlage with down growth of odontogenic epithelium (arrows).

sent for histological confirmation. Thus, the frequency of odontomas reported from these countries is probably underestimated. Ameloblastomas (A-S/Ms) on the other hand need a biopsy for confirmation of the diagnosis, and the radical treatment is often performed in a Medical Hospital. As it has been suggested that ameloblastomas are more common in Blacks than in Caucasians, it remains to be proved that the geographical variation suggested by the above data may also be based on ethnic differences. Benign odontogenic neoplasms (including hamartomatous lesions) seem to outnumber their malignant counterparts by a factor as high as 100 {531}.

Etiology

The etiology of benign and malignant odontogenic tumours is unknown. The majority of odontogenic tumours seem to arise de novo, without an apparent causative factor.

Clinical features

The large majority of odontogenic tumours occurs intraosseously within the maxillofacial skeleton, while extraosseous odontogenic tumours occur nearly always in the tooth-bearing mucosa. The clinical features of most benign odontogenic tumours are non-specific; benign odontogenic tumours show slow expansive growth with no or slight pain. In contrast, pain is the first and most common symptom followed by rapidly developing swelling in nearly all malignant odontogenic tumours. The tumour may erode or break through the cortex of the jaw bones.

Imaging

Because odontogenic tumours may be composed of soft and hard tissues, their radiographic appearance will vary from radiolucent to radiopaque. Intraoral dental (plain) radiographs are usually the first means to identify the presence of an intrabony lesion. Panoramic radiography is mandatory as a component of the diagnostic protocol. For the diagnosis of

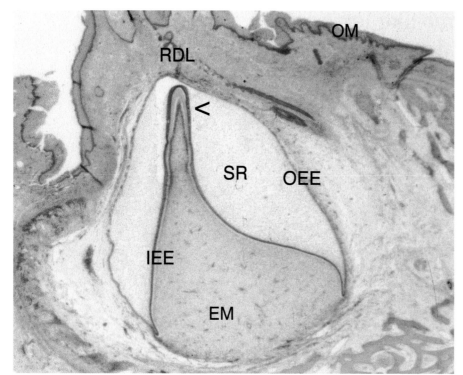

Fig. 6.2 Dental anlage with initial formation of dental hard structures (<). EM, ectomesenchyme; OM, oral mucosa. RDL, rests of dental lamina; SR, stellate reticulum; OEE, outer enamel epithelium; IEE, inner enamel epithelium.

odontogenic tumours cross-sectional imaging studies (CT, MRI) cover both topography and fine structure of the lesion, and give valuable information about tumour extension.

Precursor lesions

Developmental odontogenic cysts may contribute to the formation of certain odontogenic tumours and intraosseous squamous cell carcinoma.

Odontogenesis and genetics

Odontogenesis depends on the sequential and reciprocal interactions between cranial neural crest (CNC)-derived ectomesenchymal cells and the epithelium that lines the oral cavity {357}. Contact of these CNC-cells with oral epithelium initiates tooth development by the formation of an epithelial tooth bud with a surrounding condensation of CNC cells. It is not yet clear whether the initial odontogenic potential lies in CNC cells inducing the epithelium to form the tooth bud or the converse, CNC cells responding to an inductive stimulus from the oral epithelial lining {2897}. After these initial events, the dental epithelium has acquired the ability to instruct tooth formation when combined with CNC cells

from regions normally not contributing to odontogenesis but subsequently, this instructive potential shifts to the dental mesenchyme as exemplified by combination studies with nondental epithelium {2897}.

Experimental and family cluster studies of the molecular events associated with tooth development have resulted in the identification of over 200 genes playing a role in this area {464}. Of these, the fibroblast growth factor–8 partitions the jaw into an alveolar and a basal part, whereas sonic hedgehog is involved with the formation of the tooth bud {464}. Expression of both these genes in turn induces upregulation of additional genes, both in epithelium and ectomesenchyme as odontogenesis proceeds.

Malignant odontogenic tumours

Definition

Most malignant odontogenic tumours are generally considered the counterparts of benign odontogenic tumours, but others such as the primary intraosseous squamous cell carcinoma are not.

Classification

Malignant odontogenic tumours (MOTs) are classified as odontogenic carcinomas and odontogenic sarcomas. Odontogenic carcinosarcoma as included in the previous WHO classification {2051} and more recently discussed {2394} is not included in the present classification due to lack of evidence for its existence as an entity.

Epidemiology

Generally, MOTs are rare entities. Some of them are exceedingly rare. Odontogenic carcinomas seem to occur more frequently in the elderly {2402}.

Etiology

The etiology of MOTs is unknown.

Clinical features / Imaging

Clinical symptoms are identical to those of other malignant tumours in the maxillofacial region. Swelling, pain, bleeding, ulceration of the oral mucosa, mobility of teeth, paraesthesia or anaesthesia may be indicators of a MOT. Involvement of local lymph nodes and distant metastases may occur early in the course of the disease. Extensive jaw bone destruction with ill defined borders are characteristic and in addition a mixed radiographic pattern may be evident. Hard tissue structures may be diagnosed on plain radiographs, CTs or MRIs.

Therapy

Due to the small number of published cases of MOTs specific treatment protocols or guidelines are at present not available. Surgical resection with tumour-free margins is the therapy of choice.

Precursor lesions

In some cases MOTs have been demonstrated to develop from preexisting benign counterparts.

Prognosis and predictive factors

Generally, the prognosis for MOTs is poor.

Odontogenic / ameloblastic carcinomas

J.J. Sciubba
L.R. Eversole
P.J. Slootweg

Metastasizing ameloblastoma

Definition
Metastasizing ameloblastoma is an ameloblastoma that metastasizes in spite of a benign histologic appearance.

ICD-O code
Metastasizing (malignant)
ameloblastoma   9310/3

General features
Metastasizing ameloblastoma shows no specific features different from ameloblastomas that do not metastasize. Therefore, this diagnosis can only be made in retrospect, after the occurrence of metastatic deposits. Thus, it is clinical behaviour and not histology that justifies a diagnosis of metastasizing ameloblastoma. Ameloblastomas with atypia are ameloblastic carcinomas {1875}. Confusion may also arise through the use of the term atypical ameloblastoma to denote lesions with fatal outcome for various reasons, either metastasis, histological atypia or relentless local spread {50}. Metastatic deposits of ameloblastomas are mostly seen in the lung {1386,1439, 2405} but have also been reported at other sites.

Ameloblastic carcinoma – primary type

Definition
The ameloblastic carcinoma is a rare pri-

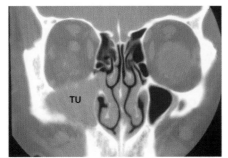

Fig. 6.3 Ameloblastic carcinoma. Large, osteodestructive tumour of the right maxillary sinus with extension into the orbit. (TU, tumour)

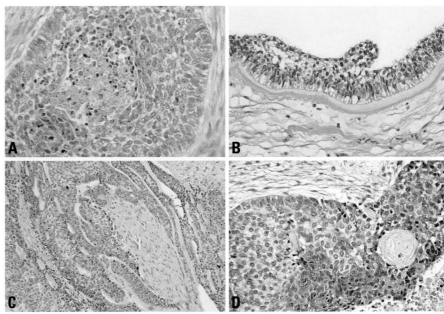

Fig. 6.4 Ameloblastic carcinoma. **A** A focus of comedonecrosis lies within an island of ameloblastic cells demonstrating cellular atypia, mitotic activity and individual cell necrosis. **B** Early carcinomatous changes are present within the lining of this cystic ameloblastic carcinoma. **C** Cords and seams of malignant cells surround and infiltrate a medium sized peripheral nerve. **D** A small peripheral nerve lies within an island of ameloblastic carcinoma. Within the island are numerous necrotic cells with pyknotic nuclei.

mary odontogenic malignancy that combines the histological features of ameloblastoma with cytological atypia. This will be the case even in the absence of metastases.

ICD-O code   9270/3

Epidemiology
The incidence of ameloblastic carcinoma is unknown, fewer than 60 cases have been reported. The reason for the high number of reported cases from China where 6.7% of all odontogenic tumours are malignant is not clear. {1569}.

Clinical features / Imaging
Approximately 2/3 of ameloblastic carcinomas involve the mandible {492,1813}. Only 19 cases have been reported to occur in the maxilla {593}. Males and females are equally affected. The posterior segments of the jaws represent the most common site. Generally, ill defined or irregularly marginated radiolucencies are characteristic. Cortical expansion often with perforation, may be present as well as infiltration into adjacent structures

Histopathology
Ameloblastic carcinoma is characterized by malignant cytologic features in combination with the overall histological pattern of an ameloblastoma. A tall columnar cellular morphology with pleomorphism, mitotic activity, focal necrosis, perineural invasion and nuclear hyperchromatism may be present. Peripheral palisading and so-called reverse or inverted nuclear polarity will be present. A stellate reticulum structure will usually be seen. Cystic spaces may be present that are lined by epithelium {497}.
Atypical cells form nests and broad ribbons which may branch and anastomose with focal areas of subtle necrosis to more obvious central, comedo necrosis-like areas. Ameloblastic carcinomas show a high proliferation index compared to benign ameloblastomas by

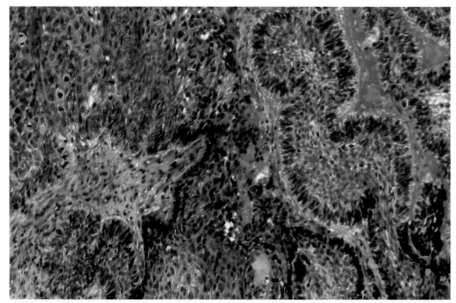

Fig. 6.5 Ameloblastic carcinoma, secondary type. Islands with atypical cells and increased mitotic activity (left) are juxtaposed to typical ameloblastoma (right) with palisading and reversed nuclear polarity of peripheral cells.

virtue of an increased index of proliferating cell nuclear antigen in addition to higher levels of aneuploidy {1315,1793}.

Differential diagnosis

The differential diagnosis includes ameloblastomas which may show an occasional mitotic figure. Other odontogenic carcinomas including primary intraosseous squamous cell carcinoma and clear cell odontogenic carcinoma are usually distinct; however, some ameloblastic carcinomas have been reported to show clear cell features and yet others may contain a spindle cell component. Metastatic carcinomas should also be considered; however, they do not display ameloblastic features.

Somatic genetics

Aneuploidy has been found to be more frequently present in the ameloblastic carcinoma and may be used as a strong predictor of malignant potential of questionable lesions {1793}. More recently 5q13 amplification was demonstrated by comparative genomic hybridization (CGH) in an ameloblastic carcinoma {1289}.

Prognosis and predictive factors

Maxillary ameloblastic carcinomas demonstrate tumour-related deaths or pulmonary metastases in over one-third of cases {593}. Mandibular counterparts

behave in a similar manner, where local recurrences are likely to precede metastases {2363}.

Ameloblastic carcinoma – secondary type (dedifferentiated), intraosseous

Definition

Ameloblastic carcinoma arises in a pre-existing benign ameloblastoma. The term "dedifferentiated ameloblastoma" has been applied when morphologic features of typical ameloblastoma were noted {1029,2405,2651}. This in turn separates metastazising ameloblastoma since cytologic atypia is not a feature of this entity.

ICD-O code   9270/3

Synonym

Carcinoma ex intraosseous ameloblastoma

Epidemiology

Dedifferentiated ameloblastoma or ameloblastic carcinoma arising within a pre-existing microscopically verified benign ameloblastoma is a very rare occurrence. Most cases arise in older individuals (7th decade) {1029,2651}, usually with a clinically proven long-standing ameloblastoma.

Clinical features / Imaging

As per the definition of the entity, a prior benign or conventional ameloblastoma must be present initially, followed by development of malignant behaviour. Often, multiple local jaw recurrences will precede this transformation, as well as prior radiation therapy {2405}. Heralding the transformation is a corresponding shift from the typical radiographic presentation of an ameloblastoma of slow growth to one of more rapid bony expansion with infiltration of tumour beyond the buccal and lingual cortices, with invasion into the adjacent soft tissues {548}.

Histopathology

Clusters or nests and islands of epithelium within a collagenous stroma are composed of a peripheral layer of polarized cells enclosing stellate to basaloid cells in the early transition or de-differentiation stage. Individual cellular features include pleomorphism, frequent mitotic figures, indistinct cell membranes, focal necrosis, loss of cellular cohesion, and infiltration along nerve bundles {548}.

Prognosis and predictive factors

Proximity of the lesion to vital structures including the orbit, cranial base and pterygomaxillary fossa are important in gaining surgical access on one hand and clear surgical margins on the other, thus impacting on survival. As with the de novo ameloblastic carcinoma, prognosis must remain guarded over an observation period of several years.

Ameloblastic carcinoma – secondary type (dedifferentiated), peripheral

Definition

Transformation of a pre-existing peripheral extraosseous ameloblastoma to a malignant cellular phenotype {1673, 1674}. Prior cases of so-called intraoral basal cell carcinomas (gingiva) may, in retrospect, be considered within this category as well {102,635,2033,2780}.

ICD-O code   9270/3

Synonym

Carcinoma ex peripheral ameloblastoma

Epidemiology

To date six cases of an ameloblastic carcinoma arising within a preexisting peripheral ameloblastoma with a 1:1 gender distribution have been reported {2033}.

Clinical features/Imaging

A gingival mass with variable surface alterations including irregularity, concavity, sessile, and pedunculated features as well as alveolar bone resorption have characterized the previously reported cases of transformed peripheral ameloblastoma. They are generally nontender, and may be associated with a developing inter-radicular radiolucency with separation of the roots of adjacent teeth {102,1674}.

Histopathology

Nests, strands and follicles of recognizable ameloblastoma-type histology within the gingival soft tissues may be noted in association with variable degrees of squamous differentiation. An extensive network of tumour islands with peripherally located columnar cells and stellate reticulum-type areas will be present. Nests of keratin, cellular and nuclear pleomorphism, and abnormal mitotic figures will extend to and invade alveolar bone and around peripheral nerves {320}.

Prognosis and predictive factors

Wide local excision with en bloc resection of the involved segment of the affected jaw bone is the treatment of choice. Long-term follow-up is mandatory {2780}.

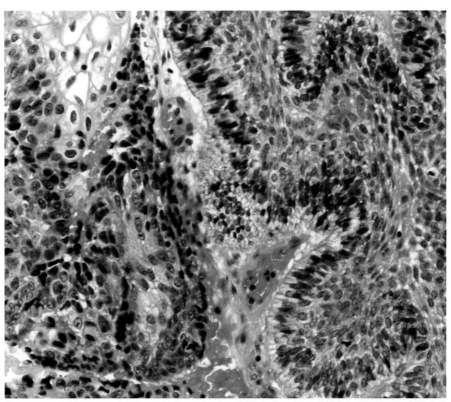

Fig. 6.6 Ameloblastic carcinoma, secondary type. Aggregates of moderately differentiated squamous cell carcinoma abutting ameloblastoma with peripheral palisading of tumour cells and central parts reminiscent of stellate reticulum.

Primary intraosseous squamous cell carcinomas

L.R. Eversole
C.H. Siar
I. van der Waal

Primary intraosseous squamous cell carcinoma - solid type

Definition
Primary intraosseous squamous cell carcinoma (PIOSCC) is a central jaw carcinoma derived from odontogenic epithelial remnants. Subcategories of PIOSCC include (1) a solid tumour that invades marrow spaces and induces osseous resorption, (2) squamous cancer arising from the lining of an odontogenic cyst and (3) a squamous cell carcinoma in association with other benign epithelial odontogenic tumours. When the tumour destroys the cortex and merges with the surface mucosa, it may be difficult to distinguish between a PIOSCC and a true carcinoma arising from the oral mucosa. Invasion from an antral primary must also be excluded.

ICD-O code   9270/3

Synonym
Primary intra-alveolar epidermoid carcinoma

Epidemiology
The male: female ratio approaches 2:1, with a mean age of 55 years, although cases have been encountered during infancy.

Etiology
These tumours arise centrally in the jaws, with no communication with the upper

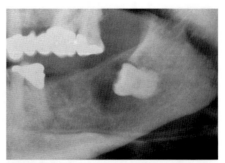

Fig. 6.7 Primary intraosseous squamous cell carcinoma, cystogenic, non-keratinizing cyst. Dentigerous cyst of a lower wisdom tooth, showing an ill defined outline.

aerodigestive tract mucosa and are therefore not subjected to exposure of the usual carcinogenic factors.

Localization
PIOSCC is more often found in the body and posterior mandible than the maxilla. Maxillary cases are most frequently seen in the anterior segment.

Clinical features
Signs and symptoms
Most cases are asymptomatic and are discovered incidentally during the course of routine dental radiographs. Facial swelling may be observed. Perineural invasion of the inferior alveolar nerve will produce paresthesia of the lip.

Imaging
Radiographically, PIOSCCs are osteolytic. The margins of the radiolucency are often irregular and noncorticated. Larger

extensive lesions may show cortical bone expansion and destruction.

Tumour spread and staging
PIOSCC spreads both regionally and distantly.

Macroscopy
Gross features of PIOSCCs are those of any carcinoma within bone.

Histopathology
PIOSCC is characterized by islands of neoplastic squamous epithelium with the features of squamous cell carcinoma. Most lesions are moderately differentiated without prominent keratinization. The stroma may or may not exhibit an inflammatory infiltrate. Metastatic squamous cell carcinoma has to be excluded. There are no specific histopathologic features that distinguish a metastatic squamous cancer from PIOSCC. When the central jaw carcinoma can be documented histologically to arise from the epithelial lining of an odontogenic cyst, primary site of origin is accepted. Mucoepidermoid carcinoma also arises from the lining of odontogenic cysts and must be included in the differential diagnosis. Special staining for mucin may be helpful.

Histogenesis
Carcinomas that arise centrally within the jaw bones putatively arise from epithelial remnants of odontogenesis that include the periradicular rests of Malassez and

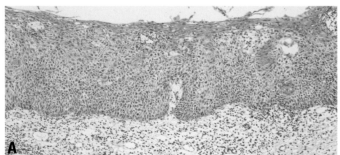
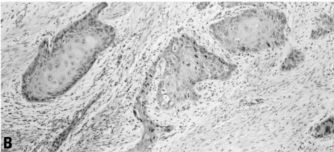

Fig. 6.8 Primary intraosseous squamous cell carcinoma, cystogenic, non-keratinizing cyst. **A** Part of the cyst wall showing epithelial dysplasia. **B** In other areas well differentiated squamous cell carcinoma was present as observed in the solid type.

the reduced enamel epithelium surrounding impacted teeth {2397}. Rarely, a central jaw squamous cell carcinoma represents dedifferentiation from a benign ameloblastoma {2651}.

Primary intraosseous squamous cell carcinoma derived from keratocystic odontogenic tumour

Definition
A squamous cell carcinoma arising within the jaws without connection to the oral mucosa in the presence of an a keratocystic odontogenic tumour (KCOT).

ICD-O code   9270/3

Epidemiology
Thirteen cases of primary intraosseous squamous cell carcinoma deriving from KCOT have been documented {1305, 1615}. Most of these lesions are encountered in older patients, 40 years and above, with male predilection.

Etiology
There are no known specific predisposing factors.

Localization
The mandible is involved much more frequently than the maxilla {1305}.

Clinical features / Imaging
Early lesions are generally insidious {1305,1615}, usually presenting as a benign odontogenic cyst and the diagnosis of carcinoma is only made after microscopic examination. In others, local symptoms relate to the effects of the lesion at specific sites i.e. pain, swelling, loosening of teeth, non-healing extraction sockets, and paraesthesia. Lesions in advanced disease stage frequently appear as overtly malignant growths with associated ulceration and induration. Regional lymphadenopathy may also be present.
Radiographically, early lesions are often indistinguishable from any odontogenic cyst. In some, the margins of the radiolucent defect appear irregular and 'ragged.' Late lesions are obviously destructive. A multilocular appearance with cortical destruction and frequent soft tissue extension characterizes these late-stage neoplasms.

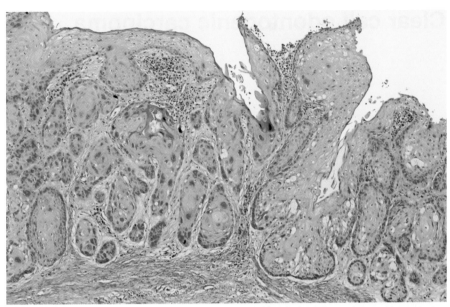

Fig. 6.9 Primary intraosseous squamous cell carcinoma (PIOSCC) derived from odontogenic cyst. The lining of the odontogenic cyst (upper left) shows severe dysplasia with transition to an invasive focally keratinized squamous cell carcinoma.

Histopathology
The histological appearance of this lesion is typically that of a keratinizing well-differentiated squamous cell carcinoma in conjunction with KCOT. The main differential diagnosis would include keratoameloblastoma, squamous odontogenic tumour, central high-grade mucoepidermoid carcinoma and metastatic lesions {1305}.

Genetics
One case of mandibular odontogenic carcinoma revealed abnormalities in a small subset of genes {34}.

Prognosis and predictive factors
Lack of information precludes definitive prognostication.

Primary intraosseous squamous cell carcinoma derived from odontogenic cysts

Definition
A squamous cell carcinoma arising within the jaws without connection to the oral mucosa, and in the presence of an odontogenic cyst other than keratocystic odontogenic tumour.

ICD-O code   9270/3

Epidemiology
There are less than fifty well-documented

cases. In a series of 28 patients the mean age was 56 years and the male to female ratio was almost 2:1.

Clinical features / Imaging
The majority occur in the mandible with symptoms of pain, paraesthesia or anaesthesia of the lower lip. The radiographic aspect may mimic any type of odontogenic cyst.

Histopathology
Histopathologically, the tumour is characterized as a cyst lined by any type of epithelium that can be seen in odontogenic cysts in association with a squamous cell carcinoma. Various degrees of dysplasia may be observed in the epithelial cyst lining. The architecture of verrucous hyperplasia or verrucous carcinoma may be present, as well.

Prognosis and predictive factors
PIOSCC associated with an impacted lower third molar seems to have a favourable prognosis; however, the number of reported cases is small.

Clear cell odontogenic carcinoma

G. Bang
H. Koppang

Definition

Clear cell odontogenic carcinoma (CCOC) is characterized by sheets and islands of vacuolated and clear cells.

ICD-O code   9341/3

Historical annotation

In the past CCOC was called clear cell ameloblastoma {2712} and clear cell odontogenic tumour {699,1004} and was considered a benign tumour in the previous WHO classification of 1992 {2051}.

Epidemiology

Only 36 cases have been reported during the last 15 years. The tumour has a strong female predilection and tends to occur in older adults, the mean age at diagnosis being close to 60 years, range 17-89 {1784}.

Localization

The most frequently affected site is the mandible.

Clinical features / Imaging

The CCOC usually causes swelling of the jaws and loosening of teeth. Aggressive tumour growth results in an ill-defined radiolucency, and root resorption may occur {114}.

Histopathology

A biphasic pattern is often exhibited. CCOC is primarily composed of a fibrous stroma with islands of epithelial cells revealing clear to faintly eosinophilic cytoplasm, well-demarcated cell membranes and irregular dark-staining nuclei. Also cords of dark-staining basaloid cells with scant eosinophilic cytoplasm may be seen {114}. In addition, ameloblastomatous islands with palisaded peripheral cells may be observed.

Mitoses and necrosis are rare. Histochemically, many of the tumour cells contain abundant delicate and coarse diastase degradable PAS-positive granules, but they are negative for mucin and amyloid {114,521}.

Immunoprofile

The clear and eosinophilic tumour cells are consistently reactive for cytokeratins 13, 14, 19, 8, 18 and EMA. They are negative for vimentin, S-100-protein, desmin, smooth muscle actin, HMB-45, alpha (1)-chymotrypsin, CD31, CD45 and GFAP {114,521,699,1172,1499}.

Differential diagnosis

Since clear cells frequently may be seen in other neoplasms in the oral and maxillofacial region, it is important to rule out lesions like salivary gland tumours, melanotic tumours, metastatic renal cell carcinoma and clear cell variant of calcifying epithelial odontogenic tumour {1172,1784,2040}.

Genetics

DNA-analysis has shown a polyploid population with DNA index of 1.93 and an S-phase of 10.2% {114}. Comparative genomic hybridization discloses consistent chromosomal aberrations in both primary and metastatic CCOC {275}.

Prognosis and predictive factors

The CCOC exhibits an aggressive growth pattern and frequently recurs. The tumour can metastasize to regional lymph nodes and lungs, as well as to bone, and tumour progression may even cause tumour related death.

Consequently, resection with tumour-free margins is the treatment of choice, and long-term follow-up is mandatory. Adjuvant radiotherapy is a rational option for tumours that have eroded cortical bone {256}.

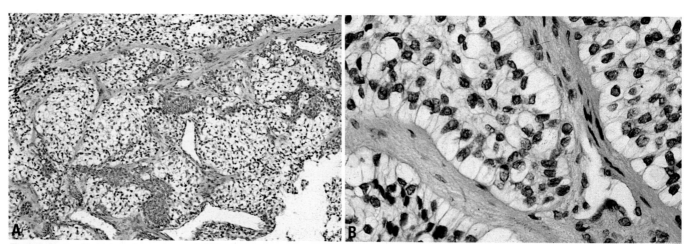

Fig. 6.10 Clear cell odontogenic carcinoma. **A** Biphasic tumour pattern with sheets of clear cells and irregular cords and strands of dark, basaloid cells, intersected by narrow bands of fibrous stroma. **B** Sheets of polygonal cells with central clear or faintly eosinophilic cytoplasm, well defined cell membrane and dark, peripheral or central nucleus. Peripheral cells abutting on narrow fibrous bands are palisaded. Tumour cells show clear cytoplasm with apical nucleus.

Ghost cell odontogenic carcinoma

T. Takata
Y. Lu

Definition
Ghost cell odontogenic carcinoma is a malignant odontogenic epithelial tumour with features of calcifying cystic odontogenic tumour and/or dentinogenic ghost cell tumour.

ICD-O code   9302/3

Synonyms
Calcifying ghost cell odontogenic carcinoma, malignant epithelial odontogenic ghost cell tumour, carcinoma arising in a calcifying odontogenic cyst, aggressive epithelial ghost cell odontogenic tumour, malignant calcifying odontogenic cyst and malignant calcifying ghost cell odontogenic tumour.

Epidemiology
Only 19 cases have been reported in the English literature and more than half of them were from Asia. The tumour occurs more commonly in men than women (male: female=2:1) and affects patients in the age range of 13-72 years with a peak incidence in the fourth decade.

Localization
The tumour occurs more commonly in the maxilla than the mandible (2:1), either at anterior or posterior area, corresponding to the site distribution of the calcifying odontogenic cyst. {297}.

Clinical features / Imaging
Clinical features include swelling, often with paraesthesia. Imaging shows a poorly demarcated, osteolytic radiolucency with some radiopaque material. Displacement of tooth roots is common and tooth impaction and root resorption are occasionally noted. Large lesions in the maxilla often destroy the sinus wall, grow into the nasal and orbital cavities, and extend to adjacent structures.

Macroscopy
A typical lesion consists of a well-circumscribed cystic portion and a solid portion with gritty consistency on cut-surface, although some are completely solid.

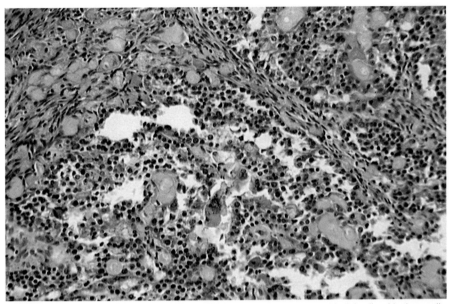

Fig. 6.11 Ghost cell odontogenic carcinoma. An admixture of the malignant epithelial cells with ghost cells is characteristic.

Histopathology
The diagnosis of the neoplasm is based on the identification of a malignant epithelial tumour containing classic benign features of calcifying cystic odontogenic tumour. The malignant component consists of rounded epithelial islands in a fibrous stroma. The epithelial cells are either small, rounded with dark nuclei or larger with vesicular nuclei. Many mitoses are seen. Ghost cells are found in varying numbers either isolated or in clusters. Dysplastic dentin may be present {1314,1568}. The relationship of the benign and malignant features appears to have two distinct forms. In the first pattern, the malignant epithelial component is physically separated from the classical benign lesion, which is either cystic or solid. The other pattern is an admixture of the malignant epithelial component with typical benign features {672,1260,1568}. PCNA labelling index is a possible parameter in differentiating the ghost cell odontogenic carcinoma from its benign counterparts. PCNA labelling indices (65.9±7.3% and 65.2±5.6%) in the malignant epithelial cells are significantly higher than in the benign neoplastic (45.8%) and cystic variants (29.3% and 11.6%) {1460,2536}. Immunohistochemical overexpression of p53 protein is demonstrated in the tumour cells {1568}.

Prognosis and predictive factors
The prognosis is unpredictable due to a wide spectrum of growth patterns. They vary from a slowly growing, locally invasive tumour to a highly aggressive and rapidly growing neoplasm with local recurrence and metastasis. The overall five-year survival rate is 73%. Recurrences are common {341,1260, 1314,1568,2536}.

Odontogenic sarcomas

R. Carlos
M. Altini
Y. Takeda

Ameloblastic fibrosarcoma

Definition
Ameloblastic fibrosarcoma (AFS) is an odontogenic tumour with a benign epithelial and a malignant ectomesenchymal component. It is regarded as the malignant counterpart of the ameloblastic fibroma (AF).

ICD-O code   9330/3

Synonym
Ameloblastic sarcoma

Epidemiology
There is a wide age range (3-89 years) with a mean age of 27.5 years at diagnosis, versus the AF (14.8 years) {2034}. Patients with AFS derived from a preexisting AF have a mean age of 33 years {1794}. Those with de novo AFS have a mean age of 22.9 years {266}. Sixty three percent of reported cases have occurred in males and 37% in females.

Etiology
The etiology of AFS is unknown. Approximately one third of AFS represents malignant transformation of a preexisting AF.

Localization
The mandible is the most commonly affected site (78%), followed by the max-illa (20%) {266}. In both jaws the posterior region is the site of predilection. Only one case of peripheral AFS has been published.

Clinical features / Imaging
Typically, AFS presents as an expansile intraosseous radiolucency with ill-defined borders {2394}. Swelling and pain are common findings. Paraesthesia has been observed {266}.

Macroscopy
AFS has a fleshy consistency, with a white to yellowish cut surface.

Histopathology
The histologic pattern of AFS resembles ameloblastic fibroma in which the epithelial tissue is benign but the connective tissue component is malignant. The epithelium is composed of budding and branching cords of small polygonal epithelial cells admixed with islands and knots. Larger islands have a border of columnar cells with hyperchromatic nuclei. A hypercellular connective tissue stroma displaying mitotically active cells surrounds the epithelial component {2394}. Recurrent tumours tend to show greater stromal cellularity and mitotic rate. In addition, the amount of the epithelial component may decrease or disappear {2394,2539}.

Prognosis and predictive factors
The biologic behaviour of AFS is that of a highly locally aggressive neoplasm with extremely low potential for distant metastasis. Of 64 cases only one had metastasis to mediastinal nodes and liver {266, 440,532,917,1794}.

Ameloblastic fibrodentino – and fibro-odontosarcoma

Definition
A tumour with histological features of ameloblastic fibrosarcoma, together with dysplastic dentin (fibro-dentinosarcoma) and/or enamel/enameloid and dentin/dentinoid (fibro-odontosarcoma).

ICD-O code   9290/3

Synonyms
Ameloblastic dentinosarcoma; ameloblastic odontosarcoma; ameloblastic sarcoma; odontogenic sarcoma.

Epidemiology
To date only fourteen cases have been reported in the literature {266,1794, 2539}. Nine cases occurred in men and four in women. The age range is 12-83 years with a peak in the third decade.

Clinical features / Imaging
Most cases present a slow growing pain-

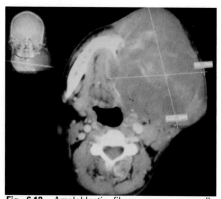

Fig. 6.12 Ameloblastic fibrosarcoma, unusually extensive, destroying the left mandible. [Courtesy Dr. A. Meneses, Istituto de Cancerologia, Mexico].

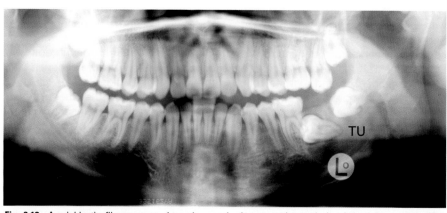

Fig. 6.13 Ameloblastic fibrosarcoma. Irregular poorly demarcated osteolysis of the left mandible (TU, tumour).

less jaw swelling. Radiographically, the lesions are radiolucent, sometimes multilocular with poorly circumscribed outlines. One or more dense opacities representing the hard tissue components may be present.

Precursor lesions
Ameloblastic fibro-odontomas are regarded as possible precursor lesions {46,1135,1794}.

Histopathology
The tumour shows the typical features of ameloblastic fibrosarcoma in addition to the formation of dental hard tissues in scattered areas {46,1462,2540,2814}.

Prognosis and predictive factors
The treatment of choice is surgical resection {46,2394}. Ameloblastic sarcomas seem to have a better prognosis than other jaw sarcomas and can generally be regarded as low-grade. Only one case has shown regional metastases. Local recurrences are more often seen {2540}.

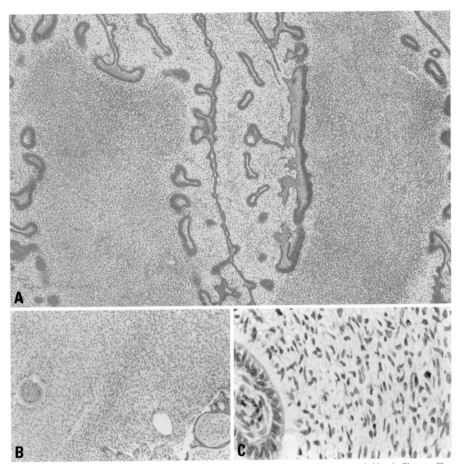

Fig. 6.14 Ameloblastic fibrosarcoma. **A** At low magnification, the tumour has an ameloblastic fibroma-like pattern. **B** Nests and cords of odontogenic epithelium in a highly cellular odontogenic ectomesenchyme. **C** Marked pleomorphism and mitotic figures in odontogenic ectomesenchyme adjacent to an epithelial island.

Ameloblastomas

D.G. Gardner
K. Heikinheimo
M. Shear
H.P. Philipsen
H. Coleman

Ameloblastoma, solid / multicystic type

Definition
The solid/multicystic ameloblastoma (A-S/M) is a slowly growing, locally invasive, epithelial odontogenic tumour of the jaws with a high rate of recurrence if not removed adequately, but with virtually no tendency to metastasize.

ICD-O code
9310/0

Synonyms
Conventional ameloblastoma; classical intraosseous ameloblastoma.

Epidemiology
Although rare, the A-S/M is the second most common odontogenic tumour. It exhibits no gender predilection and occurs over a wide age range. Most cases are diagnosed between 30 and 60 years of age, while the tumour is rare below the age of 20 years. Geographic and racial differences have been described {1431,2325}.

Etiology
The cause of A-S/M is not known. Dysregulation of several genes in normal tooth development may play a role in its histogenesis {1048}.

Localization
The tumour occurs exclusively in the jaws, rarely in the sinonasal cavities. Approximately 80% occur in the mandible, with a marked predilection for the posterior region, except in African Blacks in whom any region of the mandible may be involved, particularly the symphysis {427}. Most maxillary examples occur in the posterior region.

Clinical features / Imaging
Small A-S/Ms may be asymptomatic. More commonly, A-S/Ms present as variably sized swellings of the jaws. Pain or paraesthesia are rare. A-S/Ms may be unilocular or multilocular radiolucencies resembling cysts and they may reveal scalloped borders. An unerupted tooth may be associated with A-S/M. Resorption of the roots of adjacent teeth is common. Definitive diagnosis of A-S/Ms cannot be made radiologically, since similar radiographic features are displayed by e.g. keratocystic odontogenic tumour or myxoma. Particularly for maxillary A-S/Ms, CT-scans or MRIs are recommended.

Tumour spread and staging
A-S/Ms spread slowly by infiltration through the medullary spaces and may erode cortical bone. Eventually, it will resorb the cortical plate and may extend into adjacent tissues. Tumours of the posterior maxilla tend to obliterate the maxillary sinus and subsequently extend intracranially.

Histopathology
There are two basic histopathologic patterns, the follicular and plexiform, without clinical relevance. The follicular pattern consists of islands of odontogenic epithelium within a fibrous stroma. Typically, the basal cells of these islands are columnar, hyperchromatic, and lined up in a palisaded fashion. Typically their nuclei are displaced away from the basement membrane, and their cytoplasm is generally vacuolated. The central cells may be loosely arranged, resembling

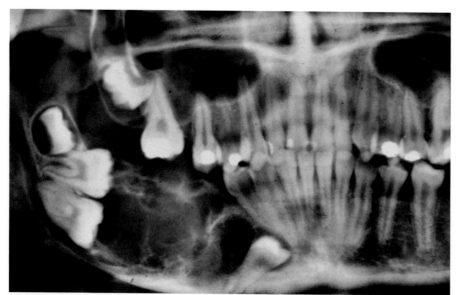

Fig. 6.15 Ameloblastoma, solid / multicystic type. Multilocular (soap bubble-like) radiolucency of the right horizontal and ascending ramus of the mandible including a number of impacted teeth.

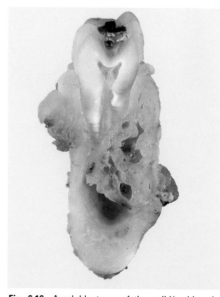

Fig. 6.16 Ameloblastoma of the solid/multicystic type consisting of friable brownish tissue.

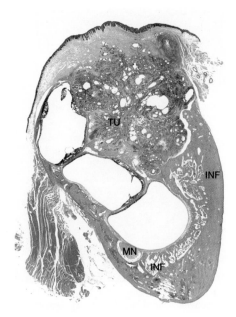

Fig. 6.17 Whole mount section of an ameloblastoma with cystic change, bone destruction and infiltration of overlying gingiva (TU, tumour, INF, intrabony infiltration, MN, mandibular nerve).

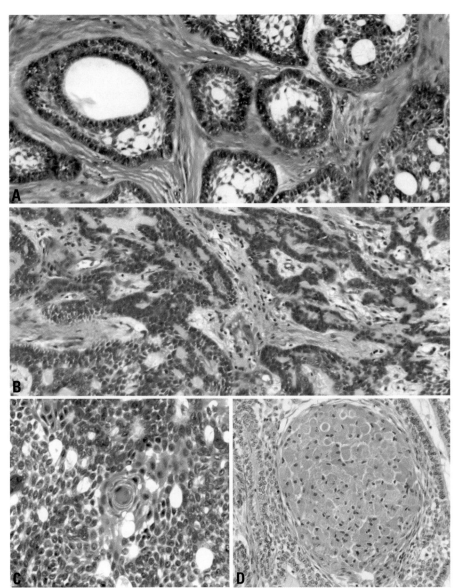

Fig. 6.18 Ameloblastoma **A** Follicular pattern with tumour island showing peripheral palisading and central cystic degeneration. **B** Plexiform pattern with anastomosing strands and cords of tumour cells. **C** Focal keratinization in acanthomatous ameloblastoma. **D** Eosinophilic granulation of cytoplasm in granular ameloblastoma.

stellate reticulum. These areas often become cystic and at times confluent. If these cells are spindle-shaped, basaloid, granular or showing squamous differentiation, the terms spindle cell ameloblastoma, basal cell ameloblastoma, granular ameloblastoma and acanthomatous ameloblastoma have been used. In addition ghost cells may be observed.

The plexiform pattern contains basal cells arranged in anastomosing strands with an inconspicuous stellate reticulum. The stroma is usually delicate, often with cyst-like degeneration.

For both histologic patterns, mitotic activity and cellular pleomorphism are rarely noted. The microscopic differential diagnosis may include ameloblastic fibroma, squamous odontogenic tumour, adenomatoid odontogenic tumour, odontogenic remnants in dental follicles, epithelial-rich odontogenic fibroma, calcifying odontogenic cyst and adenoid cystic carcinoma arising form the maxillary sinus.

Genetics

A recent study using comparative genomic hybridization described chromosomal aberrations in 2 of 17 A-S/Ms {1191}. A notably homogeneous gene profile in eight examples has been shown by cDNA array. Thirty-four of the 588 genes studied, demonstrated differ-

ences in ameloblastomas compared to tooth germs. The fos-oncogene and tumour-necrosis-factor-receptor-1 (TNFRSF-1A) were the most overexpressed genes. Ten genes, including sonic hedgehog (SHH), cadherins 12 and 13 (CDH12, and 13), plus transforming growth-factor-ß1 (TGF-ß1), were underexpressed in all ameloblastomas studied {1048}.

Prognosis and predictive factors

Long-term follow up is essential, since recurrences have been noted more than ten years after the initial treatment.

Treatment should include excision with an adequate margin of uninvolved tissues. Lesions involving the posterior maxilla, demonstrate the poorest prognosis. Radiotherapy should not be used in the first line treatment of A-S/M. Metastasizing ameloblastoma is discussed elsewhere in this volume (page 287).

Ameloblastoma, extraosseous / peripheral type

Definition

The extraosseous / peripheral ameloblastoma (A-E/P) is the extraosseous counterpart of the intraosseous solid / multicystic ameloblastoma (A-S/M).

ICD-O code   9310/0

Synonyms
Soft tissue ameloblastoma, ameloblastoma of mucosal origin, ameloblastoma of the gingiva.

Epidemiology
Extraosseous/peripheral ameloblastomas (A-E/Ps) comprise 1.3-10% of all ameloblastomas {2033}. Age range varies from 9 and 92 years with 64% of all cases occurring in the fifth through seventh decade. The mean age of patients with A-E/Ps (males: 53 years; females: 51 years) is significantly higher than for the intraosseous counterpart which has a mean age of 37 years {2149}. The male:female ratio is 1.9:1 {2149}.

Localization
A-E/Ps is located to the tooth-bearing areas (gingiva) or alveolar mucosa in edentulous areas. A mandible:maxilla ratio of 2.4:1 is noted. Multicentric origin of A-E/Ps has been reported {1075}.

Clinical features / Imaging
The A-E/P is a painless, firm and exophytic growth with a smooth, pebbly or papillary surface. Rarely, intraosseous ameloblastomas may extend to the gingival tissues and merge with the gingival epithelium, creating an exophytic A-E/P-like lesion {2473}. Apart from a superficial erosion or depression (saucerization or cupping) of the bone crest due to pressure resorption, there is rarely significant bone involvement {2149}.

Macroscopy
The gross specimen consists of a firm to spongy, pinkish-grey tissue mass..

Histopathology
The A-E/P consists of odontogenic epithelium with the same histomorphological cell types and patterns as seen in A-S/M. Some lesions are located entirely within the connective tissue of the gingiva, showing no continuity with the surface epithelium, whereas others seem to fuse with or originate from the mucosal epithelium. It is generally believed that basal cell carcinoma of the gingiva (BCCG) and A-E/P represent the same

neoplasm {861}. Squamous cells in the acanthomatous areas of A-E/Ps may show ghost cell formation, and in some parts of the tumour islands, vacuolated or clear cells occur in discrete clusters {1879,2137}. The stroma is that of a mature, fibrous connective tissue. Rare cases of malignant A-E/Ps (ameloblastic carcinomas) have been reported {2033, 2526,2649}.

Differential diagnosis
Differential diagnosis includes: (1) peripheral odontogenic fibroma. The proliferation of strands and islands of odontogenic epithelium in this tumour may be so extensive as to make the distinction from A-E/P difficult {862}, (2) peripheral variant of the squamous odontogenic tumour {2029}, and (3) odontogenic gingival epithelial hamartoma (OGEH) {103}. The present view is that A-E/P and OGEH represent the same lesion {2033}.

Histogenesis
A-E/P may arise from odontogenic epithelial remnants within the gingival lamina propria or from the basal cell layer of the gingival epithelium.

Prognosis and predictive factors
A-E/P does not show invasive behaviour and conservative excision is the treatment of choice. The recurrence rate is low (16-19%) {300,1852}. Long-term follow-up is recommended.

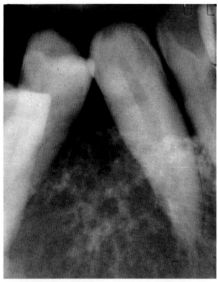

Fig. 6.19 Radiograph revealing a mixed radiolucency/radiopacity in a desmoplastic ameloblastoma of the mandible.

Ameloblastoma – desmoplastic type

Definition
Desmoplastic ameloblastoma (A-D) is a variant of ameloblastoma with specific clinical, imaging and histological features.

ICD-O code   9310/0

Synonym
Ameloblastoma with pronounced desmoplasia

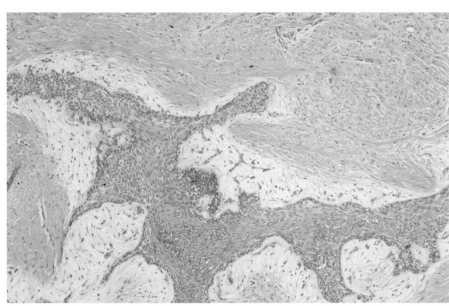

Fig. 6.20 Desmoplastic ameloblastoma. Notice irregularly shaped epithelial island surrounded by a narrow zone of loose-structured connective tissue embedded in desmoplastic stroma.

Epidemiology

A-D is similar to A-S/M regarding age and gender distribution {2035,2352}.

Localization

The maxilla: mandible ratio is 1:1. The ratio for A-S/M is 1:5.4 {2149}. The A-Ds are found predominantly in the anterior mandibular region.

Clinical features / Imaging

A painless swelling of the jaw bone represents the chief initial complaint. The size of the tumour varies between 1.0 and 8.5 cm in diameter. An extraosseous variant of A-D has not been reported. Radiographically, about 50% of A-Ds show a mottled, mixed radiolucency / radiopacity with diffuse margins, suggesting a fibro-osseous lesion. Resorption of tooth roots and bone formation may occur. The ill-defined borders of A-Ds make high-resolution CT and MRI helpful in treatment planning {2595}.

Macroscopy

The lesional tissue has a gritty consistency; the cut surface is solid in most cases.

Histopathology

In A-Ds the stromal component dominates, compressing the odontogenic epithelial components. The epithelial tumour islands are very irregular or bizarre in shape with a pointed, stellate appearance. The epithelial cells at the periphery of the islands are cuboidal with occasional hyperchromatic nuclei. Columnar cells with nuclear polarity are rarely conspicuous. The islands have a swirled, hypercellular centre with spindle-shaped or squamous, epithelial cells. Microcysts may occur centrally. Myxoid changes of the juxtaepithelial stroma are often found. Formation of metaplastic osteoid trabeculae (osteoplasia) may be present {2035}. A fibrous capsule is not present corresponding to the radiographically poorly defined tumour margin. A combination of A-D with A-S/M is known and has been termed as "hybrid lesion" {1703,2035}.

Immunoprofile

In contrast to A-S/M, marked immunoexpression of TGF-β has been observed {2537}.

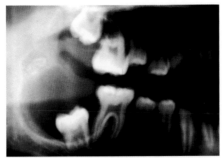

Fig. 6.21 Unicystic ameloblastoma. Panoramic radiograph mimicking dentigerous (follicular) cyst with impacted second mandibular molar.

Prognosis and predictive factors

Present knowledge leads to the recommendation to apply the same treatment modality as for A-S/M.

Ameloblastoma, unicystic type

Definition

The unicystic ameloblastoma (A-U) represents an ameloblastoma variant, presenting as a cyst.

ICD-O code   9310/0

Synonym

Cystogenic ameloblastoma

Epidemiology

Cases associated with an unerupted tooth show a mean age of 16 years as opposed to 35 years in the absence of an unerupted tooth {2030}. The mean age is significantly lower than that for A-S/M. There is no gender predilection {13}. Five to 15% of all ameloblastomas are of the unicystic type {2149}.

Localization

More than 90% of cases involve the mandible, usually the posterior region {13}.

Clinical features / Imaging

Some cases are asymptomatic, sometimes presenting as a swelling of the posterior mandible. Up to 80% are associated with an unerupted mandibular third molar. The lesion presents radiographically as a well corticated unilocular, often pericoronal radiolucency {702,1461}. Root resorption may occur {2149}. The clinical radiographic diagnosis is frequently a dentigerous (follicular) cyst.

Fig. 6.22 Schematic view of histological variants of unicystic ameloblastoma: luminal (ameloblastomatous cyst epithelium), intraluminal (protruding into cyst cavity) and mural (left and right, invading cyst wall).

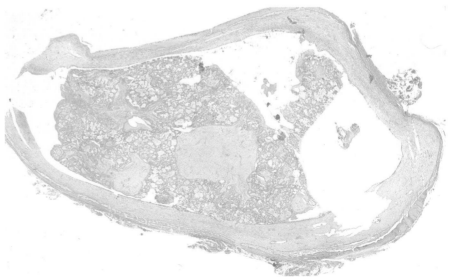

Fig. 6.23 Intraluminal variant of unicystic ameloblastoma with plexiform pattern.

Macroscopy

The lesions vary in size and, when removed intact, are typically cystic, and generally attached to an unerupted tooth at the cemento-enamel junction. The cyst wall may contain one or more tumour proliferations extending into the lumen. These proliferations and other thickened areas must be selected for microscopic examination.

Tumour spread and staging

The A-U is an expansile lesion that can destroy a significant portion of the jaw. The A-U does not usually behave as an A-S/M and does not infiltrate the surrounding bone.

Histopathology

Two histopathologic variants exist. The luminal variant is a cystic lesion lined by ameloblastomatous epithelium. In addition intraluminal extensions may occur. These extensions usually exhibit a plexiform epithelial pattern {13,865,2030}. There is no tumour infiltration into the fibrous wall {13,2030}.

The mural variant, the cyst wall is infiltrated by ameloblastomatous epithelium that exhibits either a follicular or plexiform pattern. Sometimes both variants may occur in the same lesion {13,2030}.

The mural variant of A-U may be confused with either dentigerous cysts or

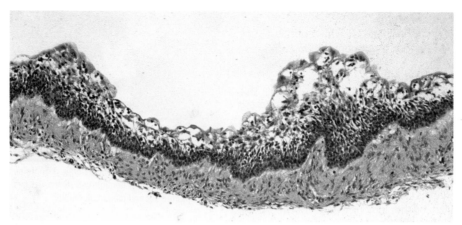

Fig. 6.24 Unicystic ameloblastoma (luminal type) showing ameloblastomatous epithelium lining the cyst wall.

dental follicles containing a lot of odontogenic epithelial remnants. These epithelial nests, however, do not show the typical histologic features of ameloblastoma: peripheral palisading and nuclear polarization.

Prognosis and predictive factors

Most A-Us are enucleated with the preoperative clinical diagnosis of dentigerous cyst and it is only on pathologic examination that their true nature is determined.

The luminal variant does not infiltrate the surrounding bone and as a result no further treatment is required for these lesions. Long-term follow up is recommended {13,2324}.

When a putative dentigerous cyst is excised and is subsequently designated as a A-U of the mural type, further treatment will depend upon the depth of epithelial invasion into the cyst wall. If invasion is limited, as confirmed by adequate sampling, careful follow-up is recommended. With deep extension of epithelium into the cyst wall, further surgical intervention must be considered, along with mandatory long-term follow up.

Squamous odontogenic tumour

P.A. Reichart

Definition
Squamous odontogenic tumour (SOT) is a locally infiltrative neoplasm consisting of islands of well-differentiated squamous epithelium in a fibrous stroma.

ICD-O code   9312/0

Epidemiology
The SOT is a rare tumour with less than 50 cases reported. The age range is between 8-74 years with a mean of 38.7 years {1170}. The gender ratio is 1.4:1 (men:women).

Etiology
The etiology of SOT is unknown.

Localization
SOT usually occurs intraosseously and probably develops in the periodontal ligament between the roots of vital erupted, permanent teeth. The mandible is affected more often than the maxilla.

Clinical features / Imaging
Mobility of teeth, local pain, swelling of the gingiva, osseous expansion or mild gingival erythema may be observed {979}. Radiographically, a unilocular or triangular radiolucency between the roots of adjacent teeth is seen. Extensive SOTs may present a multilocular pattern. The peripheral variant may produce some 'saucerization' of the underlying bone – a result of pressure from tumour

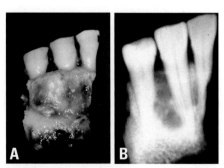

Fig. 6.25 Squamous odontogenic tumour (SOT). **A** Surgical specimen with bulging of the interdental vestibular cortical plate. **B** Surgical specimen radiograph showing multilocular radiolucency.

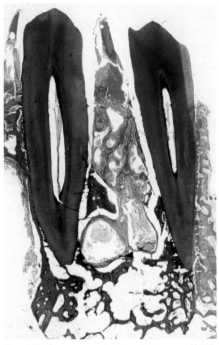

Fig. 6.26 Squamous odontogenic tumour (SOT). SOT between the roots of mandibular canine and first premolar.

expansion rather than neoplastic infiltration.

Histopathology
SOTs are composed of islands of well-differentiated squamous epithelium of varying size and shape. Islands are rounded or oval, but irregular and cord-like structures may be seen. Individual tumour islands reveal a peripheral layer of low cuboidal or flat epithelial cells. Epithelial islands may undergo central microcystic degeneration. Individual islands may contain calcified material. SOTs may be mistaken for an acanthomatous ameloblastoma, a desmoplastic ameloblastoma, a well-differentiated squamous cell carcinoma, or pseudoepitheliomatous hyperplasia.
SOT must be differentiated from so-called "squamous odontogenic tumour-like islands arising in the walls of odontogenic cysts".

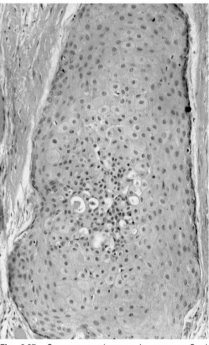

Fig. 6.27 Squamous odontogenic tumour. Oval island of well-differentiated odontogenic epithelium with central microcystic degeneration. Mitotic activity is not increased.

Prognosis and predictive factors
Conservative surgical treatment is usually sufficient. Recurrences are rare and are probably due to incomplete removal.

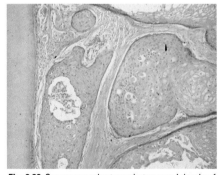

Fig. 6.28 Squamous odontogenic tumour. Islands of odontogenic epithelium without peripheral palisading close to the dental root (left).

Calcifying epithelial odontogenic tumour

T. Takata
P.J. Slootweg

Definition
The calcifying epithelial odontogenic tumour (CEOT) is a locally invasive epithelial odontogenic neoplasm, characterized by the presence of amyloid material that may become calcified.

ICD-O code 9340/0

Synonym
Pindborg tumour {2046,2047}.

Epidemiology
CEOT accounts for approximately 1% of all odontogenic tumours occurring in patients between 20 and 60 years of age, with a mean around 40 years {2031}. There is no gender predilection. Most cases are intraosseous, approximately 6% arise in extraosseous locations. Intraosseous tumours affect the mandible more often than the maxilla with a ratio of 2:1. There is a predilection for the premolar/molar region, although any site may be involved. Peripheral lesions usually occur in the anterior gingiva {1133}.

Clinical features / Imaging
The tumour presents as an asymptomatic slow-growing expansile mass of the jaw. Peripheral gingival lesions are firm painless masses. Radiographically, most CEOTs present as mixed radiolucent-radiopaque lesions, but they may show considerable variation. They may be unilocular or multilocular. In about half of the cases, an unerupted tooth, most often a mandibular third molar, is associated with the lesion. Computed tomography and magnetic resonance imaging provide useful information in the diagnosis and treatment of CEOT {507}.

Macroscopy
Macroscopic features are those of a solid tumour with various amounts of calcification. Cystic change is not seen.

Histopathology
The tumour consists of a fibrous stroma with islands and sheets of polyhedral

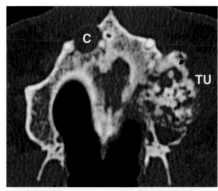

Fig. 6.29 CEOT of the left maxilla (TU) showing mixed radiolucency and radiopacities. In addition the right maxilla shows a radicular cyst (C).

epithelial cells with abundant eosinophilic cytoplasm, sharply defined cell borders and well-developed intercellular bridges. Their nuclei are frequently pleomorphic, with giant nuclei being common. Mitotic figures are rarely encountered; in case of malignant transformation, mitoses are frequent {2688}.

Eosinophilic, homogeneous hyalin material that is often calcified in the form of concentric rings is present within or around the sheets of tumour cells. Positive staining with Congo red and fluorescence with thioflavine T show this material to be amyloid.

Some tumours are amyloid-rich, while others demonstrate epithelial-predominance. Calcification is characteristic but non-calcifying variants also occur {2399,2538}. Lack of calcification is more common in extraosseous tumours. Clear cells may be present within the epithelial nests; they contain glycogen. In some cases, the clear cells make up a significant proportion of the tumour {2031}.

In a minority of cases, the CEOT may be seen in a composite relationship with the adenomatoid odontogenic tumour {2031}.

Differential diagnosis
Due to the presence of cytonuclear pleomorphism and intercellular bridges, CEOT may be mistaken for intraosseous

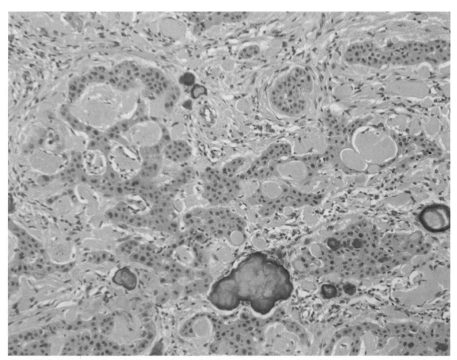

Fig. 6.30 Calcifying epithelial odontogenic tumour. The neoplasm consists of islands or sheets of polyhedral epithelial cells close to eosinophilic material in a fibrous connective tissue stroma.

squamous cell carcinoma, either primary or metastatic. The clear cell variant of the CEOT must be distinguished from clear cell odontogenic carcinoma, metastatic carcinomas composed of clear cells such as renal cell carcinoma and salivary gland malignancies including mucoepidermoid carcinoma and acinic cell carcinoma.

Prognosis and predictive factors

The CEOT is a locally invasive tumour. Small tumours may be enucleated, but larger ones require local resection. An overall recurrence rate of about 14% has been noted {803}. A relatively higher recurrence rate of 22% has been noted for the clear cell variant {1086}. Long-term follow-up is recommended.

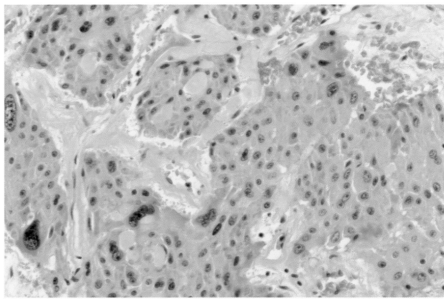

Fig. 6.31 CEOT. Giant and pleomorphic nuclei in the absence of mitoses are frequently found and do not indicate malignancy. Note intracellular homogenously dispersed eosinophilic material representing amyloid.

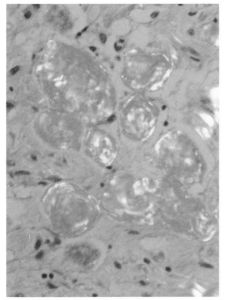

Fig. 6.32 Calcifying epithelial odontogenic tumour. Congo red staining shows green birefringence when subjected to polarized light.

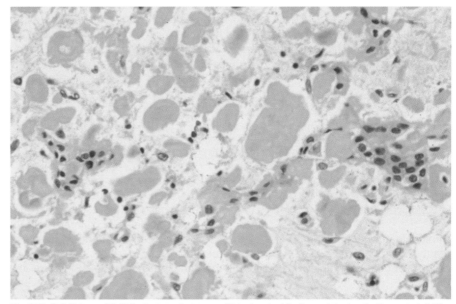

Fig. 6.33 Calcifying epithelial odontogenic tumour. Histochemical findings of the hyalin-like materiall. The material is positively stained with Congo red.

Adenomatoid odontogenic tumour

H.P. Philipsen
H. Nikai

Definition

Adenomatoid odontogenic tumour (AOT) is composed of odontogenic epithelium in a variety of histoarchitectural patterns, embedded in a mature connective tissue stroma and characterized by slow but progressive growth.

ICD-O code   9300/0

Epidemiology

The AOT accounts for 2-7% of all odontogenic tumours {2028,2032}. The age range varies between 3 and 82 years. More than two thirds are diagnosed in the second decade of life and 90% are found before the age of 30. More than half of the cases occur among teenagers {2032}. The male:female ratio is 1:1.9. In some Asian countries the ratio may reach 1:3.2 {2613}.

Localization

The AOT almost exclusively occurs intraosseously with a preference for the maxilla over the mandible with a ratio of 2.1:1. The rare peripheral type occurs almost exclusively in the anterior maxillary gingiva {2036}.

Clinical features / imaging

Intraosseous AOTs may be found in association with unerupted permanent teeth (follicular type), in particular the four canines that account for 60% with the maxillary canines alone accounting for 40%. Most AOTs are asymptomatic. When growth of the intraosseous variants causes cortical expansion, it may present as a palpable bony-hard swelling with or without slight pain. The intraosseous AOTs may cause displacement of neighbouring teeth. The peripheral variant presents as a fibroma or an epulis-like lesion of the gingiva.

Radiographically, the intraosseous, follicular AOT, shows a well-defined, unilocular radiolucency around the crown and often part of the root of an unerupted permanent tooth, mimicking a dentigerous cyst. If not associated with an unerupted tooth (extrafollicular type), AOT presents as a unilocular radiolucent lesion. In two thirds of the intraosseous variant, the radiolucency shows discrete radiopaque foci {2036}. The peripheral variant may disclose erosion (saucerization) of the alveolar bone crest.

Histopathology

At low magnification the most striking pattern is that of variably sized solid nodules of cuboidal or columnar cells of odontogenic epithelium forming nests or rosette-like structures with minimal stromal connective tissue. Between the

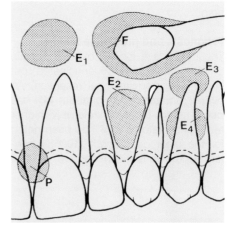

Fig. 6.34 Variants of AOT: E1-E4, extrafollicular sites; F, follicular; P, peripheral.

epithelial cells and in the centre of the rosette-like configurations, eosinophilic amorphous material ("tumour droplets") is present.

Conspicuous within the cellular areas are structures of tubular or duct-like appearanc The duct-like spaces are lined by a single row of columnar epithelial cells, with the nuclei polarized away from the luminal surface. The duct-like spaces represent pseudolumina formed by secretion of the columnar epithelial cells. The lumen may be empty or contain eosinophilic material or cellular debris. The duct-like structures may not be present in all AOTs. In addition to forming ducts, the cuboidal to columnar cells form convoluted cords in complicated patterns that often exhibit invaginations. Another characteristic cellular pattern is composed of nodules consisting of polyhedral, eosinophilic epithelial cells of squamous appearance with distinct cell boundaries and prominent intercellular bridges. The nuclei may occasionally reveal mild (degenerative) pleomorphism. These nodules may contain pools of amorphous amyloid-like material and globular masses of calcified substances. Melanin pigmentation of both lesional tissue and stroma cells has been described. Occurrence of a hyaline, dysplastic material or calcified osteodentin

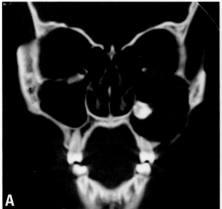 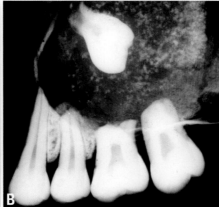

Fig. 6.33 A CT scan of AOT involving the entire maxillary sinus reaching the orbital floor. **B** Unusually large maxillary AOT. Radiograph of operation specimen showing impacted third molar in an expansile osteolysis with stippled calcifications (same case as A).

may be found in AOTs. It is likely the result of a metaplastic process, as odontogenic ectomesenchyme is not present, and thus should not be interpreted as an induction phenomenon, although in very rare cases dentin-like material containing dentinal tubules may occur. The mature connective tissue stroma of the AOT is generally loosely structured and contains thin-walled congested vessels.

CEOT-like areas found in AOTs should be considered a histological variant of AOT, as should areas of AOTs mimicking calcifying ghost cell odontogenic cysts {2888}, developing odontomas or other odontogenic tumours or hamartomas.

Prognosis and predictive factors

AOTs are cured by local excision. Recurrences are extremely rare {2032}.

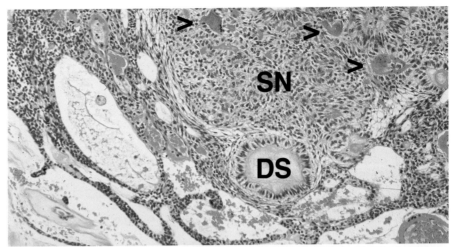

Fig. 6.35 Adenomatoid odontogenic tumour. AOT with a solid nodule of cuboidal epithelial cells (SN) containing several eosinophilic, amorphous "tumour droplets" (arrows), a duct-like structure (DS) lined by a single row of columnar epithelial cells. At the periphery strands of epithelium in a cribriform pattern.

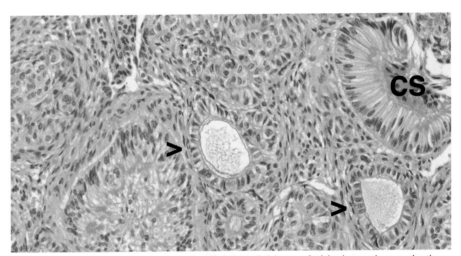

Fig. 6.36 Adenomatoid odontogenic tumour (AOT). Solid, cell-rich area of minimal stromal connective tissue showing duct-like structures (arrows), and convoluted structure (CS) of tall columnar epithelial cells.

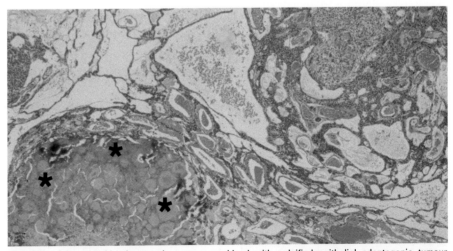

Fig. 6.37 Adenomatoid odontogenic tumour combined with calcified epithelial odontogenic tumour AOT/CEOT. The tumour shows areas of CEOT-like foci (asterisks) in an otherwise typical AOT with cribriform configurations of epithelial strands and several dilated thin-walled vessels in the sparse stroma.

Keratocystic odontogenic tumour

H.P. Philipsen

Definition

A benign uni- or multicystic, intraosseous tumour of odontogenic origin, with a characteristic lining of parakeratinized stratified squamous epithelium and potential aggressive, infiltrative behaviour. It may be solitary or multiple. The latter is usually one of the stigmata of the inherited naevoid basal cell carcinoma syndrome (NBCCS).

ICD-O code   9270/0

Synonyms

The traditional designation is odontogenic keratocyst (OKC), which stresses the benign behaviour of this lesion. However, the WHO Working Group recommends the term keratocystic odontogenic tumour (KCOT) as it better reflects its neoplastic nature. Other synonyms include odontogenic keratocystoma and primordial cyst.

Epidemiology

Keratocystic odontogenic tumours (KCOT) occur from the first to the ninth decades with a peak in the second and third decades {2323}. The mean age of patients with multiple KCOTs, with or without the NBCCS, is lower than those with single non-recurrent KCOTs. Most series have shown a preponderance in males.

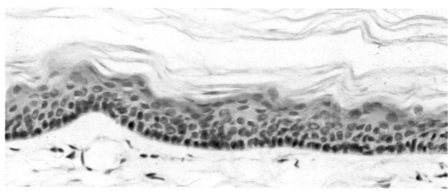

Fig. 6.38 Keratocystic odontogenic tumour. Extensive desquamation of keratinized epithelium into the lumen. Note characteristic prominence of basal cell layer.

Etiology

Recent studies have demonstrated the role of the PTCH gene in the etiology of KCOTs {110,143,471,1344,1467,1468, 1481,1854}.

Localization

The mandible is involved more frequently than the maxilla, with figures ranging from 65-83% of cases. About one-half originate at the angle of the mandible, extending anteriorly and superiorly {2323}.

Clinical features

The most important clinical feature of the KCOT is its potential for locally destructive behaviour, its recurrence rate, and its tendency to multiplicity, particularly when associated with the NBCCS. Patients may complain of pain, swelling or discharge. These tumours may reach a large size prior to discovery. KCOT may penetrate cortical bone and involve adjacent structures.

Imaging

KCOTs may appear as small, round or ovoid unilocular radiolucencies or may be larger with scalloped margins. A mandibular radiolucency may involve body, angle and ascending ramus. The radiolucencies tend to be well-demarcated with distinct sclerotic margins, but may be diffuse in parts. Maxillary lesions tend to be smaller, but more extensive involvement may occur. True multilocular mandibular lesions are not uncommon.

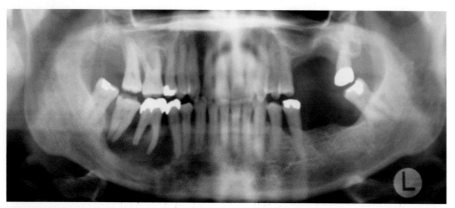

Fig. 6.39 KCOT presenting as an unilocular osteolysis mimicking radicular cyst.

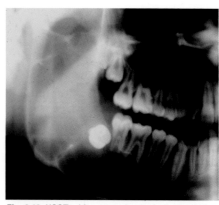

Fig. 6.40 KCOT with septated osteolysis simulating a follicular cyst.

Adjacent teeth may be displaced but root resorption occurs rarely {2323}.

CT scans may be helpful in detecting cortical perforation and assessment of soft tissue involvement. They may be of particular value in the evaluation of patients with multiple NBCCS-related KCOTs {1563}. Contrast enhanced MRI may provide more detailed information {1204, 1744}.

Macroscopy
Linings are thin and fragile, and are usually collapsed and folded.

Histopathology
The KCOTs are lined by a regular parakeratinized stratified squamous epithelium, usually about 5-8 cell layers thick and without rete ridges. There is a well-defined, often palisaded, basal layer of columnar or cuboidal cells. The nuclei of the columnar basal cells tend to be oriented away from the basement membrane and are often intensely basophilic. This is an important feature in distinguishing KCOT from jaw cysts with keratinization. The parakeratotic layers often have a corrugated surface. Desquamated keratin is present in many of the cavities. Mitotic figures are found frequently in the suprabasal layers. Some linings may show features of epithelial dysplasia {22} but malignant transformation to squamous cell carcinoma is rare {1600}.

In the presence of an intense inflammatory process, the epithelial lining loses its characteristic cellular and architectural features.

Cystic jaw lesions that are lined by orthokeratinizing epithelium do not form part of the spectrum of a keratocystic odontogenic tumour (KCOT).

Histogenesis
It is generally agreed that KCOT arises from odontogenic epithelium. The available evidence points to two main sources of the epithelium: the dental lamina or its remnants and extensions of basal cells from the overlying oral epithelium {284,2323,2478}.

Genetics
The NBCCS or *PTCH* gene has been mapped to chromosome 9q22.3-q31 {720} and probably functions as a tumour suppressor. Studies on NBCCS and sporadic KCOT have provided molecular

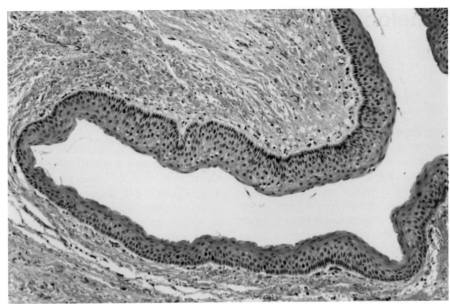

Fig. 6.41 KCOT extending into adjacent soft tissues presenting a characteristic lining with parakeratinized epithelial surface.

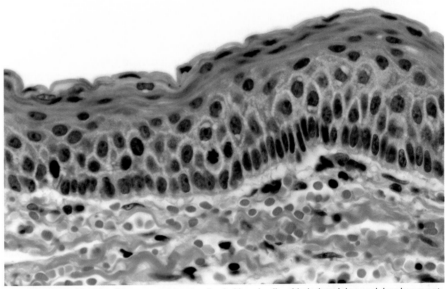

Fig. 6.42 KCOT with 5-8 cell layers, prominent palisaded basal cells with dark staining nuclei and corrugated surface with parakeratinization. Note centrally located intraepithelial suprabasal mitosis.

evidence of a two-hit mechanism in the pathogenesis of these tumours demonstrating allelic loss, at two or more loci, of 9q22 {1481,1539} leading to overexpression of bcl-1 and *TP53* in the NBCCS. This supports the concept that KCOT represents a neoplasm {1539}. There is also accumulating evidence that the PTCH gene might be a significant factor in the development of sporadic KCOT {143,1344,1467,1468,1854}. Furthermore, preliminary results have shown over-expression and amplification of genes located in 12q {1047}.

Prognosis and predictive factors
The KCOT is a potentially aggressive lesion. Patients should be carefully followed up after treatment because of the common presence of daughter cysts and a tendency for multiplicity.

Ameloblastic fibroma / fibrodentinoma

P.J. Slootweg

Definition

Ameloblastic fibroma (AF) consists of odontogenic ectomesenchyme resembling the dental papilla and epithelial strands and nests resembling dental lamina and enamel organ. No dental hard tissues are present. If there is dentin formation, the lesion is referred to as ameloblastic fibrodentinoma (AFD)

ICD-O code

Ameloblastic fibroma   9330/0
Ameloblastic fibrodentinoma
                                9271/0

Epidemiology

AF is a rare odontogenic tumour {531, 1930,2140}. The mean age is 14.8 years (range from 7 weeks to 62 years).

Localization

AF mainly occurs in the posterior mandible {2034}.

Clinical features / Imaging

Most cases of AF present as painless swelling or are discovered due to disturbances of tooth eruption. Radiographically, the tumour presents as a well-demarcated radiolucency, often in connection with a malpositioned tooth {2034}.

Histopathology

The epithelial component of AF consists of branching and anastomosing epithelial strands that form knots of varying size. These have a peripheral rim of columnar cells similar to the inner enamel epithelium that embraces a loosely arranged spindle-shaped epithelium identical to stellate reticulum. The epithelial strands lie in a myxoid cell-rich stroma with stellate-shaped fibroblasts with long slender cytoplasmic extensions resembling embryonic tooth pulp. The amount of epithelium may vary. Dental hard tissues do not form part of the histologic spectrum of AF. Mitotic figures both in epithelial and mesenchymal components may occur; if present, they should raise concern about the benign nature of the case.

The epithelial component resembles ameloblastoma. The stromal component however differs in that it is an immature cell-rich myxoid tissue with an embryonic appearance. Some AFs may contain granular cells {2034,2539}.

Rarely, tumours with the histomorphology of AF may form dysplastic dentin, and are called ameloblastic fibrodentinomas (AFD) {2051,2539}.

Histologic features similar to AF may be observed in the hyperplastic dental follicle {1313,2489}. The distinction relies on

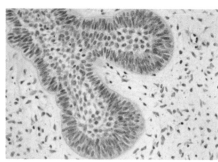

Fig. 6.43 Ameloblastic fibroma with reticular pattern of the central epithelium and palisaded peripheral cells. Inconspicuous nuclei of the ectomesenchymal stromal cells.

correlation of the histology to the radiographic appearance: a radiolucent rim surrounding an unerupted tooth, in case of a dental follicle and an expansive radiolucent jaw lesion, in case of ameloblastic fibroma.

Prognosis and predictive factors

Treatment consists of enucleation and curettage. Recurrence may occur but this does not justify initial aggressive treatment {2034}. Rarely, AF may progress to malignancy (ameloblastic fibrosarcoma).

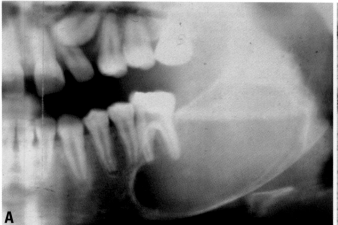
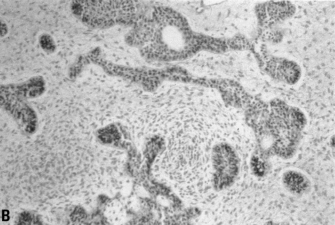

Fig. 6.44 A Ameloblastic fibroma presenting as a well demarcated osteolysis with sclerotic rim. **B** Ameloblastic fibroma with strands and islands of odontogenic epithelium showing peripheral palisading, embedded in a cell-rich ectomesenchyme resembling the dental papilla.

Ameloblastic fibro-odontoma

Y. Takeda
C.E. Tomich

Definition

Ameloblastic fibro-odontoma (AFO) is a tumour, which has the histologic features of ameloblastic fibroma (AF) in conjunction with the presence of dentin and enamel.

ICD-O code 9290/0

Epidemiology

AFO is less common than AF. The mean age is between 8-12 years. There is no gender or anatomic site predilection.

Clinical features / Imaging

AFO is often asymptomatic and may be detected as a result of failure of tooth eruption. Radiographically, AFO exhibits a well-circumscribed unilocular or multilocular radiolucency with varying levels of radiopacity depending on the extent of mineralization. AFO is often associated with an unerupted tooth.

Histopathology

AFO is composed of soft and hard tissues. The soft tissue component is iden

tical to AF; the hard tissue component consists of dental hard structures. These two components may be present in varying proportions. Odontoameloblastoma may be considered in the differential diagnosis.

Prognosis and predictive factors

The prognosis is excellent; recurrences have been rarely described.

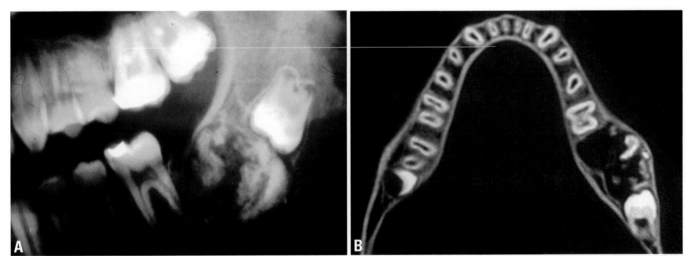

Fig. 6.45 Ameloblastic fibro-odontoma. **A** Ameloblastic fibro-odontoma of the left mandible showing radiopacities in a large translucency. The second molar is displaced and impacted. **B** CT scan of the same patient.

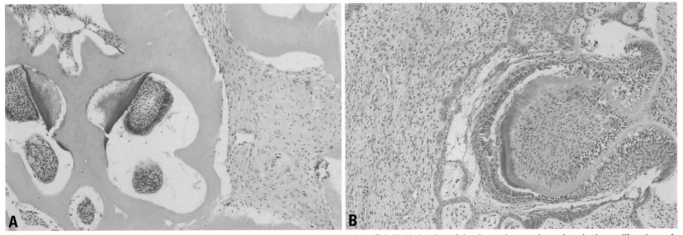

Fig. 6.46 Ameloblastic fibro-odontoma. **A** Well-formed dentin and enamel in the lesion. **B** Initial induction of dentin- and enamel-matrices in the proliferating soft tissue similar to that of ameloblastic fibroma.

Odontoma, complex type

F. Prætorius
A. Piattelli

Definition
Odontoma, complex type (OC) is a tumour-like malformation (hamartoma) in which enamel and dentin, and sometimes cementum, is present.

ICD-O code
Odontoma   9280/0
Odontoma, complex type 9282/0

Synonym
Complex composite odontoma

Epidemiology
OC is one of the most common odontogenic tumours. It is primarily diagnosed in children, adolescents, and young adults {1104,2034,1004}. There is no gender predilection.

Etiology
The etiology is unknown {2037}.

Localization
OCs occur in tooth-bearing regions, mostly in the posterior part of the mandible.

Clinical features / Imaging
OCs are painless slowly growing lesions. Growth stops when they are fully matured some reaching up to 6 cm in diameter. The majority measures less than 3 cm. Swelling of the jaw may be evident. Adjacent teeth may be displaced, and impaction of a permanent tooth is a common finding {1949A}.

Radiographically, OCs appear as a spherical or ovoid radiopacity with a fine radiating periphery, surrounded by a radiolucent zone, which may be broader in a developing complex odontoma. Differential diagnosis from a compound odontoma or even an osteoma may not be possible radiographically.

Histopathology
In mature OCs the soft tissue capsule consists of a loose connective tissue containing strands or islands of odontogenic epithelium. In developing OCs the outer part of the odontoma consists of a cell rich zone of soft tissue with formation of dentin and enamel, not resembling tooth morphology. The lesion appears as a mass of primarily tubular dentin which encloses hollow circular or oval structures with empty spaces from decalcified mature enamel, enamel-matrix producing epithelium and connective tissue. The structure of the hard dental tissue may vary. The lesion consists mainly of wavy and plicated walls of tubular or dysplastic dentin covered by enamel. Between these walls are irregular curvilinear clefts that contain enamel matrix-producing epithelium and connective tissue. Cementum is scarce except on the "root" surfaces of tooth-like structures. Scattered ghost cells may be present {2288A}.

The distinction between complex and compound odontoma is mainly based on the presence of tooth-like structures in compound odontomas. The differential diagnosis between a developing complex odontoma and an ameloblastic fibro-odontoma is sometimes impossible.

Prognosis and predictive features
Complex odontomas are treated by local excision. Recurrences have only been reported in cases of incomplete removal of developing complex odontomas {2167A}.

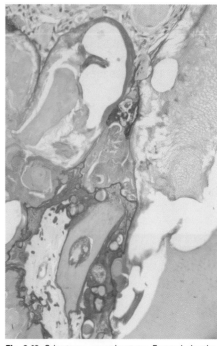
Fig. 6.48 Odontoma, complex type. Enamel, dentin, and cementum-like tissue are arranged in a haphazard pattern, in contrast to the regular structure encountered in compound odontoma.

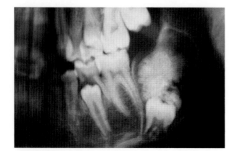
Fig. 6.47 Odontoma, complex type, with a dense radiopacity and a retained molar.

Odontoma, compound type

F. Prætorius
A. Piattelli

Definition
A tumour like malformation (hamartoma) with varying numbers of tooth-like elements (odontoids).

ICD-O code
Odontoma   9280/0
Odontoma, compound type
                         9281/0

Synonym
Compound composite odontoma

Epidemiology
Odontoma, compound type (OCp) is primarily diagnosed in children and adolescents {1104,2034} with no gender predilection. It has been reported to be the most common of all odontogenic neoplasms and tumour-like lesions.

Etiology
The etiology is unknown {2037}.

Localization
OCps may occur in any tooth-bearing area of the jaws. The anterior maxilla is most frequently affected.

Clinical features / Imaging
OCps are painless, slowly growing lesions. When fully matured, development ceases. The size usually varies

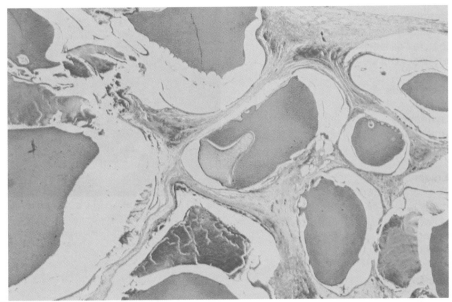

Fig. 6.50 Section of a developing compound odontoma. In a body of connective tissue several malformed tooth germs are seen cut in varying planes. This figure was used in the first edition of the WHO Histological Typing of Odontogenic Tumours published 1971 {2050}.

between 1 and 2 cm in diameter, but a diameter of up to 6 cm has been reported. Swelling of the jaw is seen in less than 10% of the cases. Many are located close to the incisal/ occlusal part of an impacted tooth, thus impeding eruption. Displacement of erupted teeth is seen in some cases. Some occur in a site where the permanent tooth is missing. Multiple OCps have been reported {1622, 103A, 2267A} and they may be part of Gardner syndrome {66}.

Peripheral lesions developing entirely within the gingival soft tissues are rare {891}.

Radiographically, the OCp appears as a collection of tooth-like structures surrounded by a radiolucent zone. Adjacent teeth may be displaced but are never resorbed.

Macroscopy
The specimen consists of a number of tooth-like structures enclosed in a fibrous capsule which is thin if the lesion has matured. In most cases the final diagnosis can be made on the basis of macroscopic examination.

Histopathology
Sections of immature, developing compound odontomas show several dysmorphic tooth germs in a loosely textured connective tissue with cords and islands of odontogenic epithelium. Much of the enamel matrix is preserved in spite of decalcification {2040A}.

Prognosis and predictive factors
OCps are treated by local excision. Recurrences have never been reported.

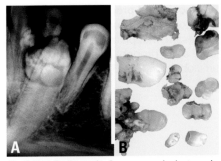

Fig. 6.49 A Radiograph of a compound odontoma in the left canine region of the mandible in a 12-year-old boy. The canine is impacted. Tooth-like structures can be identified. B Macroscopic view of the compound odontoma shown in A. Besides the deciduous canine, the connective tissue capsule and multiple tooth-like elements are seen.

Odontoameloblastoma

A. Mosqueda-Taylor

Definition
Odontoameloblastoma (OA) combines features of ameloblastoma with those of an odontoma.

ICD-O code   9311/0

Synonyms
Ameloblastic odontoma, odontoblastoma.

Epidemiology
The rare occurrence of this neoplasm precludes definite epidemiologic data {1783}. Most OAs have been diagnosed during the first three decades of life {1783}

Localization
This tumour equally affects mandible and maxilla with most of the cases occuring posterior to the canines.

Clinical features / Imaging
Presenting signs may include bone expansion, root resorption, tooth displacement and occasional pain {1288, 1783}.
Radiographically, OA appears as a well-defined unilocular or multilocular radiolucent lesion in which varying amounts of radiopaque material may be identified {1783,2594} Most cases are associated with displaced unerupted teeth.

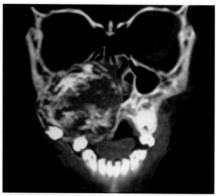

Fig. 6.51 Odontoameloblastoma. CT scan showing a well-circumscribed lesion containing abundant mineralized material and displacing unerupted teeth in a 9-year-old boy

Macroscopy
Most OAs are unencapsulated. On cut section, the lesion has a multinodular architecture with soft and hard tissue components. The amount of mineralized tissue may appear as large lobulated masses or as rudimentary teeth scattered within the soft tissue.

Histopathology
The epithelial component consists of islands and cords of odontogenic epithelium demonstrating follicular and plexiform patterns, typical of ameloblastoma. In addition to the fibrous stroma, this

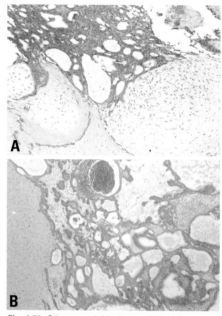

Fig. 6.52 Odontoameloblastoma. **A** Nodular masses of odontogenic mesenchyme adjacent to a proliferating epithelium that exhibits a plexiform ameloblastoma pattern. **B** Area of plexiform ameloblastoma adjacent to a nodule of odontogenic mesenchyme.

tumour shows a variable amount of cellular myxoid tissue adjacent to the epithelium, where mineralized dental tissues are formed as in odontomas {1288,1783, 2594}. Isolated small foci of ghost cells may occasionally be found {1783}

Prognosis and predictive factors
Odontoameloblastoma is a locally aggressive neoplasm similar in behaviour and prognosis to conventional ameloblastoma {966,1288,1783,2594}.

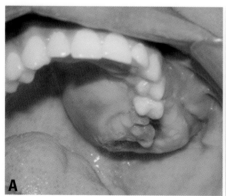
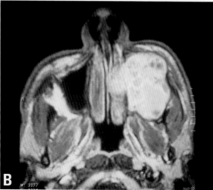

Fig. 6.53 A Odontoameloblastoma located on the left maxilla. Expansile mass in a 19-year-old man. The lesion was known to be present and progressively growing for at least 12 months. **B** Contrast-enhanced MRI of lesion shown in A, which extends up to midline. Courtesy Dr J.J. Trujillo.

Calcifying cystic odontogenic tumour

F. Prætorius
C. Ledesma-Montes

Definition

Calcifying cystic odontogenic tumour (CCOT) is a benign cystic neoplasm of odontogenic origin, characterized by an ameloblastoma-like epithelium with ghost cells that may calcify.

ICD-O code   9301/0

Synonyms

Keratinizing and calcifying odontogenic cyst, Gorlin cyst, calcifying odontogenic cyst

Epidemiology

The CCOT may present as an intraosseous or extraosseous process. The age range varies from 5-92 years without gender predilection {297,298, 1121}.

Localization

CCOT shows an equal site distribution for maxilla and mandible. Extraosseous CCOTs usually present in the incisor-cuspid area. Most of the intraosseous CCOTs also are found in the incisor-cuspid area {297}.

Clinical features / Imaging

Extraosseous CCOTs are pink to reddish, circumscribed, smooth surfaced, elevated masses, measuring up to 4 cm in diameter. They are usually asymptomatic

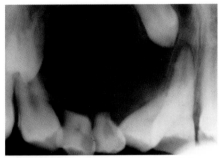

Fig. 6.54 CCOT. Radiograph of maxilla. Well-demarcated radiolucent lesion with divergence of roots and displacement of an impacted canine.

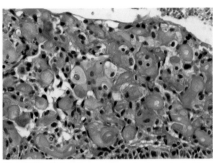

Fig. 6.55 Calcifying cystic odontogenic tumour (CCOT) with numerous ghost cells in different stages of development.

{298}. Intraosseous CCOTs present as a painless swelling {297}.

Radiographs of extraosseous CCOTs may show saucerization and sometimes displacement of adjacent teeth. Intraosseous CCOTs are generally seen as unilocular radiolucencies with a well-circumscribed border. In about 50%, a variable amount of radiopaque material is seen. Root resorption is common, as is root divergence. An associated unerupted tooth is seen in one third of the cases {297,667}.

Histopathology

In either variant the cyst wall is lined by a thin ameloblastomatous epithelium with the formation of ghost cells. These ghost cells may calcify {2538A}. Proliferation of

odontogenic epithelium in the adjacent connective tissue {1121,2077, 2315} and dysplastic dentin may be observed.

Prognosis and predictive factors

Enucleation is the appropriate treatment for most CCOTs. Recurrence has not been reported for the extraosseous type {298}. A few recurrences have been reported for the intraosseous type {297}. Features of CCOT have been described in a number of other odontogenic tumours {1099,2077}.

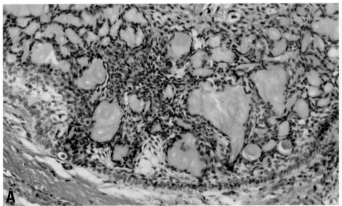
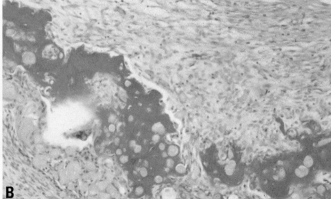

Fig. 6.56 Calcifying cystic odontogenic tumour (CCOT) **A** Cyst lining showing cuboidal or columnar basal cells with dark oval nuclei forming a palisade. The upper epithelial layers resemble the stellate reticulum of the enamel organ. Scattered ghost cells are seen. van Gieson stain. **B** Islands of proliferating odontogenic epithelium containing ghost cells in connective tissue. A band of dentinoid (red) has been formed in contact with the epithelium. Van Gieson stain.

Dentinogenic ghost cell tumour

F. Prætorius
C. Ledesma-Montes

Definition

A locally invasive neoplasm characterised by ameloblastoma-like islands of epithelial cells in a mature connective tissue stroma. Aberrant keratinization may be found in the form of ghost cells in association with varying amounts of dysplastic dentin.

ICD-O code   9302/0

Synonyms

Calcifying ghost cell odontogenic tumour, odontogenic ghost cell tumour, epithelial odontogenic ghost cell tumour, dentinoameloblastoma.

Formerly dentinogenic ghost cell tumour (DGCT) was considered a solid variant of the calcifying odontogenic cyst {297, 1121,1498,2077}.

Epidemiology

DGCT occurs as an intraosseous and less commonly as an extraosseous variant. The age range is from the second to the ninth decade. The DGCT is somewhat more common in men than in women.

Localization

DGCT may occur in any tooth-bearing area of the jaws. There is no preference for maxilla or mandible. The extraosseous variant shows a predilection for the anterior part of the jaws, while the intraosseous variant most often affects the canine to first molar region.

Clinical features / Imaging

The tumour is usually asymptomatic {1121,2527}.

The extraosseous variant presents as sessile, sometimes pedunculated, exophytic nodule of the gingival or alveolar mucosa. Many have occurred in edentulous areas. The size varies from 0.5-4.0 cm, but most are between 0.5 and 1 cm. Radiographs will show saucerization of the underlying bone in about 20% of the cases {298,1553}. Teeth in the affected area may be displaced. DGCT is slow growing.

The size of the intraosseous DGCT varies from 1 to more than 10 cm in diameter. It is usually asymptomatic. There may be bony expansion and in some cases resorption of cortical bone with extension into soft tissues. Adjacent teeth may be displaced and mobile.

Radiographs show a radiolucent to mixed radiolucent/radiopaque appearance depending on the amount of calcification. The borders are usually well-demarcated. Most are unilocular. Resorption of adjacent teeth is a common finding, and associated impacted teeth have been described {297,667}.

Histopathology

There is no difference between the microscopic features of the intra- and extraosseous variant. The tumour infiltrates the surrounding tissue. Sheets and rounded islands of odontogenic epithelium are seen in a mature connective tissue. The epithelium of the tumour islands resembles that of an ameloblastoma. Mitoses are not seen. Minor cysts may form in the epithelial islands. A characteristic feature is the transformation of the epithelial cells into ghost cells. Individual as well as large islands of ghost cells may be seen. Where basal layer cells are transformed into ghost cells the basement membrane disappears, while ghost cells extrude into the fibrous connective tissue evoking a foreign body reaction. Some ghost cells undergo calcification {723}. DGCT forms dysplastic dentin although in minute amounts. Ghost cells may be trapped in the dysplastic dentin, which in some areas may be mineralized.

DGCT can be distinguished from ameloblastoma by the presence of large numbers of ghost cells and dysplastic dentin. DGCT may be difficult to distinguish form a multicystic calcifying cystic odontogenic tumpur (CCOT). Malignant transformation of a DGCT into an odontogenic ghost cell carcinoma has been described.

Prognosis and predictive factors

The intraosseous DGCT may be aggressive with wide local resection recommended, particularly if the tumour is radiologically ill-defined. Enucleation is an appropriate treatment of the extraosseous DGCT; no recurrences have been reported, except in some intraosseous cases, and even malignant transformation has been documented.

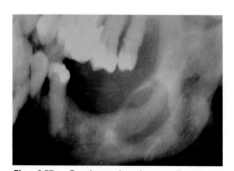

Fig. 6.57 Dentinogenic ghost cell tumour. Radiograph of right mandible with well-defined radiolucency representing a recurrence of a DGCT.

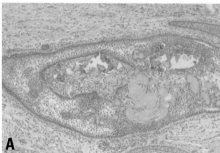
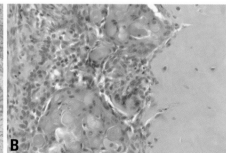

Fig. 6.58 Dentinogenic ghost cell tumour. **A** The central part of the area with stellate reticulum like epithelial cells is transformed into ghost cells, some of which are calcified. **B** A number of the stellate cells have been transformed into ghost cells. On the right dysplastic dentin (dentinoid) is seen.

Odontogenic fibroma

H.P. Philipsen
P.A. Reichart
J.J. Sciubba
I. van der Waal

Definition

The odontogenic fibroma (OF) is a rare neoplasm characterized by varying amounts of inactive-looking odontogenic epithelium embedded in a mature, fibrous stroma.

ICD-O code

9321/0

Synonyms and historical annotation

Controversy exists as to concept and definition {628}. At present the term OF is applied to two histological types of lesions: the epithelium-poor type (formerly termed simple type) and the epithelium-rich type (formerly termed complex or WHO-type).

Epidemiology

Due to lack of uniform definition, data on relative frequency are wide-ranged and inconsistent. When considering the epithelium-rich type, the age range of 15 reported cases was 11-66 years with a mean of 40 years, with a female predominance of 2.8:1 {37,522,609,620, 629, 1206,1618,2045,2270}.

Localization

Topographically, two variants can be distinguished: an intraosseous or central type (COF) described here and an extraosseous or peripheral type {530}. From the above-mentioned source of epithelium-rich cases, more were located in the mandible giving a maxilla: mandible ratio of 1:6.5 with most lesions found in the mandibular/premolar area.

Clinical features / Imaging

The epithelium-rich type presents a slow-growing, progressive but painless swelling, often with cortical expansion. In half of cases the tumour appears as a unilocular radiolucent area with well-defined often sclerotic borders. Rarely, the occurrence of calcified material may produce a mixed radiolucent / radiopaque appearance. Larger lesions show scalloping of the margins. Adjacent teeth may be displaced. Some tumours are associated with the crown of an unerupted tooth.

Histopathology

The epithelium-poor type of COF is a non-infiltrating connective tissue lesion resembling a dental follicle. It is minimally cellular with dispersed delicate collagen fibres. A considerable amount of ground substance produces a fibromyxoid quality to the background. Scattered remnants of inactive-looking odontogenic epithelium appear as small irregular islands and cords. Occasionally, variably-formed calcifications occur.

The epithelium-rich type of COF is composed of cellular, fibroblastic connective tissue interwoven with less cellular and often vascular areas. Islands or strands of inactive-looking odontogenic epithelium are an integral component; they may be sparse but are often conspicuous. This type shows foci of calcified material considered to be metaplastically produced dysplastic cementum/osteoid/dentin. A well-defined capsule is rare. Subvariants of both histological types of COF have been described {37,628, 1928}.

Histogenesis

It has been suggested {863} that the epithelium-poor type of COF is derived from the dental follicle whereas the epithelium-rich type arises from the periodontal ligament. Existence of two types of COF has been challenged {999}.

Prognosis and predictive factors

Both types of COF are benign lesions and are cured by local enucleation. Long-term follow-up studies are not available.

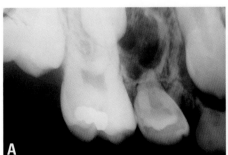
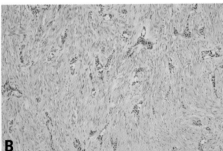
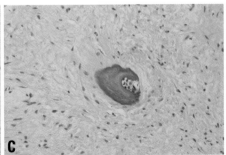

Fig. 6.59 Odontogenic fibroma, epithelium-rich type. **A** Periapical radiograph with a well outlined osteolysis with internal trabeculation. **B** Collagenous cell rich stroma with numerous strands of odontogenic epithelium without palisading of peripheral cells. **C** Calcified material encircles an epithelial island.

Odontogenic myxoma / myxofibroma

A. Buchner
E.W. Odell

Definition

Odontogenic myxoma (OM) is an intraosseous neoplasm characterized by stellate and spindle-shaped cells embedded in an abundant myxoid or mucoid extracellular matrix. When a relatively greater amount of collagen is evident, the term myxofibroma may be used.

ICD-O code   9320/0

Synonym

Odontogenic fibromyxoma

Epidemiology

The frequency of Odontogenic myxoma (OM) varies in different parts of the world between 3-20% of all odontogenic tumours {1925}. In most studies, OM is the third most frequent odontogenic tumour (after odontoma and ameloblastoma). The age range varies from 1-73 years, with a mean age of 30 years. The majority is diagnosed in the 2nd-4th decades. OM is slightly more common in females {1245}.

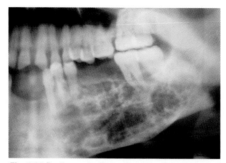

Fig. 6.60 Radiograph of an odontogenic myxoma of the mandible showing the characteristic septa crossing at right angles.

Localization

Two-thirds of OMs are located in the mandible. OMs are most common in the molar regions. Maxillary lesions tend to obliterate the maxillary sinuses as an early feature {1245}.

Clinical features / Imaging

Small OMs are asymptomatic. Large OMs cause painless expansion. Cortical perforation may occur when large. Unilateral sinonasal obliteration may mimic nasal polyposis.
Radiographically, OMs appear as uniloc-ular or multilocular radiolucency, sometimes showing a fine "soap bubble" or "honeycomb" appearance occasionally with fine trabeculations. The borders of the tumour are usually well-defined and corticated but can be poorly defined or diffuse. Root displacement occurs, as does root resorption. Larger OMs may present with periosteal reactions.
CT may reveal the fine bony septa and allows for anatomic deliniation.

Macroscopy

Gross examination reveals a grey-white mass with a typical translucent mucinous appearance. The consistency varies from gelatinous to firm, depending on the amount of collagen present and fine white bands of collagen may be visible on the cut surface.

Histopathology

OM is characterized by randomly oriented stellate, spindle-shaped and round cells with long, fine, anastomosing pale or slightly eosinophilic cytoplasmic processes extending from the centrally placed nucleus. Cells are evenly dis-

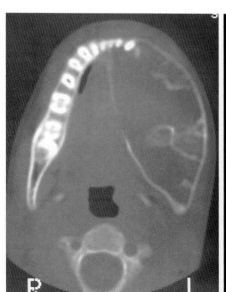
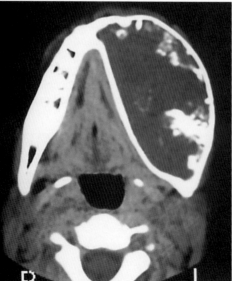
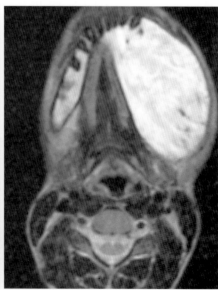

Fig. 6.61 Odontogenic myxoma of the body of the mandible showing thin expanded cortex and bony septa in bone window (left) and low soft tissue density (centre). The high proton density resulting from water bound to the myxoid stroma gives the lesion a hyperintense signal in T2 weighted magnetic resonance imaging (right). Courtesy Dr. C.J. Nortje and Dr L.J. van Rensburg.

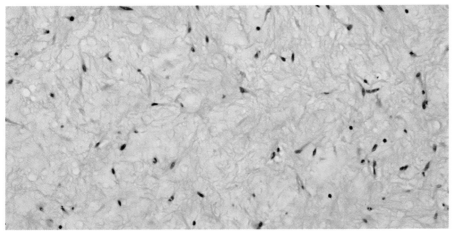

Fig. 6.66 Typical appearance of odontogenic myxoma with randomly oriented stellate, spindle-shaped and round cells with long cytoplasmic processes.

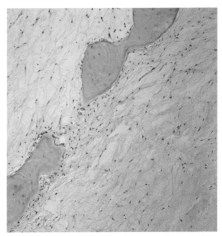

Fig. 6.64 Septum of residual lamellar bone within an odontogenic myxoma.

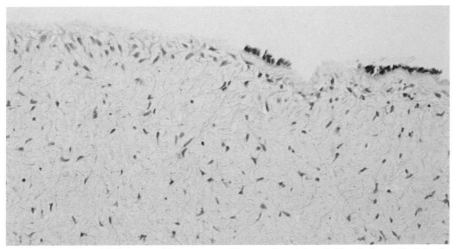

Fig. 6.63 Normal dental follicle resembling a myxoma. The smooth periphery (left) and a few epithelial cells of the reduced enamel epithelium (right) exclude myxoma histologically.

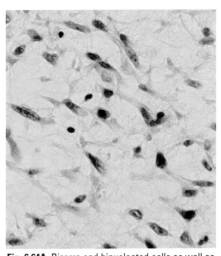

Fig. 6.64A Bizarre and binucleated cells as well as mild cellular pleomorphism may be present.

persed in an abundant mucoid or myxoid stroma that contains only a few fine collagen fibres. Binucleated cells, mild pleomorphism and mitotic figures may occur {1649}. Rests of odontogenic epithelium are not obvious in most lesions and are not required for establishing final diagnosis. Some OMs may permeate into the marrow spaces in a pseudo-malignant pattern. Some OMs have a tendency to produce collagen fibres and are designated myxofibroma. There is no evidence that these more collagenous variants behave differently.

Histochemical studies show that the ground substance is rich in acid mucopolysaccharides, primarily hyaluronic acid and, to a lesser degree, chondroitin sulphate.

OM is strikingly similar microscopically to myxoid enlarged or 'hyperplastic' dental follicle and the dental papilla of a developing tooth. Misdiagnosis of these entities should be avoided by correlation with the clinical and radiographic features {121,1313,2489}. In maxillary cases, confusion with nasal polyps is a risk. The microscopic differential diagnosis should also include myxoid nerve sheath tumours, chondromyxoid fibroma, low-grade myxoid fibrosarcoma and other myxoid sarcomas.

Somatic genetics

A study of 23 cases has shown that odontogenic myxomas are not associated with activating mutations of the Gs alpha gene {239}. Odontogenic myxoma has been reported in a single case of tuberous sclerosis {1019} but is not otherwise associated with Carney complex or any known genetic lesion. In one study

karyotypic aberrations have been demonstrated {1969A}.

Prognosis and predictive factors

The tendency of OM to permeate into marrow spaces makes effective enucleation and curettage difficult. Small lesions have been successfully treated in this way but larger lesions may require complete excision with free margins. Recurrence rates from various studies average about 25% but in spite of this, the prognosis is good. Recurrence usually follows incomplete removal within two years but may occur much later. Death may ensue due to cranial base extension {1969A}.

Cementoblastoma

I. van der Waal

Definition
A cementoblastoma is characterized by the formation of cementum-like tissue in connection with the root of a tooth.

ICD-O code   9273/0

Epidemiology
Just over a hundred cases have been reported. The age range is from 8 up to 44 years, the mean being approximately 20 years {262}. There is no distinct gender preference.

Localization
The majority of cementoblastomas are located in the mandible, particularly related to the permanent first molar; association with a primary tooth is exceptional.

Clinical features / Imaging
The most common finding is a painful swelling at the buccal and lingual/palatal aspect of the alveolar ridges. The vitality of the involved tooth remains intact. Lower-lip paresthesia or a pathologic fracture of the mandible are rarely reported {262}.
Radiographically, the tumour is well-defined and is mainly of a radiopaque or mixed-density, surrounded by a thin radiolucent zone. Root resorption, loss of root outline and obliteration of the periodontal ligament space are common findings.

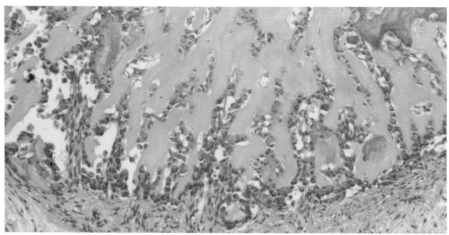

Fig. 6.65 Peripheral radiating columns of unmineralized tissue in cementoblastoma, which, seen in isolation, are difficult to distinguish from osteoblastoma or osteosarcoma. Note the rim of connective tissue at the bottom corresponds to the peripheral radiolucent zone in Fig. 6.66.

Macroscopy
The tumour consists of a rounded or nodular mass attached to one or more tooth roots and is surrounded by a grey-to-tan layer of irregular soft tissue {262}.

Histopathology
A cementoblastoma consists of dense masses of acellular cementum-like material in a fibrous, sometimes rather vascular stroma that may contain multinucleated cells. The tumour mass blends with the root of a tooth with simultaneous root resorption. In the more mature parts of the tumour, basophilic reversal lines may produce a Paget disease-like pattern. At the periphery sheets of unmineralized tissue may be seen, often being arranged in radiating columns. The differential diagnosis includes osteoblastoma, the only distinctive criterion being the true connection with the surface of the root of a tooth in case of a cementoblastoma {2400}. An important differential diagnosis is osteosarcoma. Without radiographs it is difficult to properly diagnose a cementoblastoma. The diagnosis cannot be made on the biopsy alone.

Prognosis and predictive factors
In case of incomplete removal, together with the associated tooth, recurrence is common {262}.

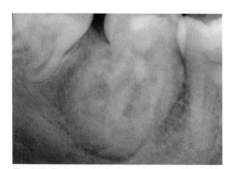

Fig. 6.66 Radiograph of cementoblastoma. The original contour of the radices are hardly recognizable anymore. Notice thin peripheral radiolucent zone.

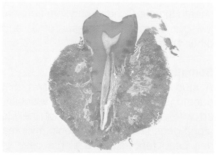

Fig. 6.67 Cementoblastoma. The root surface is largely destroyed by the cementum-like tissue, while the pulpal tissue of the tooth still remained vital.

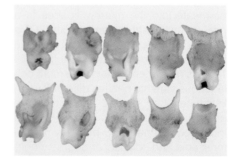

Fig. 6.68 Maxillary cementoblastoma, sliced buccopalatally. The tumour is attached to the resorbed roots of the involved teeth.

Ossifying fibroma

P. J. Slootweg
S.K. El Mofty

Definition
Ossifying fibroma (OF) is a well-demarcated lesion composed of fibrocellular tissue and mineralized material of varying appearances. Juvenile trabecular ossifying fibroma (JTOF) and juvenile psammomatoid ossifying fibroma (JPOF) are two histologic variants of ossifying fibroma.

ICD-O code   9262/0

Synonyms
Cementifying fibroma, cemento-ossifying fibroma, juvenile (active/aggressive) ossifying fibroma

Epidemiology
OF most commonly occurs in the 2nd to 4th decades and shows a predilection for females {261}. The mean age of the histological subtypes varies. In patients with JPOF it is about 20 years compared to 35 years in cases of conventional ossifying fibroma {1229}. JTOF has a still lower mean age range (8.5-12 years) {644}.

Localization
OF is mostly seen in the posterior mandible {261}. JPOF mainly occurs in the bony walls of the paranasal sinuses whereas in the JTOF the maxilla is the site of predilection {644}.

Clinical features / Imaging
OF causes expansion of the involved

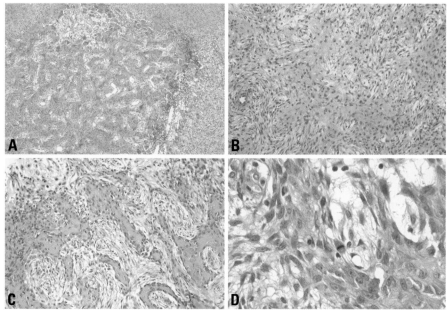

Fig. 6.69 Juvenile trabecular ossifying fibroma (JTOF). **A** The bony trabeculae may exhibit irregular mineralization and may form an anastomosing lattice. **B** At higher magnification, the gradual transition between bone and fibroblastic background tissue is clearly displayed. **C** The bony trabeculae in JTOF usually are lined by a rim of swollen osteoblasts. This feature serves to make the distinction between JTOF and fibrous dysplasia. **D** Mitotic figures, occasionally numerous, may be present.

bone {261}. Radiographs show a demarcated lesion that may have radiodense as well as radiolucent areas depending on the various contributions of soft and hard tissue components {261}.

Macroscopy
OFs are well-demarcated, firm lesions without further noteworthy macroscopical features.

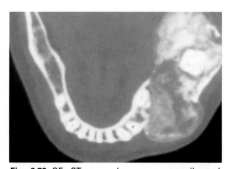

Fig. 6.70 OF. CT scan shows an expansile and demarcated mixed radiodense and radiolucent lesion of the mandible.

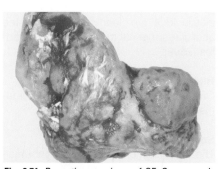

Fig. 6.71 Resection specimen of OF. Gross specimen showing jaw deformity due to expanding tumour.

Histopathology
Ossifying fibroma (OF) is composed of fibrous tissue that may vary in cellularity from areas with closely packed cells to nearly acellular parts within the same lesion. The mineralized component may consist of woven bone, lamellar bone and acellular to poorly cellular basophilic and smoothly contoured deposits thought to be cementum. Due to the presence of this cementum-like material, ossifying fibromas have also been called cemento-ossifying fibroma. However, cementum is defined as a mineralized material covering the surface of the roots of the teeth and outside this location, its distinction from bone is equivocal and without clinical relevance {261,2401}. OF may be confused with fibrous dysplasia. The most important distinguishing feature is the presence of demarcation and/or encapsulation in OF as opposed to the merging with its surroundings as shown by fibrous dysplasia. In addition, the variation in cellularity as well as in

appearances of mineralized material serves to distinguish OF from fibrous dysplasia {2401,2699}. Distinction between OF and osseous dysplasia on histologic grounds only may be problematic as both entities share the variation in stromal cellularity and appearances of mineralized material. Clinical presentation and radiographic appearance may be decisive (see osseous dysplasia).

Juvenile trabecular ossifying fibroma (JTOF) consists of cell-rich fibrous tissue containing bands of cellular osteoid without osteoblastic rimming together with slender trabeculae of immature bone containing coarse lacunae with plump osteocytes and are lined by a dense rim of enlarged osteoblasts. Sometimes these trabeculae may anastomose to form a lattice. Mitoses are present, especially in the cell-rich areas. Additional but less typical features are multinucleated giant cells, pseudocystic stromal degeneration, and haemorrhages {644,2051, 2406}.

Juvenile psammomatoid ossifying fibroma (JPOF) is characterized by a fibroblastic stroma containing small ossicles resembling psammoma bodies. The stroma varies from being loose and fibroblastic to intensely cellular with minimal intervening collagen. The mineralized material consists of spherical or curved ossicles that are acellular or show sparsely distributed cells. These ossicles should not be confused with the cementum-like deposits that are present in conventional OF. These particles have a smooth contour with sometimes a radiating fringe of collagen fibers, whereas the ossicles in JPOF have a thick irregular collagenous rim that may attain such a size that it includes multiple ossicles. The ossicles themselves may also fuse to form trabeculae showing reversal lines. Sometimes, JPOF contains deeply basophilic concentrically lamellated particles as well as irregular thread-like or thorn-like calcified strands in a hyalinized background. Other features such as trabeculae of woven bone as well as lamellar bone, pseudocystic stromal degeneration and haemorrhages result in areas similar to an aneurysmal bone cyst. Multinucleate giant cells, and mitotic figures may be present, but are not specific for this variant of ossifying fibroma. JPOF has to be distinguished from extra-

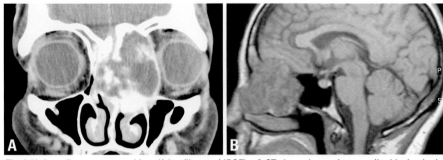

Fig. 6.72 Juvenile psammomatoid ossifying fibroma (JPOF) . **A** CT shows large circumscribed lesion in the left ethmoid region. Histology showed this lesion to be a JPOF. **B** MRI from the same case as shown in A.

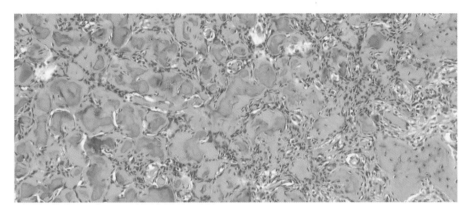

Fig. 6.73 JPOF. At high magnification, the ossicles of JPOF show a osteoid rim of varying width. The intervening stroma consists of densely packed fibroblasts.

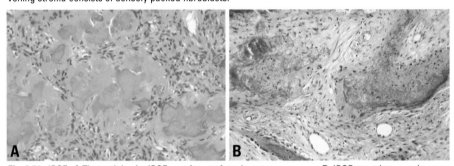

Fig. 6.74 JPOF. **A** The ossicles in JPOF may fuse to form larger aggregates. **B** JPOF may also contain more loose stromal areas. These may contain irregular deposits of collagenous material in which threadlike calcifications are present.

cranial meningioma with psammoma bodies, which demonstrates EMA positivity. Moreover, the psammomatoid ossicles in JPOF are clearly different from the acellular spherical true psammoma bodies {2599}.

Histogenesis
OFs originate from the periodontal ligament {2861}.

Somatic genetics
The following chromosomal abnormalities have been observed in OF: one case with three reciprocal translocations with the karyotype 46,XY,t(1;18)(q21;q21.3),

t(3;10)(P13;q22),t(6;11)(p22;p15), one case with alterations affecting the short arms of chromosomes X, 2, and 7 and 3 cases with identical chromosomal breakpoints occurring at bands Xq26 and 2q33, with an identical t(X;2)(q26;q33) reciprocal translocation in 2 cases and an interstitial insertion of bands 2q24.2q33 into Xq26 in the third case {528,919,2254}.

Prognosis and predictive factors
OFs continue to enlarge when left untreated. Therefore, they should be removed completely.

Fibrous dysplasia

G. Jundt

Definition
Fibrous dysplasia (FD) is a genetically-based sporadic disease of bone that may affect single or multiple bones (monostotic: MFD, polyostotic: PFD). FD occurring in multiple adjacent craniofacial bones is regarded as monostotic (craniofacial FD). FD may be part of the McCune-Albright syndrome (MAS).

Epidemiology
The monostotic form (MFD) is equally distributed in both genders and ethnic groups and is six times more common than the polyostotic: PFD {775}. PFD is more frequent in females (F/M ratio, 3:1). MFD and PFD are mainly diagnosed in children and young adults. However, in the 3% of all PFD-cases that occur in the setting of McCune-Albright syndrome, the disease may manifest in infants {775, 1018}.

Etiology
Mutations in the gene (GNAS I) encoding for the α-subunit of a signal transducing G-protein (Gs-α) lead to increased c-AMP production affecting proliferation and differentiation of preosteoblasts {472,1633,2175}.

Localization
In the jaws, FD occurs more often in the maxilla than in the mandible, and may involve adjacent bones like the zygoma or the sphenoid {93,2710}. The long tubular bones, especially the femur, followed by the flat bones of the jaws, the skull (base of skull prior to neurocranium), and the ribs, are the most frequently affected sites in the skeleton {2067}.

Clinical features
Signs and symptoms
Complaints usually consist of painless swelling often leading to facial asymmetry, occasionally accompanied by irregular café-au-lait spots. Maxillary and mandibular involvement may lead to displacement of teeth, malocclusion and, rarely, root resorption {1759}. In FD affecting the paranasal sinuses nasal obstruction may occur {2321}. Lesions extending to the orbit may cause visual impairment, while temporal bone lesions may produce hearing loss. Sometimes facial pain, headaches or facial numbness develops {140,281,1586}. Children presenting with FD, especially PFD, and irregular café-au-lait spots should be carefully examined for MAS {1002}. An

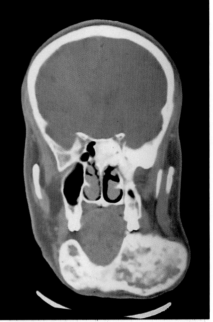

Fig. 6.76 Fibrous dysplasia. Polyostotic fibrous dysplasia (mandible, base of skull) with extreme deformity of the mandible. Frontal (coronal) CT scan, bone window.

elevation of alkaline phosphatase, even in the absence of fractures and unrelated to the extent of the disease has been noted in up to one third of FD patients {1018}.

Imaging
Three different radiographic patterns of FD involving the maxillofacial skeleton have been described: cystic (radiolucent or lytic; early lesions), sclerotic (mid-phase lesions), and mixed radiolucent/radiopaque (pagetoid: late lesions) comprising 21%, 23% and 56%, respectively {281,820,1759}. Asymmetric homogeneously radiodense opacities with "ground glass"-appearance that blend into normal bone, thin cortices and bone expansion are highly characteristic for FD and best seen on CT scans on bone windows {520}. In the jaws, superior displacement of the mandibular canal, narrowing of the periodontal ligament space and effacing of the lamina dura are findings suggestive of FD {520,1759,2024, 2572}. On MRI, signals are intermediate

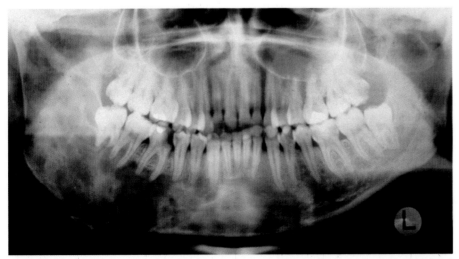

Fig. 6.75 Fibrous dysplasia of the jaw. Radiograph showing expansile osteolysis with irregular opacities of the mandible, extending into the ascending ramus up to the mandibular condyle. Partially eroded lamina dura of affected teeth.

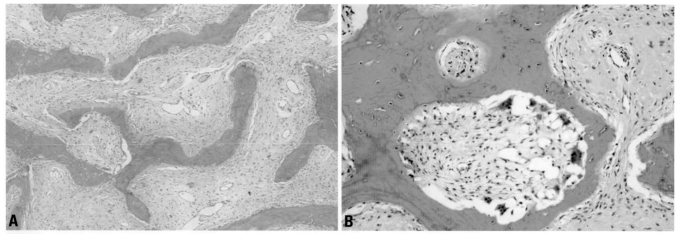

Fig. 6.77 Fibrous dysplasia. **A** Trabeculae of woven bone without osteoblastic rimming embedded in a monotonous cell rich stroma. GNAS I mutational analysis revealed arg>cys replacement. **B** Osteoclastic resorption contributes to irregular shape of trabeculae. Sharpey fibers are recognizable. GNAS I analysis revealed an arg>cys amino acid substitution.

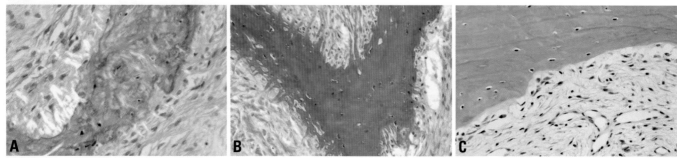

Fig. 6.78 Fibrous dysplasia. **A** Extension of Sharpey fibers from trabeculae into stroma on polarized microscopy. **B** Collagenous Sharpey fibers reaching from bone into cellular stroma. Absence of osteoblastic rimming. GNAS I analysis revealed arg>cys amino acid substitution. Van Gieson stain. **C** In long-standing fibrous dysplasia focal lamellar remodelling may occur in the absence of osteoblastic rimming. GNAS I analysis revealed arg>cys amino acid substitution.

on T1 and proton-weighted images, and heterogeneous hypointense on T2, showing a moderate to marked signal enhancement following Gd-DPTA administration {1586,1759}.

Histopathology

FD consists of cellular fibrous tissue with spindle shaped cells and immature, isolated trabeculae of woven bone generally without rimming of osteoblasts {2401, 2710}. Characteristically, bundles of collagen fibres oriented perpendicular to the bone surface, compatible with Sharpey-fibers, can be demonstrated {1018,2067,2176}. Osteoid seams are present and best visualized on undecalcified sections {210,2067}. In long standing lesions some osteoblastic rimming and "maturation" to lamellar bone may occur. This may result in parallel ordered bony trabeculae {2379,2401}. Cartilaginous foci in FD of the jaws or skull have not been documented.

Genetics

Activating mutations in the GNAS1 gene, coding for the α-subunit of the stimulatory G-Protein have been proven in MFD, PFD as well as in MAS {472,2175}. In eight of eleven cases clonal chromosomal aberrations have been described, including both structural and numeric changes. Repeated chromosomal changes have only been documented so far for trisomy 2 and rearrangements of 12p13, in three cases each {527}. These findings may suggest that FD is a neoplastic process {472,527,775}.

Prognosis and predictive factors

In most cases of FD the lesions seem to stabilize with skeletal maturation. Surgical interventions may be necessary for functional reasons or severe disfigurement {2710}. Very rarely, sarcoma development, predominantly osteosarcoma, has been reported preferentially in craniofacial bones and even in the

absence of prior irradiation {220,2213, 2522,2835}.

Osseous dysplasias

P.J. Slootweg

Definition
Osseous dysplasias (ODs) are idiopathic processes located in the periapical region of the tooth-bearing jaw areas, characterized by a replacement of normal bone by fibrous tissue and metaplastic bone.

Synonyms
Periapical cemental dysplasia, periapical osseous dysplasia, focal cemento-osseous dysplasia, periapical cementoma.

Epidemiology
OD has a predilection for middle-aged black females {261}.

Localization
OD is confined to the tooth-bearing part of the jaws.

Clinical features / Imaging
The condition occurs in various clinical forms that bear different names. When occuring in the anterior mandible and involving only a few adjacent teeth, it is called periapical osseous dysplasia. A similar limited lesion occurring in a posterior jaw quadrant is known as focal osseous dysplasia, formerly called focal cemento-osseous dysplasia {2502}. Two other types of OD are more extensive, occuring bilaterally in the mandible or even involving all 4 jaw quadrants. The first is known as florid osseous dysplasia {261,2864}. This type of OD mainly occurs in middle-aged black females. The second occurs at young age and causes considerable jaw expansion. This OD type is called familial gigantiform cementoma; it shows an autosomal dominant inheritance with variable expression but sporadic cases without a history of familial involvement have been reported {7, 2864}.

Periapical and focal OD usually are incidental radiographic findings. The involved teeth remain vital. Florid OD may give rise to symptoms in cases of concomitant infection. Jaw expansion is not a feature of ODs with the exception of the familial gigantiform cementoma and is rarely seen in florid OD.

ODs may be predominantely radiolucent, predominantly radiodense or mixed. Radiodensity tends to increase with time. In the mixed or radiodense stage of OD, a radiolucent halo usually separates the

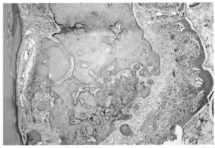

Fig. 6.80 Focal OD laterally in the periodontal ligament space between the root surface (left) and alveolar tooth socket (right). This case is more heavily mineralized than that in Fig. 6.79B.

lesions from the surrounding bone and the root surface.

Histopathology
All types of OD consist of cellular fibrous tissue, woven as well as lamellar bone and masses of cementum-like material. There is no capsule. The hard tissue component in most cases does not fuse with the root surface of the involved teeth, but may merge with the surrounding bone. Secondary inflammatory changes may occur, especially with the florid OD and the familial gigantiform cementoma. OD resembles ossifying fibroma (OF) histologically. Clinical and radiographic information is needed to make the distinction {2485}. OD may be also confused with fibrous dysplasia (FD). However, the variation in appearances of mineralized material distinguishes both lesions, fibrous dysplasia almost exclusively consisting of woven bone {2401}.

Histogenesis
Osseous dysplasia is considered to originate from the periodontal ligament {2861}.

Prognosis and predictive factors
The various forms of osseous dysplasia do not require treatment unless complications occur such as infection of sclerotic bone masses as may be encountered in florid OD or facial deformity as may be seen in familial gigantiform cementoma.

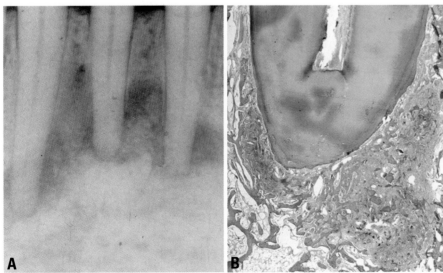

Fig. 6.79 Osseous dysplasia. **A** Dental radiograph showing partly mineralized periapical OD. **B** Focal OD presenting as a periapical fibrous lesion containing bony particles of varying appearances. Fortuitous finding in a mandible resected for treatment of squamous cell carcinoma (SCC).

Central giant cell lesion

G. Jundt

Definition
Central giant cell lesion (CGCL) is a localized benign but sometimes aggressive osteolytic proliferation consisting of fibrous tissue with haemorrhage and haemosiderin deposits, presence of osteoclast-like giant cells and reactive bone formation.

Synonyms
Central giant cell granuloma, reparative giant cell granuloma.

Epidemiology
CGCL is found in all age groups, however, most cases are diagnosed in patients under 30 years of age, with an incidence rate of 1.1/million population / year {559}. In contrast to giant cell tumour of bone, about 1/3 of patients are younger than 20 years {1239}. Women are more often affected than men (1.5-2:1) {1244}.

Localization
The mandible is more often involved than the maxilla {1244,2782}. Molar and pre-molar areas are more often affected than the anterior parts or the ascending ramus {2460}. Involvement of the condyle or maxillary sinus is rare {11, 1244}. Multifocal giant cell lesions do occur. They may be sporadic and unre-lated to other conditions (eg. hyper-parathyroidism, cherubism, Noonan syndrome) {2414,2663}.

Clinical features / Imaging
Most cases present as asymptomatic incidental findings. Some, however, pres-ent with pain or paraesthesia, swellings, or loosening of teeth. Nasal obstruction may occur {1239,2782}.
CGCL are expansile, radiolucent and often multiloculated lesions, rarely mixed with opacities, with scalloped and mostly well-defined but non-corticated borders. With increasing size, multilocularity is more often noticed {2460}. Disappea-rance of the lamina dura, root resorption or, more often, tooth displacement are additional findings {452,967,1244,2460, 2782}. Intralesional wavy bony septa are characteristic {967}. Periapical localiza-tion may mimic periapical granuloma {524}.

Histopathology
The lesion consists of spindle-shaped fibroblastic or myofibroblastic cells {643,1920}, loosely arranged in a fibrous, sometimes fibromyxoid, vascularized tis-sue with haemorrhagic areas, haemosiderin deposits, macrophages, lymphocytes, granulocytes and, rarely, plasma cells. Especially in the haemor-rhagic areas, evenly dispersed or small clusters of osteoclast-like giant cells are found {84,452,771}. In addition, travers-ing collagen bundles are present, often accompanied by metaplastic bone for-mation, giving the lesion a somewhat lob-ular appearance. Mitoses are frequently

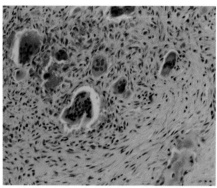

Fig. 6.81 CGCL. Clusters of multinucleated giant cells close to small foci of haemorrhage accompa-nied by mononuclear cells. Reactive bone forma-tion within the spindle cell stroma (lower right).

found {1239,2398,2839}. Since brown tumour of hyperparathyroidism is mor-phologically indistinguishable from CGCL, determination of parathormone levels may be indicated, especially in elderly patients or when multifocal lesions are present {1276,1645,2694}.

Genetics
In one case of a peripheral CGCL of the distal phalanx a cytogenetic study has been performed revealing a transloca-tion involving the X-chromosome and chromosome 4 [t(X;4)(q22;q31.3)] {310}.

Prognosis and predictive factors
Histological findings are not predictive of biological behaviour. The treatment of CGCL is careful enucleation. In case of recurrences, more extensive surgery should be considered. Administration of calcitonin (intranasal or s.c), {558,1015,1921} or glucocorticoids (intralesional) has proven effective in some cases {333,1394}. More recently, antiangiogenic therapy with interferon alpha has been successfully applied {1241}.

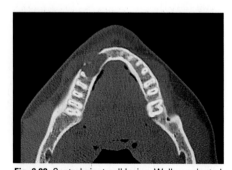

Fig. 6.82 Central giant cell lesion. Well marginated hypodense osteolysis with vestibular cortical destruction but no cortical thinning. Transversal CT scan, bone window.

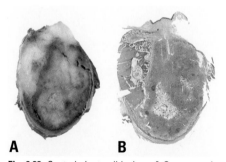

A   **B**

Fig. 6.83 Central giant cell lesion. **A** Gross speci-men with brownish friable tissue. **B** Well circum-scribed lesion, demarcated from adherent soft tis-sues (top) and mandibular bone (left).

Cherubism

G. Jundt

Definition
Cherubism is an autosomal dominant inherited disease that is characterized by a symmetrical distension of the jaws, often leading to a typical facial expression. The histology is indistinguishable from central giant cell lesion.

Epidemiology
Cherubism is a familial disease affecting 100% of males and up to 70% of females. Sporadic cases do occur {589,1237,2023}. Generally, diagnosis is made in early childhood (14 months to 4 years) or, in milder forms, in pre-adolescence. With increasing age, especially after cessation of bone growth, the lesions regress {2608}.

Localization
All four quadrants of the jaws can be involved. Usually the mandible is affected more extensively, starting at the angle

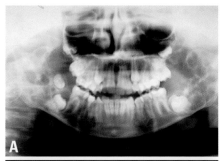

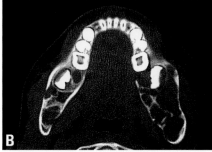

Fig. 6.84 Cherubism. **A** Bilateral expansile multilocular osteolytic lesions of both mandibular angles and the ascending ramus. To a lesser extent, both tuber maxillae are also affected. **B** CT scan showing bilateral 'soap bubble'-like expansion of mandible with intralesional bony septa. Thinned corticalis with focal perforation.

at the time of permanent molar eruption. The process may extend into the ascending ramus without affecting the condyle, and the mandibular body. In the maxilla, both tuberosities are affected initially followed by involvement of the anterior and inferior portions of the orbits {76,479}.

Clinical features / Imaging
Symmetrical swellings and an indolent clinical course are characteristic. Bilateral maxillary enlargement may lead to retraction of the facial skin including the lower eyelids, resulting in scleral exposure and the typical "looking toward Heaven" appearance (cherubs on Renaissance paintings) {479,1236}. Other consequences are tooth displacement and delay in tooth eruption, loosening of teeth, speech alterations and visual impairment. In addition, cervical lymphadenopathy is noticed {24,76,1287, 2608}.

Affected bones are expanded by bilateral, well-delineated multilocular radiolucencies with a "soap bubble" appearance. The cortices may become thinned and focally perforated. With advancing age, the initially fibrous tissue is replaced by bony structures, leading to sclerosis {76}. The diagnosis is supported by clinical presentation (bilateral enlargement of the jaws) and the typical radiological findings on panoramic or lateral views, or CT-scans {1105}.

Histopathology
Initially, fibrous tissue and giant cells resembling osteoclasts are present, giving an impression that may be almost indistinguishable from central giant cell lesion {1287,2840}. Additional features are haemosiderin deposits and stromal fibrosis {1237}. Although a rare finding, perivascular cuff-like collagen deposits are regarded as characteristic for cherubism {990}. Although the histology is not specific, the combination of clinical appearance, radiology and central giant-cell lesion-like histology is diagnostic.

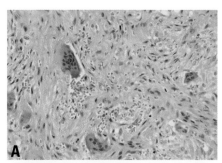

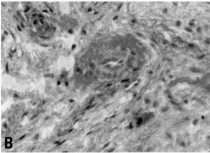

Fig. 6.85 Cherubism **A** Loosely arranged fibrous tissue with haemorrhage and few osteoclastic giant cells. **B** Cuff-like perivascular collagenous deposits. Van Gieson stain.

Genetics
Cherubism is an autosomal dominant familial disease and has been mapped to chromosome 4p16.3 {1621,2608}. Through analysis of 12 families, the mutated gene was recently identified as SH3BP2, coding for a c-Abl-binding protein. However, since the mutation was not detected in three other families, mutations in genes different from SH3BP2 cannot be ruled out {2650}.

Prognosis and predictive factors
With time, especially after puberty, the lesions regress {1286}. Before puberty, surgery should be carried out only in cases of severe functional disturbances {1362}.

Aneurysmal bone cyst

G. Jundt

Definition
Aneurysmal bone cyst (ABC) is an expansile osteolytic lesion often multilocular, with blood filled spaces separated by fibrous septa containing osteoclast-type giant cells and reactive bone.

Epidemiology
ABC has an incidence of 0.014/100.000 and occurs preferentially in patients below the age of 30 years with a peak in the second decade {1464}. Epidemiologic data for the jaws are lacking. However, ABC in the jaws is rare encompassing 1-3% of all ABCs {1239}.

Etiology
ABC may arise primarily or as a secondary event in another bone lesion, e.g. giant cell lesion or fibrous dysplasia {2483,2802}. Most lesions are believed to be reactive, however, an association with trauma is unlikely, especially for maxillary ones {150}. Cytogenetic data provide evidence that at least some ABCs are neoplastic.

Localization
ABC is more often found in the mandible {1303} with a predominance for the posterior regions including the ascending ramus {1246}. The condyle is only exceptionally affected {1787}. A more uniform distribution is noted in the maxilla {150}.

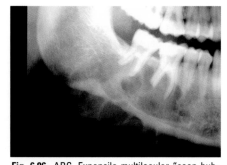

Fig. 6.86 ABC. Expansile multilocular "soap bubble"-like osteolysis with soft tissue extension transversed by intralesional bony septa. Although barely visible, the extraosseous component is well delineated. Root resorption of included teeth.

Clinical features
ABC may present with marked swelling and few symptoms. Malocclusion, tooth displacement and loosening may develop. Teeth remain vital {150,2482}. Root resorption may be present {1246}. Orbital involvement may lead to exophthalmos and diplopia. Nasal obstruction or bleeding is rare {150}.

Imaging
Unilocular or multilocular radiolucent lesions are seen. In up to 10% a mixed radiopaque-radiolucent pattern can be found. Borders are well delineated but perforations of the cortices may be present and extensions into the soft tissues do occur. On cross sectional imaging studies internal septa are visible. Fluid-fluid levels produced by sedimentation of blood cells in lesional cavities are particularly seen on MRI (gradient echo sequences or T2 weighted images) and are very characteristic {78,1246,2160}.

Histopathology
ABC is haemorrhagic, multilocular and well circumscribed. The blood-filled cavities are lined by macrophages and not by endothelial cells {39}. They represent pseudocysts since there is no epithelial lining. The septa are composed of inconspicuous fibroblasts, osteoclast-like giant cells and reactive bone or irregular osteoid are distributed parallel to the septal lining. Haemosiderin deposits are also present. Mitoses are frequently found, however, atypical forms are not seen. Necrosis may be present {1303,2802}.

Genetics
A 17p-rearrangement is a constant finding in ABC in the extracranial skeleton, most often presenting as balanced translocation with 16q but other chromosomes may also be involved {147,1072, 1894,1977,2281,2832}. One case originating in the nose revealed a (6;17)(p21;p13) translocation {2797}. Since the metaphases of the non-involved chromosomes seem to be nor-

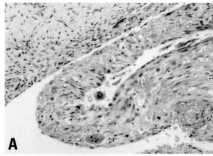

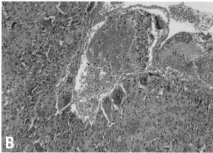

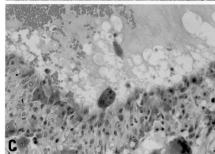

Fig. 6.87 ABC. **A** Pseudoendothelial covering of septa by macrophages and giant cells. **B** Wall of pseuodocyst delineated by macrophages and giant cells. **C** Macrophages covering the septa do not show cellular atypia. Close to the surface giant cells are seen.

mal the translocations may be regarded as resulting from acquired aberrations providing evidence, that at least some ABCs are clonal proliferations {775}. Familial cases have been reported {598, 943,2692}.

Prognosis and predictive factors
ABC can be treated with curettage {1249}. Soft tissue extension increases the risk of recurrence. Embolization has also been applied successfully {956}.

Simple bone cyst

G. Jundt

Definition
Simple bone cyst (SBC) is an intraosseous pseudocyst devoid of an epithelial lining, either empty or filled with serous or sanguinous fluid.

Synonyms
Solitary bone cyst, traumatic bone cyst, haemorrhagic bone cyst, haemorrhagic cyst, unicameral bone cyst, idiopathic bone cavity

Epidemiology
SBC is most commonly observed during the second decade of life {184}. In contrast to the long bones (male/female ratio of 2-3:1), in the jaws there is no gender predilection {1392}.

Etiology
The etiology is unknown {1752,2341}.

Localization
The mandible {1239} is almost exclusively affected {1239,1392}. Most SBCs are located in the anterior part of the mandible {1392}. Cases with bilateral lesions have been described {1990}.

Clinical features
In general, SBC is discovered incidentally. Complaints are tenderness or mild pain. Displacement of teeth or pathological fractures are very unusual {2341}. Teeth are usually vital {1006}. A history of trauma is rarely reported {1665}.

Imaging
Usually, SBC is radiolucent and unilocular with no or only slight expansion of bone and cortical thinning {1665}. Superior margins extend between the roots of teeth and are characteristically scalloped and corticated {2272}. Root resorption is an unusual finding. Intracavitary fluid has been visualized on T2 weighted MRI images {690}.
A final diagnosis is aided by finding an empty cavity at surgical exploration.

Histopathology
The lining of the cavity is made up of connective tissue covering the underlying bone with a membrane-like layer {184,1239}. Rarely, a thickened myxofibromatous wall is seen {1665,2224}. Small amounts of new bone formation and collagen deposits may be present, often described as appearing fibrin- or cementum-like. In addition, scattered giant cells and haemosiderin are also found {1006}.

Genetics
Only two genetically analyzed cases, localized in the long bones, have been reported so far. Complex clonal structural rearrangements of chromosome 4, 6, 8, 16, 21, and both 12 were demonstrated {2686}. In addition, a translocation t(16;20)(p11.2;q13) present as the sole abnormality has been described {2166}.

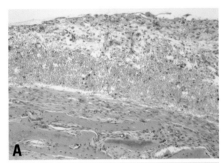

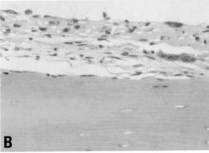

Fig. 6.89 Simple bone cyst (SBC). **A** Membrane-like fibrous covering of the cavity overlying bone. **B** Thinned corticalis covered by a membranous layer and fibroblasts on top. Focal deposition of collagen (top right).

Prognosis and predictive factors
Usually bone healing is completed within a year after surgical exploration. However, persistence following curettage may occur requiring additional treatment {789,1392}.

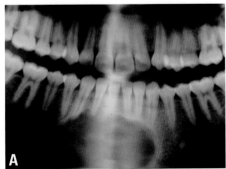

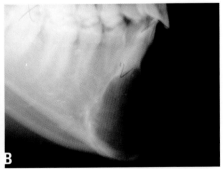

Fig. 6.88 SBC. **A** Centrally located unicameral osteolysis with sclerotic margins extending between the roots of adjacent teeth. Panoramic radiograph. **B** Expansion of mandible with thinning of corticalis.

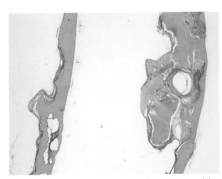

Fig. 6.90 SBC. Thinned cortical bone covered by fibrous septa.

CHAPTER 7

Tumours of the Ear

Tumours are unusual in the ear. In the external ear most of the neoplasms are those of the covering skin. Only the ceruminous glands are peculiar to the external ear, but ceruminous tumours are rare. The underlying bone contributes some swellings and neoplasms to this area. The most common tumour in the middle ear is the adenoma, which arises from low-mitotic cuboidal epithelium that may become neoplastic. The inner ear is composed of a specific inert bone, a virtually non-mitotic sensory area and nerves. Tumours that are derived from Schwann cells are the only frequent neoplasms of the inner ear, indeed of the whole temporal bone.

Diagnosis of ear tumours presents a peculiar difficulty in that the whole structure is often encased in dense bone. Although modern imaging techniques have helped greatly to identify tumours and tumour-like lesions of the ear, there is still a need for autopsy studies in this area.

WHO histological classification of tumours of the ear

Tumours of the external ear
Benign tumours of ceruminous glands
    Adenoma   8420/0
    Chondroid syringoma   8940/0
    Syringocystadenoma papilliferum   8406/0
Cylindroma   8200/0
Malignant tumours of ceruminous glands
    Adenocarcinoma   8420/3
    Adenoid cystic carcinoma   8200/3
    Mucoepidermoid carcinoma   8430/3
Squamous cell carcinoma   8070/3
Embryonal rhabdomyosarcoma   8900/3
Osteoma and exostosis   9180/0
Angiolymphoid hyperplasia with eosinophilia   9125/0

Tumours of the middle ear
Adenoma of the middle ear   8140/0

Papillary tumours
    Aggressive papillary tumour   8260/1
    Schneiderian papilloma   8121/0
    Inverted papilloma   8121/1
Squamous cell carcinoma   8070/3
Meningioma   9530/0

Tumours of the inner ear
Vestibular schwannoma   9560/0
Lipoma of the internal auditory canal   8850/0
Haemangioma   9120/0
Endolymphatic sac tumour   8140/3

Haematolymphoid tumours
B-cell chronic lymphocytic leukaemia /   9823/3
    small lymphocytic lymphoma   9670/3
Langerhans cell histiocytosis   9751/1

Secondary tumours

___
[1] Morphology code of the International Classification of Diseases for Oncology (ICD-O) {821} and the Systematized Nomenclature of Medicine (http://snomed.org). Behaviour is coded /0 for benign tumours, /3 for malignant tumours, and /1 for borderline or uncertain behaviour.

Ceruminous gland neoplasms of external auditory canal and cylindroma

L. Michaels
L.D.R. Thompson

Definition

External ear neoplasms derived from ceruminous glands are very uncommon and can be benign or malignant. Only the adenoma (ceruminoma) can be categorized as being derived specifically from ceruminous glands. Syringocystadenoma papilliferum and adenoid cystic carcinoma arising in this region can sometimes manifest an origin from ceruminous glands. These tumours are either benign or malignant.

Localization

The expected site of origin is in the superficial part of the external canal.

Clinical features

The symptoms of this lesion, like other external ear canal lesions, are conductive hearing loss and discharge. Pain and facial nerve palsy are clinical predictors of malignancy.

Epidemiology

The benign and malignant tumours occur with equal frequency in men and women with a mean age of 49 years (range 26-89 years) {569,1478,1589}.

Adenoma of ceruminous glands

ICD-O code   8420/0

Macroscopy

Gross appearances are those of a non-ulcerating superficial grey mass up to 4 cm in diameter, which is covered by skin.

Histopathology

Microscopically this neoplasm lacks a capsule. It is composed of regular oxyphil glands often with intraluminal projections. The glandular epithelium is bilayered. The outer myoepithelial layer may not be obvious in all parts of the neoplasm. In some ceruminomas, acid-fast fluorescent ceroid pigment may be found which is similar to that seen in normal ceruminal glands {2778}.
Electron microscopy. One case of ceruminous gland adenoma showed apocrine caps, microvilli, cell junctions, secretory granules, vacuoles, lipid droplets and siderosomes, the characteristic ultrastructural features of apocrine glands {2260}.

Chondroid syringoma

Definition

Benign tumour similar to the pleomorphic adenoma of salivary glands.

ICD-O code   8940/0

Synonym

Pleomorphic adenoma or mixed tumour.

Histopathology

Cartilage, myoepithelial and adenomatous structures are features of this neoplasm.

Syringocystadenoma papilliferum

Definition

Benign adnexal tumour with features similar to those seen at other sites.

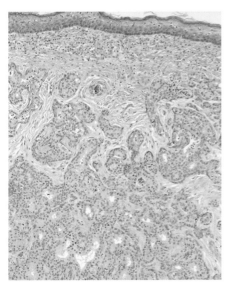

Fig. 7.1 Ceruminous adenoma. Keratinized squamous epithelium overlies a circumscribed but unencapsulated neoplastic proliferation of ceruminous glands. Note glandular and small cystic profiles.

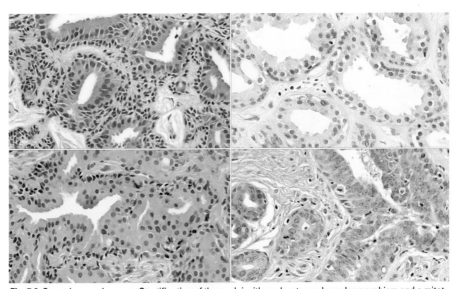

Fig. 7.2 Ceruminous adenoma. Stratification of the nuclei with moderate nuclear pleomorphism and a mitotic figure (upper left); Abundant eosinophilic-granular cytoplasm in the luminal cells which show focal decapitation secretion (upper right); glandular structures separated by fibrous connective tissue (lower left); inner luminal secretory cells subtended by basal myoepithelial cells demonstrate the dual cell population (lower right).

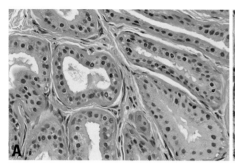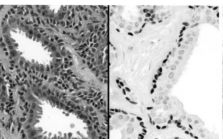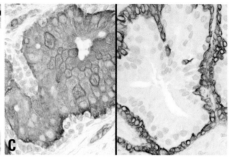

Fig. 7.3 Ceruminous adenoma. **A** Yellow-brown "ceroid" lipofuscin-like material is seen in the cytoplasm of ceruminous cells, a feature seen in modified ceruminous sweat glands and in ceruminous adenomas. **B** Glandular structures show ceruminous decapitation secretion in the luminal cells subtended by a prominent, well-defined myoepithelial cell layer (left). The myoepithelial cell nuclei are accentuated with a p63 immunoreaction (right). **C** Differential immunohistochemical staining highlights the luminal cells (CK7, left) while CK5/6 accentuated the basal cells (right).

ICD-O code	8406/0

Synonym
Hidradenoma papilliferum

Epidemiology and localization
Syringocystadenoma papilliferum is seen in children or young adults usually on the scalp or face. Occasionally it occurs in the ear canal.

Histopathology
Cystic invagination from surface epithelium. Projecting into the lumen are papillae covered by bilayered apocrine glandular epithelium which may show decapitation secretion typical of ceruminous glands.

Cylindroma

Definition
Cylindroma is a benign tumour arising from the epidermal adnexae, whether apocrine- or eccrine-derived is not conclusively known.

ICD-O code	8200/0

Synonym
Turban tumour

Localization
In the external ear the lesion may be present on the pinna or in the external canal. In these situations it may be part of a multiple "turban tumour" presentation of this neoplasm on the scalp.

Histopathology
It is composed histologically of rounded masses of small, darkly staining cells which fit together in a jig-saw-like pattern and are surrounded by pink-staining hyaline material. Extracellular hyaline globules are often present in the cellular masses. Larger cells with vesicular nuclei are also seen {2804}. In contrast to primary adenoid cystic carcinoma, cylindroma in the external canal does not have a cribriform structure, but does have larger cells with vesicular nuclei.

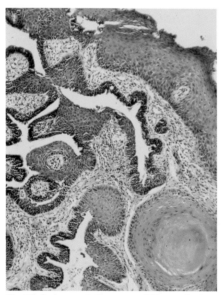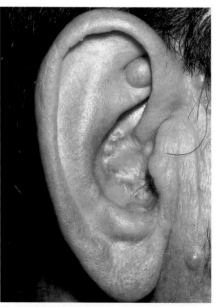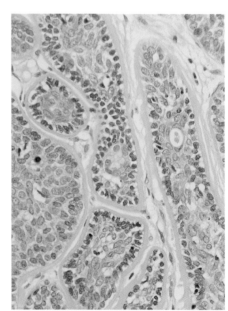

Fig. 7.4 Syringocystadenoma papilliferum of external ear canal. Note papillae lined by bilayered glandular epithelium projecting into a cystic lumen. There is also a prominent epidermoid cyst.

Fig. 7.5 Cylindroma of pinna with multiple spherical lesions on pinna, face and temporal region. From L. Michaels & H. Hellquist {1711}.

Fig. 7.6 Cylindroma of pinna showing jigsaw-like pattern of cell groups, surrounded by hyaline basement membranes.

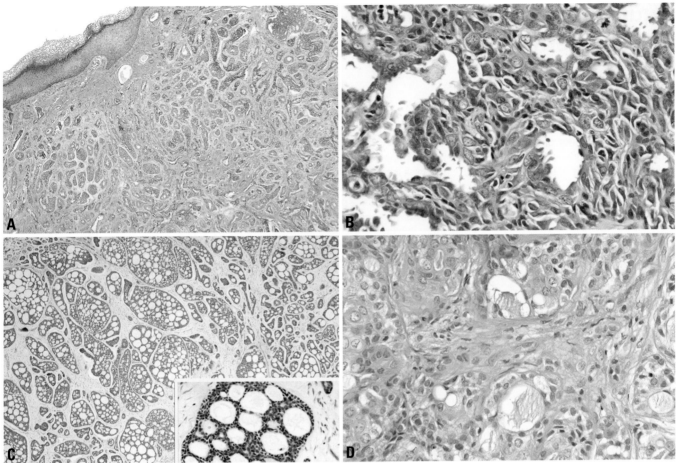

Fig. 7.7 Ceruminous adenocarcinoma. **A** An intact surface epithelium is subtended by an infiltrating "biphasic" neoplastic proliferation separated by dense fibrosis. **B** A ceruminous adenocarcinoma (NOS) demonstrating decapitation secretion in the center gland, while the remarkably atypical cells are seen in an "infiltrative" growth pattern. Note the mitotic figure in the upper right corner. **C** Adenoid cystic carcinoma. The overall cribriform ("Swiss-cheese") pattern is seen on both the low power and with the inset. **D** Mucoepidermoid carcinoma, intermediate grade. Epithelial cells and mucous cells are readily identified in this infiltrating neoplasm.

Malignant tumours of ceruminous glands

Definition
An infiltrating neoplasm derived from ceruminous glands.

ICD-O codes
Adenocarcinoma 8420/3
Adenoid cystic carcinoma
8200/3
Mucoepidermoid carcinoma
8430/3

Localization
Superficial part of the external ear canal. Origin from the adjacent parotid salivary gland should be excluded.

Histopathology
Low and high-grade adenocarcinoma
These neoplasms possess a glandular structure with evidence of apocrine dif- ferentiation and infiltration. Low-grade tumours show loss of a myoepithelial layer and infiltration. The cells of high-grade tumours are markedly atypical with increased mitotic activity and wide-spread invasion.

Adenoid cystic carcinoma
The microscopic features of these tumours are indistinguishable from those arising in salivary glands. They charac-teristically widely infiltrate adjacent tis-sues and invade nerve sheaths.

Mucoepidermoid carcinoma
The tumours arising in this location are usually low-grade and the microscopic features are similar to those arising in salivary glands.

Prognosis and predictive factors
Recurrence often complicates surgical removal of high-grade tumours. Death due to involvement of local vital struc-tures and metastases has been reported. Relentless, although often delayed recur-rence and eventual bloodstream metas-tasis, particularly to the lungs is likewise a feature of adenoid cystic carcinoma.

Squamous cell carcinoma of the external ear

L. Michaels
S. Soucek

Definition
This malignant tumour of stratified squamous epithelium arises from the normal epidermal covering of the external canal of the pinna.

ICD-O code
8070/3

Synonyms
Epidermoid carcinoma, squamous carcinoma

Epidemiology
The average age at diagnosis is 65-70 years for the pinna lesions and there is a male predominance. The age at presentation is 52-55 years for the external canal tumours which show a female predominance {1226}.

Etiology
Actinic overexposure and frostbite have been suggested as causes of the pinna lesion. The canal tumours have been linked with the same tumour type in the middle ear as possibly resulting from prolonged chronic inflammation. It is possible, however, that the clinical impression of chronic inflammation has been mistaken, the patients' symptoms being the result of an occult squamous cell carcinoma.

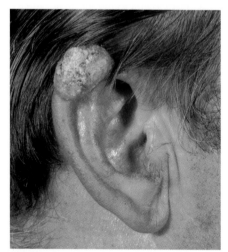

Fig. 7.8 Squamous cell carcinoma of the pinna forming a large mass with central ulceration.

Localization
The majority of squamous cell carcinomas of the external ear arise on the pinna; a lesser number arise in the external canal. The external ear sites of involvement in the pinna in a study of 52 patients are shown in Table 7.1. Rarely there is bilateral external ear involvement {2807}.

Clinical features
The pinna lesions being in an exposed position are identified early. A serious problem with the canal lesions is the delay in diagnosis because of the minimal symptoms that may be present. Pain, hearing loss and drainage of blood or pus are the main features in that group. A plaque-like or even polypoid mass may be felt or even seen.

Macroscopy
Squamous cell carcinomas arising on the pinna grossly resemble those seen elsewhere on the skin. The appearances of the canal lesions are those of a mass, sometimes warty, occluding the lumen and invading deeply into the surrounding tissues. There may be dissolution of the tympanic membrane with invasion of the middle ear. Occasionally, the well-differentiated lesions may not be detected clinically until well advanced.

Tumour spread and staging
The TNM staging for skin does not seem applicable at this site because of the presence of cartilage invasion.

Histopathology
Epidermoid carcinoma of the external ear usually shows significant degrees of keratinization. Those showing a spindle cell morphology must be differentiated from melanomas and soft tissue tumours. In the cases with a canal origin evidence of origin from canal epidermis is usually present. In cases arising deeply within the ear canal there is usually a concomitant origin from middle ear epithelium and dissolution of the tympanic membrane. The neoplasm may be so well dif-

Table 7.1 Sites of involvement of squamous cell carcinoma of the pinna in 52 patients {2336}.

Site	Number of Patients
Helix	27
Posterior auricle	11
Antihelix	6
Triangular fossa	3
Concha	3
Lobule	2

ferentiated that it can be confused with a papilloma. The association of such a neoplasm with marked desmoplasia may further delay the correct diagnosis. Verrucous carcinoma has been seen in the external ear {2456}.

Precursor lesions
Actinic keratosis may precede squamous cell carcinoma.

Prognosis and predictive factors
Squamous cell carcinoma of the pinna is an aggressive disease with a high propensity for local recurrence. Tumours confined to the external ear usually have a good outlook after surgical therapy. The outcome of the disease following surgical excision is related to the clinical stage at presentation, the higher the stage the worse the outcome {1915}. Metastatic spread of squamous carcinoma of the pinna and external auditory meatus to lymph nodes is unusual. Lesions arising in the canal have a worse prognosis because of the late diagnosis and invasion of adjacent structures.

Embryonal rhabdomyosarcoma

A. Sandison

Rhabdomyosarcoma and its variants have been comprehensively discussed in the WHO Classification of Tumours of Soft Tissue and Bone {775}. This section focuses on its occurrence as a primary tumour in the external ear canal.

Definition
A primitive malignant tumour with phenotypic and biological features of embryonic skeletal muscle.

ICD-O code   8900/3

Synonyms
Myosarcoma, embryonal sarcoma, botryoid sarcoma.

Epidemiology
Rhabdomyosarcoma is rare in any part of the body. There is a distinct group arising in the head and neck of children, often very young, with a predilection for the palate, middle ear and orbit.

Localization
Most of the tumours arise in the middle ear with extension into the external canal as an "aural polyp".

Clinical features
Embryonal rhabdomyosarcoma should be excluded in any child presenting with a polyp in the external ear canal. Advanced cases may present with aural discharge, facial weakness and swelling in the region of the ear {1116}. Extensive destruction of the bone at the base of the skull, especially the petrous bone has been described.

Histopathology
Only the embryonal subtype of rhabdomyosarcoma is recognized as occurring at this site. The characteristics of this polypoid tumour are those of rhabdomyoblasts and primitive mesenchymal cells showing a variable degree of skeletal muscle differentiation loosely arranged but with condensation beneath the epithelium (cambium layer). Yolk sac tumour has been described as a polypoid tumour presenting in the external ear canal. However, this is histologically distinct, being composed of small round blue cells arranged in a vacuolated pattern with formation of Schiller-Duval bodies and expressing alpha fetoprotein {833}. A detailed description of embryo

nal rhabdomayosarcoma including immunophenotype is given in the WHO Classification of Tumours of Soft Tissue and Bone {775}.

Histogenesis
Although it is suggested that this tumour arises from striated muscle fibres in the middle ear, it seems more likely that the origin is from undifferentiated mesenchymal cells.

Genetics
Mutations in a region mapped to the short arm of chromosome 11 (11p15) have been associated with most embryonal rhabomyosarcomas. Several genes have been mapped to this site. Complex structural and numerical chromosomal rearrangements have been associated with embryonal rhabdomyosarcoma. These are discussed in detail in the WHO Bone and Soft tissue book.

Prognosis and predictive factors
Modern chemotherapeutic schedules have dramatically improved the outcome for children with this tumour.

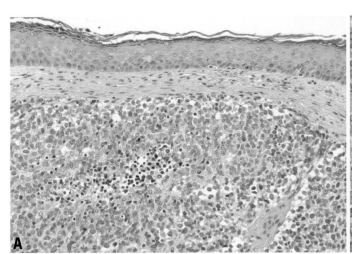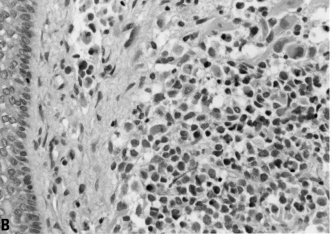

Fig. 7.9 Ear rhabdomyosarcoma. **A** A central area of necrosis is surrounded by "primitive cells" with a very high nuclear to cytoplasmic ratio. The neoplasm is separated from the surface. **B** This polypoid tumour has a "Grenz-Zone" between the neoplastic cells and the mucosal surface. The malignant cells have abundant eosinophilic cytoplasm.

Fibrous dysplasia

A. Sandison

Definition
Fibrous dysplasia (FD) is a benign localised intramedullary proliferation of trabecular woven bone admixed with fibrous tissue. It may be monostotic, involving one bone or polyostotic involving several bones.

Synonyms
Benign fibro-osseous lesion.

Epidemiology
FD affects children and adults and there is no geographical, or racial predilection. The monostotic form affects both sexes equally; the polyostotic form is more common in females by a 3:1 ratio.

Etiology
Exact etiology is uncertain. The most recent attempts to define the disorder have focused on genetics and molecular biology.

Localization
Any bone in the body can be affected. In the head and neck the skull and facial bones are affected in 10-20% of cases of monostotic disease and 50% of polyostotic cases. In cases with involvement of the temporal bone., the disease is pre-

dominantly monostotic. The tympanic, mastoid, squamous or petrous temporal bone may be involved. Other unusual sites include the internal auditory canal, the lateral semi-circular canal and the ossicles. In a retrospective analysis of patients with fibrous dysplasia affecting the skull base, Lustig et al found the temporal bone to be affected in 24% .

Clinical features
The main clinical features of disease affecting the temporal bone are: (i) progressive loss of hearing, mostly conductive but which can be sensorineural and profound in some cases, (ii) temporal bone enlargement with progressive bony occlusion of the external auditory meatus, (iii) facial nerve palsy in some patients when the process affects the seventh cranial nerve, (iv) constriction of the ear canal may result in development of an epidermoid cyst lateral to the tympanic membrane likened to cholesteatoma by Megerian et al {1698}.

Macroscopy
The affected bone is often expanded and the marrow is replaced by firm grey/tan tissue depending on the proportion of bony, fibrous and cartilaginous elements.

There may be cyst formation.

Histopathology
The lesion consists of irregular trabeculae of woven bone arising abruptly from a bland spindle cell stroma. The trabeculae may be curved and shaped like letters in the Chinese ideogram and are devoid of a rim of osteoblasts. There is no nuclear atypia and mitoses are few. The proportion of fibrous and bony tissue is variable. The lesion may include benign cartilage. Secondary changes include osteoclast giant cells, foamy histiocytes and aneurysmal bone cyst formation.

Genetics
Polyostotic fibrous dysplasia (POFD) may occur in the setting of McCune-Albright syndrome, caused by activating mutations in the complex GNAS locus on chromosome 20 {327,527,577}.

Prognosis and predictive factors
Fibrous dysplasia has rarely been associated with malignant transformation including osteogenic sarcoma, fibrosarcoma and chondrosarcoma, but the temporal bone is not one of the sites where this change has been described.

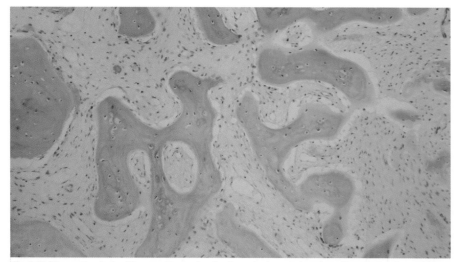

Fig. 7.10 Fibrous dysplasia of temporal bone showing irregular bony trabeculae without a rim of osteoblasts.

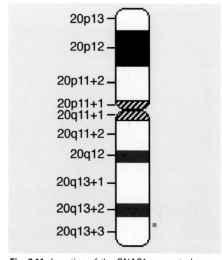

Fig. 7.11 Location of the GNAS1 gene at chromosome 20q13.2-13.3.

Osteoma and exostosis

A. Sandison
T. Beale

Definition
Benign bony enlargement of the deeper portion of the external auditory meatus. There are two distinct forms. Exostosis is more common than osteoma.

ICD-O code
Osteoma   9180/0

Synonyms
Osteochondroma, osteocartilaginous exostosis.

Etiology
Exostosis appears to be related to trauma such as repeated exposure to cold water; in swimmers there appears to be an association with development of exostoses of the tympanic bone {769}. Exostoses have also been observed in individuals who routinely use stethoscopes, eg cardiologists {550}. The etiology of osteoma is not clear.

Localization
Osteoma is a very rare lesion, which is a single, unilateral, spherical mass on a distinct pedicle arising in the region of the tympanosquamous or tympanomastoid suture line. It has only occasionally been described outside the external auditory canal and the middle ear, developing in the mastoids, temporal bone internal auditory canal, glenoid fossa eustachian tube, petrous apex and styloid process.

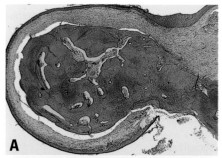

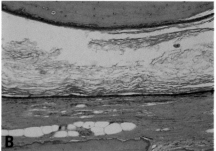

Fig. 7.12 A Osteoma of deep external canal. From L. Michaels & H. Hellquist {1711}. **B** Exostosis of deep external canal. Note thin epidermal layer on the exostosis above and on the canal skin below and their proximity to the bone. In deeper sections, the exostosis merges gradually with the deep canal bone without pedunculation.

Exostoses are common, broad-based lesions, often bilateral and symmetrical which are usually situated deeper in the ear canal than osteomas. In the bony portion of the normal external auditory meatus there are no adnexal structures and subcutaneous tissue and perios-

teum combine to form a thin layer. Therefore the distance between the epidermal surface and underlying bone is small, which may explain the propensity for exostoses of the tympanic bone to develop in those who swim frequently in cold water {2121}.

Clinical features
Symptoms are usually those of ear canal obstruction. Osteoma and exostosis are often associated with infection of the external canal on the tympanic membrane side. Surgical removal may be required to enhance drainage as well as to relieve the conducting hearing loss.

Histopathology
The osteoma is a spherical, pedunculated lesion composed of cortical lamellar bone on the outside overlying trabecular bone with intervening marrow spaces. The trabecular bone may show appositional woven bone formation. Normal squamous epithelium of the ear canal is often seen on the surface. The exostosis does not usually show marrow spaces. Both these lesions are distinct from the recently described benign fibro-osseous lesion of the superficial external canal {2121}.

Prognosis and predictive factors
These are benign lesions with no potential for malignant transformation.

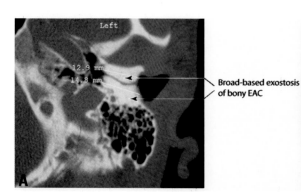

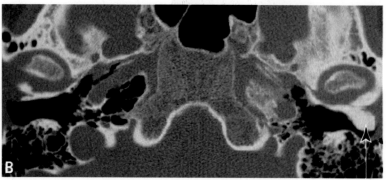

Fig. 7.13 A Exostosis. Coronal CT scan showing broad-based exostosis of deep external canal. **B** Osteoma. Axial CT scan showing a pedunculated osteoma of one external canal originating from the bone of deep external canal (arrow).

Angiolymphoid hyperplasia with eosinophilia

K. Henry

Definition
A benign vascular tumour with well formed, but immature, blood vessels, the majority of which are lined by plump, epithelioid (histiocytoid) endothelial cells. Subcutaneous examples are usually associated with a muscular artery. Most cases have a prominent inflammatory component in which eosinophils are a conspicuous feature.

Synonyms
Epithelioid haemangioma (ICD-O 9125/0), nodular angioblastic hyperplasia with eosinophilia and lymphofolliculosis, subcutaneous angioblastic lymphoid hyperplasia with eosinophilia and inflammatory angiomatoid nodule.

Epidemiology
There is a wide age range with a peak in the third to fifth decades and women are affected more often than men {759, 1945}.

Etiology
Whether angiolymphoid hyperplasia with eosinophilia is a reactive lesion rather than a neoplasm is still debated. Features cited as supporting a reactive process include a history of trauma (10 % of cases), its relationship around a larger vessel showing evidence of damage and the prominent inflammatory component {759,1945}.

Localization
The lesion occurs most frequently on the head, particularly the forehead and scalp (often in the distribution of the superficial temporal artery) and in the skin of the ear and the peri-auricular area. Other common sites are the distal parts of the extremities, especially the digits. Other skin surfaces may be involved and occurrences in oral mucous membranes, pharynx and orbit have been reported {759,1945}. Deep-seated sites are rare, as are an origin in a large vessel.

Clinical features
Most patients present with a nodule which has been present for a year or less; sometimes the lesion may have been present for as long as 15 years.

In the skin, including that of the ear, the lesions which are often painful or pruritic, appear as dome shaped erythematous or hyperpigmented papules or nodules which may be excoriated and bleed easily. The pre-excision diagnosis is usually that of an angioma or epidermal cyst. There may be several nodules and these can become chronic and coalesce into confluent plaques. There is very little tendency for spontaneous resolution but systemic spread has never been reported. In some patients there is a peripheral blood eosinophilia.

Macroscopy
The lesions are usually 0.5-2.0 cm in diameter; they rarely exceed 5.0 cm. Those lesions which contain blood, resemble a haemangioma but in most cases the appearances are rather non-specific. Sub-cutaneous nodules may resemble a lymph node because of circumscription and a peripheral inflammatory/lymphoid reaction.

Histopathology
Histologically, there are both vascular

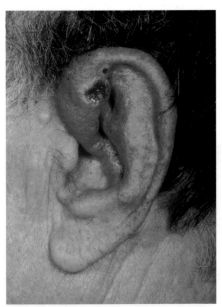

Fig. 7.14 Angiolymphoid hyperplasia with eosinophilia. Lesions were present in the upper helices of both ears in this elderly man.

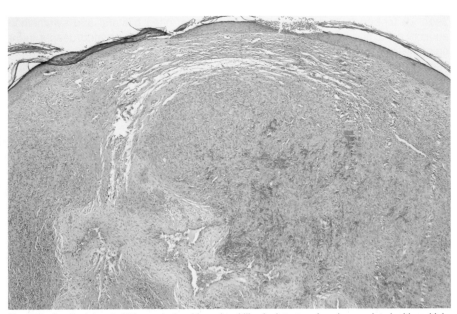

Fig. 7.15 Ear Angiolymphoid hyperplasia with eosinophilia. An intact surface is associated with multiple lobules of inflammatory elements with increased vascularity.

Table 7.2 Clinical and histological features of angiolymphoid hyperplasia with eosinophilia (ALH E) and Kimura disease.

	Angiolymphoid hyperplasia with eosinophilia	Kimura disease .
Clinical		
Sex,Age most often	Women , 3rd and 5th decades	Men, young to middle age
Geographical	Worldwide	Most common in Far East, occasionally in Europe
Skin/subcutis	Red brown papules	Large disfiguring masses.
Common sites	Forehead, scalp, ears	Submandibular, parotid, preauricular.
Regional lymph nodes	Not involved	Often involved
Eosinophilia	Sometimes	Almost always
Raised IgE	Never	Always
Prognosis	Excellent. May recur.	Excellent. Relapses common
Histopathology		
Small vessels	Numerous, immature. May lack lumina or appear as solid groups. May show relation to a larger vessel.	Numerous. Thin walled. Resemble HEVs No association with a large vessel
Endothelium	Histiocytoid/epithelioid May be vacuolated.	No special features
Connective tissue	Variable numbers of eosinophils, lymphocytes Numerous mast cells	Oedematous; rich in eosinophils, plasma cells Numerous mast cells
Lymphoid follicles	Sometimes present	Always present
Germinal centres	Normal, activated No IgE on FDCs	Polykaryocytes common May contain eosinophils. May be follicle lysis Deposition of IgE on FDCs

HEVs: high endothelial venules
FDCs: follicular dendritic cells

and inflammatory cellular components. There is a prominent proliferation of small, capillary sized blood vessels. Often there is a vaguely lobular pattern due to clustering of the capillary sized vessels around a medium sized thicker walled vessel. The vessels are lined by plump, epithelioid (histiocytoid) endothelial cells. The vessels look immature and may lack well-defined lumina; sometimes they appear as solid groups of cells. The nuclei of the endothelial cells are large, there is a finely distributed chromatin pattern and often there are central nucleoli. The cytoplasm may appear vacuolated. An inflammatory cell infiltrate with numerous eosinophils, mast cells and lymphocytes is present, though the numbers of eosinophils may vary considerably from case to case. In the peripheral zones of deeper lesions, formation of lymphoid follicles is often present. In deep seated lesions, there is commonly an associated larger blood vessel, usually a muscular artery; and the lining endothelial cells may also appear epithelioid. Dermal lesions are less well circumscribed and demarcated from the surrounding tissue then deeper lesions.

Immunoprofile
The epithelioid endothelial cells express CD31 and Factor VIII. CD34 is also expressed but usually only weakly. Immunostaining for actin can be helpful in demonstrating an intact myopericytic layer around the immature vessels. Mast cells are demonstrated by immunostaining with mast cell tryptase, CD117 (C kit) or IgE (since mast cells bear receptors for IgE).

Prognosis and predictive factors
While there is no metastatic potential for this tumour, local recurrences following excision occur in up to one third of patients {1945}. The reasons for this are not clear. The recurrences might be the result of incomplete excision, re-growth from a persisting underlying vascular anomaly or merely a reflection of its neoplastic potential. Whatever the reason, follow-up after complete local excision is indicated.
Angiolymphoid hyperplasia must be distinguished from Kimura disease {450, 1322} with which it has been confused in

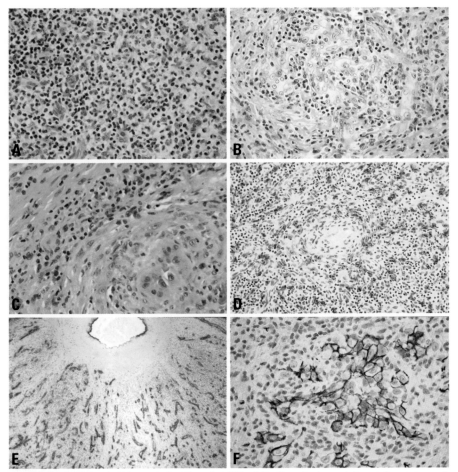

Fig. 7.16 Ear. Angiolymphoid hyperplasia with eosinophilia. **A** Capillary sized vessels in an inflammatory cell infiltrate of lymphocytes and eosinophils. **B** High power view of vessels showing their immature appearance, plump histiocytoid endothelial cells and absence of lumina. Note the surrounding eosinophils. **C** Endothelial cell hyperplasia within the central vessel. There is some associated fibrosis and eosinophils are present in the surrounding inflammatory infiltrate. **D** Numerous mast cells, revealed by their receptor to IgE, surround the medium and small sized blood vessels. **E** Factor VIII immunostaining shows arcades of capillary sized vessels in relation to a central muscular artery (this lesion involved the lip). **F** Immunohistochemistry. Membrane expression of CD31 by the histiocytoid endothelial cells.

the past since the two diseases were considered to represent the same disease process {2750}.

Kimura disease

Kimura disease is a chronic inflammatory condition of unknown etiology which presents as large, deep and often disfig-uring, subcutaneous masses in the pre-auricular, parotid and submandibular regions. Often, there is enlargement of regional lymph nodes {1390}. Occasionally, only lymph nodes are involved. There is a peripheral blood eosinophilia and raised levels of IgE and the histological features are distinctive {1385}.

Kimura disease is endemic in the Far East where it affects predominantly young to middle aged men with an age range of 11-80 years. However, the disease also occurs sporadically in Caucasians in the Western World {1069}. Histologically, the subcutaneous masses are found to be composed of lymphoid follicles surrounded by oedematous connective tissue rich in eosinophils and containing numerous thin walled blood vessels resembling high endothelial venules (HEVs). Infiltration of the germinal centres with eosinophils and follicle lysis is a frequent finding as is the presence of polykaryocytes. The polykaryocytes (cells with multilobed nuclei resulting from endoreduplication) in Kimura disease are derived from follicular dendritic cells {1069}. There is deposition of IgE on the processes of the follicular dendritic cells and there are also numerous mast cells, the latter well shown by immunostaining with antibody to IgE since mast cells bear receptor for IgE {1067}. Plasma cells may also be prominent. The disease is self-limiting with an excellent prognosis, though the lesions may recur.

The etiology is unknown. The raised levels of IgE, the IgE deposition in germinal centres and eosinophilia suggest the disease may be atopic in nature; and that the allergic response is results from lymphocyte-mediated interleukin-5 {680}.

Idiopathic pseudocystic chondromalacia

L. Michaels

Definition
A non-neoplastic swelling of the pinna resulting from localized accumulation of fluid within elastic cartilage.

Synonym
Endochondral pseudocyst

Epidemiology
The lesion occurs mainly in young and middle-aged adults, although it has been reported in children. Minor degrees of this lesion may be present in any damaged ear cartilage.

Etiology
Minor trauma from repeated rubbing of the auricle may play a part {592}. The fluid may exude from undamaged perichondrial vessels that cannot be absorbed by the damaged perichondrial vessels. Small pseudocysts of the elastic cartilage of the pinna may also be seen in the vicinity of inflammatory or neoplastic lesions of that region.

Localization
This condition occurs in any part of the ear cartilage.

Clinical features
The patient complains of painless swelling of a part of the ear cartilage.

Macroscopy
The gross appearance is one of a localized swelling of the auricular cartilage. The cut surface shows a well-defined cavity in the cartilage which is distended with yellowish watery fluid {1043}.

Histopathology
Microscopically the cavity shows a lining of degenerated cartilage on one surface; on the other surface the cartilage is normal.

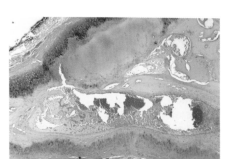

Fig. 7.17 Idiopathic pseudocystic chondromalacia. The cartilage shows multiple cystic cavities in various stages of organization. Hemorrhage is present in the lower cavity.

Immunoprofile
There is no expression in the cells lining the cyst-like spaces for CD 31 or cytokeratins indicating that this is an accumulation of fluid in the elastic cartilage rather than an epithelial cyst or a vascular pseudocyst.

Chondrodermatitis nodularis chronica helicis

L. Michaels

Definition
A non-neoplastic ulcerating nodule on the helix of the ear, which always involves the underlying cartilage.

Synonym
Winkler disease

Epidemiology
The condition occurs in the third or fourth decades in both sexes.

Etiology
Scleroderma-like changes in the vessels lead to the obstruction of small arteries of the perichondrium which comprise the primary lesions leading to cartilage necrosis {242}. The acute inflammation and epidermal ulceration are secondary to the nearby cartilage necrosis.

Localization
The lesion occurs in the helix of the auricle, less commonly in the antihelix.

Clinical features
A small exquisitely painful ulcerating nodule forms on the auricle, usually in the superior portion of the helix.

Macroscopy
The nodule on the helix is ulcerated in its centre and shows cornified edges. Extruded necrotic cartilage may be seen in the floor of the ulcer.

Histopathology
There is ulceration of the skin of the auricle and complete necrosis of the superficial region of the elastic cartilage of the auricle. A piece of necrotic cartilage infiltrated by neutrophils and bacterial colonies may be present in the floor of the ulcer. The perichondrium of the elastic cartilage shows obstructive thickening of small arteries. Epidermis at the edge of the ulcerated lesion is hyperplastic.

Prognosis and predictive factors
The lesion is usually cured by surgical removal of the painful nodule.

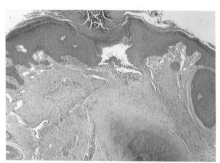

Fig. 7.18 Chondrodermatitis nodularis helicis. The epidermis at the edge of the ulcerated lesion is hyperplastic. The ulcer overlies the cartilage, with fibrosis and inflammatory elements present. Small foci of fibrinoid necrosis are noted.

Cholesterol granuloma and cholesteatoma

L. Michaels
S. Soucek
T. Beale

Cholesterol granuloma

Definition

Cholesterol granuloma is a foreign body giant cell reaction to crystals of cholesterol deposited in the middle ear cleft. It is accompanied by chronic otitis media.

Etiology

Cholesterol granuloma arises from haemorrhage derived from the inflammatory tissue of cholesterol granuloma, the red cell membranes becoming degenerated to cholesterol.

Localization

The main site of cholesterol granuloma is the middle ear cleft. This includes the tympanic cavity and mastoid air cells. Pneumatized air cells at the apex of the temporal bone may also be the seat of an expanding destructive lesion of this type.

Clinical features

The tympanomastoid lesions do not, in themselves, produce symptoms. Symptoms of chronic otitis media may be present, however. Cholesterol granulomas of the petrous apex may grow and even invade the cochlea and into the cerebellopontine angle, producing a tumour like mass with hearing loss and life-threatening symptoms.

Macroscopy

Yellow nodules are seen in tympanic cavity and mastoid in this condition. The petrous apex lesions appear cystic, the contents being altered blood.

Histopathology

The yellow tympanomastoid lesions are composed microscopically of cholesterol crystals (dissolved away to leave empty clefts in paraffin-embedded histological sections) surrounded by foreign body type giant cells and other chronic inflammatory cells. Such cholesterol granulomas are almost always found in the midst of haemorrhage in the middle ear mucosa. Hemosiderin is often present within macrophages among the cells surrounding the cholesterol granuloma. The contents of petrous apex cystic lesions are altered blood, and cholesterol clefts with a foreign body giant cell reaction. The wall of such lesions shows granulation tissue with haemosiderin. Remains of low cuboidal (middle ear) epithelium and bone, representing the wall of a pneumatized air cell, may be seen in biopsies of this condition {49,1062}.

Cholesteatoma of the middle ear and petrous apex

Cholesteatoma is a misnomer being neither cholesterol containing nor a neoplasm. Cholesteatoma is a cystic or "open" mass of keratin squames with a living "matrix". Although it is not a neoplastic lesion, especially in the middle ear cleft, it may act like one in that it has a propensity to destroy tissue and to recur after excision.

Acquired cholesteatoma of the middle ear

Definition

A cholesteatoma associated with a perforated tympanic membrane is acquired.

Epidemiology

This entity is seen mainly in older children and young adults.

Etiology

It seems likely that the acquired cholesteatoma is derived from entry of external ear canal epidermis into the middle ear. Most cases are associated with severe otitis media in which entry of stratified squamous epithelium from the external ear epidermis through the tympanic membrane occurs. In some cases, it follows blast injury with perforation of the tympanic membrane at the time of the injury {1377}. Acquired cholesteatoma is also known to follow retraction

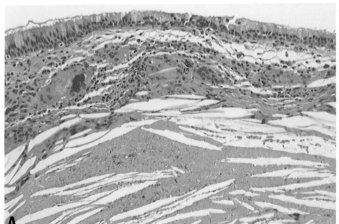
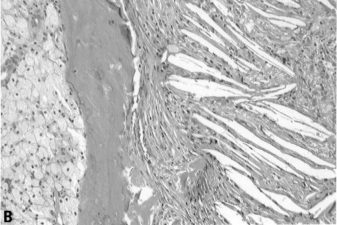

Fig. 7.19 Ear cholesterol granuloma. **A** An intact respiratory-type epithelium overlies the cholesterol clefts and foreign-body type giant cells seen in a cholesterol granuloma. **B** Innumerable histiocytes are seen adjacent to bone with areas of cholesterol cleft formation and inflammatory response.

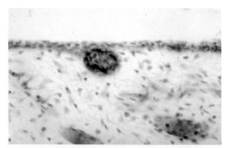

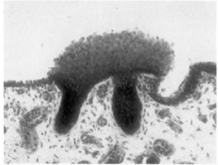

Fig. 7.20 Cholesteatoma. Two epidermoid formations, (cell rests) in the fetal middle ear. The upper was found in a 17 gestational week fetus, the lower in a 37 gestational week fetus. These structures are agreed to be precursors of congenital cholesteatoma.

pocket of the tympanic membrane where it is not due to obstruction of the mouth of a retraction pocket, but rather to the deep ingrowth of a band of stratified squamous epithelium from the fundus of the retraction pocket into the middle ear {2751}.

Localization
The main site of origin of this lesion is the upper posterior part of the middle ear.

Clinical features
The patient presents with a foul-smelling aural discharge and conductive hearing loss. On examination of the tympanic membrane there is, in most cases, a perforation of the superior or posterosuperior margin.

Macroscopy
The cholesteatoma is seen as a pearly grey structure in the middle ear cavity associated with severe chronic otitis media.

Histopathology
Acquired cholesteatoma is usually "open" rather than "closed" or cystic. The pearly material of the cholesteatoma consists of dead, fully differentiated anucleate keratin squames. This is the

corneal layer of the squamous cell epithelium. As in any normal stratified epithelium there are one to three basal layers of cells above which is a prickle (malpighian or spinous) layer composed of five or six rows of cells with intercellular bridges. The deeper layers of the epithelium of the cholesteatoma matrix frequently show evidence of increased proliferation reflected by down-growths into the underlying sub-epidermal connective tissue.

Immunoprofile
The excessive activity has been confirmed by: (a) the strong expression of cytokeratin 16, a marker for hyperproliferative keratinocytes, by cholesteatoma, but its absence in middle ear and external ear epithelium, except in the annulus region of the external tympanic membrane epithelium {278}, (b) the strong expression of MIB-1, an antigen related to Ki-67, which also indicates hyperproliferative activity {2494}, (c) counts of silver-stained argyrophil nucleolar organizer regions, a technique which likewise displays proliferative activity, shows significantly larger numbers of these structures in the nuclei of acquired cholesteatoma as compared with those of the epidermis of the deep external auditory meatal skin {2496}, (d) acquired cholesteatomatous epithelium shows an abnormally high concentration of IL-1, TGF-alpha, EGF-R and 4F2, all being growth factors {2495} indicating greater growth and differentiating activity than is present in normal epidermis.

Genetics
Acquired cholesteatoma does not show DNA aneuploidy nor does it possess an inherent genetic instability, a critical fea-

ture of all malignant lesions {33}.

Congenital cholesteatoma of the middle ear

Definition
Congenital cholesteatoma is defined in clinical practice as a cholesteatoma of the middle ear which exists in the presence of an intact tympanic membrane, the implication being that severe chronic otitis media, which normally produces a perforation of the tympanic membrane, has not led to its development.

Epidemiology
This lesion is found in infants and young children.

Etiology
Small colonies of cells confirmed by immunohistochemistry as being epidermoid in nature are found near the tympanic membrane on the lateral anterior superior surface of the middle ear in every temporal bone after 15 weeks gestation. These "epidermoid formations", are derived from the actively growing epidermis of the eardrum. They increase significantly in size with increasing age and at the same time show increasing epidermoid differentiation {1502}. In normal development, the epidermoid colonies disappear by the first post partum year. However, if one of them does not resolve, but continues to grow, this will become a congenital cholesteatoma.

Localization
The majority of cases are found in the antero-superior part of the middle ear.

Clinical features
In early lesions there are no symptoms,

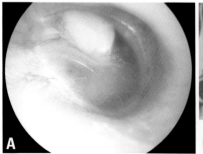

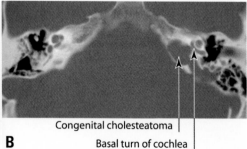

Congenital cholesteatoma

Basal turn of cochlea

Fig. 7.21 Cholesteatoma. **A** Otoscopic photograph of congenital cholesteatoma seen as a small cyst behind the ear drum in the anterosuperior part of the middle ear. **B** Coronal CT scan of petrous bone. Note the soft tissue mass with a scalloped margin eroding the petrous bone and adjacent bony cochlea suggestive of congenital cholesteatoma of middle ear.

the cholesteatoma being discovered by routine otoscopy. In later cases, the lesion is much larger and symptoms may resemble those of acquired cholesteatoma.

Macroscopy

In most cases a spherical whitish cyst in the anterosuperior part of the tympanic cavity is seen, behind an intact tympanic membrane. In 10% of congenital cholesteatomas the lesion is "open", the desquamated squames entering the tympanic cavity.

Histopathology

The matrix of congenital cholesteatoma is epidermis, comprising a single row of basal cells, several rows of malpighian cells and a thin granular layer. The surface of dead, keratinous squames merges with the keratinous contents of the cyst, or keratinous lamellae in the case of the open type.

Immunoprofile

Immunostaining shows similar features to those of acquired cholesteatoma.

Prognosis and predictive factors

If removed early, when small, congenital cholesteatoma can be considered as cured. If left, or not diagnosed, until later in life, the problems of middle ear damage and recurrence become similar to those of acquired cholesteatoma.

Cholesteatoma of the petrous apex

Definition

An epidermoid cyst arising in the region of the petrous apex. It bears no relation to cholesteatoma of the middle ear.

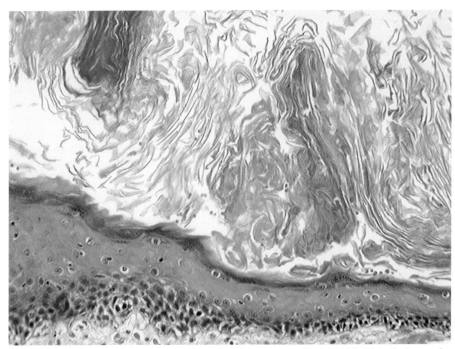

Fig. 7.22 Cholesteatoma. A squamous epithelium sheds abundant keratinaceous debris into the lumen of a cholesteatoma.

Etiology

It is probably of congenital origin, but no cell rest has been discovered from which it might arise.

Clinical features

This lesion usually presents with facial palsy and hearing loss, due to involvement of the seventh and eighth cranial nerves, respectively, in the cerebellopontine angle {564}.

Histopathology

The histological appearance is similar to that of middle ear cholesteatomas.

Adenoma of the middle ear

L. Michaels
S. Soucek

Definition
Adenoma is a benign glandular neoplasm showing variable differentiation along neuroendocrine and mucin-secreting pathways.

ICD-O code   8140/0

Synonyms
Middle ear adenomatous tumour, neuroendocrine adenoma of the middle ear, carcinoid of the middle ear.

Epidemiology
This is an uncommon neoplasm, but among the most frequent ones arising in the middle ear. There is an approximately equal sex distribution, with an age range of 20-80 years, and a mean age of 45 years {2623}.

Localization
The tumour arises anywhere in the middle ear cavity, sometimes extending into the mastoid. In one reported case it arose from the epitympanic part of the tympanic membrane {75}. In a small number of cases it may be found to have spread through the tympanic membrane {2623}.

Clinical features
Patients complain of muffled hearing with a pressure sensation in the affected ear. Otoscopy shows an intact tympanic membrane in the first stage with a dark brown-reddish coloured structure behind it. Tumour may later expand and involve the ossicular chain causing conductive hearing loss and may penetrate the tympanic membrane. Treatment is surgical. The tumour is usually easily removed, but if ossicles are entrapped reconstructive surgery is needed.

Macroscopy
The neoplasm has been described as being white, yellow, grey or reddish brown at operation and, unlike paraganglioma, is usually not vascular. Although not encapsulated it seems to peel away from the walls of the surrounding middle ear with ease, although ossicles may sometimes be surrounded by the tumour and may even show destruction.

Histopathology
Adenoma is formed by closely apposed small glands with a "back to back" appearance. In some places a solid or trabecular arrangement is present. Sheet-like, disorganized areas are seen in which the glandular pattern appears to be lost. This may be artefactual and related to the effects of the trauma used in taking the biopsy specimen, on the delicate structure of the cells, but the appearance may erroneously lead one to suspect malignancy. The cells are regular, cuboidal or columnar and may enclose luminal secretion. A distinct and predominant "plasmacytoid" appearance of the epithelial cells of the neoplasm may be displayed {2164}. The small central nuclei rarely contain nucleoli and show no significant mitotic activity. No myoepithelial layer is seen. Periodic acid-Schiff and Alcian blue stains may be positive for mucoprotein secretion in the gland lumina and in the cytoplasm of the tumour cells.

Soon after adenoma of the middle ear was described in 1976 {588,1160}, it was

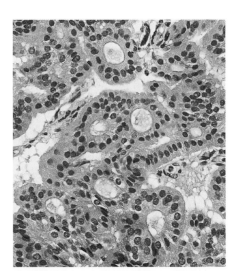

Fig. 7.23 Adenoma of the middle ear. High-power view. From L. Michaels & H. Hellquist {1711}.

reported that some glandular tumours of the middle ear, otherwise apparently identical to an adenoma, showed neuroendocrine features as shown by Grimelius positivity, the presence of numerous membrane-bound granules on electron microscopy, and expression of immunohistochemical markers for neuroendocrine activity. The concept of "carcinoid tumour" evolved, i.e. that this was a distinct neoplasm with significant neuroendocrine differentiation. As with carcinoids in other locations, it was considered to have malignant potential. It is now clear that most, probably all, middle ear adenomas express neuroendocrine markers {2623,2727}.

Immunoprofile
Neuroendocrine markers such as synaptophysin, chromogranin, and various polypeptides, are demonstrated in addition to cytokeratins {2623}.

Electron microscopy
Ultrastructural examination of five cases showed basally situated cells and solid tumour containing neuroendocrine granules which were positive for neuroendocrine markers. This is in contrast to apically situated dark cells which contained mucous granules and were negative for neuroendocrine markers {2727}.

Precursor lesions
The lesions arise from the lining epithelium of the middle ear. Under appropriate stimuli such as otitis media, this epithelium has the potential for glandular differentiation. However, neuroendocrine differentiation has not been demonstrated in either normal or "metaplastic" glandular epithelium.

Genetics
There has so far been no study of molecular genetic aspects of this tumour. This neoplasm does not occur in families.

Prognosis and predictive factors
There have been a few recurrences after incomplete local surgical excision.

Papillary tumours of the middle ear

L. Michaels
A. Sandison
G.L. Davis

Aggressive papillary tumour

Definitions
Tumour with a papillary, non-stratified epithelial pattern showing invasive behaviour.

ICD-O code   8260/1

Synonyms
Primary adenocarcinoma of the middle ear of papillary type, aggressive papillary tumour of temporal bone, papillary adenoma.

Epidemiology
Forty-six cases with this neoplasm were collected from the literature in 1994 {843}. Some of these had been reported as low-grade adenocarcinoma of probable endolymphatic sac origin {1038}. Review of each of the case reports in these two studies, together with cases reported more recently, reveals a total of 24 cases in which the middle ear was involved, comprising 17 females and 7 males. The age-range at time of diagnosis was between 16 and 55 years with a median age of 33 and a mean age of 34 years. In many of the cases, however, the patient had already suffered symptoms subsequently ascribable to the tumour for some years when the diagnosis was made, so that the age of onset may be considerably younger than is suggested.

Localization
The tumour is found in any area of the middle ear, including the mastoid process and air cells and may fill the tympanic cavity. In all of the described cases, except two {519,2481} there was extensive invasion outside the middle ear, involving the apical portion of the petrous bone in most and in a few the tumour reached the cerebellopontine angle and the cerebellum.
It has been suggested that cases of aggressive papillary middle ear tumour with widespread involvement of the temporal bone may arise from a primary papillary adenocarcinoma of the endo-

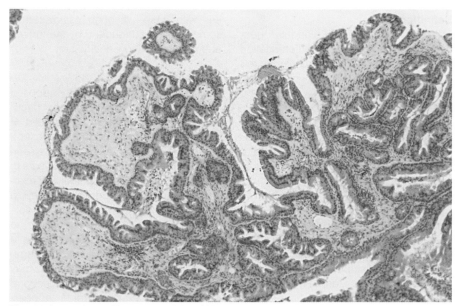

Fig. 7.24 Aggressive papillary tumour of the middle ear.

lymphatic sac {1038}. The frequent association of papillary tumours in the middle ear with apical petrous bone neoplasia of the same type, the similarity of the histological appearances of the neoplasms in the two regions and the association of some cases of papillary tumours in both regions with von Hippel-Lindau disease would seem to favour this concept, but an origin in the middle ear in some cases of this neoplasm has not been definitely excluded. This would explain the presence of the neoplasm in the middle ear only in two described cases. In the single description of the pathological changes of aggressive papillary tumour of the middle ear in an autopsied temporal bone, widespread deposits of tumour at inner ear sites are depicted, but no mention is made of involvement of the endolymphatic sac or duct {2355}. Whatever the site or sites of origin of this tumour it should be recognized that papillary epithelial tumour of the middle ear is frequently an aggressive neoplasm, in contrast to the non-papillary adenoma of the middle ear which is quite benign {1741}.

Clinical features
In most cases of this neoplasm clinical and audiological features point to a middle ear lesion. Suspicion of a neoplasm of the middle ear is enhanced by the otoscopic features in a few cases. Indeed, the tympanic membrane has been perforated by the tumour, which is seen to lie in the external canal in some cases. On imaging the medial parts of the petrous temporal bone show, in the great majority of cases, areas of involvement by a lytic lesion, representing an invasive neoplasm which may extend posteriorly outside the temporal bone and invade the cerebellum {843}. Fifteen percent of patients with aggressive papillary tumour of middle ear have been found to possess neoplasms or other manifestations of Von Hippel-Lindau syndrome. There may be a family history of this condition in the patient without its actual physical manifestations {843}.

Histopathology
The middle ear cleft, including the mastoid air cells, is usually filled with the papillary tumour. Bone invasion is often seen. A papillary glandular pattern is present

Table 7.3 Histopathology of Schneiderian-type or inverted papillomas of the middle ear described in the literature

Literature source	Histological description given	Possible alternative diagnosis
1. Stone et al. {2480}	"Inverted papilloma" and high grade carcinoma	Squamous cell carcinoma of middle ear
2. Kaddour et al {1242}	"Transitional cell papilloma" Inverted papilloma in nose	Inverted papilloma derived from nasal tumour
3. Roberts et al {2184}	Entirely papillary	Papilloma of middle ear
4. Seshul et al {2308}	Malignant change in inverted papilloma	Squamous cell carcinoma of middle ear
5. Wenig {2757} Case 1 "	Epidermoid papilloma" with "inverted" and "cylindric cell papilloma"	Papilloma of middle ear
6. Wenig {2757} Case 2	"Epidermoid papilloma" with exophytic and endophytic growth	Papilloma of middle ear
7. Wenig {2757} Case 3	"Epidermoid papilloma" with features of "cylindric cell papilloma"	Papilloma of middle ear
8. Wenig {2757} Case 4	"Epidermoid papilloma" with features of "cylindric cell papilloma"	Papilloma of middle ear
9. Wenig {2757} Case 5	"Epidermoid papilloma" with features of "cylindric cell papilloma"	Papilloma of middle ear
10. Jones et al {1234}	Squamous epithelium with areas of carcinoma in-situ	Squamous carcinoma of middle ear
11. Chhetri et al {423}	Papillary with areas of squamous epithelium adjacent to respiratory epithelium	Papilloma of middle ear

with complex interdigitating papillae lying loosely or infiltrating fibrous connective tissue. The papillae are lined by a single layer of low, cuboidal to columnar epithelial cells with uniform nuclei, eosinophilic cytoplasm and indistinct cell borders. Thyroid follicle-like areas may be present, similar to those seen in endolymphatic sac carcinoma.

Immunoprofile

Markers for cytokeratin, epithelial membrane antigen and S100 are positive. The absence of thyroglobulin must be determined to exclude metastatic papillary carcinoma of the thyroid. Markers for CK7, CK20 and carcinoembryonic antigen may also be useful to exclude metastatic deposits from lung and colon.

Genetics

The genetic aspects of von Hippel-Lindau disease are described below. In view of the association of some cases of that condition with aggressive papillary middle ear tumours it is suggested that the clinical assessment of each case with

the latter neoplasm should include an investigation for the gene mutations of von Hippel-Lindau disease.

Schneiderian-type papilloma

Schneiderian epithelium refers to the normal respiratory-type ciliated epithelium of the nose and paranasal sinuses. Schneiderian papillomas are tumours of the nose and paranasal sinuses that are stated to be derived from this epithelium. Three such types of papillomas are described: inverted (endophytic), exophytic (fungiform, everted) and oncocytic (cylindric cell). Intermediate types are said to be found between the three forms {1741}. It has, however, been denied that such intermediate forms exist and it is suggested that the three types are each separate and distinct entities of the nose and paranasal sinuses {1714}. Of the three histological forms only inverted papilloma is characteristically a sinonasal neoplasm. The other two types of Schneiderian-type papilloma may be

seen at other sites. Low-grade squamous carcinoma in the nose may sometimes be mistaken for inverted papilloma {1710}.

Fourteen cases of middle ear tumours purportedly resembling Schneiderian-type papilloma have been found in the literature. Each of these cases is listed in Table 7.3; wherever possible the histological appearances are summarized in the table; in some insufficient or no histological description was given. In two cases only were the features of inverted papilloma depicted: in Case 1 the term "inverted" and in Case 2 the term "endophytic" were used to describe the neoplasm. "Inverted" or "endophytic" features comprised only a portion of the tumours in the two cases. In Case 2 {1242} the term transitional cell papilloma was used. This is a term that has frequently been applied to describe everted squamous cell papilloma. In this case inverted papilloma was found in the nasal cavity and it was suggested that the papillomas might have spread from there to the middle ear by way of the

Eustachian tube. In Cases 1, 4 and 10 "inverted papilloma" were found in the middle ear concomitantly with in situ or invasive squamous carcinoma and it seems possible that the "inverted papilloma" areas might have been, in reality, areas of low grade squamous carcinoma.

We would suggest that a good case has not been made for the occurrence of inverted papilloma in the middle ear. Some of the lesions may have been papillomas of the middle ear as described above. In Case 2 inverted papilloma could conceivably have colonized the middle ear from the nasal cavity. Further detailed descriptions of the entity are required to justify the diagnosis of such a diagnostic category in this situation.

Inverted papilloma

Definition
Papillary neoplasm of the middle ear which is histologically identical to that occurring in the sinonasal region.

ICD-O code   8121/1

Localization
Middle ear. Also occurs in association with similar papillomas of the upper respiratory tract, either by direct continuity or in a multicentric fashion.

Clinical features
It usually presents as chronic otitis media.

Macroscopy
Polypoid tumour filling the middle ear cavity.

Prognosis and predictive factors
Thus far, these tumours have shown no evidence of invasion but recurrences are common {2757}.

Choristoma

L. Michaels

Definition
A choristoma in contrast to a hamartoma, is composed of tissues which are not normally present in the part of the body where it is found. Choristomas are occasionally seen in the middle ear. They are composed of one or other of two types of tissue: salivary gland or glial tissue.

Salivary gland choristoma

Localization
This lesion usually occurs as a mass in the middle ear attached posteriorly in the region of the oval window. There are usually absent or malformed ossicles {1093}.

Histopathology
Salivary gland choristomas consist as a rule of lobulated mixed mucous and serous elements like the normal submandibular or sublingual gland, but unlike the parotid gland.

Glial choristoma

Clinical features
In this lesion, masses composed of glial tissue are identified in biopsy material from the middle ear. A bony deficit with consequent herniation of brain tissue into the middle ear should be ruled out by imaging {1257}.

Histopathology
Glial masses are present, composed largely of astrocytic cells with large amounts of glial fibrils.

Immunoprofile
The identity of the tissue as glial may be confirmed by immunohistochemical staining for glial acidic fibrillary protein.

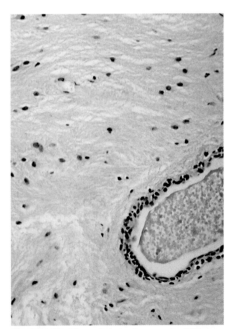

Fig. 7.25 Fibrillary glial choristoma of middle ear with a metaplastic gland..

Squamous cell carcinoma of the middle ear

L. Michaels
S. Soucek
T. Beale

Definition
A malignant tumour composed of stratified squamous epithelium arising from the cuboidal and / or pseudostratified epithelium of the middle ear.

ICD-O code
8070/3

Synonyms
Epidermoid carcinoma, squamous carcinoma

Epidemiology
The disease affects males and females equally, with an age range of 34-85 years and an average age of 60 years.

Etiology
An origin from long-term chronic inflammation of the middle ear has been suggested. However, malignant neoplasia in its earlier stages has clinical features similar to those of chronic otitis media. Moreover biopsy is not usually carried out during surgery when a diagnosis only of otitis media has been made. Therefore, longstanding squamous carcinoma of the middle ear may go undiagnosed.

Localization
The neoplasm soon expands to involve much of the middle ear. There is extension by tumour through the bone on the medial wall of the Eustachian tube to infiltrate the perineurium of nerves in the carotid canal. The tumour also penetrates the thin layer of bone between the posterior mastoid air cells and the dura with subsequent invasion along the dura and into the internal auditory meatus. Bilateral squamous cell carcinomas of the middle ear have been described {1713}.

Clinical features
This tumour is usually advanced at presentation. The patient usually complains of pain in the ear, bleeding and a serosanguinous discharge from the ear canal. In those cases with a concomitant external canal carcinoma a plaque-like or even polypoid mass may be felt or even seen in the canal. Seventh nerve palsy is an important sign indicating infiltration beyond the middle ear.

Macroscopy
A tumour fills the middle ear and may extend into the mastoid air cells and along the pathways described above.

Histopathology
The neoplasm is a keratinizing squamous cell carcinoma with a variable degree of differentiation. Atypical change and even carcinoma in situ may be seen in some parts of the middle ear epithelium adjacent to the tumour. The tumour arises from malignant stratified squamous epithelium and in certain areas an origin directly from basal layers of cuboidal or columnar epithelium may be seen.

Precursor lesions
There is no evidence of a relationship to cholesteatoma or the epidermoid cell rests which normally occur in the middle ear during development.

Prognosis and predictive factors
The prognosis is uniformly poor and does not correlate with degree of tumour differentiation.

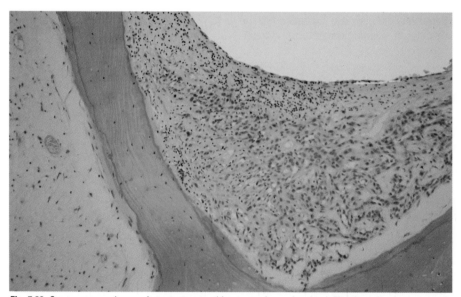

Fig. 7.26 Squamous carcinoma. Autopsy temporal bone specimen showing infiltration of squamous carcinoma of middle ear into mastoid air cell.

Meningioma of the middle ear

L. Michaels
S. Soucek

Definition
Meningioma is a benign tumour usually forming intracerebrally, but sometimes seen involving bony structures around the brain including the middle ear. It arises from the pia-arachnoid cells of the meninges.

ICD-O code   9530/0

Epidemiology
Meningioma of the middle ear affects women more than men, shows an age range of between 10 and 80 years with a mean age of 49.6 years. Female patients present at an older age (women 52.0 years, men 44.8 years) {2597}.

Localization
Meningiomas occur at a number of sites in the temporal bone, including the internal auditory meatus, the jugular foramen, the geniculate ganglion region and the roof of the Eustachian tube {1830}. The most common temporal bone site for primary meningioma is in the middle ear cleft. In a recent study (36 patients), most tumours involved the middle ear, but a few involved adjacent structures such as the external canal or temporal bone. Only two showed extension from CNS on imaging {2597}.
In neurofibromatosis type 2 (NF-2 see below), meningioma-like masses occur commonly in the internal auditory canal and cerebellopontine angle.

Clinical features
Patients present clinically with hearing change, otitis media, pain, and/or dizziness / vertigo.

Macroscopy
Gross appearances are those of a granular mass with a gritty consistency.

Histopathology
Microscopically the neoplasm in the middle ear shows the same histological features of any of the well-described subtypes of intracranial meningioma. The most common variety seen in the middle ear is the meningothelial type, in which the tumour cells form masses of epithelioid, regular cells often disposed into whorls. Occasionally, fibroblastic and psammatous variants are seen.

Immunoprofile
Histological diagnosis may be difficult because the typical features of meningioma are absent. Under these circumstances immunocytochemistry is of diagnostic value. Vimentin and epithelial membrane antigen are expressed in the majority of meningiomas and cytoker- atins are uniformly negative. Expression of S-100 protein identifies spindle cell tumours as of neurogenic origin, thus excluding spindle cell meningioma.

Prognosis and predictive factors
Although Nager's review of temporal bone meningiomas (1964) indicated that only two out of 30 patients survived a 5-year period {1830}, more recent experience of middle ear meningiomas signals a better outlook after careful local excision (5-y survival, 83%).

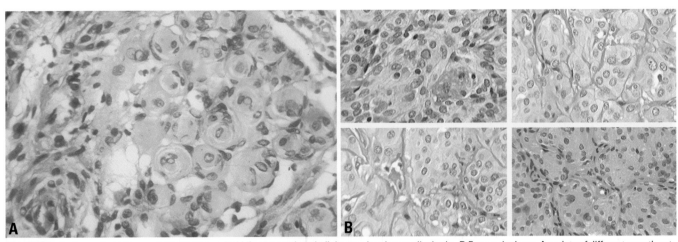

Fig. 7.27 Meningioma of middle ear. **A** Meningioma of middle ear, meningothelial type, showing small whorls. **B** Ear meningioma. A variety of different growth patterns can be seen, but the meningothelial nature of the neoplasm is always maintained..

Vestibular schwannoma

L. Michaels
T. Beale
A. Sandison
S. Soucek

Definition
A benign nerve sheath tumour arising in the internal auditory canal.

ICD-O code   9560/0

Synonyms
Acoustic neuroma, acoustic neurinoma. neurilemmoma

Epidemiology
Vestibular schwannoma is the most common neoplasm of the temporal bone. Unilateral vestibular schwannoma accounts for 5-10% of all intracranial tumours and for most of the cerebellopontine angle tumours. It is found in about 0.8% of consecutive adult necropsies {1475}. The age at presentation is the fifth or sixth decade. It also is seen in younger people in association with neurofibromatosis type 2.

Etiology
Solitary vestibular schwannoma occurs sporadically, and does not seem to be associated with a gene mutation. The etiology is unknown.

Localization
Vestibular schwannoma was formerly considered to arise most commonly at the glial-neurilemmal junction of the eighth cranial nerve. Such a site of origin has now become doubtful {2834}. In one study of five temporal bones with small vestibular schwannomas, the tumour arose more peripherally {2834}. The vestibular division of the nerve is usually affected. Rarely, the cochlear division is the source of the neoplasm. Growth takes place from the site of origin of the tumour, both centrally onto the cerebellopontine angle and peripherally along the canal. Vestibular schwannoma is usually unilateral, but may be bilateral, in which case the condition is neurofibromatosis 2.

Clinical features
Progressive unilateral hearing loss (90% of patients) and tinnitus (70% of patients) are the clinical manifestations, due to cochlear involvement. Less common symptoms are: headache, vertigo, facial pain and facial weakness. The neoplasm may grow slowly for years without causing symptoms and may be first diagnosed only at post-mortem. Diagnosis is usually made by MRI scanning. In small, slowly growing tumours, an option for management is non-surgical, using MRI scanning at intervals to observe growth. Surgical removal may be carried out by drilling from the external canal through the temporal bone or by craniotomy and middle fossa approach to the internal auditory meatus, or by stereotactically guided gamma knife surgery.

Macroscopy
The neoplasm is of variable size and shape. Small tumours either do not widen the canal at all or produce only a small indentation in the bone.
The larger tumours often have a mushroom shape with two components, the stalk - a narrower, elongated part in the canal - and an expanded part in the region of the cerebellopontine angle. The bone of the internal auditory canal is widened funnel-wise as the neoplasm grows.
The tumour surface is smooth and lobulated. The cut surface is yellowish, often with areas of haemorrhage and cysts. A multicystic vestibular schwannoma has been described {1804}. The vestibular division of the eighth nerve may be identified on the surface of the tumour and attached to it while the cochlear division is often stretched by the neoplasm, but not attached to it.

Histopathology
Vestibular schwannoma is a neoplasm of the nerve sheath / Schwann cells. This tumour typically shows closely packed spindle cells, often with palisaded nuclei and Verocay bodies (Antoni A areas) and less cellular areas with a loose reticular pattern and microcystic degeneration sometimes containing numerous xanthoma cells (Antoni B). The degree of cellularity of the neoplasm can be high or low. The spindle cells frequently are moderately pleomorphic, but mitotic figures are rare. The presence of pleomorphism does not necessarily denote a malignant tendency, but in rare cases undoubted malignant changes can appear associated with an increased growth rate {120}. Thrombosis and necrosis may be present focally.
Tumour extension into the modiolus or vestibule along cochlear or vestibular nerve branches may be present even in solitary vestibular schwannomas, although more common in NF-2. Granular or homogeneous fluid exudate is usually present in the perilymphatic spaces of the cochlea and vestibule. This may arise as a result of pressure by the neoplasm on veins draining the cochlea and vestibule in the internal auditory meatus. Hydrops of the endolymphatic system may occur and in larger tumours there is atrophy of spiral ganglion cells and nerve fibres in the basilar membrane.

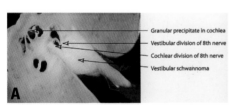
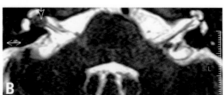

Granular precipitate in cochlea
Vestibular division of 8th nerve
Cochlear division of 8th nerve
Vestibular schwannoma

Fig. 7.28 Vestibular schwannoma. **A** Microsliced autopsy temporal bone. The neoplasm arises from the vestibular division of the eighth nerve and compresses the cochlear division. Note the granular deposit lining the cochlea, a feature of most larger vestibular schwannomas. From L. Michaels & H. Hellquist {1711}. **B** Axial T2 post-contrast MRI scan of the posterior fossa showing a well-defined intracanalicular vestibular schwannoma (arrow). Note the eighth cranial nerve leading into the tumour.

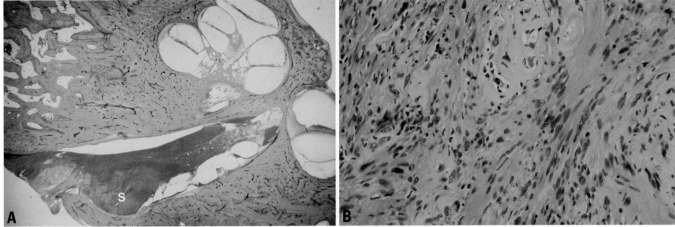

Fig. 7.29 Vestibular schwannoma. **A** Small vestibular schwannoma (S) in autopsy temporal bone specimen. It is arising from the vestibular division of the eighth nerve and causing a small indentation only of the bony wall of the internal canal. There is exudate in the vestibule, but not in the cochlea. From L. Michaels & H. Hellquist {1711}. **B** Vestibular schwannoma showing Antoni A appearance and hyaline blood vessels.

Immunoprofile

These tumours express diffuse, strong nuclear positivity for S-100 protein. Vimentin expression is also usually positive though not specific. These findings are common to both unilateral vestibular schwannoma and the schwannomas of NF2. Glial fibrillary acidic protein and neurone specific enolase markers may also be expressed. The tumours are consistently negative for CD34, a marker widely used for the diagnosis of solitary fibrous tumours, unless there are widespread degenerative changes {2625}.

The proliferation marker Ki67 has demonstrated that tumours 18 mm or smaller in diameter have lower proliferation indices and growth rates, than tumours larger than 18 mm {186}. The proliferation index in vestibular schwannoma associated with NF-2 is higher than in solitary vestibular schwannomas {17}.

Electron microscopy

Schwann cells are identified as the cell of origin by their Interdigitating slender cytoplasmic processes covered with a continuous layer of basal lamina {434}. Extensive degeneration of the vestibular sensory organ as detected ultrastructurally is brought about by growth of the neoplasm from the vestibular division of the eighth nerve. Even small tumours may cause this change {2241}.

Genetics

Ninety five per cent of vestibular schwannomas are unilateral and are sporadic. Less than 5% of tumours are bilateral and therefore associated with the NF2 gene. The risk that a unilateral tumour is the first indication of NF2 is closely related to the age of the patient. Young patients under the age of 25 are at high risk of developing contralateral tumours and NF2 while patients with unilateral tumours who are over the age of 55 have virtually no risk of developing NF2. There is no increased incidence of unilateral vestibular schwannoma or NF2 in the offspring of patients with unilateral vestibular schwannoma {1595}.

Prognosis and predictive factors

Size is an important aspect in the prognosis of cases of vestibular schwannoma. Tumours 18 mm or smaller in diameter have lower proliferation indices and growth rates than tumours larger than 18 mm {186}.

Microneuromas and Paget disease of bone

Definition

Small non-neoplastic tumours composed of masses of intertwined bundles of nerve fibres and Schwann cells, which are sometimes observed near the cochlea or vestibule in the temporal bones of cases of Paget disease of bone. It is likely that they are the result of pressure by the growth of the pagetic bone on the nerve fibres with their regeneration and the production of traumatic neuromas {2275}.

Neurofibromatosis type 2

A. Sandison
L. Michaels
G.L. Davis

Definition

An autosomal dominant disorder characterized by a high incidence of bilateral vestibular schwannomas as well as schwannomas of other cranial and peripheral nerves, and other benign intracranial and intraspinal tumours.

Synonym

Bilateral acoustic neuroma, bilateral vestibular schwannoma

Epidemiology

The condition usually presents clinically in the first or second decade of life.

Localization

Bilateral vestibular schwannoma is characteristic of neurofibromatosis type 2. The tumours usually arise from the superior vestibular branch of the 8th cranial nerve. In addition, schwannomas of other cranial and peripheral nerves do occur as well as a wide variety of other benign intracranial and intraspinal tumours including schwannoma of other cranial and peripheral nerves, meningiomas, ependymomas, spinal neurofibromas, and gliomas. Juvenile posterior subcapsular cataract is also found.

Clinical features

Vestibular schwannomas in NF2 patients grow more rapidly than sporadic unilateral tumours. Infiltration of the cochlear and facial nerves occurs, making it more dif-

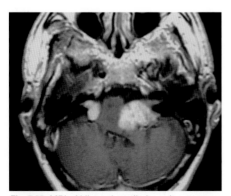

Fig. 7.30 MRI of bilateral vestibular schwannomas in a 32 year old man with NF2.

ficult to preserve hearing and facial nerve function after surgery. Screening of the relatives of affected subjects is necessary. Affected relatives of these patients often have normal audiograms and normal auditory brain stem responses in the presence of a schwannoma, and it has been recommended that the screening of relatives of NF2 patients should be by magnetic resonance image scanning with gadolinium (Gd-DTPA) enhancement {1326}.

In contrast to NF2, neurofibromatosis type 1 or von Recklinghausen disease is characterized by dermal neurofibromas. However, otological manifestations of neurofibromatosis were recorded in 6.5% of children with NF1, involving external ear canal, middle ear and eighth cranial nerve {2415}.

Macroscopy

The gross appearance of the vestibular schwannomas in neurofibromatosis 2 is similar to that of sporadic vestibular schwannoma.

Tumour spread and staging

There is invasion of the facial nerve in the internal auditory canal and also invasion of the modiolus and bony vestibular wall in some cases {2354}.

Histopathology

Vestibular schwannomas in NF2 are similar to those of sporadic vestibular schwannoma.

Immunoprofile

The degree of labelling with the proliferation marker Ki67 is higher in cases of NF2 that in those of solitary vestibular schwannoma {17}. Otherwise, the immunoprofile is identical.

Genetics

NF2 is an autosomal dominant condition. About 50% of patients have NF2 as a result of a new mutation and 50% inherit the disease from an affected parent. The children of an affected person have a 50% chance of inheriting the disease

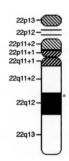

Fig. 7.31 Neurofibromatosis type 2. Schematic representation showing the localisation of the NF2 gene on the long arm of chromosome 22.

and prenatal diagnosis is available.

The gene for NF2 is a suppressor gene which has been mapped to the long arm of chromosome 22 (22q12). It codes for a protein which has been called by two names; MERLIN which stands for moezin-ezrin radixin like protein because it resembles the family of cytoskeletal associated proteins and SCHWANNOMIN because of its role in preventing schwannoma formation. It is a membrane-associated protein believed to inhibit cell growth and motility and preserve cell shape as well as anchoring the cell cytoskeleton to the surrounding matrix. Studies aimed at identifying germline mutations in patients with NF2 found mutations in up to 2/3 of cases. A wide variety of mutations have been found in all exons of the NF2 gene apart from exons 16 and 17. Ninety per cent of the mutations are predicted to truncate the gene product by introducing a stop codon, a frameshift with premature termination or a splicing alteration. This suggests that loss of the protein's function is necessary for tumourigenesis {1595}.

A family on the Isle of Man, Great Britain, with inherited salivary gland neuroendocrine carcinoma and amelogenesis imperfecta {1712} also displayed vestibular schwannoma in two male sibs, bilateral in one. Molecular genetic analysis has not yet been carried out, but it is likely that the disease process in this family is genetically related to NF2.

Lipoma of the internal auditory canal

L. Michaels

Definition
A benign tumour of adipocytes, important in this situation because it can mimic vestibular schwannoma.

ICD-O code 8850/0

Localization
Either in the cerebellopontine angle or in the internal auditory canal.

Clinical features
The most frequent associated symptoms are of cochleovestibular origin, such as hearing loss, dizziness and unilateral tinnitus. Other associated symptoms involve the facial nerve or the trigeminal nerve. Complete resection is associated with cranial nerve damage {2557}. The lesion may be mistaken clinically for a schwannoma, but magnetic resonance imaging can distinguish between the two entities. Where there is doubt, frozen section diagnosis of an incisional biopsy should be carried out to avoid the risk of damage to the 7th or 8th cranial nerve or their branches which may pass through the tumour.

Macroscopy
There may be erosion of the walls of the internal auditory canal as with vestibular schwannoma, and lipoma may appear similar to the latter at operation.

Histopathology
The tumour is similar to lipomas elsewhere except that 7th or 8th cranial nerve or their branches may be present among the adipocytes {2375}.

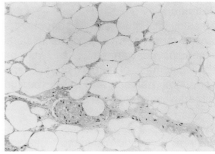

Fig. 7.32 Lipoma of the internal auditory canal showing a nerve branch amid the adipocytes. From Michaels & Hellquist, Ear, Nose & Throat Histopathology, Springer Verlag, London, 1991 {1711}.

Haemangioma

A. Sandison

Definition
A benign tumour of blood vessels.

ICD-O code 9120/0

Synonyms
Cavernous haemangioma, vascular tumour, vascular malformation.

Etiology
Little is known about these rare tumours. Only 43 cases were reported in the world literature up to the year 2000 {2313}. They are thought to arise from the dense vascular networks around the geniculate ganglion and Scarpa ganglion, which may account for the site predilection.

Localization
Haemangioma of the temporal bone occur most frequently at two sites, the internal auditory meatus and the geniculate ganglion {1669}. Cavernous haemangioma arising in the cerebellopontine angle can mimic vestibular schwannoma, which occur more commonly at this site.

Clinical features
Patients may present with hearing loss or facial paralysis due to VIIth cranial nerve involvement, which usually happens at an early stage, before the tumour reaches 1 cm diameter. Symptoms are suggestive of haemangioma if they are disproportionate to the size of the lesion as seen on imaging, or fluctuate with hormonal changes such as occur in pregnancy. MRI imaging shows a lesion that enhances with gadolinium and which may contain areas of microcalcification.

Histopathology
The lesions are composed of irregular dilated vascular spaces with collagenous walls lined by a single layer of endothelium.

Prognosis and predictive factors
Although they are benign lesions, haemangiomas enlarge and do not spontaneously involute. Early surgical intervention is recommended to best preserve facial nerve function.

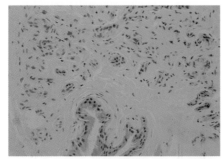

Fig. 7.33 Capillary haemangioma of the auditory canal.

Endolymphatic sac tumour

L. Michaels
T. Beale
A. Sandison
S. Soucek

Definition
Endolymphatic sac tumour (ELST), a non-metastasizing adenocarcinoma of endolymphatic sac origin, is a slowly-growing tumour which widely invades the petrous bone.

ICD-O code   8140/3

Synonyms
Heffner tumour {1038}, low grade adeno-carcinoma of endolymphatic sac origin (LGAES), aggressive papillary middle ear tumour (APMET).

Epidemiology
A rare neoplasm of adults. Although ELST is extremely rare in the general population. An association with von Hippel-Lindau disease (VHL) is established {1696}.

Etiology
The mutations in the VHL gene have been implicated in the development of ELST.

Localization
At an early stage of its growth, the neoplasm is sited within the endolymphatic sac {970,1026}. At a later stage, it destroys much of the petrous bone, including the middle ear and extends to the posterior fossa into the cerebellopontine angle {1038,2767}.

Clinical features
Tinnitus, hearing loss and vertigo, similar or identical to the symptoms of Ménière disease, are present in about one third of patients. It is presumed that early obstruction of the endolymphatic sac leads to hydrops of the endolymphatic system of the labyrinth. As the tumour spreads, facial nerve paralysis and/or cerebellar disorders may develop. Imaging reveals a lytic temporal bone lesion, appearing to originate from the region between the internal auditory canal and sigmoid sinus (which is the approximate position of the endolymphatic sac). There is eventually prominent extension into the posterior cranial cavity and invasion of the middle ear.

Histopathology
In most cases, ELST has a variable papillary-glandular appearance, the papillary proliferation being covered by a single row of low cuboidal cells. The vascular nature of the papillae in some cases has given the tumour a histological resemblance to choroid plexus papilloma. Some cases show areas of dilated glands containing secretion which resembles colloid. Such thyroid-like areas may even dominate the histological pattern. A few cases show a clear cell predominance resembling carcinoma of the prostate and renal cell carcinoma.
Despite controversy surrounding the origin of so-called "aggressive papillary middle ear tumour" (APMET see above) {844}, current evidence suggests that it is ELST with extension into the middle ear.

Immunoprofile
These tumours express cytokeratin and some express glial fibrillic acidic protein. Specific markers for metastases including thyroglobulin and prostate-specific antigen are negative.

Genetics
The gene responsible for Von Hippel Lindau (VHL) has been mapped to the short arm of chromosome 3 (3p 25-26). Mutations in this gene have been reported in patients with ELST. The gene is thought to be a tumour suppressor gene since genetic analysis of tumours in patients with VHL disease supported Knudson's hypothesis that an inherited mutation in one allele, followed by somatic mutation and loss of function of the second allele were required for tumourigenesis. In the case of sporadic tumours, tumourigenesis results from somatic mutation in both alleles of the tumour suppressor gene. A germline mutation of the VHL gene and somatic mutation of the wild type allele have been shown in ELST from VHL patients and somatic mutations in the VHL gene have been demonstrated in sporadic ELST. The rarity of ELST has meant that analysis of the tumours for specific mutations has been difficult. Hamazaki et al reported the genetic analysis of a case of ELST which

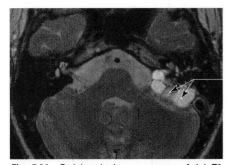

Fig. 7.34 Endolymphatic sac tumour. Axial T2 weighted MRI scan of the posterior fossa. The white area represents fluid within the endolymphatic sac and the grey area the solid component of the endolymphatic sac tumour.

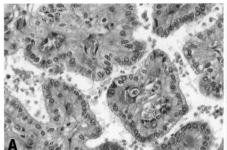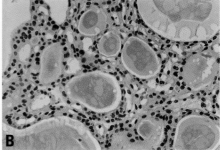

Fig. 7.35 Endolymphatic sac tumour. **A** Mild atypical nuclei are identified at the luminal surface of the papillary projections. Thin fibrovascular cores are present. **B** Endolymphatic sac tumour showing thyroid-like glandular pattern.

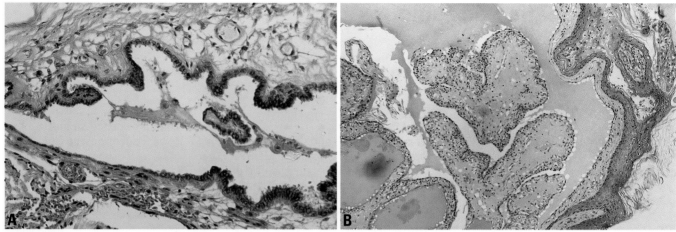

Fig. 7.36 A Normal endolymphatic sac showing papillary pattern of lining. **B** Endolymphatic sac tumour showing papillary pattern.

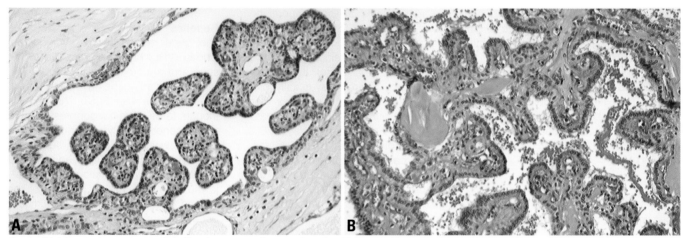

Fig. 7.37 Endolymphatic sac tumour. **A** A dilated space contains a number of papillary projections, although it is lined by the same morphologically bland-appearing nuclei. **B** Simple papillary projections with areas of sclerosis. The cuboidal cells have an increased nuclear to cytoplasmic ratio.

occurred in the absence of VHL disease {984}. This showed a nucleic acid substitution of G to T in nucleotide 546 in the VHL gene which resulted in an amino acid substitution (Trp to Cys codon117). An identical mutation has been reported in other VHL families. This suggests that the VHL gene is associated with ELST tumourigenesis with or without VHL disease.

Prognosis and predictive factors

The tumour grows slowly over many years and is not known to metastasize. Many tumours have already attained a large size at presentation. It is important to screen all patients with VHL for ELST by imaging so that small tumours may be detected early and completely excised {1696}. Likewise, all patients with ELST should be screened for the VHL gene.

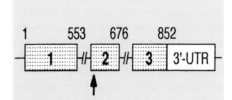

Fig. 7.38 Endolymphatic sac tumour. Schematic representation of the VHL gene and site of mutations in ELST. The arrow indicates the site of mutation in exon 2. The 3' untranslated region (3'-UTR) is unshaded. Nucleotides are numbered according to the VHL cDNA sequence. From Hamazki et al. {984}
.

Haematolymphoid tumours

K. Henry

These tumours, in the WHO classification of haematological malignancies {1197}, are primarily stratified according to lineage into myeloid, lymphoid, histiocytic/dendritic cell and mast cell neoplasms. In each category, neoplasms are defined according to morphology, immunophenotype, genetic features and clinical syndromes. For each type of neoplasm a cell of origin is proposed.

Ear lymphomas

Lymphomas occurring in and around the ear are rare compared to other sites. They may involve the pre- and retro-auricular lymph nodes, temporal bone or skin and soft tissue.Those lymphomas affecting the pre-auricular lymph nodes are predominantly disseminated or nodal.

Lymphomas of bone tend to occur with persistence of red marrow. With the exception of plasma cell tumours such as plasma cell myeloma (synonyms: multiple myeloma, myelomatosis) and plasmacytoma (synonym: solitary plasmacytoma of bone), both of which can involve the squamous and petrous temporal bone, lymphomas are extremely rare in the temporal bone. The mastoid process, part of the temporal bone, contains air cells and lacks marrow.

B-cell chronic lymphocytic leukaemia/small lymphocytic lymphoma (B-CLL / SLL)

ICD-O code	9823/3

Of those lymphomas resulting in cutaneous lesions of the head and neck, including the ears, the most common is B-cell chronic lymphocytic leukaemia/ small lymphocytic lymphoma. Leukaemic infiltrates in the skin or leukaemia cutis are not rare. Lesions on the face including ears have been recognized for several decades as heralding the onset of B-CLL / SLL {352,353,2071,2265}. They are included in the section on 'Cutaneous involvement in primary extra-cutaneous B-cell lymphomas' in the WHO

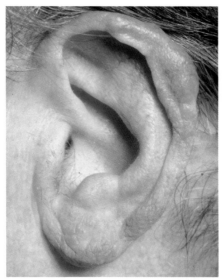

Fig. 7.39 B-CLL / SLL. Leukaemia cutis. A middle aged man presenting with infiltrates in the skin of the right and left ears including the ear lobes. The skin of his nose tip was also involved.

Classification of Skin Tumours.
The B-CLL infiltrates may appear as macules, plaques, papules, nodules, ulcers and even bullous lesions. Such infiltrates occur at sites of previous herpes simplex or herpes zoster have been well documented {354}. Leukaemic infiltrates have also been observed at sites typical of lymphadenosis benigna cutis

(earlobe, nipple, scrotum), a Borrelia burgdorferi-associated cutaneous B-cell pseudolymphoma {352}, now called Borrelia-associated lymphocytoma cutis. Most cases of B-CLL with cutaneous infiltrates are not associated with decreased survival; those associated with a poor prognosis have exhibited progression of the underlying disease to a high-grade large B-cell lymphoma (Richter syndrome) {353,2884}.

Histiocytic and dendritic cell neoplasms

Histiocytic and dendritic cell neoplasms are derived from the phagocytic and accessory cells, which have a major role in the processing and presentation of antigen to lymphocytes and which are bone marrow derived. The origin of the B-antigen presenting follicular dendritic cells remains to be established. They are not of bone marrow origin; an origin from either a fixed stromal/mesenchymal cell or from blood vessel endothelium are the two favoured options {1068}.
Histiocytic and dendritic cell neoplasms are rare. Of these tumours, only Langerhans cell histiocytosis has a significant incidence of ear disease by virtue of involvement of the temporal bone and middle ear.

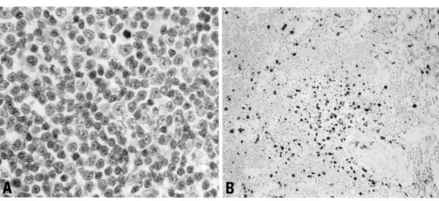

Fig. 7.40 A B-CLL/ SLL, biopsy of ear lobe. High power view of a proliferation centre. Admixed with small lymphocytes, are the proliferating larger prolymphocytes with small nuclei and para-immunoblasts with prominent nucleoli. **B** Nuclear expression of Ki 67 showing a higher proliferation index in a proliferation centre than in the surrounding small lymphocytic component.

Langerhans cell histiocytosis

K. Henry

Definition

Langerhans cell histiocytosis (LCH) is a neoplastic proliferation of Langerhans cells, with expression of CD1a, S100 and the presence of Birbeck granules by ultrastructural examination.

ICD-O code   9751/1

Synonyms

Histiocytosis X, Langerhans cell granulomatosis.Clinical variants have been referred to as Letterer-Siwe disease, Hand-Schuller-Christian disease and solitary eosinophilic granuloma of bone.

Epidemiology

LCH is rare {1511}. The incidence is about 5 per million with most cases occurring in children {1887}. Bone involvement in LCH counts for less than 1% of all bone lesions. There is a wide distribution of age from a few months to the 9th decade of life {1066}. Males are affected more often than females and the disease is more common in Whites of northern European origin than Blacks.

Etiology

This is unknown. There may be an association with a history of neonatal infection but there is no evidence of viral involvement {1672}.

Localization

Three overlapping syndromes are recognised {1511}.
Unifocal disease occurs in the majority of patients and usually involves bone (solitary eosinophilic granuloma). It is the bones of skull which are particularly affected, followed in frequency by the femur, pelvic bones and ribs.
Less commonly, unifocal disease is confined to a lymph node, skin or lung. LCH involving lungs in adults is nearly always associated with smoking and is thought to represent a different, possibly reactive disease {2684A}. In multifocal, unisystem disease (Hand-Schuller-Christian disease), several sites in one organ, almost always bone, are affected.

In multifocal, multisystem disease (Letterer-Siwe disease) many organs are involved such as bones, skin, liver, spleen, lymph nodes and bone marrow. Any bone may be involved, with the highest frequency occurring in the bones of the skull in children {1511}.
In temporal bone disease the lesion involves the medial part of the external auditory meatus {2099}.

Clinical features

Pain and swelling of the affected area is the most common presentation. In children with temporal bone involvement, the presenting features can simulate those of otitis media and mastoiditis because of otorrhoea and mastoid and facial swelling. Radiologically, early lytic lesions can suggest an aggressive disease process. Mutifocal unisystem disease is usually confined to young children, and the multiple destructive bone lesions are often associated with adjacent soft tissue masses. With skull bone involvement there may also be exophthalmos and diabetes insipidus if the pituitary is affected and tooth loss, if the jaw bones are involved. Multifocal multisystem system disease usually occurs in infants and in addition to bone lesions, there are fever, skin involvement, hepatosplenomegaly and pancytopaenia because of bone marrow involvement.

Macroscopy

The involved tissue is soft and usually red. If haemorrhage and necrosis are present, the colour may be yellow due to the presence of lipid and many eosinophils.

Histopathology

Crucial to the diagnosis is the recognition of the Langerhans cell. It is the nuclear appearances which are so distinctive; the nuclei are folded or grooved resembling a coffee bean or lobulated and indented. The nuclear chromatin is finely dispersed, nucleoli are inconspicuous and the nuclear membranes are thin. Mitotic activity is quite variable; some-

times there are up to 6 mitoses per sq. mm. In bone lesions Langerhans cells are found in nests and clusters. Necrosis is often present and should not be interpreted as suggesting aggressive disease. Admixed with the Langerhans cells are eosinophils, sometimes in large numbers, lymphocytes, neutrophils and plasma cells. Multinucleated osteoclast-like giant cells and lipid laden foamy macrophages can usually be identified. In old lesions foamy macrophages are numerous and there is significant fibrosis. The appearances of the lesions are so characteristic that the diagnosis can be made on cytological preparations, including touch preparations.

Immunoprofile

Neoplastic Langerhans cells resemble normal Langerhans cells in their expression of CD1a {675} and S-100 protein, the latter being expressed in both nuclei and cytoplasm {1835}. They also express CD4, vimentin, HLA DR and placental alkaline phosphatase (PLAP). CD68 and lysozyme are variably and only weakly expressed; and there is no expression of the follicular dendritic cell markers CD21 or CD35. Immunostaining for Ki67 shows a proliferation index of between 2% and 25%.
While their phenotype resembles that of normal Langerhans cells it is not identical, for in contrast their normal counterparts do not express placental alkaline phosphatase (PLAP) and also show differences in the expression of adhesion molecules {557}.

Electron microscopy

As in normal Langerhans cells, neoplastic Langerhans cells contain the unique cytoplasmic organelle called the Birbeck or Langerhans granule. 'Granule' is something of a misnomer, since the characteristic shape is that of a tennis racket or long necked flask. These structures, which vary in length from 200-400 nanometres, are pentalaminar rods measuring 33 nanometres in width with a vesicular expansion at one end. They

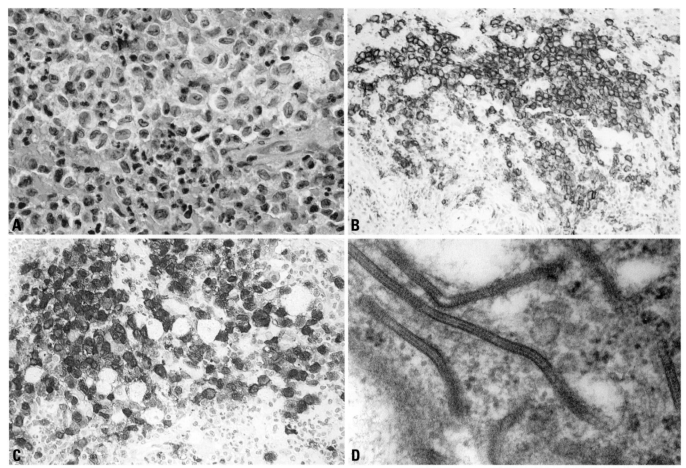

Fig. 7.41 A Langerhans cell histiocytosis, presenting as chronic otitis media due to involvement of the mastoid bone. High power view showing the distinctive Langerhans cells with their grooved and folded nuclei and some eosinophils. **B** Langerhans cell histiocytosis, immunohistochemistry. Strong membrane expression of CD1a by neoplastic Langerhans cells. Note that in contrast to their normal counterparts they lack the long cytoplasmic extensions. **C** Langerhans cell histiocytosis, immunohistochemistry. Strong expression for S100 in nuclei as well as cytoplasm. **D** Langerhans cell histiocytosis, ultrastructure. High magnification showing the pentalaminar rod shaped structure of Birbeck granules.

arise from the cell membrane {1066}. Their function is unknown.

Genetics
In all of the clinical syndromes/variants of LCH, studies of the X-linked androgen receptor gene have demonstrated that the proliferation of Langerhans cells is clonal {2796,2873}.

Prognosis and predictive factors
It is the demonstration that Langerhans cell histiocytosis represents a clonal proliferation that has led to its acceptance as a neoplastic disorder. However, the prognosis for patients with either monostotic or limited polyostotic disease is good. Death is rare in LCH and is associated with disseminated forms of the disease. Thus the clinical outcome directly relates to the number of organs affected {946}. The overall survival of patients with unifocal disease is 95% dropping to 75% with 2 organs involved and with further drops with increasing organ involvement. In about 10% of patients there is progression of unifocal lesions to multifocal disease. The presence of cytological atypia or an increased mitotic rate does not appear to correlate with prognosis {2181}.

Secondary tumours

G.L. Davis

Definition

Neoplasms which originate from sites other than within the structures of the ear i.e. external auditory canal, middle ear and temporal bone. These may be metastatic via blood or lymphatic channels from non-contiguous sites, or spread directly from a contiguous site by invasion of surrounding tissues or extension along / through existing channels.

Epidemiology

Secondary neoplasms in the ear / temporal bone are rare, amounting to 5-6% of 2,528 benign and malignant ear neoplasms compiled from surgical pathology accessions from four institutions {549}. Among the 1,781 ear neoplasms listed from the U.S. Armed Forces Institute of Pathology, only 31 (1.74%) had "metastasized" to the ear, most of these to the middle ear.

However, post-mortem histologic studies of temporal bones reveal metastatic cancer in 47 (22%) of 212 cancer patients {895}, virtually all of whom had had disseminated disease. The epidemiology of metastases involving the temporal bone is virtually identical to that cited for the skeletal system {775}.

Incidence and mortality

Virtually all patients with metastases to the ear/temporal bone have a known primary malignancy elsewhere and wide-spread metastatic diesease. Breast is by far the most common malignancy metastasizing to the temporal bone, followed by lung/bronchus, prostate, melanoma and thyroid. In spite of the frequency of metastases of renal carcinoma to bone, metastasis to the temporal bone appears to be rare, although a recent review reported renal origin in 9% of cases {1748}.

However among 12 patients with occult carcinoma found incidentally at autopsy only one had distant metastases: prostate carcinoma with widespread bone metastases including temporal bone. Among 18 patients, "adequately treated" and clinically free of cancer, none had residual cancer at autopsy, including temporal bone {895}.

Metastasis through direct extension

Direct extension into the ear / temporal bone occurs from the upper aero-digestive tract via the Eustachian tube and middle ear, and from the posterior fossa of the skull via the internal auditory canal. Direct invasion through bone and soft tissues occurs through the skull base and about the external ear in the parotid area. Head and neck primary tumours, excluding thyroid, account for the largest number (22%) of secondary tumours involving the ear by direct extension and/or invasion..

Localization

Blood borne metastases tend to localize to the petrous ridge (83%) and mastoid (28%) and are usually bilateral, multiple and associated with metastases to other bones.

Contiguous spread via existing channels: anteriorly from the upper aerodigestive tract to the middle ear (21%) via the Eustachian tube (14.5%); posteriorly from the brain and meninges via the internal auditory meatus (28%) to the inner ear.

Invasion of bone and soft tissue with extension into the base of the skull and external auditory canal and middle ear and mastoid occurs with paragan-gliomas and malignancies of the parotid gland.

Table 7.5 Temporal bone metastatic sites from 47 patients who died with malignancy University of Minnesota. From T.I. Gloria-Cruz et al. {895}.

Petrous apex	83%
Mastoid	27.6%
Internal auditory canal	27.6%
Middle ear	21.1%
Facial nerve	19.7%
Eustachian tube	14.5%
Osseous labyrinth	
Otic capsule	13.2%
Cochlea	10.5%
Vestibule	9.2%
External ear	9.2%
Membranous labyrinth	
Cochlear duct	7.9%
Saccule	3.9%
Utricle	3.9%
Semicircular canals	3.0%

Clinical features

Metastases to the temporal bone generally occur late in the course of the disease. Signs and symptoms in 101 patients with a history of malignant neoplasm included hearing loss (28%), vertigo (10%) facial palsy (9%), tinnitus (7%), otalgia (5%), otorrhea (2%), external canal mass (2%), nystagmus (2), no symptoms (36%) {895,1863}.

Histopathology

The secondary tumours maintain the phenotype of the primary. Since these secondary tumours occur in late stages of known malignant disease, evaluation of the unknown primary is rarely undertaken. Poorly differentiated malignancies invading the external auditory canal from a parotid lesion require consideration of parotid carcinoma, melanoma and adenocarcinoma of the canal. Biopsy of secondary temporal bone lesions, except for cerebellopontine angle tumours, is rarely undertaken and their origin is inferred by imaging studies, a history of malignancy or pathologic or cytologic studies of contiguous lesions.

Table 7.4 Site(s) of origin of tumours metastatic to temporal bone {895,1863}. Age range, 2 - 87 years.

Site	Total number (%)	
Breast	27	(22%)
Head and neck incl. brain (7) and choroid plexus (1)	26	(21%)
Lung/bronchi	12	(10%)
Prostate	10	(8%)
Malignant melanoma	7	(6%)
Unknown origin	7	(6%)
Thyroid	5	(4%)
Miscellaneous other sites	9	(23%)
Total	123	

CHAPTER 8

Tumours of the Paraganglionic System

The paraganglionic system develops early in gestation and is of neural crest origin. It consists of two components – the adrenal medulla and a diffuse collection of extra – adrenal paraganglia.

The extra-adrenal paraganglia are specialized collections of neuroendocrine cells that migrate in close association with the cranial nerves, large blood vessels, and autonomic nerves and ganglia. They vary in size from those that are just barely visible, such as the carotid bodies, to those that are apparent at the microscopic level, such as the laryngeal paraganglia.

As a group, neoplasms of the extra-adrenal paraganglia (paragangliomas) are uncommon and occur most often above the clavicles. Since paragangliomas are discussed in depth in the WHO Classification of Tumours of Endocrine Organs {577}, they are only briefly summarized in this chapter.

Tumours of the paraganglionic system: Introduction

L. Barnes
L.L.Y. Tse
J.L. Hunt
L. Michaels

Introduction

The extra-adrenal paraganglia can be divided into sympathetic and parasympathetic types. Although they are indistinguishable at the cellular level, they differ in their anatomic distribution and secretory products The sympathetic paraganglia are found primarily in the axial regions of the trunk along the prevertebral and paravertebral sympathetic chains and in connective tissue in or near pelvic organs. In contrast, parasympathetic paraganglia are localized almost exclusively in the head and neck along the branches of the glossopharyngeal and vagus nerves.

Although both types of paraganglia produce catecholamines, clinical signs of excess production are usually associated with those that are of sympathetic origin. Tumours associated with significant amounts of epinephrine (adrenaline) are almost always of sympathetic origin. Those lesions that occur in patients with hypoxemia, in contrast, are typically parasympathetic in origin. Overlaps in secretory expression, however, do occur. Parasympathetic paragangliomas, in contrast to their sympathetic counterparts, are also more often familial and less likely to be malignant Paragangliomas of the head and neck are found primarily at the bifurcation of the common carotid artery, in the middle ear – temporal bone, along the course of

Table 8.1 WHO Classification and ICD-O codes of paragangliomas of the head and neck region. For paragangliomas outside the head and neck region, see WHO Classification of Tumours of Endocrine Organs {577}.

Carotid body paraganglioma	8692/1
Jugulotympanic paraganglioma	8690/1
Vagal paraganglioma	8693/1
Laryngeal paraganglioma	8693/1
Miscellaneous paragangliomas	8693/1

[1] Morphology code of the International Classification of Diseases for Oncology (ICD-O) {821} and the Systematized Nomenclature of Medicine (http://snomed.org). Behaviour is coded /0 for benign tumours, /3 for malignant tumours, and /1 for borderline or uncertain behaviour.

Table 8.2 Classification of paraganglia and their main secretory products.

Paraganglion	Secretion
1. Adrenal medulla	80% epinephrine (adrenaline)
2. Extra-adrenal Sympathetic	90% norepinephrine (noradrenaline)
Parasympathetic	Dopamine

the vagus nerve, and exceptionally, in the orbit, nasal cavity, paranasal sinuses, nasopharynx, larynx, trachea and thyroid.

Anatomy
Carotid body paraganglia

Carotid body paraganglia are paired, bilateral, usually symmetrical aggregates of specialized neuroendocrine tissue located at the bifurcation of the common carotid artery along its posteromedial wall, either within or immediately external to the adventitia. They are anchored to the artery by a band of fibrovascular tissue referred to as the ligament of Mayer. Each measures about 3-7 mm in greatest dimension and weighs 3-15 mg {894, 1034,2231,2879}. They function as chemoreceptors sensitive to changes in oxygen tension, carbon dioxide content and hydrogen ion concentration.

Jugulotympanic paraganglia

Small paraganglia with a structure similar to the carotid body have been described in the ear {957}. More than 50% of these structures are situated in relation to the jugular bulb; a minority are found under the mucosa of the middle ear in the region of the medial promontory wall. The tumours arising from these paraganglia form the more frequent jugular paraganglioma (glomus jugulare) and the less frequent tympanic paraganglioma (glomus tympanicum), respectively.

Vagal paraganglia

The vagus nerve (from the Latin "vagus" meaning wandering and meandering)

Table 8.3 Comparison of sympathetic and parasympathetic paragangliomas.

Feature	Sympathetic	Parasympathetic
Location	Abdomen	Head and Neck
Functional status	Occasional	Uncommon
Familial history	Uncommon	Common
Malignancy	14-50%*	1-13%*

*Varies according to site of origin of the paraganglioma.

arises from 8-10 rootlets on the lateral border of the medulla that converge to form a cord on entering the jugular foramen. It is the longest cranial nerve and has a superior ganglion, which lies within the jugular foramen, and just below this, a middle ganglion. A third, much larger ganglion, known as the ganglion nodosa, lies more inferiorly. It is approximately 2.5 cm long and lies high in the neck, just behind the internal carotid artery.

Vagal paraganglia do not form a discrete "body" as seen at the carotid artery bifurcation, but rather consist of 6-7 small, dispersed aggregates of paraganglionic tissue. They may be found within (intravagal), or adjacent to (juxtavagal), the vagus nerve, usually at the level of the nodose ganglion. In rare instances, paraganglionic tissue may be found in sites just above or below the nodose ganglion. Their function is unknown, but they may have a role as a chemoreceptor and moderator of the cardiopulmonary system.

Laryngeal paraganglia

The larynx contains two pairs of paraganglia that are divided into two groups: superior and inferior. The superior paraganglia are between 0.1 mm and 0.3 mm in diameter. They occur bilaterally in the upper one-third of the false cord, adjacent to the superior margin of the thyroid cartilage, in close proximity to the superior laryngeal artery and nerve {2731}. The inferior paraganglia are also bilateral but larger than the superior group, averaging 0.3- 0.4mm in diameter {1331}.

Table 8.4 Differential diagnosis of paraganglioma of the head and neck.

Stain	Paraganglioma	Carcinoid	Medullary Thyroid Carcinoma	Anaplastic Carcinoma	Melanoma	Renal Cell Carcinoma
Synaptophysin	+	+	+	−	−	−
Keratin	−	+	+	+	−	+
HMB-45	−	−	−	−	+	−
Renal cell carcinoma antigen	−	−	−	−	−	+
Calcitonin	−	−/+	+	−	−	−
Thyroid transcription factor	−	−	+	−	−	−
Congo red (amyloid)	−	−	+	−	−	−

They characteristically occur between the inferior border of the thyroid cartilage and cricoid cartilage or between the cricoid cartilage and first tracheal ring in relationship to the inferior laryngeal artery and nerve.

Aberrant and accessory paraganglia are described {1331,2878}. Occasionally, paraganglia may even be found within nerves rather than adjacent to them. This is especially so regarding the recurrent laryngeal nerve {525}. The physiological role of the laryngeal paraganglia is also unknown. They may possibly serve as extracarotid chemoreceptors or have some effect on respiration via the larynx.

Terminology

The preferred terminology for tumours of the extradrenal paraganglia is "paraganglioma", prefaced by the anatomic site of origin, for instance, carotid body paraganglioma {1412}. If the tumour is functional or malignant, it would be designated, for example, as a functional carotid body paraganglioma or a malignant carotid body paraganglioma. Although the adrenal medulla is technically a paraganglion, a tumour arising from this site is still regarded as a phaeochromocytoma rather than a paraganglioma.

Diagnostic procedures

Computed tomography (CT) with contrast medium and magnetic resonance imaging (MRI) with gadolinium are invaluable in defining the location, size and extent of a paraganglioma {1587, 2124}. The typical CT appearance of a carotid body and vagal paraganglioma is that of a homogenous, hypervascular, well-defined soft tissue mass. If there has been haemorrhage or focal thrombosis, a heterogenous pattern of enhancement

will be seen. CT scans of jugulotympanic paragangliomas may also show expansion and erosion of the jugular foramen. As the tumour expands, it may destroy the surrounding bony labyrinth and ossicular chain and extend into the region of the cerebellopontine angle {2124}.

MRI characteristics of all paragangliomas are similar. A well-defined hypointense mass with areas of signal void is typically seen on T1-weighed images {1587}. A "salt and pepper" pattern is commonly seen in all lesions larger than 2 cm. This pattern is usually seen on T2-weighed images and is due to areas of high vascularity associated with haemorrhage or slow blood perfusion. In addition to providing superior definition, MRI can also detect much smaller paragangliomas than CT scans.

Octreotide scintigraphy is an important adjunct. It can be used not only to confirm the diagnosis of a neuroendocrine neoplasm, but also to detect additional occult tumours, to separate postoperative changes from residual or recurrent disease and for screening patients at risk for familial paragangliomas {1398,1587}. Ultrasound has a limited role in the evaluation of head and neck paragangliomas. It is useful in the evaluation and follow-up of carotid body paragangliomas and to some extent vagal paragangliomas. Its use in the detection and assessment of jugulotympanic paragangliomas is limited because of the surrounding bone.

Although non-invasive imaging has almost universally replaced angiography as the primary radiographic procedure for diagnosing paragangliomas, angiography still remains an important component in the management of these

patients, especially in regards to preoperative embolization to reduce the blood supply of the tumour.

Genetics

It is commonly stated that about 10% of all paragangliomas of the head and neck are familial and inherited as an autosomal dominant trait with genomic imprinting {951,1670,2665}. There is no tumour when the gene is inherited from the mother. Paternal transmission of the gene, however, results in tumour(s) in children even if the father is clinically unaffected. Some investigators are of the opinion that because of skipping of generations after maternal transmission of the gene, that the incidence of familial paragangliomas is vastly underestimated and may be as high as 50% of all cases {2678}.

Genetic linkage analyses of several large families with hereditary paragangliomas have identified three loci associated with these tumours – paraganglioma 1 (PGL1) on chromosome 11q23, PGL2 on chromosome 11q13.1 and PGL3 on chromosome 1q21-q23 {1080,1634,1897}. Studies have identified the PGL1 gene as SDHD and the PGL3 gene as SDHC, both of which encode mitochondrial respiratory chain proteins {181,182,889}.

In a study of 8 patients with sporadic (non-familial) paragangliomas of the head and neck, 3 exhibited deletions at chromosome 11q, 2 at 11q22-23 and 1 at 11q13 {213}. This suggests that sporadic and familial paragangliomas may share a similar molecular-genetic pathogenesis. It is now possible through genetic analysis to identify early on those patients who are at risk for familial paragangliomas, with the possibility of gene therapy on the horizon {2025}.

Carotid body paraganglioma

L. Barnes
L.L.Y. Tse
J.L. Hunt

Introduction

A neuroendocrine neoplasm derived from carotid body paraganglia composed of chief and sustentacular cells arranged in a characteristic (Zellballen) pattern.

ICD-O code

8692/1

Synonyms

Carotid body tumour, chemodectoma, glomus tumour, non-chromaffin paraganglioma, neuroendocrine tumour.

Age and sex distribution

They occur primarily in adults averaging 40-50 years of age and are rare in children. At sea level, the sex distribution ranges from 1:1-1:4 in favour of females {136,951,1410,1869,2155}. However, at altitudes above 2000 meters, there is a female predominance of 8.3:1 {2188}. It has been postulated that the monthly loss of blood through menstruation in women and a larger pulmonary capacity and greater enthusiasm for sports and athletic conditioning in men may allow males to escape chronic hypoxia and account for this wide gender gap {2188}.

Etiology

Familial inheritance and chronic hypoxia are the only known risk factors.

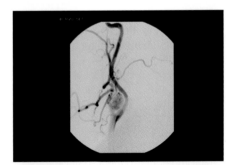

Fig. 8.1 Carotid body paraganglioma. Angiogram shows a hypervascular mass at the bifurcation of the common carotid artery with separation of the internal and external carotid arteries. Courtesy of Drs. Jim Rabinov and Hugh Curtin, Department of Radiology, Massachusetts General Hospital, Boston, MA, USA.

Localization

The tumours occur at the bifurcation of the common carotid artery with no significant lateralization to either side of the neck. As they enlarge, they may become adherent, invade or incorporate the external and/or internal carotid arteries.

Clinical features

Although uncommon, carotid body paragangliomas are regarded as the most common paraganglioma of the head and neck.

Signs and symptoms

The typical presentation is that of a slowly enlarging, asymptomatic mass deep to the anterior border of the sternocleidomastoid muscle just below the angle of the mandible. The tumour can be moved from side to side but with little or no movement in a vertical plane (Fontaine's sign). Occasionally, it may be associated with pain, hoarseness, dysphagia, Horner's syndrome, headache, syncope, bruit or thrill. Functional tumours with catecholamine – induced hypertension are exceptional {509}.

Infrequently, the tumour may be bilateral or associated with paragangliomas in other sites (usually a vagal or jugulotympanic paraganglioma) or occur in combination with a phaeochromocytoma, a well-differentiated thyroid carcinoma or a component of multiple endocrine neoplasia syndrome or Carney triad {481,509, 1391,1422,1430}. Hereditary deficiencies of clotting factors VII and X have also been observed in a few patients with familial carotid body paragangliomas {1376}.

Imaging

Carotid body paragangliomas appear on angiography as hypervascular masses at the carotid artery bifurcation with eventual splaying of the internal and external carotid arteries.

Macroscopy

The tumours are usually between 2.0 and 6.0 cm (average 3.8 cm) and are firm,

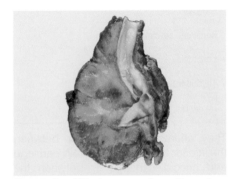

Fig. 8.2 Carotid body paraganglioma. Cut surface showing encasement of a segment of external carotid artery which had to be sacrificed.

rubbery, well circumscribed, and invested by a thin, sometimes focally thickened fibrous capsule. On cut surface, most have a variegated yellow, tan, pink, red or brown appearance with areas of fibrosis and haemorrhage. A few are homogenously tan-pink or yellow-brown. A large artery, usually the external carotid, is occasionally seen occurring through the tumour or attached peripherally.

Histopathology

These highly vascular tumours are composed of two cell types, chief and sustentacular, arranged in a characteristic alveolar or Zellballen pattern. The chief cells (type I cells, epithelioid cells) are more numerous and contain catecholamine-bound neurosecretory granules as seen ultrastructurally. The sustentacular cells (type II cells, supporting cells) are devoid of neurosecretory granules and are characteristically located at the periphery of the Zellballen.

The chief cells often show considerable nuclear enlargement and hyperchromatism and contain cytoplasm that varies from pink to clear, to amphophilic and which may be vacuolated. Spindle-shaped chief cells are uncommon and mitoses are sparse to absent. Vascular and perineural invasion are infrequent and have no prognostic significance.

Immunoprofile

The chief cells express synaptophysin,

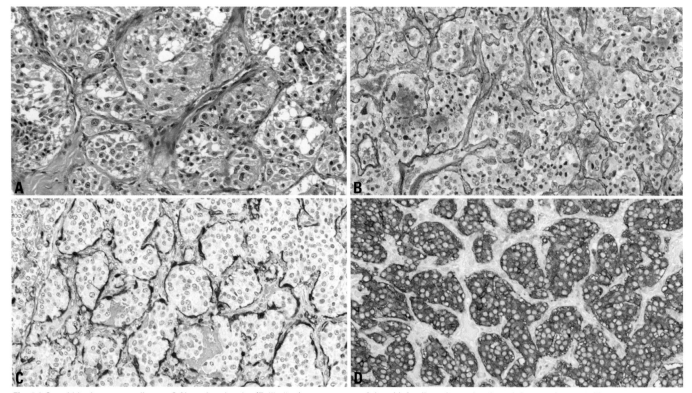

Fig. 8.3 Carotid body paraganglioma. **A** Note the alveolar (Zellballen) arrangement of the chief cells, anisonucleosis and the prominent capillary network around each group of cells. **B** Reticulin stain accentuates the alveolar (Zellballen) arrangement of chief cells. **C** S-100 protein highlights the peripheral layer of sustentacular cells surrounding each group of cells. **D** The chief cells are strongly positive for synaptophysin; sustentacular cells are negative.

chromogranin and neuron-specific eno-lase. They are negative for cytokeratin, carcinoembryonic antigen, S-100 protein and calcitonin. The sustentacular cells express S-100 protein and glial fibrillary acidic protein.

Malignant carotid body paraganglioma

Paragangliomas are divided into non-invasive (circumscribed, encapsulated), locally invasive and metastatic categories. Some locally invasive tumours may even cause the death of the patient. Although clinically malignant, these tumours are still regarded as locally invasive. A tumour is considered malignant only if there is metastasis to regional lymph nodes or to more distant sites, such as the lungs and bones.

The incidence of malignant (metastasizing) carotid body paragangliomas ranges from 2-13% {136}. Unfortunately, the clinical behaviour cannot be predicted on the basis of routine histology. Such features as nuclear pleomorphism, mitotic activity, necrosis and vascular – perineural invasion are unreliable prognosticators and have been found in benign as well as malignant tumours {136}. Other findings such as DNA ploidy, absence of sustentacular cells, number of expressed neuropeptides, assessment of argyrophilic nucleolar organizer regions and proliferative markers (PNCA, Ki-67) show no consistent correlation with histological behaviour {661,871,1335,1336, 1382, 1526,2678,2748,136,}.

Sporadic (non-familial) carotid body paragangliomas are more likely to be malignant than those that are familial – 12% versus 2.5% {951}. Metastases may be apparent at the time of initial therapy or may not become apparent until 20 years later {1967}.

Surgery with or without adjuvant irradiation is used for local disease. Chemotherapy, however, is largely ineffective {1656}. The overall 5-year relative survival is 59.5%. If the metastases are confined to regional lymph nodes, the 5-year survival is 76.8% but decreases to 11.8% for patients with distant metastases {1451}.

Differential diagnosis

The differential diagnosis includes carcinoid, medullary thyroid carcinoma, anaplastic carcinoma, metastatic melanoma and renal cell carcinoma. Immunostains are useful in separating these tumours.

Genetics

One-third of familial carotid body paragangliomas are bilateral, as opposed to 4% bilateral sporadic (non-familial) cases {951}. These may appear synchronously or asynchronously.

C-myc, bcl-2 and c-jun are abnormally expressed in some tumours and may contribute to tumourigenesis {2719, 2721}. Overexpression of TP53, however, does not appear to be an etiologic factor {2720}.

Prognosis and predictive factors

Carotid body paragangliomas are slowly growing tumours with a median growth of 0.83 mm per year and a median doubling time of 7.13 years {1205}.

Surgery, often with sacrifice of one or more branches of the carotid arterial system, is the treatment of choice. Somewhere between 0-10% of tumours will recur. This is not necessarily a sign of malignancy but rather inadequate excision and regrowth.

Jugulotympanic paraganglioma

L. Michaels
S. Soucek
T. Beale
A. Sandison

Definition

A neoplasm arising from one or other of the paraganglia situated in the vicinity of the jugular bulb or on the medial promontory wall of the middle ear.

ICD-O code   8690/1

Synonyms

Jugulotympanic chemodectoma, glomus jugulare tumour, jugular glomus tumour, glomus tympanicum tumour, tympanic glomus tumour.

Epidemiology

Solitary jugulotympanic paragangliomas arise predominantly in females. The age range is between 13 and 85 years with a mean age of about 50 years. The familial type occurs predominantly in men.

Localization

Most jugulotympanic paragangliomas arise from the paraganglion situated in the wall of the jugular bulb. A minority arise from the paraganglion situated near the middle ear surface of the promontory. The distinction between jugular and tympanic paragangliomas can easily be made in the patient by modern imaging methods with which the jugular neoplasm is identified as arising from the jugular bulb region and shows evidence of invasion of the petrous bone, while the tympanic neoplasm is confined to the middle ear. Jugulotympanic paragangliomas may also be multicentric or coexist with tumours of other types. They may be bilateral in the same patient and coexist with carotid body paragangliomas which may also be bilateral {1949}. They may also coexist with adrenal gland pheochromocytomas.

Clinical features

Most patients present with conductive hearing loss. Pain in the ear, facial palsy, haemorrhage, and tinnitus are also described. On examination, a red vascular mass is seen either behind the intact tympanic membrane or sprouting through the latter into the external canal. Surgical approach to the mass at biopsy often results in severe bleeding.

Etiology

The etiology of the solitary type is unknown. In the multiple familial type there is evidence of a gene mutation on chromosome 11.

Macroscopy

The neoplasm is an irregular reddish mass. In the jugular variety, the petrous temporal bone and the middle ear space are largely replaced by red, firm material as far as the tympanic membrane. The otic capsule is rarely invaded by paraganglioma.

Investigation of a paraganglioma in an autopsy temporal bone by the microslicing method, showed the shape of the jugular bulb to be retained, but the lumen was completely filled by neoplasm. The tumour invaded the apical region of the petrous temporal bone and the middle ear space was completely filled by neoplasm as far as the tympanic membrane. However, the surgical specimen is usually fragmented.

Histopathology

The histological appearances of the jugular and tympanic paragangliomas are similar, resembling that of the carotid body paraganglioma. Epithelioid, small, uniform cells, with finely granular cytoplasm are separated by numerous blood vessels. The tumour cells often form clusters or "Zellballen" with peripheral flattened cells. Nuclei are usually uniform and small, but diagnosis is sometimes made difficult by the presence of bizarre or multinucleate cells which, however, do not indicate malignancy. A prominent fibrous stroma is sometimes present.

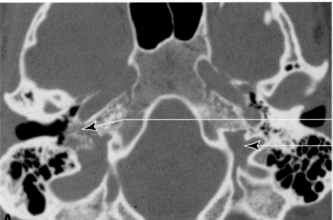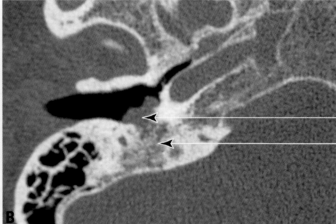

Fig. 8.4 Jugulotympanic paragangliomas. **A** Axial CT scan of petrous bone. On the right side, there is erosion of the cortex of the jugular foramen in keeping with a jugular paraganglioma (upper arrow). Note the normal jugular foramen (lower arrow) on the left. **B** Axial CT scan of petrous bone. Soft tissue mass in the posterior or hypotympanum (upper arrow). The adjacent permeative erosion (lower arrow) suggests that this is a tympanic paraganglioma.

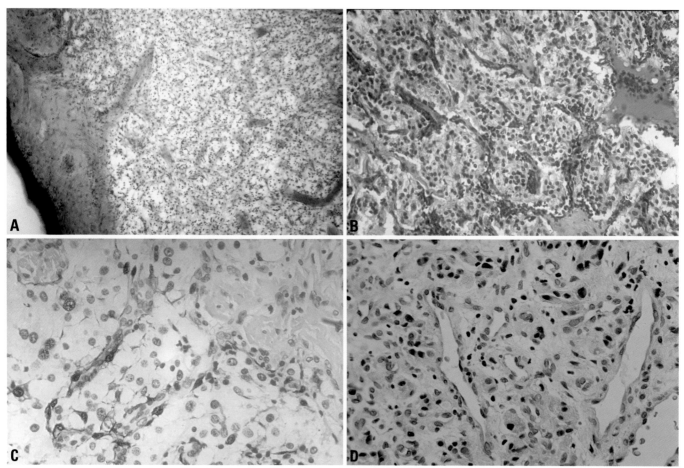

Fig. 8.5 Jugulotympanic paragangliomas. **A** Section of autopsy case of jugulotympanic paraganglioma showing tumour behind tympanic membrane. **B** Histological appearance of jugulotympanic paraganglioma. **C** Jugulotympanic paraganglioma showing numerous sustentacular cells (S100 protein). **D** Jugulotympanic paraganglioma showing bizarre cells some of which are multinucleate.

Immunoprofile

The immunoprofile of these tumours has been covered in an earlier section (Immunoprofile p. 364-365).

Electron microscopy

Paragangliomas shows membrane-bound, electron-dense neurosecretory granules in the cytoplasm of the tumour cells consistent with catecholamine content {2277}.

Prognosis and predictive factors

Jugulotympanic paraganglioma is a neoplasm of slow growth. The jugular variety infiltrates the petrous bone, but distant metastasis is rare. Radiation therapy, and in some cases surgery, offers a high rate of cure for the localized neoplasms.

Vagal paraganglioma

L. Barnes
L.L.Y. Tse
J.L. Hunt

Definition
A neuroendocrine neoplasm derived from paraganglia found within or adjacent to the vagus nerve usually in the vicinity of the ganglion nodosum.

ICD-O code   8693/1

Synonyms
Vagal body paraganglioma, glomus tumour, glomus vagale, chemodectoma, non-chromaffin paraganglioma, neuroendocrine tumour.

Epidemiology
Age and Sex distribution
Vagal body paragangliomas are more common in women (64%) and occur over a broad age range (19-86 years) with an average of 45-55 years {215,282,689, 1410,1411,1736,1868,2659}.

Etiology
Most are sporadic. Some are related to familial inheritance. Although chronic hypoxia may lead to hyperplasia of vagal paraganglia, there is no conclusive evidence, in contrast to the carotid body paraganglioma, that it leads to the development of a vagal paraganglioma {1409}.

Localization
The tumours typically occur in the rostral portion of the vagus nerve in the vicinity of the ganglion nodosum. In a review of 99 vagal paragangliomas in which the side of origin was indicated, 56% arose on the right side of the neck, 39% on the left side and 5% were bilateral {2879}.

Clinical features
The vagal paraganglioma is the third most frequent paraganglioma of the head and neck, exceeded in frequency only by the carotid body and jugulotympanic paragangliomas. It characteristically presents as a slowly enlarging, asymptomatic mass at the angle of the mandible and/or as a bulge in the lateral oropharyngeal wall. As it increases in size, deficits of cranial nerves IX, X, XI

Table 8.5 Vagal paraganglioma: clinico-pathologic features*

Average age (n=139)	45 – 55 years (range 19 – 86 years)
Gender (n=139)	64% female (range 50 – 85%)
Multicentric tumours (n=124)	33% (range 10 – 46%)
Familial history (n=124)	17% (range 0 – 47%)
Functional tumours (n=139)	3.6% (range 0 – 11%)
Local recurrence (n=126)	8% (range 0 – 20%)
Malignant tumours (n=139)	7% (range 0 – 16%)
*Data based on references {215,282,689,1410,1411,1736,1868,2659}.	

and XII and the cervical sympathetic chain are common, resulting in unilateral vocal cord dysfunction, dysphagia, atrophy of the tongue, shoulder weakness and Horner syndrome. At the time of diagnosis, anywhere from 35-65% of patients may manifest one or more cranial nerve deficits.

Functional tumours with catecholamine-induced hypertension are distinctly uncommon, occurring in only 3.6% of all tumours.

Imaging
Vagal paragangliomas are highly vascular and are located in the suprahyoid neck, well above the level of the carotid bifurcation and typically displace both external and internal carotid arteries anteromedially.

Macroscopy
The tumours are fusiform or circular and abut directly onto the base of the skull. They usually range from 2.0-6.0 cm and are firm, rubbery, well circumscribed and surrounded by a thin, sometimes focally thickened fibrous capsule. In a few instances, they may be poorly defined and locally infiltrative.

On cut surface, they have a variegated yellow, tan, pink, red or brown appearance with fibrosis and haemorrhage or they may be uniformly homogenous. A portion of one or more large nerves, usually the vagus, is often attached.

Histopathology
The histopathology, immunoprofile, ultrastructural features and differential diagnosis are similar to those previously

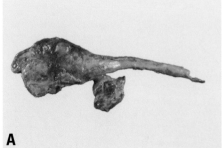 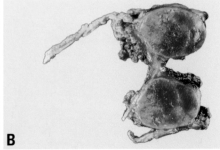

Fig. 8.6 Vagal paraganglioma. **A** Note the expanded portion of the vagus nerve which represents the neoplasm. A small group of lymph nodes is attached at the center of the specimen. **B** Cross section shows a spongy, focal haemorrhagic tan surface. A segment of vagus nerve is attached.

described for the carotid body paraganglioma.

Malignant vagal paraganglioma
Overall 7% of vagal paragangliomas are malignant by virtue of metastases. In one review of 15 malignant vagal paragangliomas, 73% were associated with cervical lymph node metastasis and 27% with distant metastases (lung, bone, liver and brain) {1050}. Most metastases are apparent either at or within four years of diagnosis.

Genetics
Patients with sporadic (non-familial) vagal paragangliomas may have more than one paraganglioma and should always be evaluated for this possibility. The incidence of finding multiple tumours in this population varies according to the thoroughness of the examination and the length of follow-up. When multiple, the tumours may appear synchronously or asynchronously. In a collective review of 124 vagal paragangliomas, 33% were associated, either at the time of diagnosis or on follow-up, with additional paragangliomas, usually a carotid body or,

less frequently, a jugulotympanic paraganglioma. Seventeen percent of patients also had a family history of paragangliomas.
DNA analysis of 10 vagal paragangliomas utilizing image analysis, revealed 5 to be diploid, 4 diploid – tetraploid and 1 aneuploid {137}. DNA abnormalities are, therefore, common in these tumours and cannot be used to predict prognosis.

Prognosis and predictive factors
Vagal paragangliomas are slowly growing with an estimated median growth rate of one millimetre per year and a median doubling time of 8.89 years {1205}.
Options for treatment include surgical resection, radiation, and, in selected cases due to their slow growth rate, even observation. Most clinicians favour surgery. Almost invariably, the vagus nerve and sometimes even other cranial nerves, have to be sacrificed. In those instances where the nerve is preserved, function typically remains permanently impaired. Failure to remove the nerve may also predispose the patient for future recurrence.

Radiation is used for elderly patients who are poor operative risks or for those unfortunate individuals who have bilateral vagal paragangliomas (the larger tumour is preferentially excised while the smaller one is irradiated).
Following surgery, 8% of vagal paragangliomas will develop local recurrence. The tumour may recur as early as 12 months after therapy or as late as 22 years. Local recurrence is not necessarily a sign of malignancy but often results from inadequate excision.

Laryngeal paraganglioma

L. Barnes
L.L.Y. Tse
J. Hunt

Definition

A neuroendocrine neoplasm derived from either the superior or inferior paraganglia of the larynx composed of chief and sustentacular cells arranged in a characteristic organoid (Zellballen) pattern.

ICD-O code   8693/1

Synonyms

Glomus tumour, chemodectoma, nonchromaffin paraganglioma, neuroendocrine tumour.

Age and sex distribution

Laryngeal paragangliomas are rare, with only 62 cases identified in a critical review of the world literature in 1994 {125,739}. They are three times more common in women and have been described in patients from 5-83 years of age (median 44 years) {739,2586}.

Etiology

Other than a familial inheritance, there are no known risk factors.

Localization

The vast majority (82%) occur in the supraglottic larynx, presumably arising from the superior pair of laryngeal paraganglia, and present as a submucosal mass in the region of the aryepiglottic fold – false vocal cord {125}. Only 15% occur in the subglottis and 3% in the glottis. The right side of the larynx is more often involved than the left by a ratio of 2.3:1 {125}.

Clinical features

Most patients present with more than one complaint and have been symptomatic for an average of 26 months (median 23 months; range 3 weeks to 12 years) {125}. The major symptom, by far, is hoarseness. Others, in decreasing order of frequency, are dysphagia, dyspnea, stridor, dysphonia, sore-painful throat, neck mass, haemoptysis, coughing, shortness of breath, foreign body sensation in the throat, and otalgia. Bruits and pulsation are usually absent.

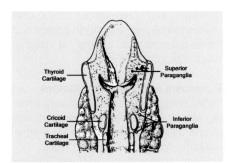

Fig. 8.7 Diagram of the larynx showing location of laryngeal paraganglia.

Functional laryngeal paragangliomas are exceptional with only one possible case report {1438}. The patient, a 25-year-old woman with a supraglottic paraganglioma had sinus tachycardia and hypertension, which disappeared following surgical removal of the tumour. Neither the patient nor the tumour was evaluated for hormone production. Other alleged functional tumours that have been reported are probably atypical carcinoids {1184,1240,2691}.

Imaging

Very few laryngeal paragangliomas have been evaluated preoperatively with angiograms. Of those that have, the blood supply of supraglottic paragangliomas has been from the superior thyroid artery, superior laryngeal artery or a branch of the external carotid artery {125,149,1123,1357,2236}. An angiogram of a single case of a subglottic paraganglioma showed the blood supply was via the thyrocervical trunk {1940}.

Macroscopy

The tumours characteristically present as a well-circumscribed, tan, brown or reddish-brown 0.5-6.0 cm (average 2.6 cm) submucosal mass {125}. Cut surface varies from smooth to multinodular, with or without areas of fibrosis.

Histopathology

Histopathology, immunoprofile, ultrastructural features and differential diagnosis are similar to those of the carotid body paraganglioma.

Malignant laryngeal paraganglioma

Although commonly stated that 25% of all laryngeal paragangliomas are malignant {851,2413,2779}, a critical review of these cases has revealed that almost all of these are examples of atypical carcinoids incorrectly labelled as malignant paragangliomas {125}.

Current studies indicate that only about 2% of all laryngeal paragangliomas are malignant {739}. Only a single acceptable case has been reported. This involved a 36 year-old woman with a paraganglioma of the larynx that metastasized to the lumbar spine 16 years after the diagnosis {96,2212}.

Genetics

Laryngeal paragangliomas may be associated with paragangliomas in other sites {125}. The most frequent association is with a carotid body paraganglioma {1020,2236,2679}. Cases have also been described associated with a jugulotympanic and a tracheal paraganglioma {510,1328}. Another example has been reported in a 35 year-old man with a family history of carotid body paragangliomas who presented with a subglottic paraganglioma {254}.

DNA analysis of two laryngeal paragangliomas has shown both to be diploid {125}.

Prognosis and predictive factors

Surgery is the treatment of choice, preferably through an external approach {739}. Endoscopic excision should be avoided (even for small lesions) because bleeding, which may be diffuse, may be difficult to control. Preoperative angiography and embolization, in an attempt to devascularize the tumour, is not essential since the superior thyroid artery can easily be ligated prior to resection. An elective neck dissection is not warranted. Seventeen per cent of patients have developed local recurrence from 1-16 years after initial excision {125}.

Contributors

Dr. Susan L. ABBONDANZO
Dept. of Hematopathology
Armed Forces Institute of Pathology
6825 16th Street NW
Washington, DC 20306-6000
USA
Tel. +1 202 782 1723
Fax. +1 202 782 9157
Abbondan@afip.osd.mil

Dr. Lucía ALÓS
Dept. Anatomia Patologica
Hospital Clínic de Barcelona
Villarroel, 170
08036 Barcelona
SPAIN
Tel. +34 93 227 5450
Fax. +34 93 227 5717
lalos@clinic.ub.es

Dr. Mario ALTINI
Division of Oral Pathology
Private Bag 3
Wits 2050
SOUTH AFRICA
Tel. +27 11 717 2139
Fax. +27 11 717 2146
altinim@dentistry.wits.ac.za

Dr. Paul L. AUCLAIR *
Maine Medical Center
Dept. of Pathology
22 Bramhall Street
Portland, ME 04102
USA
Tel. +1 207 871 4025
Fax. +1 207 871 6360
auclap@mmc.org

Dr. Gisle BANG
5207 S?fteland
Norway
Tel. +47 5 6307076
Fax. +47 5 5973158
gunnvor.oijordsbakken@gades.uib.no

Dr. Leon BARNES *
Dept. of Pathology, Room A608
University of Pittsburgh Medical Center
200 Lothrop Street
Pittsburgh, PA 15213
USA
Tel. +1 412 647 3735
Fax. +1 412 647 6251
barnesel@msx.upmc.edu

---

* The asterisk indicates participation
in the Working Group Meeting on the
WHO Classification of Head and Neck
Tumours that was held in Lyon,
France, July 16-19, 2003.

Dr. Timothy J. BEALE
Royal National Throat, Nose & Ear
Hospital
Gray's Inn Road
London WC
UNITED KINGDOM
Tel. +44 20 7915 1441
Fax. +44 20 7915 1668
timothy.beale@royalfree.nhs.uk

Dr. Franco BERTONI *
Istituto Rizzoli
Anatomia Patologica
Via di Barbiano 1/10
40136 Bologna
ITALY
Tel. +39 051 6366591
Fax. +39 051 6366592
franco.bertoni@ior.it

Dr. Wojciech BIERNAT *
Neuropathology and Molecular Pathology
Medical University of Gdansk
ul. Debinki 1
80-211 Gdansk
POLAND
Tel. +48 58 349 1531
Fax. +48 58 349 1535
biernat@amg.gda.pl

Dr. Paolo BOFFETTA
Gene-Environment Epidemiology Group
Int. Agency for Research on Cancer
150 Cours Albert Thomas
69008 Lyon
FRANCE
Tel. 04 72 73 84 41
Fax. 04 72 73 83 20
boffetta@iarc.fr

Dr. Jerry E. BOUQUOT
Dept. of Diagnostic Sciences, Room 3.094J
Univ. of Texas at Houston Dental Branch
6516 M.D. Anderson Blvd.
Houston, TX 77030
USA
Tel. +1 713 792 4000
Fax. +1 713 792 2383
bouquot@aol.com

**Dr. Margaret S. BRANDWEIN-
GENSLER ***, Dept. of Pathology
Albert Einstein College of Medicine
Montefiore Medical Ctr. - Moses Division
111 East 210 Street
Bronx, NY 10467-2401, USA
Tel. +1 718 920 2456
Fax. + 1 718 882 8461
margie_brandwein@Yahoo.com

Dr. Robert B. BRANNON
Oral Pathology Dept.- Box 144
LSU School of Dentistry
1100 Florida Av.
New Orleans, LA 70119-2799
USA
Tel. +1 504 619 8551
Fax. +1 504 619 8751
rbrann@lsuhsc.edu

Dr Freddie BRAY
The Cancer Registry of Norway
Montebello
0310 Oslo
NORWAY
Tel. +47 23 33 39 83
Fax. +47 22 45 13 70
freddie.bray@kreftregisteret.no

Dr. John J. BUCHINO
Dept. of Pathology, Kosair Childrens
Hospital, University of Louisville
PO Box 35070
Louisville, KY 40232
USA
Tel. +1 502 629 7900
Fax. +1 502 629 7906
johnbuchino@louisville.edu

Dr. Amos BUCHNER
Chairman Dept. of Oral Pathology
School of Dental Medicine
Tel Aviv University
Tel Aviv
ISRAEL
Tel. +972 3 6419415
Fax. +972 3 6409250
buchner@post.tau.ac.il

Dr. Joseph CALIFANO *
Dept. of Otolaryngology
Johns Hopkins Medical Institutions
601 N. Caroline Street, 6th Floor
Baltimore, MD 21287-0910
USA
Tel. +1 410 955 6420
Fax. +1 410 955 8510
jcalifa@jhmi.edu

Dr. Eduardo CALONJE
Dept. of Diagnostic Dermatopathology
St John's Institute of Dermatology
St Thomas Hospital
London SE1 7EH
UNITED KINGDOM
Tel. + 44 20 7188 6408
Fax. + 44 20 7188 6382
jamie.calonje@kcl.ac.uk

Dr. Antonio CARDESA *
Dept. Anatomia Patologica
Hospital Clinic/ University of Barcelona
Villarroel 170
Barcelona, 08036
SPAIN
Tel. +34 93 227 5450
Fax. +34 93 227 5717
acardesa@clinic.ub.es

Dr. Roman CARLOS
Centro de Medicina Oral de Guatemala
16 calle 4-53 zona 10
Edificio Marbella, Of. 4-E
Guatemala City 01010
GUATEMALA
Tel. +502 363 0769/0770
Fax. +502 337 0705
roman@guate.net

Dr. John K.C. CHAN *
Dept. of Pathology
Queen Elizabeth Hospital
Wylie Road
Kowloon, Hong Kong
SAR CHINA
Tel. +852 2958 6830
Fax. +852 2385 2455
jkcchan@ha.org.hk

Dr. Alexander Chak-Lam CHAN
Dept of Pathology
Queen Elizabeth Hospital
30 Gascoigne Road
Kowloon, Hong Kong
SAR CHINA
Tel. +852 2958 6823
Fax. +852 2385 2455
chancl@ha.org.hk

Dr. Wah CHEUK
Dept. of Pathology
Queen Elizabeth Hospital
Wylie Road
Kowloon, Hong Kong
SAR CHINA
Tel. +852 2958 6835
Fax. +852 2385 2455
cheuk_wah@hotmail.com

Dr. Michael M.C. CHEUNG
Dept. of Clinical Oncology
Queen Elizabeth Hospital 11/F, Block R
Gascoigne Road
Kowloon, Hong Kong
SAR CHINA
Tel. +852 2958 6441
Fax. +852 2359 4782
michaelmccheung@hkcr.org

Dr. Hedley G. COLEMAN
Division of Oral Pathology,
Private Bag 3
Wits 2050
SOUTH AFRICA
Tel. +27 11 717 2139
Fax. +27 11 717 2146
colemanhg@dentistry.wits.ac.za

Dr. Hugh D. CURTIN
Dept. of Radiology
Massachusetts Eye and Ear Infirmary
243 Charles Street
Boston, MA 02114
USA
Tel. +1 617 573 3842
Fax. +1 617 573 3490
hdcurtin@meei.harvard.edu

Dr. Gustave L. DAVIS *
Dept. of Pathology, P.O. Box 208023
Yale University School of Medicine
310 Grant Street, 250 BML
New Haven, CT 06520-8023
USA
Tel. +1 203 785 5486
Fax. +1 203 737 1064
gustave.davis@yale.edu

Dr. Vera Cavalcanti DE ARAUJO
Centro de Pesquisas Odontolgicas So
Leopoldo Mandic
Rua Jos?? Rocha Junqueira 13
Ponte Preta - Campinas SP 3041-445
SP BRAZIL
Tel. +55 19 3237 3611
Fax. +55 19 3237 3611
veraa@slmandic.com.br

Dr. Louis P. DEHNER
Division of Anatomic Pathology
Washington University Medical Center
660 South Euclid Avenue, Box 8118
St Louis, MO 63110
USA
Tel. +1 314 362 0150
Fax. +1 314 362 0327
dehner@path.wustl.edu

Dr. Pavel DULGUEROV
Division of Head and Neck Surgery
Geneva University Hospital
24 Rue Micheli-du-Crest
1211 Geneva 14
SWITZERLAND
Tel. +41 22 372 8285
Fax. +41 22 372 8240
pavel.dulguerov@hcuge.ch

Dr. Samir K. EL MOFTY
Dept of Pathology
Washington University School of Medicine
660 South Euclid Ave, Box # 8118
St. Louis, MO 63110
USA
Tel. +1 314 362 2681
Fax. +1 314 747 2040
elmofty@path.wustl.edu

Dr. Adel K. EL-NAGGAR *
Dept. of Pathology Box 85
The University of Texas
MD Anderson Cancer Center
Houston,TX 77030
USA
Tel. +1 713 792 3109
Fax. +1 713 792 5532
anaggar@mdanderson.org

Dr. Gary ELLIS *
Oral & Maxillofacial Pathology
ARUP Laboratories
500 Chipeta Way
Salt Lake City, Utah 84108-1221
USA
Tel. +1 801 583 2787 ext 3123
Fax. +1 801 584 5207
gellis@aruplab.com

Dr Cosme EREO
Servicio de Anatoma Patolgica
Hospital de Basurto. UPV/EHU
Avd de Montevideo, 18
48013 Bilbao
SPAIN
Tel. +34 944 006033
Fax. +34 944 006302
cereno@hbas.osakidetza.net

Dr. Lewis Roy EVERSOLE
Dept of Pathology and Medicine
School of Dentistry, Room 408
Univ. of the Pacific, 2155 Webster Street
San Francisco, CA 94115
USA
Tel. +1 415 929 6560
Fax. +1 415 929 6662
leversol@SF.UOP.EDU

Dr. John W. EVESON *
Dept. of Oral and Dental Science
Bristol Dental Hospital and School
Lower Maudlin Street
Bristol BS1 2LY
UNITED KINGDOM
Tel. +44 117 928 4304/5
Fax. +44 117 928 4428
j.w.eveson@bristol.ac.uk

Dr. Julie C. FANBURG-SMITH
Dept. of Soft Tissue Pathology
Armed Forces Institute of Pathology
Building 54, Room GO90
14th Street and Alaska Avenue, N.W.
Washington, DC 20306-6000, USA
Tel. +1 202 782 2788
Fax. +1 202 782 9182
fanburg@afip.osd.mil

Dr Jacques FERLAY
Descriptive Epidemiology Group
Int. Agency for Research on Cancer
150 Cours Albert Thomas
69372 Lyon cedex 08 Lyon
FRANCE
Tel. +33 4 72 73 84 90
Fax. +33 4 72 73 86 50
ferlay@iarc.fr

Dr. Jorge A. FERREIRO
Dept. of Pathology
Abbott Northwestern Hospital
800 East 28th Street
Minneapolis,MN 55407
USA
Tel. +1 612 863 4685
Fax. +1 612 863 8375
jorgeferreiro@hotmail.com

Dr. Isabel FONSECA
Servio de Patologia Morfolgica
Instituto Portugus de Oncologia de
Francisco Gentil
Rua Professor Lima Basto
1099-023 Lisboa, PORTUGAL
Tel. +351 21 7229825
Fax. +351 21 7200475
nop36473@mail.telepac.pt

Dr. William FOO
Hong Kong Cancer Registry
c/o Dept. of Clinical Oncology
Queen Elizabeth Hospital
30 Gascoigne Road
Kowloon, Hong Kong, SAR CHINA
Tel. +852 2958 6231
Fax. +852 2359 4782
foow@ha.org.hk

Dr. Silvia FRANCESCHI
Unit of Field and Intervention Studies
Int. Agency for Research on Cancer
150 Cours Albert Thomas
69372 Lyon cedex 08
FRANCE
Tel. +33 4 72 73 84 02
Fax. +33 4 72 73 83 45
franceschi@iarc.fr

Dr. Alessandro FRANCHI
Dept. of Human Pathology and Oncology,
University of Florence
Viale G.B. Morgagni 85
50134 Florence
ITALY
Tel. +39 055 4478102
Fax. +39 055 4379868
alessandro.franchi@unifi.it

Dr. Henry F. FRIERSON, JR.
Dept of Pathology
PO Box 800214
University of Virginia Medical Center
Charlottesville, VA 22908
USA
Tel. 1 434 982 4404
Fax. 1 434 924 8767
hff@virginia.edu

Dr. Nina GALE *
Institute of Pathology, Faculty of
Medicine, University of Ljubljana
Korytkova 2
1000 Ljubljana
SLOVENIA
Tel. +386 1 543 71 02
Fax. +386 1 543 71 01
nina.gale@mf.uni-lj.si

Dr Yan GAO
Dept. of Oral Pathology
Peking University School of Stomatology
22 South Ave. Zhonguancun Haidian Dist.
100081 Beijing
CHINA
Tel. +86 106 217 9977 ext 2214
Fax. +86 106 217 3402
gaoyan0988@263.net

Dr. David G. GARDNER
8961 East 29th Ave
Denver, CO 80238
USA
Tel. +1 303 377 3445
dnhgardner@msn.com

Dr. Douglas R. GNEPP *
Dept. of Pathology
Rhode Island Hospital
593 Eddy Street
 Providence, RI 02903
USA
Tel. +1 401 444 8513
Fax. +1 401 444 8514
dgnepp@lifespan.org

Dr. Robert K. GOODE
Dept. of Oral & Maxillofacial Pathology
(Suite 646, DHS), Tufts University
1 Kneeland St.
Boston, MA 02111
USA
Tel. +1 617 636 6510
Fax. +1 617 636 6780
robert.goode@tufts.edu

Dr. Kristiina HEIKINHEIMO
Dept of Oral and Maxillofacial Surgery
Institute of Dentistry, University of Turku
Lemminkisenkatu 2
FIN-20520 Turku 52
FINLAND
Tel. +358 2 333 8212
Fax. +358 2 333 8356
heikinhe@netlife.fi

Dr. Kristin HENRY *
Dept. of Histopathology
Imperial College London
Charing Cross Hospital
Fulham Palace Road
London W6 8RF, UNITED KINGDOM
Tel. +44 20 8846 7133
Fax. +44 20 8846 1364
k.henry@imperial.ac.uk

Dr. Dolly P. HUANG
Dept. of Anatomical & Cellular Pathology
The Chinese University of Hong Kong
Hong Kong
SAR CHINA
Tel. +852 2632 2350
Fax. +852 2637 6274
waisinhuang@cuhk.edu.hk

Dr Jennifer L. HUNT
Dept. of Pathology, PUH A610.2, University
of Pittsburgh
200 Lothrop Street
Pittsburgh, PA 15213
USA
Tel. +1 412 647 9051
Fax. +1 412 647 6251
huntjl@upmc.edu

Dr. Andrew G. HUVOS
Dept. of Pathology
Memorial Sloan-Kettering Cancer Center
1275 York Avenue
New York, NY 10021
USA
Tel. +1 212 639 5905
Fax. +1 212 717 3203
huvosa@mskcc.org

Dr. K. Thorsten JÄKEL
Gemeinschaftspraxis Pathologie
Richtweg 19
D-28195 Bremen
GERMANY
Tel. +49 40 42 803 3173
Fax. +49 40 42 803 2556
jaekel@pathologie-bremen.de

Dr. Wei-Hua JIA
Cancer Center, Sun Yat-Sen University
651 Dongfeng Road East
Guangzhou 510060
CHINA
Tel. +86 20 8734 3181
Fax. +86 20 8734 3392
jiaweihua@163.net

Dr. Newell W. JOHNSON *
Oral and Maxillofacial Medicine and
Pathology, GKT Dental Institute
Caldecot Road
London, SE5 9RW
UNITED KINGDOM
Tel. +44 20 7346 3608
Fax. +44 20 7346 3624
newell.johnson@kcl.ac.uk

Dr. Gernot JUNDT *
Dept. of Pathology
University Hospital Basel
Schoenbeinstrasse 40
CH-4003 Basel
SWITZERLAND
Tel. +41 61 265 2867
Fax. +41 61 265 3194
gernot.jundt@unibas.ch

Dr. Silloo B. KAPADIA
Dept. of Pathology, H179, P.O. Box 850,
The Milton S. Hershey Medical Center
Penn State University School of Medicine
Hershey, PA 17033
USA
Tel. +1 717 531 8246
Fax. +1 717 531 7741
skapadia@att.net

Dr. Paul KLEIHUES *
Dept. of Pathology
University Hospital Zurich
Schmelzbergstr. 12
8091 Zurich
SWITZERLAND
Tel. +41 1 25 53 516
Fax. +41 1 255 2525
paul.kleihues@usz.ch

Dr Sakari KNUUTILA
Haartman Institute and HUSLAB
Haartmaninkatu 3, 4th flr (Box 21)
University of Helsinki
FIN-00014 Helsinki
FINLAND
Tel. +358 9 191 26527
Fax. +358 9 191 26788
sakari.knuutila@helsinki.fi

Dr. Hanna StrØmme KOPPANG
Dept. of Pathology and Forensic
Odontology, Institute of Clinical Dentistry
University of Oslo
Box 1109 Blindern
0317 Oslo, NORWAY
Tel. +47 228 52353
Fax. +47 228 52351
hanna@odont.uio.no

Dr. Tseng-tong KUO
Dept. of Pathology
Chang Gung Memorial Hospital
199 Tun Hwa North Road
Taipei
TAIWAN / CHINA
Tel. +886 3 328 1200 ext. 2727
Fax. +886 3 328 0147
ttkuo@cgmh.org.tw

Dr. Kimihide KUSAFUKA
Division of Pathology
Shizuoka Cancer Center
1007 Shimo-Nagakubo, Nagaizumi-cho
Suntou-gun
Shizuoka 411-8777, JAPAN
Tel. +81 55 989 5222
Fax. +81 55 989 5783
k.kusafuka@scchr.jp

Dr. Janez LAMOVEC
Dept. of Pathology
Institute of Oncology
Zaloska 2
SI-1000 Ljubljana
SLOVENIA
Tel. +386 1 5224 454
Fax. +386 1 5879 400
jlamovec@onko-i.si

Dr. Constantino LEDESMA-MONTES
Laboratorio de Patologa.
Facultad de Odontologa, UNAM
MEXICO 04510, D.F.
Tel. +52 55 5622 5562
Fax. +52 55 5550 3497
cledezma@servidor.unam.mx
cotita@avantel.net

Dr. Anne W.M. LEE *
Dept. of Clinical Oncology
Pamela Youde Nethersole Eastern Hosp.
3 Lok Man Road
Chai Wan, Hong Kong
SAR CHINA
Tel. +852 25954173
Fax. +852 29045216
awmlee@ha.org.hk

Dr. Jean E. LEWIS
Dept. of Pathology
Mayo Clinic
200 First Street, SW
Rochester, MN 55905
USA
Tel. +1 507 288 6878
Fax. +1 507 284 1599
lewis.jean2@mayo.edu

Dr T.J. LI
Dept. of Oral Pathology
Peking University School of Stomatology
22 South Ave. Zhonguancun Haidian Dist.
100081 Beijing
CHINA
Tel. +86 106 217 9977 ext 2203
Fax. +86 106 217 3402
litiejun22@vip.sina.com

Dr. Kwok- Wai LO
Dept. of Anatomical & Cellular Pathology
Prince of Wales Hospital
The Chinese University of Hong Kong
Shatin, N.T. Hong Kong
SAR CHINA
Tel. +852 263 22178
Fax. +852 263 76274
kwlo@cuhk.edu.hk

Dr. Thomas LoNING
Institut für Oralpathologie
Universitätsklinikum Eppendorf
Martinistr. 52
20246 Hamburg
GERMANY
Tel. +49 40 42 803 2536
Fax. +49 40 42 803 25 56
loening@uke.uni-hamburg.de

Dr. Yong LU
Endocyte, Inc.
1205 Kent Ave.
West Lafayette, IN 47906
USA
Tel. (765) 463-7175
Fax. (765) 463-9271
info@endocyte.com

Dr. Yong LU
Faculty of Dentistry
University of Toronto
124 Edward Street
Toronto, ON M5G 1G6
CANADA
Tel. +1 416 597 8251
Fax. +1 416 597 8251
yong.lu@utoronto.ca

Dr. Yong LU
Dept. of Oral Pathology,
Sichuan University, Renminnanlu 3-14
Chengdu, Sichuan, 610041
CHINA
Tel. +86 28 8550 1465
Fax. +86 28 8558 2167
ylu222@yahoo.com

Dr. Mario A. LUNA
Dept. Of Pathology
M.D. Anderson Cancer Center
1515 Holcombe Blvd. Box 85
Houston, TX 77030
USA
Tel. +1 713 792 3138
Fax. +1 713 745 4427
mluna@mdanderson.org

Dr. D. Gordon MACDONALD *
Glasgow Dental Hospital & School
378 Sauchiehall Street
Glasgow G2 3JZ - Scotland
UNITED KINGDOM
Tel. +44 141 211 9745/9746
Fax. +44 141 353 1593
d.g.macdonald@dental.gla.ac.uk

Dr. Peter McCARRON
Dept of Epidemiology & Public Health
Queen's University, Belfast
Mulhouse Building, Grosvenor Road
Belfast BT12 6BJ
UNITED KINGDOM
Tel. +44 28 9063 2746
Fax. +44 28 9023 1907
peter.mccarron@qub.ac.uk

Dr. Leslie MICHAELS *
Dept. of Histopathology
Royal Free & UCL Medical School
Rockefeller Building, University Street
London WC1E 6JS
UNITED KINGDOM
Tel. +44 20 7679 6038
Fax. +44 20 7387 3674
l.michaels@ucl.ac.uk

Dr. Michal MICHAL
Sikls Dept. of Pathology
Medical Faculty Hospital
Alej Svobody 80
304 60 Pilsen, CZECH REPUBLIC
Tel. +420 603 886 633
+420 37 7104 630
Fax. +420 37 710 4650
michal@medima.cz

Dr. Adalberto MOSQUEDA-TAYLOR
Departamento de Atención a la Salud
Univ. Autonoma Metropol. Xochimilco
Calzada del Hueso 1100
MEXICO, D.F 04960
Tel. +52 54 83 72 06
Fax. +52 54 83 72 06
mosqueda@correo.xoc.uam.mx

Dr. Alfons NADAL
Hospital Clinic
Universitat de Barcelona
Villarroel, 170
08036 Barcelona
SPAIN
Tel. +34 9322 75535
Fax. +34 9322 75717
anadal@clinic.ub.es

Dr. Toshitaka NAGAO *
Dept. of Diagnostic Pathology
Tokyo Medical University
6-7-1 Nishishinjuku, Shinjuku-ku
Tokyo 160-0023
JAPAN
Tel. +81 3 5339 3773
Fax. +81 3 3342 2062
nagao-t@tokyo-med.ac.jp

Dr. Hiromasa NIKAI
Hiroshima University
2-26-26 Koi-Higashi, Nishi-ku
Hiroshima 733-0811
JAPAN
Tel. +81 82 272 2560
Fax. +81 82 272 2560
nikai@hiroshima-u.ac.jp

Dr. Edward W. ODELL
Dept. of Oral Pathology
Guy's Hospital, Floor 28 Tower
London SE1 9RT
UNITED KINGDOM
Tel. +44 20 7188 4378
Fax. +44 20 7188 4375
edward.odell@kcl.ac.uk

Dr. Kerry D. OLSEN
Mayo Clinic - West 5
200 First Street, SW
Rochester, MN 55905
USA
Tel. +1 507 284 3542
Fax. +1 507 284 8855
olsen.kerry@mayo.edu

Dr. Bayardo PEREZ-ORDONEZ
Dept. of Pathology
Princess Margaret Hospital
610 University Avenue
Toronto, ON M5G 2M9
Canada
Tel. +1 416 946 2104
Fax. +1 416 946 6579
bayardo.perez-ordonez@uhn.on.ca

Dr. Hans Peter PHILIPSEN *
Edif. El Condor, Apt. 30
San Pedro de Alcantara
29670 Guadalmina Alta
SPAIN
Tel. +34 95 288 2010
Fax. +34 95 288 2010
philipsen@telefonica.net

Dr. Adriano PIATTELLI
Dpt. of Oral Pathology and Medicine
University of Chieti-Pescara
Via dei Vestini 31
66100 Chieti, ITALY
Tel. +39 0871 3554073/4083
Fax. +39 0871 3554076
apiattelli@unich.it

Dr. Ben Z. PILCH *
Dept. of Pathology
Massachusetts General Hospital
Fruit Street
Boston, MA 02114-2696
USA
Tel. +1 617 573 3159
Fax. +1 617 573 3389
bpilch@partners.org

Dr. Finn PRAETORIUS *
Dept. of Oral Pathology
University of Copenhagen
20 Norre Alle
2200 Copenhagen N
DENMARK
Tel. +45 23254836
Fax. +45 35326722
fp@odont.ku.dk

Dr. Manju L. PRASAD
Dept. of Pathology
UMass Memorial Medical Center
55 Lake Ave North
Worcester, MA 01655
USA
Tel. +1 508 334 2144
Fax. +1 508 856 2968
prasadm@ummhc.org

Dr. Kunnambath RAMADAS *
Dept. of Radiation Oncology
Regional Cancer Centre
Trivandrum
INDIA
Tel. +91 471 244 2541
Fax. +91 471 255 2388
ramdasrcc@rediffmail.com
tocsrcc@md4.vsnl.net.in

Dr. Peter A. REICHART *
Zentrum für Zahnmedizin
Charite, Campus Virchow Klinikum
Augustenburger Platz 1
13353 Berlin
GERMANY
Tel. +49 30 45 0 56 26 02
Fax. +49 30 45 0 56 29 01
peter-a.reichart@charite.de

Dr. Kiyoshi SAITO
Dept. of Neurosurgery
Nagoya University
65 Tsurumai, Showa-ku
Nagoya, 466-8550
JAPAN
Tel. +81 52 744 2353
Fax. +81 52 744 2360
kiyoshis@med.nagoya-u.ac.jp

Dr. Ann SANDISON *
Dept. of Histopathology
Charing Cross Hospital
Fulham Palace Road
London W6 8RF
UNITED KINGDOM
Tel. +44 020 8846 7139
Fax. +44 020 8846 1364
asandison@hhnt.org

Dr. Marco SANTUCCI
Dept. of Human Pathology & Oncology
University of Florence Medical School
Careggi Hospital
V.le G.B. Morgagni 85
50134 Florence, ITALY
Tel. +39 055 447 8105
Fax. +39 055 437 9868
marco.santucci@unifi.it

Dr. Patricia A. SCHACHERN
Room 226 LRB
2001 Sixth St SE
Minneapolis, MN 55455
USA
Tel. +1 612 626 9876
Fax. +1 612 626 9871
schac002@umn.edu

Dr. Stephan SCHMID
ENT Dept.
University Hospital Zürich
Frauenklinikstrasse 24
8091 Zürich
SWITZERLAND
Tel. +41 1 255 59 00
Fax. +41 1 255 41 64
stephan.schmid@usz.ch

Dr. James J. SCIUBBA *
Dept. of Otolaryngology, Head & Neck
Surgery, Johns Hopkins Medical Center
601 N. Caroline St., Rm 6243
Baltimore, MD 21287-9150
USA
Tel. +1 410 955 0406
Fax. +1 410 955 0035
jsciubb@jhmi.edu

Dr. Ratnam K. SHANMUGARATNAM
Dept. of Pathology
National University Hospital
Lower Kent Ridge Road
Singapore 119074
SINGAPORE
Tel. +65 6772 4312
Fax. +65 6778 0671
patshanm@nus.edu.sg

Dr. Mervyn SHEAR
19 Disa Road
Murdock Valley
Simon's Town 7975
SOUTH AFRICA
Tel. +27 21 786 1172
Fax. +27 21 786 3447
shear@iafrica.com

Dr. Masaki SHIMONO
Dept. of Pathology
Tokyo Dental College
1-2-2 Masago, Mihama-ku
Chiba 261-8502
JAPAN
Tel. +81 43 270 3781
Fax. +81 43 270 3784
shimono@tdc.ac.jp

Dr. Chong Huat SIAR
Dept. of Oral Pathology, Oral Medicine &
Periodontology
University of Malaya
50603 Kuala Lumpur
MALAYSIA
Tel. +603 7967 4859
Fax. +603 7967 4531
siarch@um.edu.my

Dr. David SIDRANSKY
Brady Urological Institute
Dept. of Oncology, Pathology, & Urology
John Hopkins Univ. School of Medicine
720 Rutland Ave Ross 818
Baltimore, MD 21205, USA
Tel. +1 410 502 5155
Fax. +1 410 614 1411
dsidrans@jhmi.edu

Dr. Roderick H.W. SIMPSON *
Dept. of Pathology
Royal and Devon Exeter Hospital
Church Lane, Heavitree
Exeter EX2 5DY, UNITED KINGDOM
Tel. +44 1392 402941/2942
Fax. +44 1392 402964
roderick.simpson@virgin.net

Dr. Alena SKÁLOVÁ *
Dept. of Pathology, Medical Faculty Hosp.
Dr. E. Benee 13
305 99 Pilsen
CZECH REPUBLIC
Tel. +420 377 402545
Fax. +420 377 402634
skalova@fnplzen.cz
skalova@medima.cz

Dr. Lee J. SLATER
Scripps Oral Pathology Service
5190 Governor Drive Suite 106
San Diego, CA 92122-2848
USA
Tel. +1 858 784 0600
Fax. +1 858 784 0604
leeslater@earthlink.net

Dr. Pieter J. SLOOTWEG *
Radboud Univ. Nijmmegen Medical Centre
Dept. of Pathology, HP 437
P.O. Box 9101
6500 HB Nijmegen
THE NETHERLANDS
Tel. +31 31 2436 14314
Fax. +31 31 2435 40520
p.slootweg@pathol.umcn.nl

Dr. Jorge SOARES
Serviço de Patologia Morfolgica
Inst. Portugues de Oncologia F. Gentil
Rua Prof. Lima Basto
1099-023 Lisboa
PORTUGAL
Tel. +351 217229825
Fax. +351 217229825
jorge-soares@mail.telepac.pt

Dr. Leslie SOBIN *
Hepatic & Gastrointestinal Pathology,
Armed Forces Institute of Pathology
14th Street and Alaska Avenue
Washington, DC 20306
USA
Tel. +1 202 782 2880
Fax. +1 202 782 9020
sobin@afip.osd.mil

Dr. Sava SOUCEK
ENT & Audiology Dept.
St. Marys Hospital
Praed Street
London W2 1NY
UNITED KINGDOM
Tel. +44 20 7886 6028
Fax. +44 20 7886 1847
s.soucek@ic.ac.uk

Dr. Paul M. SPEIGHT
Dept. of Oral Pathology
University of Sheffield
Claremont Crescent
Sheffield S10 2TA
UNITED KINGDOM
Tel. +44 114 271 7951
Fax. +44 114 271 7894
p.speight@sheffield.ac.uk

Dr. Göran STENMAN
Dept. of Pathology, The Lundberg
Laboratory for Cancer Research
Göteborg University
413 45 Gothenburg,
SWEDEN
Tel. +46 31 342 2922
Fax. +46 31 820 525
goran.stenman@llcr.med.gu.se

Dr. Kai Hua SUN
Dept. of Oral Pathology
Peking University School of Stomatology
22 South Ave., Zhonguancun Haidain Dist.
100081 Beijing
CHINA
Tel. +86 106 261 79977 ext 2202
Fax. +86 106 217 3402
gaoyan0988@263.net

Dr. Takashi TAKATA
Dept. of Oral Maxillofacial Pathobiology
Graduate School of Biomedical Sciences
Hiroshima University
1-2-3 Kasumi, Minami-ku, Hiroshima
JAPAN, 734-8553
Tel. +81 82 257 5631
Fax. +81 82 257 5619
ttakata@hiroshima-u.ac.jp

Dr. Yasunori TAKEDA
Dept. of Oral Pathology, School of
Dentistry, Iwate Medical University
19-1 Uchimaru
Morioka 020-8505
JAPAN
Tel. +81 19 651 5111
Fax. +81 19 621 3321
ytakeda@iwate-med.ac.jp

Dr. Lester D.R. THOMPSON *
Dept. of Pathology
Woodland Hills Medical Center
5601 De Soto Avenue
Woodland Hills, CA 91367
USA
Tel. +1 818 719 2613
Fax. +1 818 719 2309
lester.d.thompson@kp.org

Dr. Charles E. TOMICH
Oral & Maxillofacial Pathology
Dermatopathology Laboratory
9292 North Meridian Street - Suite 210
Indianapolis, IN 46260
USA
Tel. +1 317 843 2204
Fax. +1 317 843 2478
cjtomich@aol.com

Dr. William Y.W. TSANG
Dept. of Pathology
Queen Elizabeth Hospital
30 Gascoigne Road
Kowloon, Hong Kong
SAR CHINA
Tel. +852 2958 6834
Fax. +852 2385 2455
tsangyw@ha.org.hk

Dr. Loretta L.Y. TSE *
Dept. of Pathology, Rm20, 10th FL, Block M
Queen Elizabeth Hospital
30 Gascoigne Road
Hong Kong
SAR CHINA
Tel. +852 295 86887
Fax. +852 238 52455
llytse@netvigator.com

Dr. K. Krishnan UNNI
Pathology Dept.
Mayo Clinic
200 First St, SW
Rochester, MN 55905
USA
Tel. +1 507 284 1193
Fax. +1 507 284 1599
balzum.debbie@mayo.edu

Dr. Mark L. URKEN
Dept. of Otolaryngology
Mount Sinai School of Medicine
New York , NY 10029
USA
Tel. + 1 212 241 9410
Fax. + 1 212 428 4088
mark.urken@mssm.edu

Dr. Isaac VAN DER WAAL*
Dept. Oral and Maxillofacial
Surgery/Pathology, P.O. Box 7057
VU University Medical Centre
1007 MB Amsterdam
THE NETHERLANDS
Tel. +31 20 444 1023 or 4039
Fax. +31 20 444 1024 or 4046
i.vanderwaal@vumc.nl

Dr. Jacqueline E. VAN DER WAL
Dept. of Pathology
University Hospital Groningen
P.O. Box 30.001
9700 RB Groningen
THE NETHERLANDS
Tel. +31 50 3614683
Fax. +31 50 3632510
j.e.van.der.wal@path.azg.nl

Dr. Bruce M. WENIG *
Dept. of Pathology and Laboratory
Medicine, Beth Israel Medical Center/
St Lukes & Roosevelt Hospitals
First Ave. at 16th Street, 11 Silver, Rm 34
New York, NY 10003, USA
Tel. +1 212 420 4031
Fax. +1 212 420 3449
bwenig@bethisraelny.org

Dr. William H. WESTRA
Dept. of Pathology, The Weinberg
Building, Room 2242
The Johns Hopkins Medical Institutions
401 N. Broadway
Baltimore, MD 21231, USA
Tel. + 1 410 955 2163
Fax. + 1 410 955 0115
wwestra@jhmi.edu

Dr. Timothy Tak-Chun YIP
Dept. of Clinical Oncology, Queen
Elizabeth Hospital, Rm. 1305, Block R, 13/F
30 Gascoigne Road
Kowloon, Hong Kong
SAR CHINA
Tel. + 852 295 86284
Fax. + 852 261 85526
yiptct@hotmail.com

Dr. Yi- Xin ZENG
Cancer Center
Sun Yan-sen University
651 Dongfeng Road East
Guangzhou 510060
CHINA
Tel. +86 20 87343333
Fax. +86 20 87343295
yxzeng@gzsums.edu.cn

Dr. Nina ZIDAR
Institute of Pathology
Faculty of Medicine, University of
Ljubljana
Korytkova 2
1000 Ljubljana
SLOVENIA
Tel. + 386 1 543 7149
Fax. + 386 1 543 7101
nina.zidar@mf.uni-lj.si

Source of charts and photographs

1.

1.1-1.5	Dr. H.D. Curtin
1.6-1.8	Dr L.D.R. Thompson
1.9A,B	Dr. J.K.C. Chan
1.10A-C	Dr. H.F. Frierson, Jr
1.11-1.012	Dr. A. Franchi
1.13-1.015	Dr. B.M. Wenig
1.16A	Dr L.D.R. Thompson
1.16B-1.17A	Dr. J.K.C. Chan
1.17B,C	Dr L.D.R. Thompson
1.18	Dr. J.K.C. Chan
1.19-1.21	Dr L.D.R. Thompson
1.22-1.26	Dr. B. Perez-Ordone
1.27	Dr. H.D. Curtin
1.28A-1.29	Dr. L. Barnes
1.29C	Dr L.D.R. Thompson
1.29D-1.30B	Dr. L. Barnes
1.31	Dr L.D.R. Thompson
1.32A,B	Dr. L. Barnes
1.32C,D	Dr L.D.R. Thompson
1.33A	Dr. B.M. Wenig
1.33B	Dr L.D.R. Thompson
1.33C,D	Dr. B.M. Wenig
1.34-1.35	Dr. J.K.C. Chan
1.36A-1.40B	Dr L.D.R. Thompson
1.41A,B	Dr. J.K.C. Chan
1.42A	Dr L.D.R. Thompson
1.42B-1.43A	Dr. J.K.C. Chan
1.43B-1.45B	Dr L.D.R. Thompson
1.46-1.48	Dr. J.K.C. Chan
1.49A-1.52A	Dr L.D.R. Thompson
1.52B-1.53B	Dr. J.K.C. Chan
1.54A-1.59B	Dr L.D.R. Thompson
1.60	Dr. K.K. Unni
1.61	Dr. D. Davidson, Pathology Medical Services, Lincoln, Nebraska.
1.62A-C	Dr L.D.R. Thompson
1.63-1.66	Dr. K.K. Unni
1.67-1.69B	Dr. G. Jundt
1.70A,B,C	Dr. F. Bertoni
1.71A,B	Dr. L.P. Dehner
1.72A,B	Dr L.D.R. Thompson
1.72C	Dr. P.A. Reichart
1.73A,B	Dr. L.P. Dehner
1.74-1.75	Dr. M.M.C. Cheung
1.76A-1.80C	Dr. J.K.C. Chan
1.81A-C	Dr. S.B. Kapadia
1.82A-1.83D	Dr. J.K.C. Chan
1.84A,B	Dr L.D.R. Thompson
1.85A,B	Dr. H.D. Curtin
1.86A-1.87A	Dr. J.K.C. Chan
1.87B-1.88A	Dr L.D.R. Thompson
1.88B,C	Dr. J.K.C. Chan

1.89A-D	Dr. B.M. Wenig
1.90A,B	Dr. S.B. Kapadia
1.90C	Dr L.D.R. Thompson
1.90D	Dr. S.B. Kapadia
1.91A-1.92B	Dr L.D.R. Thompson
1.93A,B	Dr. M. Prasad
1.94A	Dr L.D.R. Thompson
1.94B	Dr. S.B. Kapadia
1.94C,D	Dr L.D.R. Thompson
1.95	Dr. J.K.C. Chan
1.96A,B	Dr. A. Cardesa
1.97A-C	Dr L.D.R. Thompson
1.98A-C	Dr. M.A. Luna
1.99A	Dr. L. Barnes
1.99B,C	Dr L.D.R. Thompson

2.

2.1	Dr. J.K.C. Chan
2.1A	Dr. J. Ferlay
2.2A,B	Dr. A.W.M. Lee
2.3	Dr. W. Foo
2.4-2.5	Dr. A.W.M. Lee
2.6-2.19	Dr. J.K.C. Chan
2.20	Dr. D.P. Huang
2.21	Dr. A.W.M. Lee
2.22	Dr. Y.-X. Zeng
2.23A	Dr. T. Kuo
2.23B	Dr. J.K.C. Chan
2.24-2.25D	Dr. B.M. Wenig
2.26A,B	Dr. J.K.C. Chan
2.27-2.30	Dr L.D.R. Thompson
2.20A	Dr. J.K.C. Chan

3.

3.1A-3.2B	Dr. L. Barnes
3.3	Dr. J.A.M. de Groot
3.5	Dr. J. Ferlay
3.6	World Cancer Report. IARC Press 2003
3.7A,B	Dr. A. Cardesa
3.8	Dr. P.J. Slootweg
3.9	Dr L.D.R. Thompson
3.10A,B	Dr. A. Cardesa
3.11	Dr L.D.R. Thompson
3.12	Dr. A. Cardesa
3.13-3.15A	Dr L.D.R. Thompson
3.15B-3.16B	Dr. A. Cardesa
3.16C	Dr L.D.R. Thompson
3.16D,E	Dr. A. Cardesa
3.16F	Dr L.D.R. Thompson
3.17-3.19A	Dr. A. Cardesa
3.19B	Dr L.D.R. Thompson
3.19C-3.20	Dr. A. Cardesa
3.21A	Dr L.D.R. Thompson
3.21B-D	Dr. A. Cardesa
3.22A-D	Dr L.D.R. Thompson
3.23A	Dr. A. Cardesa
3.23B-3.24	Dr. A. Cardesa
3.25A,B	Dr L.D.R. Thompson
3.26A,B	Dr. A. Cardesa

3.27	Dr. J.K.C. Chan
3.28-3.37	Dr. L. Barnes
3.38-3.45B	Dr N. Gale
3.46-3.47	Dr. J. Eveson
3.48-3.49B	Dr L.D.R. Thompson
3.50A-C	Dr L.D.R. Thompson
3.51	Dr L.D.R. Thompson
3.52-3.54F	Dr. B.M. Wenig
3.55-3.56D	Dr. L. Barnes
3.57	Dr L.D.R. Thompson
3.58A-3.59C	Dr. L. Barnes
3.60A,B	Dr. J.K.C. Chan
3.61A-3.63D	Dr. J.E. Lewis
3.64	Dr. L. Barnes
3.65	Dr. J.E. Lewis
3.66	Dr L.D.R. Thompson
3.67A	Dr. L. Barnes
3.67B	Dr L.D.R. Thompson
3.68A-3.71D	Dr. B.M. Wenig
	Dr. L. Barnes

4.

4.1	Dr. J. Eveson
4.2-4.3	From Globocan 2000
4.4A-D	Dr. F. Levi, Lausanne
4.5A,B	Dr. K. Ramadas
4.5C-D	Dr. P.A. Reichart
4.6A-4.12B	Dr. P.J. Slootweg
4.13A-C	Dr. J.K.C. Chan
4.14A-4.15D	Dr. G. MacDonald
4.16A	Dr. J. Eveson
4.16B	Dr. A.K. El-Naggar
4.16C,D	Dr. J. Eveson
4.17-4.20	Dr. P.A. Reichart
4.21A-D	Dr. E. Odell
4.22A	Dr P. Fleming / Dr. J. Eveson
4.22B-4.24	Dr. E. Odell
4.25-4.27D	Dr. P. Speight
4.28	Dr. T. Löning
4.29A,B	Dr. K.T. Jäkel
4.30-4.31B	Dr. E. Odell
4.32A-C	Dr. J. Eveson
4.33	Dr. P.A. Reichart
4.34A-D	Dr. J. Eveson
4.35-4.44B	Dr. I. Van der Waal
4.45A-4.55	Dr. J.K.C. Chan
4.56-4.58D	Dr. P. Speight

5.

5.0	Dr. J. Eveson
5.1-5.4	Dr. G.Ellis
5.5A,B	Dr. T. Nagao
5.6A,B	Dr. R.K. Goode
5.6C,D	Dr. T. Nagao
5.7-5.8B	Dr. A.K. El-Naggar
5.9A-C	Dr. M.A. Luna
5.10A	Dr. T. Nagao
5.10B	Dr. I. Fonseca
5.11A,B	Dr. T. Nagao

5.12A,B	Dr. I. Fonseca
5.12C	Dr. T. Nagao
5.13A-5.14D	Dr. G.Ellis
5.15A	Dr. T. Nagao
5.15B	Dr. G.Ellis
5.16A	Dr. T. Nagao
5.16B-5.17B	Dr. G.Ellis
5.18A	Dr. T. Nagao
5.18B	Dr. D.R. Gnepp
5.19A,B	Dr. P.L. Auclair
5.19C	Dr. T. Nagao
5.20A-C	Dr. M.S. Brandwein
5.21-5.22B	Dr. K.H. Sun
5.23A,B	Dr. T. Nagao
5.23C	Dr. M.S. Brandwein
5.24A	Dr. T. Nagao
5.24B	Dr. M.S. Brandwein
5.25A-C	Dr. T. Nagao
5.26	Dr. M.S. Brandwein
5.27A-5.28D	Dr. P.L. Auclair
5.29A	Dr. A. Skalova
5.29B	Dr. K.T. Jäkel
5.30A-5.31D	Dr. A. Skalova
5.32A,B	Dr. T. Nagao
5.33A	Dr. D.R. Gnepp
5.33B	Dr. T. Nagao
5.34	Dr. D.R. Gnepp
5.35A	Dr. T. Nagao
5.35B-5.36	Dr. D.R. Gnepp
5.37A-B	Dr. J.E. Lewis
5.38-5.43	Dr. T. Nagao
5.44-5.46	Dr. J.K.C. Chan
5.47A	Dr. T. Nagao
5.47B	Dr. M.S. Brandwein
5.48-5.51D	Dr. T. Nagao
5.52-5.55B	Dr. G. Stenman
5.56A-D	Dr. T. Nagao
5.57A,B	Dr. A. Cardesa
5.58-5.60B	Dr. V.C. De Arajo
5.61A-5.63	Dr. J. Eveson
5.64A-5.65	Dr. T. Nagao
5.66	Dr. D.R. Gnepp
5.67A	Dr. T. Nagao
5.67B	Dr. D.R. Gnepp
5.68A,B	Dr. T. Nagao
5.69A-5.73B	Dr. R.B. Brannon
5.74-5.76B	Dr. A. Skalova
5.77A,B	Dr. T. Nagao
5.78A,B	Dr. E. Odell
5.78C	Dr L.D.R. Thompson
5.79A-5.81C	Dr. S.L. Abbondanzo
5.82	Dr. T. Löning
	Dr. T. Nagao

6.

6.1-6.2	Dr. P.A. Reichart
6.3-6.4D	Dr. J.J. Sciubba
6.5-6.6	Dr. G. Jundt
6.7-6.8B	Dr. I. Van der Waal
6.9	Dr. G. Jundt
6.10A,B	Dr. G. Bang

The copyright remains with the authors. Requests for permission to reproduce figures or charts should be directed to the respective contributor. For addresses see Contributors List.

6.11	Dr. T. Takata
6.12	Dr. A. Meneses
6.13	Dr. R. Carlos
6.14A	Dr. L.J. Slater
6.14B,C	Dr. R. Carlos
6.15-6.18D	Dr. G. Jundt
6.19-6.20	Dr. H.P. Philipsen
6.21-6.29	Dr. P.A. Reichart
6.30	Dr. T. Takata
6.31	Dr. G. Jundt
6.32-6.33	Dr. T. Takata
6.33-6.34	Dr. P.A. Reichart
6.35-6.36	Dr. H. Nikai
6.37	Dr. T. Takata
6.38	Dr. P.A. Reichart
6.39	Dr. G. Jundt
6.40	Dr. P.A. Reichart
6.41-6.44B	Dr. G. Jundt
6.45A,B	Dr. P.A. Reichart
6.46A,B	Dr. Y. Takeda
6.47-6.48	Dr. I. Van der Waal
6.49A-6.50	Dr. F. Praetorius
6.51	Dr. R. Carlos
6.52A,B	Dr. A.Mosqueda Taylor
6.53A,B	Dr. J.J. Trujillo, Oral and Maxillofacial Surgery, Hospital Juárez de México, Mexico City
6.54	Dr. F. Praetorius
6.55	Dr. G. Jundt
6.56A-6.57	Dr. F. Praetorius
6.58 A	Dr. F. Praetorius
6.58B	Dr. G. Jundt
6.59A	Dr. J.J. Sciubba
6.59B,C	Dr. G. Jundt
6.60	Dr L.D.R. Thompson
6.61	Dr CJ Nortje and Dr LJ van Rensburg, Univ. of the Western Cape, South Africa
6.62-6.64	Dr. E. Odell
6.64A	Dr. G. Jundt
6.65-6.67	Dr. I. Van der Waal
6.68-6.74B	Dr. P.J. Slootweg
6.75-6.78	Dr. G. Jundt
6.79-6.80	Dr. P.J. Slootweg
6.81-6.90	Dr. G. Jundt

7.

7.1-7.3C	Dr L.D.R. Thompson
7.4-7.6	Dr. L. Michaels
7.7A-D	Dr L.D.R. Thompson
7.8	Dr. L. Michaels
7.9A,B	Dr L.D.R. Thompson
7.10-7.13B	Dr. L. Michaels
7.14	Dr. K. Henry
7.15-7.16A	Dr L.D.R. Thompson
7.16B-F	Dr. K. Henry
7.17-7.19B	Dr L.D.R. Thompson
7.20-7.21B	Dr. L. Michaels
7.22	Dr L.D.R. Thompson
7.23-7.27A	Dr. L. Michaels

7.27B	Dr L.D.R. Thompson
7.28A-7.30	Dr. L. Michaels
7.31	Dr. A. Sandison
7.32-7.34	Dr. L. Michaels
7.35A	Dr L.D.R. Thompson
7.35B-7.36B	Dr. L. Michaels
7.37A,B	Dr L.D.R. Thompson
7.38	Dr. L. Michaels
7.39-7.41D	Dr. K. Henry

8.

8.1-8.3D	Dr. L. Barnes
8.4A-8.5D	Dr. L. Michaels
8.6-8.7	Dr. L. Barnes

References

1. Anon. (1985). Tobacco habits other than smoking; betel-quid and areca-nut chewing; and some related nitrosamines. IARC Working Group. Lyon, 23-30 October 1984. IARC Monogr Eval Carcinog Risk Chem Hum 37: 1-268.

2. Anon. (1993). Immunoglobulin gene rearrangement in low-grade B-cell MALT lymphomas of salivary gland, myoepithelial sialadenitis and Sjogren's syndrome. J Pathol 169 suppl: 123A.

3. Anon. (1997). Recommendations for the reporting of specimens containing laryngeal neoplasms. Association of Directors of Anatomic and Surgery Pathology. Mod Pathol 10: 384-386.

4. Abbey LM, Page DG, Sawyer DR (1980). The clinical and histopathologic features of a series of 464 oral squamous cell papillomas. Oral Surg Oral Med Oral Pathol 49: 419-428.

5. Abbondanzo SL, Wenig BM (1995). Non-Hodgkin's lymphoma of the sinonasal tract. A clinicopathologic and immunophenotypic study of 120 cases. Cancer 75: 1281-1291.

6. Abdelkader M, Riad M, Williams A (2001). Aggressive fibromatosis of the head and neck (desmoid tumours). J Laryngol Otol 115: 772-776.

7. Abdelsayed RA, Eversole LR, Singh BS, Scarbrough FE (2001). Gigantiform cementoma: clinicopathologic presentation of 3 cases. Oral Surg Oral Med Oral Pathol Oral Radiol Endod 91: 438-444.

8. Abemayor E, Newman A, Bergstrom L, Dudley J, Magidson JG, Ljung BM (1984). Teratomas of the head and neck in childhood. Laryngoscope 94: 1489-1492.

9. Abrams AM, Melrose RJ (1978). Acinic cell tumors of minor salivary gland origin. Oral Surg Oral Med Oral Pathol 46: 220-233.

10. Abramson AL, Steinberg BM, Winkler B (1987). Laryngeal papillomatosis: clinical, histopathologic and molecular studies. Laryngoscope 97: 678-685.

11. Abu-El-Naaj I, Ardekian L, Liberman R, Peled M (2002). Central giant cell granuloma of the mandibular condyle: a rare presentation. J Oral Maxillofac Surg 60: 939-941.

12. Ackerman LV (1948). Verrucous carcinoma of the oral cavity. Surgery 670-678.

13. Ackermann GL, Altini M, Shear M (1988). The unicystic ameloblastoma: a clinicopathological study of 57 cases. J Oral Pathol 17: 541-546.

14. Adair CF, Thompson LDR, Wenig BM, Heffner DK (1996). Chondro-osseous and respiratory epithelial hamartomas of the sinonasal tract and nasopharynx. Lab Invest 74.

15. Aden KK, Adams GL, Niehans G (1988). Adenosquamous Carcinoma of the Larynx and Hypopharynx with Five New Case Presentations. Trans Am Laryngol Assoc 216-221.

16. Agathanggelou A, Niedobitek G, Chen R, Nicholls J, Yin W, Young LS (1995). Expression of immune regulatory molecules in Epstein-Barr virus-associated nasopharyngeal carcinomas with prominent lymphoid stroma. Evidence for a functional interaction between epithelial tumor cells and infiltrating lymphoid cells. Am J Pathol 147: 1152-1160.

17. Aguiar PH, Tatagiba M, Samii M, Dankoweit-Timpe E, Ostertag H (1995). The comparison between the growth fraction of bilateral vestibular schwannomas in neurofibromatosis 2 (NF2) and unilateral vestibular schwannomas using the monoclonal antibody MIB 1. Acta Neurochir (Wien) 134: 40-45.

18. Aguilera NS, Kapadia SB, Nalesnik MA, Swerdlow SH (1995). Extramedullary plasmacytoma of the head and neck: use of paraffin sections to assess clonality with in situ hybridization, growth fraction, and the presence of Epstein-Barr virus. Mod Pathol 8: 503-508.

19. Aguilera NS, Uusaf M, Wenig BM, Abbondanzo SL (1998). The blastic variant of mantle cell lymphoma arising in Waldeyer's tonsillar ring. J Laryngol Otol 112: 991-994.

20. Aguirre JM, Echebarria MA, Martinez-Conde R, Rodriguez C, Burgos JJ, Rivera JM (1998). Warthin tumor. A new hypothesis concerning its development. Oral Surg Oral Med Oral Pathol Oral Radiol Endod 85: 60-63.

21. Ahlbom HE (1936). Simple achlorhydric anaemia, plummer-vinson syndrome and carcinoma of the mouth, pharynx, and oesophagus in women. Brit Med J 2: 331-333.

22. Ahlfors E, Larsson Å, Sjogren S (1984). The odontogenic keratocyst: a benign cystic tumor? J Oral Maxillofac Surg 42: 10-19.

23. Ahmad R, Mayol BR, Davis M, Rougraff BT (1999). Extraskeletal Ewing's sarcoma. Cancer 85: 725-731.

24. Ahmadi AJ, Pirinjian GE, Sires BS (2003). Optic neuropathy and macular chorioretinal folds caused by orbital cherubism. Arch Ophthalmol 121: 570-573.

25. Akyol MU, Sozeri B, Kucukali T, Ogretmenoglu O (1998). Laryngeal pleomorphic rhabdomyosarcoma. Eur Arch Otorhinolaryngol 255: 307-310.

26. Al Khafaji BM, Nestok BR, Katz RL (1998). Fine-needle aspiration of 154 parotid masses with histologic correlation: ten-year experience at the University of Texas M. D. Anderson Cancer Center. Cancer 84: 153-159.

27. al Otieschan AA, Saleem M, Manohar MB, Larson S, Atallah A (1998). Malignant schwannoma of the parapharyngeal space. J Laryngol Otol 112: 883-887.

28. al Saleem T, Tucker GFJr, Peale AR, Norris CM (1970). Cartilaginous tumors of the larynx. Clinical-pathologic study of ten cases. Ann Otol Rhinol Laryngol 79: 33-41.

29. al Sarraf M, LeBlanc M, Giri PG, Fu KK, Cooper J, Vuong T, Forastiere AA, Adams G, Sakr WA, Schuller DE, Ensley JF (1998). Chemoradiotherapy versus radiotherapy in patients with advanced nasopharyngeal cancer: phase III randomized Intergroup study 0099. J Clin Oncol 16: 1310-1317.

30. Alameda F, Fontane J, Corominas JM, Lloreta J, Serrano S (2000). Reactive vascular lesion of nasal septum simulating angiosarcoma in a cocaine abuser. Hum Pathol 31: 239-241.

31. Albeck H, Bentzen J, Ockelmann HH, Nielsen NH, Bretlau P, Hansen HS (1993). Familial clusters of nasopharyngeal carcinoma and salivary gland carcinomas in Greenland natives. Cancer 72: 196-200.

32. Albeck H, Nielsen NH, Hansen HE, Bentzen J, Ockelmann HH, Bretlau P, Hansen HS (1992). Epidemiology of nasopharyngeal and salivary gland carcinoma in Greenland. Arctic Med Res 51: 189-195.

33. Albino AP, Kimmelman CP, Parisier SC (1998). Cholesteatoma: a molecular and cellular puzzle. Am J Otol 19: 7-19.

34. Alevizos I, Blaeser B, Gallagher G, Ohyama H, Wong DT, Todd R (2002). Odontogenic carcinoma: a functional genomic comparison with oral mucosal squamous cell carcinoma. Oral Oncol 38: 504-507.

35. Allen Chan KC, Dennis Lo YM (2002). Circulating EBV DNA as a tumor marker for nasopharyngeal carcinoma. Semin Cancer Biol 12: 489-496.

36. Allen CM, Damm D, Neville B, Rodu B, Page D, Weathers DR (1994). Necrosis in benign salivary gland neoplasms. Not necessarily a sign of malignant transformation. Oral Surg Oral Med Oral Pathol 78: 455-461.

37. Allen CM, Hammond HL, Stimson PG (1992). Central odontogenic fibroma, WHO type. A report of three cases with an unusual associated giant cell reaction. Oral Surg Oral Med Oral Pathol 73: 62-66.

38. Allen MSJr, Fitz-Hugh GS, Marsh WLJr (1974). Low-grade papillary adenocarcinoma of the palate. Cancer 33: 153-158.

39. Alles JU, Schulz A (1986). Immunocytochemical markers (endothelial and histiocytic) and ultrastructure of primary aneurysmal bone cysts. Hum Pathol 17: 39-45.

40. Allon D, Kaplan I, Manor R, Calderon S (2002). Carcinoma cuniculatum of the jaw: a rare variant of oral carcinoma. Oral Surg Oral Med Oral Pathol Oral Radiol Endod 94: 601-608.

41. Alos L, Cardesa A, Bombi JA, Mallofre C, Cuchi A, Traserra J (1996). Myoepithelial tumors of salivary glands: a clinicopathologic, immunohistochemical, ultrastructural, and flow-cytometric study. Semin Diagn Pathol 13: 138-147.

42. Alos L, Carrillo R, Ramos J, Baez JM, Mallofre C, Fernandez PL, Cardesa A (1999). High-grade carcinoma component in epithelial-myoepithelial carcinoma of salivary glands clinicopathological, immunohistochemical and flow-cytometric study of three cases. Virchows Arch 434: 291-299.

43. Alos L, Castillo M, Nadal A, Caballero M, Mallofre C, Palacin A, Cardesa A (2004). Adenosquamous carcinoma of the head and neck: criteria for diagnosis in a study of 12 cases. Histopathology 44: 570-579.

44. Aloulou S, Farhat H, Bosq J, Vanel D, Ribrag V, Turhan AG, Girinsky T, Ferme C (2002). Hodgkin's disease primarily involving the oropharynx: case report and review of the literature. Hematol J 3: 164-167.

45. Alrawi M, McDermott M, Orr D, Russell J (2003). Nasal chondromesynchymal hamartoma presenting in an adolescent. Int J Pediatr Otorhinolaryngol 67: 669-672.

46. Altini M, Thompson SH, Lownie JF, Berezowski BB (1985). Ameloblastic sarcoma of the mandible. J Oral Maxillofac Surg 43: 789-794.

47. Alvarez-Canas C, Rodilla IG (1996). True malignant mixed tumor (carcinosarcoma) of the parotid gland. Report of a case with immunohistochemical study. Oral Surg Oral Med Oral Pathol Oral Radiol Endod 81: 454-458.

48. Alvarez-Mendoza A, Calderon-Elvir C, Carrasco-Daza D (1999). Diagnostic and therapeutic approach to sialoblastoma: report of a case. J Pediatr Surg 34: 1875-1877.

49. Amedee RG, Marks HW, Lyons GD (1987). Cholesterol granuloma of the petrous apex. Am J Otol 8: 48-55.

50. Ameerally P, McGurk M, Shaheen O (1996). Atypical ameloblastoma: report of 3 cases and a review of the literature. Br J Oral Maxillofac Surg 34: 235-239.

51. Amin HH, Petruzzelli GJ, Husain AN, Nickoloff BJ (2001). Primary malignant melanoma of the larynx. Arch Pathol Lab Med 125: 271-273.

52. Amin KS, Ehsan A, McGuff HS, Albright SC (2002). Minimally differentiated acute myelogenous leukemia (AML-M0) granulocytic sarcoma presenting in the oral cavity. Oral Oncol 38: 516-519.

53. Amir R, Danahey D, Ferrer K, Maffee M (2002). Inflammatory myofibroblastic tumor presenting with tracheal obstruction in a pregnant woman. Am J Otolaryngol 23: 362-367.

54. Ampil FL, Misra RP (1987). Factors influencing survival of patients with adenoid cystic carcinoma of the salivary glands. J Oral Maxillofac Surg 45: 1005-1010.

55. Anand VK, Osborne CM, Harkey HLI (1993). Infiltrative clival pituitary adenoma of ectopic origin. Otolaryngol Head Neck Surg 108: 178-183.

56. Anaya JM, McGuff HS, Banks PM, Talal N (1996). Clinicopathological factors relating malignant lymphoma with Sjogren's syndrome. Semin Arthritis Rheum 25: 337-346.

57. Andersen PE, Cambronero E, Shaha AR, Shah JP (1996). The extent of neck disease after regional failure during observation of the N0 neck. Am J Surg 172: 689-691.

58. Anderson JR, Armitage JO, Weisenburger DD (1998). Epidemiology of the non-Hodgkin's lymphomas: distributions of the major subtypes differ by geographic locations. Non-Hodgkin's Lymphoma Classification Project. Ann Oncol 9: 717-720.

59. Anderson LG, Talal N (1972). The spectrum of benign to malignant lymphoproliferation in Sjogren's syndrome. Clin Exp Immunol 10: 199-221.

60. Andl T, Kahn T, Pfuhl A, Nicola T, Erber R, Conradt C, Klein W, Helbig M, Dietz A, Weidauer H, Bosch FX (1998). Etiological involvement of oncogenic human papillomavirus in tonsillar squamous cell carcinomas lacking retinoblastoma cell cycle control. Cancer Res 58: 5-13.

61. Annino DJJr, Domanowski GF, Vaughan CW (1991). A rare cause of nasal obstruction: a solitary neurofibroma. Otolaryngol Head Neck Surg 104: 484-488.

62. Ansari-Lari MA, Hoque MO, Califano J, Westra WH (2002). Immunohistochemical p53 expression patterns in sarcomatoid carcinomas of the upper respiratory tract. Am J Surg Pathol 26: 1024-1031.

63. Ansell SM, Habermann TM, Hoyer JD, Strickler JG, Chen MG, McDonald TJ (1997). Primary laryngeal lymphoma. Laryngoscope 107: 1502-1506.

64. Anson BJ (1966). Morris' Human Anatomy. 12th ed. McGraw Hill: New York.

65. Antonescu CR, Terzakis JA (1997). Multiple malignant cylindromas of skin in association with basal cell adenocarcinoma with adenoid cystic features of minor salivary gland. J Cutan Pathol 24: 449-453.

66. Antoniades K, Eleftheriades I, Karakasis D (1987). The Gardner syndrome. Int J Oral Maxillofac Surg 16: 480-483.

67. Araujo VC, Martins MT, Salmen FS, Araujo NS (1999). Extranodal follicular dendritic cell sarcoma of the palate. Oral Surg Oral Med Oral Pathol Oral Radiol Endod 87: 209-214.

68. Arber DA, Weiss LM, Albujar PF, Chen YY, Jaffe ES (1993). Nasal lymphomas in Peru. High incidence of T-cell immunophenotype and Epstein-Barr virus infection. Am J Surg Pathol 17: 392-399.

69. Archard HO, Heck HW, Stanley HR (1965). Focal epithelial hyperplasia: an unusual mucosal lesion found in Indian children. Oral Surg Oral Med Oral Pathol 201-212.

70. Archer KF, Hurwitz JJ, Balogh JM, Fernandes BJ (1989). Orbital nonchromaffin paraganglioma. A case report and review of the literature. Ophthalmology 96: 1659-1666.

71. Ardekian L, Manor R, Peled M, Laufer D (1999). Malignant oncocytoma of the parotid gland: case report and analysis of the literature. J Oral Maxillofac Surg 57: 325-328.

72. Argani P, Perez-Ordonez B, Xiao H, Caruana SM, Huvos AG, Ladanyi M (1998). Olfactory neuroblastoma is not related to the Ewing family of tumors: absence of EWS/FLI1 gene fusion and MIC2 expression. Am J Surg Pathol 22: 391-398.

73. Armstrong LR, Preston EJ, Reichert M, Phillips DL, Nisenbaum R, Todd NW, Jacobs IN, Inglis AF, Manning SC, Reeves WC (2000). Incidence and prevalence of recurrent respiratory papillomatosis among children in Atlanta and Seattle. Clin Infect Dis 31: 107-109.

74. Armstrong RW, Imrey PB, Lye MS, Armstrong MJ, Yu MC, Sani S (2000). Nasopharyngeal carcinoma in Malaysian Chinese: occupational exposures to particles, formaldehyde and heat. Int J Epidemiol 29: 991-998.

75. Arnold B, Zietz C, Muller-Hocker J,

Wustrow TP (1996). Adenoma of the middle ear mucosa. Eur Arch Otorhinolaryngol 253: 65-68.

76. Arnott DG (1978). Cherubism—an initial unilateral presentation. Br J Oral Surg 16: 38-46.

77. Asare-Owusu L, Shotton JC, Schofield JB (1999). Adjuvant radiotherapy for primary mucosal malignant melanoma of the larynx. J Laryngol Otol 113: 932-934.

78. Asaumi J, Konouchi H, Hisatomi M, Matsuzaki H, Shigehara H, Honda Y, Kishi K (2003). MR features of aneurysmal bone cyst of the mandible and characteristics distinguishing it from other lesions. Eur J Radiol 45: 108-112.

79. Assimakopoulos D, Kolettas E, Zagorianakou N, Evangelou A, Skevas A, Agnantis NJ (2000). Prognostic significance of p53 in the cancer of the larynx. Anticancer Res 20: 3555-3564.

80. Assimakopoulos D, Patrikakos G (2002). The role of gastroesophageal reflux in the pathogenesis of laryngeal carcinoma. Am J Otolaryngol 23: 351-357.

81. Astor FC, Donegan JO, Gluckman JL (1985). Unusual anatomic presentations of inverting papilloma. Head Neck Surg 7: 243-245.

82. Astrom AK, Voz ML, Kas K, Roijer E, Wedell B, Mandahl N, Van de Ven W, Mark J, Stenman G (1999). Conserved mechanism of PLAG1 activation in salivary gland tumors with and without chromosome 8q12 abnormalities: identification of SII as a new fusion partner gene. Cancer Res 59: 918-923.

83. Auclair PL (1994). Tumor-associated lymphoid proliferation in the parotid gland. A potential diagnostic pitfall. Oral Surg Oral Med Oral Pathol 77: 19-26.

84. Auclair PL, Cuenin P, Kratochvil FJ, Slater LJ, Ellis GL (1988). A clinical and histomorphologic comparison of the central giant cell granuloma and the giant cell tumor. Oral Surg Oral Med Oral Pathol 66: 197-208.

85. Auclair PL, Ellis GL (1996). Atypical features in salivary gland mixed tumors: their relationship to malignant transformation. Mod Pathol 9: 652-657.

86. Auclair PL, Goode RK, Ellis GL (1992). Mucoepidermoid carcinoma of intraoral salivary glands. Evaluation and application of grading criteria in 143 cases. Cancer 69: 2021-2030. **87.** Auclair PL, Langloss JM, Weiss SW, Corio RL (1986). Sarcomas and sarcomatoid neoplasms of the major salivary gland regions. A clinicopathologic and immunohistochemical study of 67 cases and review of the literature. Cancer 58: 1305-1315.

88. Aughton DJ, Sloan CT, Milad MP, Huang TE, Michael C, Harper C (1990). Nasopharyngeal teratoma ('hairy polyp'), Dandy-Walker malformation, diaphragmatic hernia, and other anomalies in a female infant. J Med Genet 27: 788-790.

89. Aust MR, Olsen KD, Lewis JE, Nascimento AG, Meland NB, Foote RL, Suman VJ (1997). Angiosarcomas of the head and neck: clinical and pathologic characteristics. Ann Otol Rhinol Laryngol 106: 943-951.

90. Austin DF, Reynolds P (1996). Laryngeal cancer. In: Cancer Epidemiology and Prevention, Schottenfeld D, Fraumeni JFJr, eds., 2nd ed. Oxford University Press: New York , pp. 619-636.

91. Autio-Harmainen H, Paakko P, Alavaikko M, Karvonen J, Leisti J (1988). Familial occurrence of malignant lym-

phoepithelial lesion of the parotid gland in a Finnish family with dominantly inherited trichoepithelioma. Cancer 61: 161-166.

92. Auvinen A, Hietanen M, Luukkonen R, Koskela RS (2002). Brain tumors and salivary gland cancers among cellular telephone users. Epidemiology 13: 356-359.

93. Awange DO (1992). Fibrous dysplasia of the jaws: a review of literature. East Afr Med J 69: 205-209.

94. Axell T (1976). A prevalence study of oral mucosal lesions in an adult Swedish population. Odontol Revy 27: 1-103.

95. Azarschab P, Stembalska A, Loncar MB, Pfister M, Sasiadek MM, Blin N (2003). Epigenetic control of E-cadherin (CDH1) by CpG methylation in metastasising laryngeal cancer. Oncol Rep 10: 501-503.

96. Azevedo-Gamas A, Gloor F (1968). [A very unusual case of tumor of the larynx. Unexpected anatomopathologic diagnosis]. Ann Otolaryngol Chir Cervicofac 85: 329-335.

97. Azzimonti B, Hertel L, Aluffi P, Pia F, Monga G, Zocchi M, Landolfo S, Gariglio M (1999). Demonstration of multiple HPV types in laryngeal premalignant lesions using polymerase chain reaction and immunohistochemistry. J Med Virol 59: 110-116.

98. Azzopardi JG, Evans DJ (1971). Malignant lymphoma of parotid associated with Mikulicz disease (benign lymphoepithelial lesion). J Clin Pathol 24: 744-752.

99. Baarsma EA (1980). The median nasal sinus and dermoid cyst. Arch Otorhinolaryngol 226: 107-113.

100. Baba Y, Tsukuda M, Mochimatsu I, Furukawa S, Kagata H, Satake K, Koshika S, Nakatani Y, Hara M, Kato Y, Nagashima Y (2001). Reduced expression of p16 and p27 proteins in nasopharyngeal carcinoma. Cancer Detect Prev 25: 414-419.

101. Baden E, Al Saati T, Caveriviere P, Gorguet B, Delsol G (1987). Hodgkin's lymphoma of the oropharyngeal region: report of four cases and diagnostic value of monoclonal antibodies in detecting antigens associated with Reed-Sternberg cells. Oral Surg Oral Med Oral Pathol 64: 88-94.

102. Baden E, Doyle JL, Petriella V (1993). Malignant transformation of peripheral ameloblastoma. Oral Surg Oral Med Oral Pathol 75: 214-219.

103. Baden E, Moskow BS, Moskow R (1968). Odontogenic gingival epithelial hamartoma. J Oral Surg 26: 702-714.

103A. Bader G (1967). Odontomatosis (multiple odontomas). Oral Surg Oral Med Oral Pathol 23, 770-773.

104. Bahler DW, Miklos JA, Swerdlow SH (1997). Ongoing Ig gene hypermutation in salivary gland mucosa-associated lymphoid tissue-type lymphomas. Blood 89: 3335-3344.

105. Bahler DW, Swerdlow SH (1998). Clonal salivary gland infiltrates associated with myoepithelial sialadenitis (Sjogren's syndrome) begin as nonmalignant antigen-selected expansions. Blood 91: 1864-1872.

106. Baillie EE, Batsakis JG (1974). Glandular (seromucinous) hamartoma of the nasopharynx. Oral Surg Oral Med Oral Pathol 38: 760-762.

107. Baiocco R, Palma O, Locatelli G (1995). Squamous carcinoma of the epiglottis with sebaceous differentiation. Report of a case. Pathologica 87: 531-533.

108. Balaram P, Sridhar H, Rajkumar T, Vaccarella S, Herrero R, Nandakumar A, Ravichandran K, Ramdas K, Sankaranarayanan R, Gajalakshmi V,

Munoz N, Franceschi S (2002). Oral cancer in southern India: the influence of smoking, drinking, paan-chewing and oral hygiene. Int J Cancer 98: 440-445.

109. Balazic J, Masera A, Poljak M (1997). Sudden death caused by laryngeal papillomatosis. Acta Otolaryngol Suppl 527: 111-113.

110. Bale AE, Gailani MR, Leffell DJ (1995). The Gorlin syndrome gene: a tumor suppressor active in basal cell carcinogenesis and embryonic development. Proc Assoc Am Physicians 107: 253-257.

111. Ball DW, Azzoli CG, Baylin SB, Chi D, Dou S, Donis-Keller H, Cumaraswamy A, Borges M, Nelkin BD (1993). Identification of a human achaete-scute homolog highly expressed in neuroendocrine tumors. Proc Natl Acad Sci U S A 90: 5648-5652.

112. Ballantyne AJ (1970). Malignant melanoma of the skin of the head and neck. An analysis of 405 cases. Am J Surg 120: 425-431.

113. Baloch ZW, LiVolsi VA (2000). Warthin-like papillary carcinoma of the thyroid. Arch Pathol Lab Med 124: 1192-1195.

114. Bang G, Koppang HS, Hansen LS, Gilhuus-Moe O, Aksdal E, Persson PG, Lundgren J (1989). Clear cell odontogenic carcinoma: report of three cases with pulmonary and lymph node metastases. J Oral Pathol Med 18: 113-118.

115. Banik S, Howell JS, Wright DH (1985). Non-Hodgkin's lymphoma arising in adenolymphoma—a report of two cases. J Pathol 146: 167-177.

116. Banks ER, Frierson HFJr, Covell JL (1992). Fine needle aspiration cytologic findings in metastatic basaloid squamous cell carcinoma of the head and neck. Acta Cytol 36: 126-131.

117. Banks ER, Frierson HFJr, Mills SE, George E, Zarbo RJ, Swanson PE (1992). Basaloid squamous cell carcinoma of the head and neck. A clinicopathologic and immunohistochemical study of 40 cases. Am J Surg Pathol 16: 939-946.

118. Banoczy J (1977). Follow-up studies in oral leukoplakia. J Maxillofac Surg 5: 69-75.

119. Bansberg SF, Olsen KD, Gaffey TA (1989). Lymphoepithelioma of the oropharynx. Otolaryngol Head Neck Surg 100: 303-307.

120. Bari ME, Forster DM, Kemeny AA, Walton L, Hardy D, Anderson JR (2002). Malignancy in a vestibular schwannoma. Report of a case with central neurofibromatosis, treated by both stereotactic radiosurgery and surgical excision, with a review of the literature. Br J Neurosurg 16: 284-289.

121. Barker BF (1999). Odontogenic myxoma. Semin Diagn Pathol 16: 297-301.

122. Barker BF, Carpenter WM, Daniels TE, Kahn MA, Leider AS, Lozada-Nur F, Lynch DP, Melrose R, Merrell P, Morton T, Peters E, Regezi JA, Richards SD, Rick GM, Rohrer MD, Slater L, Stewart JC, Tomich CE, Vickers RA, Wood NK, Young SK (1997). Oral mucosal melanomas: the WESTOP Banff workshop proceedings. Western Society of Teachers of Oral Pathology. Oral Surg Oral Med Oral Pathol Oral Radiol Endod 83: 672-679.

123. Barnes C, Sexton M, Sizeland A, Tiedemann K, Berkowitz RG, Waters K (2001). Laryngo-pharyngeal carcinoma in childhood. Int J Pediatr Otorhinolaryngol 61: 83-86.

124. Barnes L (1986). Intestinal-type adenocarcinoma of the nasal cavity and paranasal sinuses. Am J Surg Pathol 10: 192-202.

125. Barnes L (1991). Paraganglioma of the larynx. A critical review of the literature. ORL J Otorhinolaryngol Relat Spec 53: 220-234.

126. Barnes L (2000). Diseases of the larynx, hypopharynx and esophagus. In: Surgical Pathology of the Head and Neck, Barnes L, ed., 2nd ed. Marcel Dekker: New York .

127. Barnes L (2002). Schneiderian papillomas and nonsalivary glandular neoplasms of the head and neck. Mod Pathol 15: 279-297.

128. Barnes L, Appel BN, Perez H, El Attar AM (1985). Myoepithelioma of the head and neck: case report and review. J Surg Oncol 28: 21-28.

129. Barnes L, Bedetti C (1984). Oncocytic Schneiderian papilloma: a reappraisal of cylindrical cell papilloma of the sinonasal tract. Hum Pathol 15: 344-351.

130. Barnes L, Brandwein M, Som PM (2001). Diseases of the nasal cavity, paranasal sinuses, and nasopharynx. In: Surgical Pathology of the Head and Neck, Surgical Pathology of the Head and Neck, 2nd ed. Marcel Dekker Inc: New York, Basel , pp. 522-523.

131. Barnes L, Brandwein M, Som PM (2001). Surgical Pathology of the Head and Neck. 2nd ed. Marcel Dekker Inc: New York.

132. Barnes L, Ferlito A, Altavilla G, MacMillan C, Rinaldo A, Doglioni C (1996). Basaloid squamous cell carcinoma of the head and neck: clinicopathological features and differential diagnosis. Ann Otol Rhinol Laryngol 105: 75-82.

133. Barnes L, Kanbour A (1988). Malignant fibrous histiocytoma of the head and neck. A report of 12 cases. Arch Otolaryngol Head Neck Surg 114: 1149-1156.

134. Barnes L, Rao U, Contis L, Krause J, Schwartz A, Scalamogna P (1994). Salivary duct carcinoma. Part II. Immunohistochemical evaluation of 13 cases for estrogen and progesterone receptors, cathepsin D, and c-erbB-2 protein. Oral Surg Oral Med Oral Pathol 78: 74-80.

135. Barnes L, Rao U, Krause J, Contis L, Schwartz A, Scalamogna P (1994). Salivary duct carcinoma. Part I. A clinicopathologic evaluation and DNA image analysis of 13 cases with review of the literature. Oral Surg Oral Med Oral Pathol 78: 64-73.

136. Barnes L, Taylor SR (1990). Carotid body paragangliomas. A clinicopathologic and DNA analysis of 13 tumors. Arch Otolaryngol Head Neck Surg 116: 447-453.

137. Barnes L, Taylor SR (1991). Vagal paragangliomas: a clinical, pathological, and DNA assessment. Clin Otolaryngol 16: 376-382.

138. Barnes L, Yunis EJ, Krebs FJI, Sonmez-Alpan E (1991). Verruca vulgaris of the larynx. Demonstration of human papillomavirus types 6/11 by in situ hybridization. Arch Pathol Lab Med 115: 895-899.

139. Barona de Guzman R, Martorell MA, Basterra J, Armengot M, Montoro A, Montoro J (1993). Analysis of DNA content in supraglottic epidermoid carcinoma. Otolaryngol Head Neck Surg 108: 706-710.

140. Barontini F, Maurri S, Sita D (1986). Peripheral ophthalmoplegia as the only sign of late-onset fibrous dysplasia of the skull. J Clin Neuroophthalmol 6: 109-112.

141. Barr FG, Galili N, Holick J, Biegel JA, Rovera G, Emanuel BS (1993).

Rearrangement of the PAX3 paired box gene in the paediatric solid tumour alveolar rhabdomyosarcoma. Nat Genet 3: 113-117.

142. Barra S, Talamini R, Proto E, Bidoli E, Puxeddu P, Franceschi S (1990). Survival analysis of 378 surgically treated cases of laryngeal carcinoma in south Sardinia. Cancer 65: 2521-2527.

143. Barreto DC, Gomez RS, Bale AE, Boson WL, De Marco L (2000). PTCH gene mutations in odontogenic keratocysts. J Dent Res 79: 1418-1422.

144. Barrett AW, Bennett JH, Speight PM (1995). A clinicopathological and immuno-histochemical analysis of primary oral mucosal melanoma. Eur J Cancer B Oral Oncol 31B: 100-105.

145. Barrett AW, Morgan M, Ramsay AD, Farthing PM, Newman L, Speight PM (2002). A clinicopathologic and immunohistochemical analysis of melanotic neuroectodermal tumor of infancy. Oral Surg Oral Med Oral Pathol Oral Radiol Endod 93: 688-698.

146. Barton JH, Osborne BM, Butler JJ, Meoz RT, Kong J, Fuller LM, Sullivan JA (1984). Non-Hodgkin's lymphoma of the tonsil. A clinicopathologic study of 65 cases. Cancer 53: 86-95.

147. Baruffi MR, Neto JB, Barbieri CH, Casartelli C (2001). Aneurysmal bone cyst with chromosomal changes involving 7q and 16p. Cancer Genet Cytogenet 129: 177-180.

148. Barzan L, Talamini R, Politi D, Minatel E, Gobitti C, Franchin G (2002). Squamous cell carcinoma of the hypopharynx treated with surgery and radiotherapy. J Laryngol Otol 116: 24-28.

149. Basset JM, Paraire F, Francois M, Fleury P (1982). [Two further cases of rare laryngeal tumors. Lipoma and chemodectoma (author's transl)]. Ann Otolaryngol Chir Cervicofac 99: 151-158.

150. Bataineh AB (1997). Aneurysmal bone cysts of the maxilla: a clinicopathologic review. J Oral Maxillofac Surg 55: 1212-1216.

151. Batra PS, Kern RC, Pelzer HJ, Haines GKI (2001). Leiomyosarcoma of the sinonasal tract: report of a case. Otolaryngol Head Neck Surg 125: 663-664.

152. Batsakis JG (1983). Pathology consultation. Carcinoma ex lymphoepithelial lesion. Ann Otol Rhinol Laryngol 92: 657-658.

153. Batsakis JG, Brannon RB (1981). Dermal analogue tumours of major salivary glands. J Laryngol Otol 95: 155-164.

154. Batsakis JG, El Naggar AK, Luna MA (1992). Epithelial-myoepithelial carcinoma of salivary glands. Ann Otol Rhinol Laryngol 101: 540-542.

155. Batsakis JG, El Naggar AK, Luna MA (1994). Hyalinizing clear cell carcinoma of salivary origin. Ann Otol Rhinol Laryngol 103: 746-748.

156. Batsakis JG, Frankenthaler R (1992). Embryoma (sialoblastoma) of salivary glands. Ann Otol Rhinol Laryngol 101: 958-960.

157. Batsakis JG, Huser J (1990). Squamous carcinomas with glandlike (adenoid) features. Ann Otol Rhinol Laryngol 99: 87-88.

158. Batsakis JG, Hybels RD, El Naggar AK (1993). Solitary fibrous tumor. Ann Otol Rhinol Laryngol 102: 74-76.

159. Batsakis JG, Luna MA (1991). Basaloid salivary carcinoma. Ann Otol Rhinol Laryngol 100: 785-787.

160. Batsakis JG, Luna MA, Byers RM

(1985). Metastases to the larynx. Head Neck Surg 7: 458-460.

161. Batsakis JG, Luna MA, El Naggar AK (1990). Histopathologic grading of salivary gland neoplasms: II. Acinic cell carcinomas. Ann Otol Rhinol Laryngol 99: 929-933.

162. Batsakis JG, Luna MA, El Naggar AK (1991). Basaloid monomorphic adenomas. Ann Otol Rhinol Laryngol 100: 687-690.

163. Batsakis JG, Mackay B, Ordonez NG (1984). Enteric-type adenocarcinoma of the nasal cavity. An electron microscopic and immunocytochemical study. Cancer 54: 855-860.

164. Batsakis JG, Pinkston GR, Luna MA, Byers RM, Sciubba JJ, Tillery GW (1983). Adenocarcinomas of the oral cavity: a clinicopathologic study of terminal duct carcinomas. J Laryngol Otol 97: 825-835.

165. Batsakis JG, Regezi JA, Solomon AR, Rice DH (1982). The pathology of head and neck tumors: mucosal melanomas, part 13. Head Neck Surg 4: 404-418.

166. Batsakis JG, Rice DH (1981). The pathology of head and neck tumors: vasoformative tumors, part 9A. Head Neck Surg 3: 231-239.

167. Batsakis JG, Rice DH (1981). The pathology of head and neck tumors: vasoformative tumors, part 9B. Head Neck Surg 3: 326-339.

168. Batsakis JG, Rice DH, Howard DR (1982). The pathology of head and neck tumors: spindle cell lesions (sarcomatoid carcinomas, nodular fasciitis, and fibrosarcoma) of the aerodigestive tracts, Part 14. Head Neck Surg 4: 499-513.

169. Batsakis JG, Rice DH, Solomon AR (1980). The pathology of head and neck tumors: squamous and mucous-gland carcinomas of the nasal cavity, paranasal sinuses, and larynx, part 6. Head Neck Surg 2: 497-508.

170. Batsakis JG, Suarez P (2000). Mucosal melanomas: a review. Adv Anat Pathol 7: 167-180.

171. Batsakis JG, Suarez P (2000). Papillary squamous carcinoma: will the real one please stand up? Adv Anat Pathol 7: 2-8.

172. Batsakis JG, Suarez P (2000). Sarcomatoid carcinomas of the upper aerodigestive tracts. Adv Anat Pathol 7: 282-293.

173. Batsakis JG, Suarez P (2001). Schneiderian papillomas and carcinomas: a review. Adv Anat Pathol 8: 53-64.

174. Batsakis JG, Suarez P, El Naggar AK (1999). Proliferative verrucous leukoplakia and its related lesions. Oral Oncol 35: 354-359.

175. Battifora H (1976). Spindle cell carcinoma: ultrastructural evidence of squamous origin and collagen production by the tumor cells. Cancer 37: 2275-2282.

176. Bauer WH, Fox RA (1945). Adenomyoepithelioima (cylindroma) of palatal mucous glands. Arch Pathol 39: 96-102.

177. Baujat B, Attal P, Racy E, Quillard J, Parker F, Evennou A, Bobin S (2001). Chondromyxoid fibroma of the nasal bone with extension into the frontal and ethmoidal sinuses: report of one case and a review of the literature. Am J Otolaryngol 22: 150-153.

178. Bauman NM, Smith RJ (1996). Recurrent respiratory papillomatosis. Pediatr Clin North Am 43: 1385-1401.

179. Baumgartner WA, Mark JB (1980). Metastatic malignancies from distant sites to the tracheobronchial tree. J Thorac Cardiovasc Surg 79: 499-503.

180. Bayasit YA, Kanlikama M, Bakir K, Ucak R, Mumbuc S, Ozer E (2001). Malignant Mixed Tumours of the Larynx : a Case Report. Rev Laryngol Otol Rhinol (Bord) 249-251.

181. Baysal BE (2001). Genetics of familial paragangliomas: past, present, and future. Otolaryngol Clin North Am 34: 863-79, vi.

182. Baysal BE, Ferrell RE, Willett-Brozick JE, Lawrence EC, Myssiorek D, Bosch A, van der Mey A, Taschner PE, Rubinstein WS, Myers EN, Richard CWI, Cornelisse CJ, Devilee P, Devlin B (2000). Mutations in SDHD, a mitochondrial complex II gene, in hereditary paraganglioma. Science 287: 848-851.

183. Bazan V, Zanna I, Migliavacca M, Sanz-Casla MT, Maestro ML, Corsale S, Macaluso M, Dardanoni G, Restivo S, Quintela PL, Bernaldez R, Salerno S, Morello V, Tomasino RM, Gebbia N, Russo A (2002). Prognostic significance of p16INK4a alterations and 9p21 loss of heterozygosity in locally advanced laryngeal squamous cell carcinoma. J Cell Physiol 192: 286-293.

184. Beasley JDI (1976). Traumatic cyst of the jaws: report of 30 cases. J Am Dent Assoc 92: 145-152.

185. Beck JC, McClatchey KD, Lesperance MM, Esclamado RM, Carey TE, Bradford CR (1995). Presence of human papillomavirus predicts recurrence of inverted papilloma. Otolaryngol Head Neck Surg 113: 49-55.

186. Bedavanija A, Brieger J, Lehr HA, Maurer J, Mann WJ (2003). Association of proliferative activity and size in acoustic neuroma: implications for timing of surgery. J Neurosurg 98: 807-811.

187. Bedi GC, Westra WH, Gabrielson E, Koch W, Sidransky D (1996). Multiple head and neck tumors: evidence for a common clonal origin. Cancer Res 56: 2484-2487.

188. Begin LR, Rochon L, Frenkiel S (1991). Spindle cell myoepithelioma of the nasal cavity. Am J Surg Pathol 15: 184-190.

189. Beham-Schmid C, Beham A, Jakse R, Aubock L, Hofler G (1998). Extranodal follicular dendritic cell tumour of the nasopharynx. Virchows Arch 432: 293-298.

190. Beham A, Fletcher CD, Kainz J, Schmid C, Humer U (1993). Nasopharyngeal angiofibroma: an immunohistochemical study of 32 cases. Virchows Arch A Pathol Anat Histopathol 423: 281-285.

191. Beitler AJ, Ptaszynski K, Karpel JP (1996). Upper airway obstruction in a woman with AIDS-related laryngeal Kaposi's sarcoma. Chest 109: 836-837.

192. Bellacosa A, Almadori G, Cavallo S, Cadoni G, Galli J, Ferrandina G, Scambia G, Neri G (1996). Cyclin D1 gene amplification in human laryngeal squamous cell carcinomas: prognostic significance and clinical implications. Clin Cancer Res 2: 175-180.

193. Belsky JL, Tachikawa K, Cihak RW, Yamamoto T (1972). Salivary gland tumors in atomic bomb survivors, Hiroshima-Nagasaki, 1957 to 1970. JAMA 219: 864-868.

194. Belsky JL, Takeichi N, Yamamoto T, Cihak RW, Hirose F, Ezaki H, Inoue S, Blot WJ (1975). Salivary gland neoplasms following atomic radiation: additional cases and reanalysis of combined data in a fixed population, 1957-1970. Cancer 35: 555-559.

195. Benhamou CA, Laraqui N, Touhami M, Chekkoury A, Benchakroun Y, Samlali R, Kahlain A (1992). [Tobacco and cancer of the larynx: a prospective survey of 58 patients]. Rev Laryngol Otol Rhinol (Bord) 113: 285-288.

196. Benjamin B, Parsons DS (1988). Recurrent respiratory papillomatosis: a 10 year study. J Laryngol Otol 102: 1022-1028.
197. Benowitz LI, Routtenberg A (1987). A membrane phosphoprotein associated with neural development, axonal regeneration, phospholipid metabolism and synaptic plasticity. Trends Neurosci 10: 527-532.
198. Berge JK, Kapadia SB, Myers EN (1998). Osteosarcoma of the larynx. Arch Otolaryngol Head Neck Surg 124: 207-210.
199. Bergensen PJ, Kennedy PJ, Kneale KL (1987). Metastatic tumours of the parotid region. Aust NZ J Surg 57: 23-26.
200. Berkower AS, Biller HF (1988). Head and neck cancer associated with Bloom's syndrome. Laryngoscope 98: 746-748.
201. Berkowitz RG, Mahadevan M (1999). Unilateral tonsillar enlargement and tonsillar lymphoma in children. Ann Otol Rhinol Laryngol 108: 876-879.
202. Bernstein JM, Montgomery WW, Balogh KJr (1966). Metastatic tumors to the maxilla, nose, and paranasal sinuses. Laryngoscope 76: 621-650.
203. Berry JA, Wolf JS, Gray WC (2002). Squamous cell carcinoma arising in a lymphangioma of the tongue. Otolaryngol Head Neck Surg 127: 458-460.
204. Berthelet E, Shenouda G, Black MJ, Picariello M, Rochon L (1994). Sarcomatoid carcinoma of the head and neck. Am J Surg 168: 455-458.
205. Berthelsen A, Andersen AP, Jensen TS, Hansen HS (1984). Melanomas of the mucosa in the oral cavity and the upper respiratory passages. Cancer 54: 907-912.
206. Bertoni F, Dallera P, Bacchini P, Marchetti C, Campobassi A (1991). The Istituto Rizzoli-Beretta experience with osteosarcoma of the jaw. Cancer 68: 1555-1563.
207. Bertoni F, Unni KK, Beabout JW, Ebersold MJ (1992). Giant cell tumor of the skull. Cancer 70: 1124-1132.
208. Betuel H, Camoun M, Colombani J, Day NE, Ellouz R, de The G (1975). The relationship between nasopharyngeal carcinoma and the HL-A system among Tunisians. Int J Cancer 16: 249-254.
209. Bialas M, Sinczak A, Choinska-Stefanska A, Zygulska A (2002). EBV-positive lymphoepithelial carcinoma of salivary gland in a woman of a non-endemic area—a case report. Pol J Pathol 53: 235-238.
210. Bianco P, Riminucci M, Majolagbe A, Kuznetsov SA, Collins MT, Mankani MH, Corsi A, Bone HG, Wientroub S, Spiegel AM, Fisher LW, Robey PG (2000). Mutations of the GNAS1 gene, stromal cell dysfunction, and osteomalacic changes in non-McCune-Albright fibrous dysplasia of bone. J Bone Miner Res 15: 120-128.
211. Bielamowicz S, Calcaterra TC, Watson D (1993). Inverting papilloma of the head and neck: the UCLA update. Otolaryngol Head Neck Surg 109: 71-76.
212. Biggar RJ (2001). AIDS-related cancers in the era of highly active antiretroviral therapy. Oncology (Huntingt) 15: 439-448.
213. Bikhazi PH, Messina L, Mhatre AN, Goldstein JA, Lalwani AK (2000). Molecular pathogenesis in sporadic head and neck paraganglioma. Laryngoscope 110: 1346-1348.
214. Bilal H, Handra-Luca A, Bertrand JC, Fouret PJ (2003). P63 is expressed in basal and myoepithelial cells of human normal and tumor salivary gland tissues. J Histochem Cytochem 51: 133-139.
215. Biller HF, Lawson W, Som P, Rosenfeld R (1989). Glomus vagale tumors. Ann Otol Rhinol Laryngol 98: 21-26.
216. Billings KR, Fu YS, Calcaterra TC, Sercarz JA (2000). Hemangiopericytoma of the head and neck. Am J Otolaryngol 21: 238-243.
217. Binder WJ, Som P, Kaneko M, Biller HF (1980). Mucoepidermoid carcinoma of the larynx. A case report and review of the literature. Ann Otol Rhinol Laryngol 89: 103-107.
218. Bisceglia M, Cardone M, Fantasia L, Cenacchi G, Pasquinelli G (2001). Mixed tumors, myoepitheliomas, and oncocytomas of the soft tissues are likely members of the same family: a clinicopathologic and ultrastructural study. Ultrastruct Pathol 25: 399-418.
219. Blackledge FA, Anand VK (2000). Tracheobronchial extension of recurrent respiratory papillomatosis. Ann Otol Rhinol Laryngol 109: 812-818.
220. Blackwell JB (1993). Mesenchymal chondrosarcoma arising in fibrous dysplasia of the femur. J Clin Pathol 46: 961-962.
221. Blackwell KE, Calcaterra TC, Fu YS (1995). Laryngeal dysplasia: epidemiology and treatment outcome. Ann Otol Rhinol Laryngol 104: 596-602.
222. Blackwell KE, Fu YS, Calcaterra TC (1995). Laryngeal dysplasia. A clinicopathologic study. Cancer 75: 457-463.
223. Blanck C, Eneroth CM, Jakobsson PA (1970). Oncocytoma of the parotid gland: neoplasm or nodular hyperplasia? Cancer 25: 919-925.
224. Blanck C, Eneroth CM, Jakobsson PA (1971). Mucus-producing adenopapillary (non-epidermoid) carcinoma of the parotid gland. Cancer 28: 676-685.
225. Bleiweiss IJ, Huvos AG, Lara J, Strong EW (1992). Carcinosarcoma of the submandibular salivary gland. Immunohistochemical findings. Cancer 69: 2031-2035.
226. Block MS, Gross BD (1982). Epidermolysis bullosa dystrophica recessive: oral surgery and anesthetic considerations. J Oral Maxillofac Surg 40: 753-758.
227. Blot WJ, McLaughlin JK, Devesa SS, Fraumeni JF (1996). Cancers of the oral cavity and pharynx. In: Cancer Epidemiology and Prevention, Schottenfeld D, Fraumeni JFJr, eds., 2nd ed. Oxford University Press: New York , pp. 666-680.
228. Blot WJ, McLaughlin JK, Winn DM, Austin DF, Greenberg RS, Preston-Martin S, Bernstein L, Schoenberg JB, Stemhagen A, Fraumeni JFJr (1988). Smoking and drinking in relation to oral and pharyngeal cancer. Cancer Res 48: 3282-3287.
229. Boccon-Gibod LA, Grangeponte MC, Boucheron S, Josset PP, Roger G, Berthier-Falissard ML (1996). Salivary gland anlage tumor of the nasopharynx: a clinicopathologic and immunohistochemical study of three cases. Pediatr Pathol Lab Med 16: 973-983.
230. Bockmuhl U, Wolf G, Schmidt S, Schwendel A, Jahnke V, Dietel M, Petersen I (1998). Genomic alterations associated with malignancy in head and neck cancer. Head Neck 20: 145-151.
231. Bombi JA, Riverola A, Bordas JM, Cardesa A (1991). Adenosquamous carcinoma of the esophagus. A case report. Pathol Res Pract 187: 514-519.
232. Bomer DL, Arnold GE (1971). Malignant tumors of the minor salivary glands. Acta Otolaryngol .
233. Bondeson L, Andreasson L, Olsson M, Rausing A (1997). Salivary gland anlage tumor: cytologic features in a case examined by fine-needle aspiration. Diagn Cytopathol 16: 518-521.
234. Boniuk M, Zimmerman LE (1968). Sebaceous carcinoma of the eyelid, eyebrow, caruncle, and orbit. Trans Am Acad Ophthalmol Otolaryngol 72: 619-642.
235. Bonner RA, Mukai K, Oppenheimer JH (1979). Two unusual variants of Nelson's syndrome. J Clin Endocrinol Metab 49: 23-29.
236. Borg MF, Benjamin CS, Morton RP, Llewellyn HR (1993). Malignant lympho-epithelial lesion of the salivary gland: a case report and review of the literature. Australas Radiol 37: 288-291.
237. Borit A, Blanshard TP (1979). Sphenoidal pituitary adenoma. Hum Pathol 10: 93-96.
238. Bosetti C, Talamini R, Levi F, Negri E, Franceschi S, Airoldi L, La Vecchia C (2002). Fried foods: a risk factor for laryngeal cancer? Br J Cancer 87: 1230-1233.
239. Boson WL, Gomez RS, Araujo L, Kalapothakis E, Friedman E, De Marco L (1998). Odontogenic myxomas are not associated with activating mutations of the Gs alpha gene. Anticancer Res 18: 4415-4417.
240. Boston M, Derkay CS (2003). Recurrent respiratory papillomatosis. Clin Pulm Med 10-16.
241. Bottomley WK, Gabriel SA, Corio RL, Jacobson RJ, Rothchild N (1987). Histiocytosis X: report of an oral soft tissue lesion without bony involvement. Oral Surg Oral Med Oral Pathol 63: 228-231.
242. Bottomley WW, Goodfield MD (1994). Chondrodermatitis nodularis helicis occurring with systemic sclerosis—an under-reported association? Clin Exp Dermatol 19: 219-220.
243. Bouquot JE, Gnepp DR (1991). Laryngeal precancer: a review of the literature, commentary, and comparison with oral leukoplakia. Head Neck 13: 488-497.
244. Bouquot JE, Kurland LT, Weiland LH (1979). Primary salivary epithelial neoplasms in Rochester, Minnesota population. J Dent Res 58: 419.
245. Bouquot JE, Kurland LT, Weiland LH (1991). Laryngeal keratosis and carcinoma in the Rochester, MN, population 1935-1984. Cancer Detect Prev 15: 83-91.
246. Bouquot JE, Weiland LH, Kurland LT (1989). Metastases to and from the upper aerodigestive tract in the population of Rochester, Minnesota, 1935-1984. Head Neck 11: 212-218.
247. Boyle P, Macfarlane GJ, Zheng T, Maisonneuve P, Evstifeeva T, Scully C (1992). Recent advances in epidemiology of head and neck cancer. Curr Opin Oncol 4: 471-477.
248. Braakhuis BJ, Tabor MP, Leemans CR, van der Waal I, Snow GB, Brakenhoff RH (2002). Second primary tumors and field cancerization in oral and oropharyngeal cancer: molecular techniques provide new insights and definitions. Head Neck 24: 198-206.
249. Bradford CR, Wolf GT, Carey TE, Zhu S, Beals TF, Truelson JM, McClatchey KD, Fisher SG (1999). Predictive markers for response to chemotherapy, organ preservation, and survival in patients with advanced laryngeal carcinoma. Otolaryngol Head Neck Surg 121: 534-538.
250. Brandsma JL, Steinberg BM, Abramson AL, Winkler B (1986). Presence of human papillomavirus type 16 related sequences in verrucous carcinoma of the larynx. Cancer Res 46: 2185-2188.
251. Brandwein M, Al Naeif NS, Manwani D, Som P, Goldfeder L, Rothschild M, Granowetter L (1999). Sialoblastoma: clinicopathological/immunohistochemical study. Am J Surg Pathol 23: 342-348.
252. Brandwein M, Huvos AG, Dardick I, Thomas MJ, Theise ND (1996). Noninvasive and minimally invasive carcinoma ex mixed tumor: a clinicopathologic and ploidy study of 12 patients with major salivary tumors of low (or no?) malignant potential. Oral Surg Oral Med Oral Pathol Oral Radiol Endod 81: 655-664.
253. Brandwein M, LeBenger J, Strauchen J, Biller H (1990). Atypical granular cell tumor of the larynx: an unusually aggressive tumor clinically and microscopically. Head Neck 12: 154-159.
254. Brandwein M, Levi G, Som P, Urken ML (1992). Paraganglioma of the inferior laryngeal paraganglia. A case report. Arch Otolaryngol Head Neck Surg 118: 994-996.
255. Brandwein M, Moore S, Som P, Biller H (1992). Laryngeal chondrosarcomas: a clinicopathologic study of 11 cases, including two "dedifferentiated" chondrosarcomas. Laryngoscope 102: 858-867.
256. Brandwein M, Said-Al-Naief N, Gordon R, Urken M (2002). Clear cell odontogenic carcinoma: report of a case and analysis of the literature. Arch Otolaryngol Head Neck Surg 128: 1089-1095.
257. Brandwein MS, Huvos AG (1991). Oncocytic tumors of major salivary glands. A study of 68 cases with follow-up of 44 patients. Am J Surg Pathol 15: 514-528.
258. Brandwein MS, Ivanov K, Wallace DI, Hille JJ, Wang B, Fahmy A, Bodian C, Urken ML, Gnepp DR, Huvos A, Lumerman H, Mills SE (2001). Mucoepidermoid carcinoma: a clinicopathologic study of 80 patients with special reference to histological grading. Am J Surg Pathol 25: 835-845.
259. Brandwein MS, Jagirdar J, Patil J, Biller H, Kaneko M (1990). Salivary duct carcinoma (cribriform salivary carcinoma of excretory ducts). A clinicopathologic and immunohistochemical study of 12 cases. Cancer 65: 2307-2314.
260. Brandwein MS, Rothstein A, Lawson W, Bodian C, Urken ML (1997). Sinonasal melanoma. A clinicopathologic study of 25 cases and literature meta-analysis. Arch Otolaryngol Head Neck Surg 123: 290-296.
261. Brannon RB, Fowler CB (2001). Benign fibro-osseous lesions: a review of current concepts. Adv Anat Pathol 8: 126-143.
262. Brannon RB, Fowler CB, Carpenter WM, Corio RL (2002). Cementoblastoma: an innocuous neoplasm? A clinicopathologic study of 44 cases and review of the literature with special emphasis on recurrence. Oral Surg Oral Med Oral Pathol Oral Radiol Endod 93: 311-320.
263. Brannon RB, Fowler CB, Hartman KS (1991). Necrotizing sialometaplasia. A clinicopathologic study of sixty-nine cases and review of the literature. Oral Surg Oral Med Oral Pathol 72: 317-325.
264. Brannon RB, Sciubba JJ, Giulani M (2001). Ductal papillomas of salivary gland origin: A report of 19 cases and a review of the literature. Oral Surg Oral Med Oral Pathol Oral Radiol Endod 92: 68-77.
265. Braun IF, Levy S, Hoffman JCJr (1985). The use of transarterial microembolization in the management of hemangiomas of the perioral region. J Oral Maxillofac Surg 43: 239-248.
266. Bregni RC, Taylor AM, Garcia AM (2001). Ameloblastic fibrosarcoma of the

mandible: report of two cases and review of the literature. J Oral Pathol Med 30: 316-320.

267. Bremer JW, Bryan NH, De Sando LW, Ljones GC (1986). Angiofibroma: treatment trends in 150 patients during 40 years. Laryngoscope 222-231.

268. Brennan JA, Boyle JO, Koch WM, Goodman SN, Hruban RH, Eby YJ, Couch MJ, Forastiere AA, Sidransky D (1995). Association between cigarette smoking and mutation of the p53 gene in squamous-cell carcinoma of the head and neck. N Engl J Med 332: 712-717.

269. Bressac-de-Paillerets B, Avril MF, Chompret A, Demenais F (2002). Genetic and environmental factors in cutaneous malignant melanoma. Biochimie 84: 67-74.

270. Bridge JA, Kanamori M, Ma Z, Pickering D, Hill DA, Lydiatt W, Lui MY, Colleoni GW, Antonescu CR, Ladanyi M, Morris SW (2001). Fusion of the ALK gene to the clathrin heavy chain gene, CLTC, in inflammatory myofibroblastic tumor. Am J Pathol 159: 411-415.

271. Bridge JA, Liu J, Weibolt V, Baker KS, Perry D, Kruger R, Qualman S, Barr F, Sorensen P, Triche T, Suijkerbuijk R (2000). Novel genomic imbalances in embryonal rhabdomyosarcoma revealed by comparative genomic hybridization and fluorescence in situ hybridization: an intergroup rhabdomyosarcoma study. Genes Chromosomes Cancer 27: 337-344.

272. Bridge JA, Neff JR, Bhatia PS, Sanger WG, Murphey MD (1990). Cytogenetic findings and biologic behavior of giant cell tumors of bone. Cancer 65: 2697-2703.

273. Briele HA, Walker MJ, Das Gupta TK (1985). Melanoma of the head and neck. Clin Plast Surg 12: 495-504.

274. Briggs J, Evans JN (1967). Malignant oxyphilic granular-cell tumor (oncocytoma) of the palate. Review of the recent literature and report of a case. Oral Surg Oral Med Oral Pathol 23: 796-802.

275. Brinck U, Gunawan B, Schulten HJ, Pinzon W, Fischer U, Fuzesi L (2001). Clear-cell odontogenic carcinoma with pulmonary metastases resembling pulmonary meningothelial-like nodules. Virchows Arch 438: 412-417.

276. Brito H, Vassallo J, Altemani A (2000). Detection of human papillomavirus in laryngeal squamous dysplasia and carcinoma. An in situ hybridization and signal amplification study. Acta Otolaryngol 120: 540-544.

277. Brodsky L, Yoshpe N, Ruben RJ (1983). Clinical-pathological correlates of congenital subglottic hemangiomas. Ann Otol Rhinol Laryngol Suppl 105: 4-18.

278. Broekaert D, Coucke P, Leperque S, Ramaekers F, Van Muijen G, Boedts D, Leigh I, Lane B (1992). Immunohistochemical analysis of the cytokeratin expression in middle ear cholesteatoma and related epithelial tissues. Ann Otol Rhinol Laryngol 101: 931-938.

279. Brookes GB, Rose PE (1983). Malignant fibrous histiocytoma of the ethmoid sinus. J Laryngol Otol 97: 279-289.

280. Brookstone MS, Huvos AG (1992). Central salivary gland tumors of the maxilla and mandible: a clinicopathologic study of 11 cases with an analysis of the literature. J Oral Maxillofac Surg 50: 229-236.

281. Brown EW, Megerian CA, McKenna MJ, Weber A (1995). Fibrous dysplasia of the temporal bone: imaging findings. AJR Am J Roentgenol 164: 679-682.

282. Browne JD, Fisch U, Valvanis A (1993). Surgical therapy of glomus vagale tumours. Skull Base Surg 3: 192.

283. Browne K, Gee JB (2000). Asbestos exposure and laryngeal cancer. Ann Occup Hyg 44: 239-250.

284. Browne RM, Smith AJ (1991). Pathogenesis of odontogenic cysts. In: Investigative Pathology of the Odontogenic Cyst, Browne RM, ed., 1st ed. CRC Press: Boca Raton , pp. 88-109.

285. Brownson RC, Chang JC (1987). Exposure to alcohol and tobacco and the risk of laryngeal cancer. Arch Environ Health 42: 192-196.

286. Broyles EN (1943). The anterior commissure tendon. Ann Otol Rhinol Laryngol 52: 342-345.

287. Brugere J, Guenel P, Leclerc A, Rodriguez J (1986). Differential effects of tobacco and alcohol in cancer of the larynx, pharynx, and mouth. Cancer 57: 391-395.

288. Bruner JM (1987). Peripheral nerve sheath tumors of the head and neck. Semin Diagn Pathol 4: 136-149.

289. Bryan RL, Bevan IS, Crocker J, Young LS (1990). Detection of HPV 6 and 11 in tumours of the upper respiratory tract using the polymerase chain reaction. Clin Otolaryngol 15: 177-180.

290. Bryne M, Jenssen N, Boysen M (1995). Histological grading in the deep invasive front of T1 and T2 glottic squamous cell carcinomas has high prognostic value. Virchows Arch 427: 277-281.

291. Bryne M, Koppang HS, Lilleng R, Kjaerheim A (1992). Malignancy grading of the deep invasive margins of oral squamous cell carcinomas has high prognostic value. J Pathol 166: 375-381.

292. Bryne M, Koppang HS, Lilleng R, Stene T, Bang G, Dabelsteen E (1989). New malignancy grading is a better prognostic indicator than Broders' grading in oral squamous cell carcinomas. J Oral Pathol Med 18: 432-437.

293. Brynes RK, Almaguer PD, Leathery KE, McCourty A, Arber DA, Medeiros LJ, Nathwani BN (1996). Numerical cytogenetic abnormalities of chromosomes 3, 7, and 12 in marginal zone B-cell lymphomas. Mod Pathol 9: 995-1000.

294. Brzoska PM, Levin NA, Fu KK, Kaplan MJ, Singer MI, Gray JW, Christman MF (1995). Frequent novel DNA copy number increase in squamous cell head and neck tumors. Cancer Res 55: 3055-3059.

295. Bschorer R, Lingenfelser T, Kaiserling E, Schwenzer N (1993). Malignant lymphoma of the mucosa-associated lymphoid tissue (MALT)—consecutive unusual manifestation in the rectum and gingiva. J Oral Pathol Med 22: 190-192.

296. Buchino JJ (1995). Salivary gland anlage tumor: a newly recognized clinicopathologic entity of uncertain histogenesis. Adv Anat Pathol 2: 98.

297. Buchner A (1991). The central (intraosseous) calcifying odontogenic cyst: an analysis of 215 cases. J Oral Maxillofac Surg 49: 330-339.

298. Buchner A, Merrell PW, Hansen LS, Leider AS (1991). Peripheral (extraosseous) calcifying odontogenic cyst. A review of forty-five cases. Oral Surg Oral Med Oral Pathol 72: 65-70.

299. Buchner A, Merrell PW, Leider AS, Hansen LS (1990). Oral focal mucinosis. Int J Oral Maxillofac Surg 19: 337-340.

300. Buchner A, Sciubba JJ (1987). Peripheral epithelial odontogenic tumors: a review. Oral Surg Oral Med Oral Pathol 63: 688-697.

301. Buchwald C, Franzmann MB, Jacobsen GK, Juhl BR, Lindeberg H (1997). Carcinomas occurring in papillomas of the nasal septum associated with human papilloma virus (HPV). Rhinology 35: 74-78.

302. Buchwald C, Franzmann MB, Tos M (1995). Sinonasal papillomas: a report of 82 cases in Copenhagen County, including a longitudinal epidemiological and clinical study. Laryngoscope 105: 72-79.

303. Buchwald C, Lindeberg H, Pedersen BL, Franzmann MB (2001). Human papilloma virus and p53 expression in carcinomas associated with sinonasal papillomas: a Danish Epidemiological study 1980-1998. Laryngoscope 111: 1104-1110.

304. Buell P (1973). Race and place in the etiology of nasopharyngeal cancer: a study based on California death certificates. Int J Cancer 11: 268-272.

305. Bullerdiek J, Haubrich J, Meyer K, Bartnitzke S (1988). Translocation t(11;19)(q21;p13.1) as the sole chromosome abnormality in a cystadenolymphoma (Warthin's tumor) of the parotid gland. Cancer Genet Cytogenet 35: 129-132.

306. Bullerdiek J, Wobst G, Meyer-Bolte K, Chilla R, Haubrich J, Thode B, Bartnitzke S (1993). Cytogenetic subtyping of 220 salivary gland pleomorphic adenomas: correlation to occurrence, histological subtype, and in vitro cellular behavior. Cancer Genet Cytogenet 65: 27-31.

307. Bunker ML, Locker J (1989). Warthin's tumor with malignant lymphoma. DNA analysis of paraffin-embedded tissue. Am J Clin Pathol 91: 341-344.

308. Burch JD, Howe GR, Miller AB, Semenciw R (1981). Tobacco, alcohol, asbestos, and nickel in the etiology of cancer of the larynx: a case-control study. J Natl Cancer Inst 67: 1219-1224.

309. Burch WM, Kramer RS, Kenan PD, Hammond CB (1985). Cushing's disease caused by an ectopic pituitary adenoma within the sphenoid sinus. N Engl J Med 312: 587-588.

310. Buresh CJ, Seemayer TA, Nelson M, Neff JR, Dorfman HD, Bridge J (1999). t(X;4)(q22;q31.3) in giant cell reparative granuloma. Cancer Genet Cytogenet 115: 80-81.

311. Burns BF, Dardick I, Parks WR (1988). Intermediate filament expression in normal parotid glands and pleomorphic adenomas. Virchows Arch A Pathol Anat Histopathol 413: 103-112.

312. Burrows PE, Laor T, Paltiel H, Robertson RL (1998). Diagnostic imaging in the evaluation of vascular birthmarks. Dermatol Clin 16: 455-488.

313. Burt RD, Vaughan TL, McKnight B, Davis S, Beckmann AM, Smith AG, Nisperos B, Swanson GM, Berwick M (1996). Associations between human leukocyte antigen type and nasopharyngeal carcinoma in Caucasians in the United States. Cancer Epidemiol Biomarkers Prev 5: 879-887.

314. Burt RD, Vaughan TL, Nisperos B, Swanson M, Berwick M (1994). A protective association between the HLA-A2 antigen and nasopharyngeal carcinoma in US Caucasians. Int J Cancer 56: 465-467.

315. Burton DM, Heffner DK, Patow CA (1992). Granular cell tumors of the trachea. Laryngoscope 102: 807-813.

316. Byrne MN, Sessions DG (1990). Nasopharyngeal craniopharyngioma. Case report and literature review. Ann Otol Rhinol Laryngol 99: 633-639.

317. Cairns P, Polascik TJ, Eby Y, Tokino K, Califano J, Merlo A, Mao L, Herath J, Jenkins R, Westra W, Rutter JL, Buckler A, Gabrielson E, Tockman M, Cho KR, Hedrick L, Bova GS, Isaacs W, Koch W, Schwab D, Sidransky D (1995). Frequency of homozygous deletion at p16/CDKN2 in primary human tumours. Nat Genet 11: 210-212.

318. Califano J, van der Riet P, Westra W, Nawroz H, Clayman G, Piantadosi S, Corio R, Lee D, Greenberg B, Koch W, Sidransky D (1996). Genetic progression model for head and neck cancer: implications for field cancerization. Cancer Res 56: 2488-2492.

319. Califano J, Westra WH, Meininger G, Corio R, Koch WM, Sidransky D (2000). Genetic progression and clonal relationship of recurrent premalignant head and neck lesions. Clin Cancer Res 6: 347-352.

320. Califano L, Maremonti P, Boscaino A, De Rosa G, Giardino C (1996). Peripheral ameloblastoma: report of a case with malignant aspect. Br J Oral Maxillofac Surg 34: 240-242.

321. Callender T, El Naggar AK, Lee MS, Frankenthaler R, Luna MA, Batsakis JG (1994). PRAD-1 (CCND1)/cyclin D1 oncogene amplification in primary head and neck squamous cell carcinoma. Cancer 74: 152-158.

322. Callender TA, Weber RS, Janjan N, Benjamin R, Zaher M, Wolf P, el Naggar A (1995). Rhabdomyosarcoma of the nose and paranasal sinuses in adults and children. Otolaryngol Head Neck Surg 112: 252-257.

323. Cammoun M, Ellouz R, Behi J, Attia RB (1978). Histological types of nasopharyngeal carcinoma in an intermediate risk area. IARC Sci Publ 13-26.

324. Campbell WGJr, Priest RE, Weathers DR (1985). Characterization of two types of crystalloids in pleomorphic adenomas of minor salivary glands. A light-microscopic, electron-microscopic, and histochemical study. Am J Pathol 118: 194-202.

325. Campbell WM, McDonald TJ, Unni KK, Laws ERJr (1980). Nasal and paranasal presentations of chordomas. Laryngoscope 90: 612-618.

326. Canalis RF, Jenkens HA, Hemenway WG, Lincoln C (1978). Nasopharyngeal rhabdomyosarcoma. A clinical perspective. Arch Otolaryngol 104: 122-126.

327. Candeliere GA, Glorieux FH, Prud'homme J, St Arnaud R (1995). Increased expression of the c-fos proto-oncogene in bone from patients with fibrous dysplasia. N Engl J Med 332: 1546-1551.

328. Canioni D, Arnulf B, Asso-Bonnet M, Raphael M, Brousse N (2001). Nasal natural killer lymphoma associated with Epstein-Barr virus in a patient infected with human immunodeficiency virus. Arch Pathol Lab Med 125: 660-662.

329. Cantarella G, Neglia CB, Civelli E, Roncoroni L, Radice F (2001). Spindle cell lipoma of the hypopharynx. Dysphagia 16: 224-227.

330. Carbone A, Micheau C (1982). Pitfalls in microscopic diagnosis of undifferentiated carcinoma of nasopharyngeal type (lymphoepithelioma). Cancer 50: 1344-1351.

331. Carinci F, Marzola A, Hassanipour A (1999). Granular cell tumor of the parotid gland. A case report. Int J Oral Maxillofac Surg 28: 383-384.

332. Carlos R, Sedano HO (1994). Multifocal papilloma virus epithelial hyperplasia. Oral Surg Oral Med Oral Pathol 77:

631-635.

333. Carlos R, Sedano HO (2002). Intralesional corticosteroids as an alternative treatment for central giant cell granuloma. Oral Surg Oral Med Oral Pathol Oral Radiol Endod 93: 161-166.

334. Carney JA, Boccon-Gibod L, Jarka DE, Tanaka Y, Swee RG, Unni KK, Stratakis CA (2001). Osteochondromyxoma of bone: a congenital tumor associated with lentigines and other unusual disorders. Am J Surg Pathol 25: 164-176.

335. Carney ME, O'Reilly RC, Sholevar B, Buiakova OI, Lowry LD, Keane WM, Margolis FL, Rothstein JL (1995). Expression of the human Achaete-scute 1 gene in olfactory neuroblastoma (esthesioneuroblastoma). J Neurooncol 26: 35-43.

336. Carrau RL, Petruzzelli G, Cass SP (1995). Adenoid cystic carcinoma of the nasopharynx. Otolaryngol Head Neck Surg 112: 501-502.

337. Carter RL, Barr LC, O'Brien CJ, Soo KC, Shaw HJ (1985). Transcapsular spread of metastatic squamous cell carcinoma from cervical lymph nodes. Am J Surg 150: 495-499.

338. Caselitz J, Seifert G, Grenner G, Schmidtberger R (1983). Amylase as an additional marker of salivary gland neoplasms. An immunoperoxidase study. Pathol Res Pract 176: 276-283.

339. Casler JD, Conley JJ (1992). Surgical management of adenoid cystic carcinoma in the parotid gland. Otolaryngol Head Neck Surg 106: 332-338.

340. Castellanos JL, Lally ET (1982). Acinic cell tumor of the minor salivary glands. J Oral Maxillofac Surg 40: 428-431.

341. Castle JT, Arendt DM (1999). Aggressive (malignant) epithelial odontogenic ghost cell tumor. Ann Diagn Pathol 3: 243-248.

342. Castle JT, Thompson LD, Frommelt RA, Wenig BM, Kessler HP (1999). Polymorphous low grade adenocarcinoma: a clinicopathologic study of 164 cases. Cancer 86: 207-219.

343. Catalano PJ, Brandwein M, Shah DK, Urken ML, Lawson W, Biller HF (1996). Sinonasal hemangiopericytomas: a clinicopathologic and immunohistochemical study of seven cases. Head Neck 18: 42-53.

344. Cattaruzza MS, Maisonneuve P, Boyle P (1996). Epidemiology of laryngeal cancer. Eur J Cancer B Oral Oncol 32B: 293-305.

345. Cavalcanti MG, Ruprecht A, Quets J (1999). Evaluation of maxillofacial fibrosarcoma using computer graphics and spiral computed tomography. Dentomaxillofac Radiol 28: 145-151.

346. Cavazzana AO, Schmidt D, Ninfo V, Harms D, Tollot M, Carli M, Treuner J, Betto R, Salviati G (1992). Spindle cell rhabdomyosarcoma. A prognostically favorable variant of rhabdomyosarcoma. Am J Surg Pathol 16: 229-235.

347. Cawson RA, Gleeson MJ, Eveson JW (1997). Pathology and Surgery of the Salivary Glands. ISIS Medical Media: Oxford.

348. Cazorla M, Hernandez L, Nadal A, Balbin M, Lopez JM, Vizoso F, Fernandez PL, Iwata K, Cardesa A, Lopez-Otin C, Campo E (1998). Collagenase-3 expression is associated with advanced local invasion in human squamous cell carcinomas of the larynx. J Pathol 186: 144-150.

349. Cecchetto G, Carli M, Alaggio R, Dall'Igna P, Bisogno G, Scarzello G, Zanetti I, Durante G, Inserra A, Siracusa F, Guglielmi M (2001). Fibrosarcoma in pediatric patients: results of the Italian Cooperative Group studies (1979-1995). J Surg Oncol 78: 225-231.

350. Cerilli LA, Holst VA, Brandwein MS, Stoler MH, Mills SE (2001). Sinonasal undifferentiated carcinoma: immunohistochemical profile and lack of EBV association. Am J Surg Pathol 25: 156-163.

351. Cerilli LA, Swartzbaugh JR, Saadut R, Marshall CE, Rumpel CA, Moskaluk CA, Frierson HFJr (1999). Analysis of chromosome 9p21 deletion and p16 gene mutation in salivary gland carcinomas. Hum Pathol 30: 1242-1246.

352. Cerroni L, Hofler G, Back B, Wolf P, Maier G, Kerl H (2002). Specific cutaneous infiltrates of B-cell chronic lymphocytic leukemia (B-CLL) at sites typical for Borrelia burgdorferi infection. J Cutan Pathol 29: 142-147.

353. Cerroni L, Zenahlik P, Hofler G, Kaddu S, Smolle J, Kerl H (1996). Specific cutaneous infiltrates of B-cell chronic lymphocytic leukemia: a clinicopathologic and prognostic study of 42 patients. Am J Surg Pathol 20: 1000-1010.

354. Cerroni L, Zenahlik P, Kerl H (1995). Specific cutaneous infiltrates of B-cell chronic lymphocytic leukemia arising at the site of herpes zoster and herpes simplex scars. Cancer 76: 26-31.

355. Chadburn A, Cesarman E, Knowles DM (1997). Molecular pathology of posttransplantation lymphoproliferative disorders. Semin Diagn Pathol 14: 15-26.

356. Chadburn A, Chen JM, Hsu DT, Frizzera G, Cesarman E, Garrett TJ, Mears JG, Zangwill SD, Addonizio LJ, Michler RE, Knowles DM (1998). The morphologic and molecular genetic categories of posttransplantation lymphoproliferative disorders are clinically relevant. Cancer 82: 1978-1987.

357. Chai Y, Jiang X, Ito Y, Bringas PJr, Han J, Rowitch DH, Soriano P, McMahon AP, Sucov HM (2000). Fate of the mammalian cranial neural crest during tooth and mandibular morphogenesis. Development 127: 1671-1679.

358. Chambers EF, Norman D, Dedo HH, Ferrell LD (1982). Primary nasopharyngeal chemodectoma. Neuroradiology 23: 285-288.

359. Chan AC, Chan KW, Chan JK, Au WY, Ho WK, Ng WM (2001). Development of follicular dendritic cell sarcoma in hyaline-vascular Castleman's disease of the nasopharynx: tracing its evolution by sequential biopsies. Histopathology 38: 510-518.

360. Chan AS, To KF, Lo KW, Ding M, Li X, Johnson P, Huang DP (2002). Frequent chromosome 9p losses in histologically normal nasopharyngeal epithelia from southern Chinese. Int J Cancer 102: 300-303.

361. Chan AS, To KF, Lo KW, Mak KF, Pak W, Chiu B, Tse GM, Ding M, Li X, Lee JC, Huang DP (2000). High frequency of chromosome 3p deletion in histologically normal nasopharyngeal epithelia from southern Chinese. Cancer Res 60: 5365-5370.

362. Chan AT, Lo YM, Zee B, Chan LY, Ma BB, Leung SF, Mo F, Lai M, Ho S, Huang DP, Johnson PJ (2002). Plasma Epstein-Barr virus DNA and residual disease after radiotherapy for undifferentiated nasopharyngeal carcinoma. J Natl Cancer Inst 94: 1614-1619.

363. Chan AT, Teo ML, Lee WY, Kwan WH, Choi PH, Johnson PJ (1998). The significance of keratinizing squamous cell histology in Chinese patients with nasopharyngeal carcinoma. Clin Oncol (R Coll Radiol) 10: 161-164.

364. Chan CW, Nicholls JM, Sham JS, Dickens P, Choy D (1992). Nasopharyngeal carcinoma in situ in nasopharyngeal carcinoma. J Clin Pathol 45: 898-901.

365. Chan J, Gannon FH, Thompson LD (2003). Malignant giant cell tumor of the sphenoid. Ann Diagn Pathol 7: 100-105.

366. Chan JK (1998). Kuttner tumor (chronic sclerosing sialadenitis) of the submandibular gland: an underrecognized entity. Adv Anat Pathol 5: 239-251.

367. Chan JK, Cheuk W, Shimizu M (2001). Anaplastic lymphoma kinase expression in inflammatory pseudotumors. Am J Surg Pathol 25: 761-768.

368. Chan JK, Fletcher CD, Nayler SJ, Cooper K (1997). Follicular dendritic cell sarcoma. Clinicopathologic analysis of 17 cases suggesting a malignant potential higher than currently recognized. Cancer 79: 294-313.

369. Chan JK, Hui PK, Ng CS, Yuen NW, Kung IT, Gwi E (1989). Epithelioid haemangioma (angiolymphoid hyperplasia with eosinophilia) and Kimura's disease in Chinese. Histopathology 15: 557-574.

370. Chan JK, Ng CS, Lo ST (1987). Immunohistological characterization of malignant lymphomas of the Waldeyer's ring other than the nasopharynx. Histopathology 11: 885-899.

371. Chan JK, Sin VC, Wong KF, Ng CS, Tsang WY, Chan CH, Cheung MM, Lau WH (1997). Nonnasal lymphoma expressing the natural killer cell marker CD56: a clinicopathologic study of 49 cases of an uncommon aggressive neoplasm. Blood 89: 4501-4513.

372. Chan JK, Suster S, Wenig BM, Tsang WY, Chan JB, Lau AL (1997). Cytokeratin 20 immunoreactivity distinguishes Merkel cell (primary cutaneous neuroendocrine) carcinomas and salivary gland small cell carcinomas from small cell carcinomas of various sites. Am J Surg Pathol 21: 226-234.

373. Chan JK, Tsang WY, Hui PK, Ng CS, Sin VC, Khan SM, Siu LL (1997). T- and T/natural killer-cell lymphomas of the salivary gland: a clinicopathologic, immunohistochemical and molecular study of six cases. Hum Pathol 28: 238-245.

374. Chan JK, Tsang WY, Ng CS (1994). Follicular dendritic cell tumor and vascular neoplasm complicating hyaline-vascular Castleman's disease. Am J Surg Pathol 18: 517-525.

375. Chan JK, Tsang WY, Ng CS, Tang SK, Yu HC, Lee AW (1994). Follicular dendritic cell tumors of the oral cavity. Am J Surg Pathol 18: 148-157.

376. Chan JK, Yip TT, Tsang WY, Ng CS, Lau WH, Poon YF, Wong CC, Ma VW (1994). Detection of Epstein-Barr viral RNA in malignant lymphomas of the upper aerodigestive tract. Am J Surg Pathol 18: 938-946.

377. Chan JK, Yip TT, Tsang WY, Poon YF, Wong CS, Ma VW (1994). Specific association of Epstein-Barr virus with lymphoepithelial carcinoma among tumors and tumorlike lesions of the salivary gland. Arch Pathol Lab Med 118: 994-997.

378. Chan KH, Gu YL, Ng F, Ng PS, Seto WH, Sham JS, Chua D, Wei W, Chen YL, Luk W, Zong YS, Ng MH (2003). EBV specific antibody-based and DNA-based assays in serologic diagnosis of nasopharyngeal carcinoma. Int J Cancer 105: 706-709.

379. Chan MK, McGuire LJ, King W, Li AK, Lee JC (1992). Cytodiagnosis of 112 salivary gland lesions. Correlation with histologic and frozen section diagnosis. Acta Cytol 36: 353-363.

380. Chan MK, McGuire LJ, Lee JC (1989). Fine needle aspiration cytodiagnosis of nasopharyngeal carcinoma in cervical lymph nodes. A study of 40 cases. Acta Cytol 33: 344-350.

381. Chan SH, Chew CT, Prasad U, Wee GB, Srinivasan N, Kunaratnam N (1985). HLA and nasopharyngeal carcinoma in Malays. Br J Cancer 51: 389-392.

382. Chan SH, Day NE, Kunaratnam N, Chia KB, Simons MJ (1983). HLA and nasopharyngeal carcinoma in Chinese—a further study. Int J Cancer 32: 171-176.

383. Chan YF, Ma LT, Yeung CK, Lam KH (1988). Parapharyngeal inflammatory pseudotumor presenting as fever of unknown origin in a 3-year-old girl. Pediatr Pathol 8: 195-203.

384. Chandler JR, Goulding R, Moskowitz L, Quencer RM (1984). Nasopharyngeal angiofibromas: staging and management. Ann Otol Rhinol Laryngol 93: 322-329.

385. Chang-Lo M (1977). Laryngeal involvement in Von Recklinghausen's disease: a case report and review of the literature. Laryngoscope 87: 435-442.

386. Chang AE, Karnell LH, Menck HR (1998). The National Cancer Data Base report on cutaneous and noncutaneous melanoma: a summary of 84,836 cases from the past decade. The American College of Surgeons Commission on Cancer and the American Cancer Society. Cancer 83: 1664-1678.

387. Chang AR, Liang XM, Chan AT, Chan MK, Teo PM, Johnson PJ (2001). The use of brush cytology and directed biopsies for the detection of nasopharyngeal carcinoma and precursor lesions. Head Neck 23: 637-645.

388. Chang EZ, Lee WC (1985). Surgical treatment of pleomorphic adenoma of the parotid gland: report of 110 cases. J Oral Maxillofac Surg 43: 680-682.

389. Chang F, Wang L, Syrjanen S, Syrjanen K (1992). Human papillomavirus infections in the respiratory tract. Am J Otolaryngol 13: 210-225.

390. Chang HW, Chan A, Kwong DL, Wei WI, Sham JS, Yuen AP (2003). Detection of Hypermethylated RIZ1 Gene in Primary Tumor, Mouth, and Throat Rinsing Fluid, Nasopharyngeal Swab, and Peripheral Blood of Nasopharyngeal Carcinoma Patient. Clin Cancer Res 9: 1033-1038.

391. Chang KL, Kamel OW, Arber DA, Horyd ID, Weiss LM (1995). Pathologic features of nodular lymphocyte predominance Hodgkin's disease in extranodal sites. Am J Surg Pathol 19: 1313-1324.

392. Chang Y, Cesarman E, Pessin MS, Lee F, Culpepper J, Knowles DM, Moore PS (1994). Identification of herpesvirus-like DNA sequences in AIDS-associated Kaposi's sarcoma. Science 266: 1865-1869.

393. Chao MW, Smith JG, Laidlaw C, Joon DL, Ball D (1998). Results of treating primary tumors of the trachea with radiotherapy. Int J Radiat Oncol Biol Phys 41: 779-785.

394. Charafe-Jauffret E, Bertucci F, Ramuz O, Devilard E, Gaulard P, Brousset P, Houlgatte R, Hassoun J, Birnbaum D, Xerri L (2003). Characterization of Hodgkin's lymphoma-like undifferentiated carcinoma of the nasopharyngeal type as a particular UCNT subtype mimicking Hodgkin's lymphoma. Int J Oncol 23: 97-103.

395. Charoenrat P, Pillai G, Patel S, Fisher

C, Archer D, Eccles S, Rhys-Evans P (2003). Tumour thickness predicts cervical nodal metastases and survival in early oral tongue cancer. Oral Oncol 39: 386-390.

396. Chaturvedi P, Rodrigues G, Sanghvi VD (1999). Pseudo-malignant laryngeal nodule (inflammatory myofibroblastic tumour). Histopathology 34: 272-273.

397. Chau Y, Hongyo T, Aozasa K, Chan JK (2001). Dedifferentiation of adenoid cystic carcinoma: report of a case implicating p53 gene mutation. Hum Pathol 32: 1403-1407.

398. Chaudhry AP, Cutler LS, Leifer C, Satchidanand S, Labay G, Yamane G (1986). Histogenesis of acinic cell carcinoma of the major and minor salivary glands. An ultrastructural study. J Pathol 148: 307-320.

399. Chaudhry AP, Cutler LS, Satchidanand S, Labay G, Raj MS, Lin CC (1983). Glycogen-rich tumor of the oral minor salivary glands. A histochemical and ultrastructural study. Cancer 52: 105-111.

400. Chaudhry AP, Labay GR, Yamane GM, Jacobs MS, Cutler LS, Watkins KV (1984). Clinico-pathologic and histogenetic study of 189 intraoral minor salivary gland tumors. J Oral Med 39: 58-78.

401. Chaudhry AP, Vickers RA, Gorlin RJ (1961). Intraoral minor salivary gland tumors. An analysis of 1414 cases. Oral Surg Oral Med Oral Pathol 14: 1194-1226.

402. Chen AY, Matson LK, Roberts D, Goepfert H (2001). The significance of comorbidity in advanced laryngeal cancer. Head Neck 23: 566-572.

403. Chen CL, Hsu MM (2000). Second primary epithelial malignancy of nasopharynx and nasal cavity after successful curative radiation therapy of nasopharyngeal carcinoma. Hum Pathol 31: 227-232.

404. Chen CL, Su IJ, Hsu MM, Hsu HC (1991). Granulomatous nasopharyngeal carcinoma: with emphasis on difficulty in diagnosis and favorable outcome. J Formos Med Assoc 90: 353-356.

405. Chen CL, Wen WN, Chen JY, Hsu MM, Hsu HC (1993). Detection of Epstein-Barr virus genome in nasopharyngeal carcinoma by in situ DNA hybridization. Intervirology 36: 91-98.

406. Chen I, Tu H (2000). Pleomorphic adenoma of the parotid gland metastasizing to the cervical lymph node. Otolaryngol Head Neck Surg 122: 455-457.

407. Chen KT (1983). Clear cell carcinoma of the salivary gland. Hum Pathol 14: 91-93.

408. Chen KT (1985). Carcinoma arising in monomorphic adenoma of the salivary gland. Am J Otolaryngol 6: 39-41.

409. Chen KT, Weinberg RA (1984). Intramuscular lipoma of the larynx. Am J Otolaryngol 5: 71-72.

410. Chen SY, Brannon RB, Miller AS, White DK, Hooker SP (1978). Acinic cell adenocarcinoma of minor salivary glands. Cancer 42: 678-685.

411. Chen XM (1990). [Papillary cystadeno-carcinoma of the salivary glands: clinico-pathologic analysis of 22 cases]. Zhonghua Kou Qiang Yi Xue Za Zhi 25: 102-4, 126.

412. Chen Y, Chan SH (1994). Polymorphism of T-cell receptor genes in nasopharyngeal carcinoma. Int J Cancer 56: 830-833.

413. Chen YJ, Ko JY, Chen PJ, Shu CH, Hsu MT, Tsai SF, Lin CH (1999). Chromosomal aberrations in nasopharyngeal carcinoma analyzed by comparative genomic hybridization. Genes Chromosomes Cancer 25: 169-175.

414. Chen YK, Lin LM, Lin CC, Chen CH (2003). Keratoacanthoma of the tongue: A diagnostic problem. Otolaryngol Head Neck Surg 128: 581-582.

415. Cheng YJ, Chien YC, Hildesheim A, Hsu MM, Chen IH, Chuang J, Chang J, Ma YD, Luo CT, Hsu WL, Hsu HH, Huang H, Chang JF, Chen CJ, Yang CS (2003). No association between genetic polymorphisms of CYP1A1, GSTM1, GSTT1, GSTP1, NAT2, and nasopharyngeal carcinoma in Taiwan. Cancer Epidemiol Biomarkers Prev 12: 179-180.

416. Chervenak FA, Isaacson G, Blakemore KJ, Breg WR, Hobbins JC, Berkowitz RL, Tortora M, Mayden K, Mahoney MJ (1983). Fetal cystic hygroma. Cause and natural history. N Engl J Med 309: 822-825.

417. Chessin H, Urdaneta N, Smith H, Van Gilder J (1976). Chromophobe adenoma manifesting as a nasopharyngeal mass. Arch Otolaryngol 102: 631-633.

418. Cheuk W, Chan JK, Ngan RK (1999). Dedifferentiation in adenoid cystic carcinoma of salivary gland: an uncommon complication associated with an accelerated clinical course. Am J Surg Pathol 23: 465-472.

419. Cheung F, Pang SW, Hioe F, Cheung KN, Lee A, Yau TK (1998). Nasopharyngeal carcinoma in situ: two cases of an emerging diagnostic entity. Cancer 83: 1069-1073.

420. Cheung MM, Chan JK, Lau WH, Foo W, Chan PT, Ng CS, Ngan RK (1998). Primary non-Hodgkin's lymphoma of the nose and nasopharynx: clinical features, tumor immunophenotype, and treatment outcome in 113 patients. J Clin Oncol 16: 70-77.

421. Cheung MM, Chan JK, Lau WH, Ngan RK, Foo WW (2002). Early stage nasal NK/T-cell lymphoma: clinical outcome, prognostic factors, and the effect of treatment modality. Int J Radiat Oncol Biol Phys 54: 182-190.

422. Cheung MM, Chan JK, Wong KF (2003). Natural killer cell neoplasms: a distinctive group of highly aggressive lymphoma/leukemia. Semin Hematol 40: 221-232.

423. Chhetri DK, Rawnsley JD, Calcaterra TC (2000). Carcinoma of the buccal mucosa. Otolaryngol Head Neck Surg 123: 566-571.

424. Chhieng DC, Cangiarella JF, Cohen JM (2000). Fine-needle aspiration cytology of lymphoproliferative lesions involving the major salivary glands. Am J Clin Pathol 113: 563-571.

425. Chiang AK, Chan AC, Srivastava G, Ho FC (1997). Nasal T/natural killer (NK)-cell lymphomas are derived from Epstein-Barr virus-infected cytotoxic lymphocytes of both NK- and T-cell lineage. Int J Cancer 73: 332-338.

426. Chiang AK, Tao Q, Srivastava G, Ho FC (1996). Nasal NK- and T-cell lymphomas share the same type of Epstein-Barr virus latency as nasopharyngeal carcinoma and Hodgkin's disease. Int J Cancer 68: 285-290.

427. Chidzonga MM (1996). Ameloblastoma in children. The Zimbabwean experience. Oral Surg Oral Med Oral Pathol Oral Radiol Endod 81: 168-170.

428. Chiesa F, Mauri S, Tradati N, Calabrese L, Giugliano G, Ansarin M, Andrle J, Zurrida S, Orecchia R, Scully C (1999). Surfing prognostic factors in head and neck cancer at the millennium. Oral Oncol 35: 590-596.

429. Childers EL, Ellis GL, Auclair PL (1996). An immunohistochemical analysis of anti-amylase antibody reactivity in acinic cell adenocarcinoma. Oral Surg Oral Med Oral Pathol Oral Radiol Endod 81: 691-694.

430. Childers EL, Furlong MA, Fanburg-Smith JC (2002). Hemangioma of the salivary gland: a study of ten cases of a rarely biopsied/excised lesion. Ann Diagn Pathol 6: 339-344.

431. Childs CC, Parham DM, Berard CW (1987). Infectious mononucleosis. The spectrum of morphologic changes simulating lymphoma in lymph nodes and tonsils. Am J Surg Pathol 11: 122-132.

432. Chin KW, Billings KR, Ishiyama A, Wang MB, Wackym PA (1995). Characterization of lymphocyte subpopulations in Warthin's tumor. Laryngoscope 105: 928-933.

433. Ching AS, Khoo JB, Chong VF (2002). CT and MR imaging of solitary extramedullary plasmacytoma of the nasal tract. AJNR Am J Neuroradiol 23: 1632-1636.

434. Chitale AR, Murthy AK, Desai AP, Lalitha VS (1991). Peripheral nerve sheath tumours: an ultrastructural study of 30 cases. Indian J Cancer 28: 1-8.

435. Cho KJ, El Naggar AK, Mahanupab P, Luna MA, Batsakis JG (1995). Carcinoma ex-pleomorphic adenoma of the nasal cavity: a report of two cases. J Laryngol Otol 109: 677-679.

436. Cho KJ, El Naggar AK, Ordonez NG, Luna MA, Austin J, Batsakis JG (1995). Epithelial-myoepithelial carcinoma of salivary glands. A clinicopathologic, DNA flow cytometric, and immunohistochemical study of Ki-67 and HER-2/neu oncogene. Am J Clin Pathol 103: 432-437.

437. Choi HR, Batsakis JG, Callender DL, Prieto VG, Luna MA, El Naggar AK (2002). Molecular analysis of chromosome 16q regions in dermal analogue tumors of salivary glands: a genetic link to dermal cylindroma? Am J Surg Pathol 26: 778-783.

438. Choi PC, To KF, Lai FM, Lee TW, Yim AP, Chan JK (2000). Follicular dendritic cell sarcoma of the neck: report of two cases complicated by pulmonary metastases. Cancer 89: 664-672.

439. Cholewa D, Waldschmidt J (1998). Laser treatment of hemangiomas of the larynx and trachea. Lasers Surg Med 23: 221-232.

440. Chomette G, Auriol M, Guilbert F, Delcourt A (1983). Ameloblastic fibrosarcoma of the jaws—report of three cases. Clinico-pathologic, histoenzymological and ultrastructural study. Pathol Res Pract 178: 40-47.

441. Chomette G, Auriol M, Vaillant JM (1984). Acinic cell tumors of salivary glands. Frequency and morphological study. J Biol Buccale 12: 157-169.

442. Chong VF, Fan YF (1996). Skull base erosion in nasopharyngeal carcinoma: detection by CT and MRI. Clin Radiol 51: 625-631.

443. Chong VF, Fan YF (1999). Parotid gland involvement in nasopharyngeal carcinoma. J Comput Assist Tomogr 23: 524-528.

444. Chow TL, Chow TK, Lui YH, Sze WM, Yuen NW, Kwok SP (2002). Lymphoepithelioma-like carcinoma of oral cavity: report of three cases and literature review. Int J Oral Maxillofac Surg 31: 212-218.

445. Christiansen MS, Mourad WA, Hales ML, Oldring DJ (1995). Spindle cell malignant lymphoepithelial lesion of the parotid gland: clinical, light microscopic, ultrastructural, and in situ hybridization findings in one case. Mod Pathol 8: 711-715.

446. Chu PG, Chang KL, Wu AY, Weiss LM (1999). Nasal glomus tumors: report of two cases with emphasis on immunohisto-chemical features and differential diagnosis. Hum Pathol 30: 1259-1261.

447. Chua DT, Sham JS, Kwong DL, Tai KS, Wu PM, Lo M, Yung A, Choy D, Leong L (1997). Volumetric analysis of tumor extent in nasopharyngeal carcinoma and correlation with treatment outcome. Int J Radiat Oncol Biol Phys 39: 711-719.

448. Chua DT, Sham JS, Wei WI, Ho WK, Au GK (2001). The predictive value of the 1997 American Joint Committee on Cancer stage classification in determining failure patterns in nasopharyngeal carcinoma. Cancer 92: 2845-2855.

449. Chui RT, Liao SY, Bosworth H (1985). Recurrent oncocytoma of the ethmoid sinus with orbital invasion. Otolaryngol Head Neck Surg 93: 267-270.

450. Chun SI, Ji HG (1992). Kimura's disease and angiolymphoid hyperplasia with eosinophilia: clinical and histopathologic differences. J Am Acad Dermatol 27: 954-958.

451. Chung YF, Khoo ML, Heng MK, Hong GS, Soo KC (1999). Epidemiology of Warthin's tumour of the parotid gland in an Asian population. Br J Surg 86: 661-664.

452. Chuong R, Kaban LB, Kozakewich H, Perez-Atayde A (1986). Central giant cell lesions of the jaws: a clinicopathologic study. J Oral Maxillofac Surg 44: 708-713.

453. Cianfriglia F, Di Gregorio DA, Manieri A (1999). Multiple primary tumours in patients with oral squamous cell carcinoma. Oral Oncol 35: 157-163.

454. Cichowski K, Jacks T (2001). NF1 tumor suppressor gene function: narrowing the GAP. Cell 104: 593-604.

455. Clark JL, Unni KK, Dahlin DC, Devine KD (1983). Osteosarcoma of the jaw. Cancer 51: 2311-2316.

456. Claros P, Dominte G, Claros A, Castillo M, Cardesa A, Claros A (2002). Parotid gland mucoepidermoid carcinoma in a 4-year-old child. Int J Pediatr Otorhinolaryngol 63: 67-72.

457. Claudio PP, Howard CM, Fu Y, Cinti C, Califano L, Micheli P, Mercer EW, Caputi M, Giordano A (2000). Mutations in the retinoblastoma-related gene RB2/p130 in primary nasopharyngeal carcinoma. Cancer Res 60: 8-12.

458. Clausen F, Poulson H (1963). Metastatic carcinoma of the jaws. Acta Pathol Microbiol Scand 57: 361-374.

459. Cleary KR, Batsakis JG (1990). Undifferentiated carcinoma with lymphoid stroma of the major salivary glands. Ann Otol Rhinol Laryngol 99: 236-238.

460. Cleveland DB, Goldberg KM, Greenspan JS, Seitz TE, Miller AS (1996). Langerhans' cell histiocytosis: report of three cases with unusual oral soft tissue involvement. Oral Surg Oral Med Oral Pathol Oral Radiol Endod 82: 541-548.

461. Cloos J, Braakhuis BJ, Steen I, Copper MP, de Vries N, Nauta JJ, Snow GB (1994). Increased mutagen sensitivity in head-and-neck squamous-cell carcinoma patients, particularly those with multiple primary tumors. Int J Cancer 56: 816-819.

462. Cloos J, Nieuwenhuis EJ, Boomsma DI, Kuik DJ, van der Sterre ML, Arwert F, Snow GB, Braakhuis BJ (1999). Inherited susceptibility to bleomycin-induced chromatid breaks in cultured peripheral blood lymphocytes. J Natl Cancer Inst 91: 1125-1130.

463. Coates HL, Pearson BW, Devine KD, Unni KK (1977). Chondrosarcoma of the nasal cavity, paranasal sinuses and nasopharynx. Trans Am Acad Ophthalmol Otolaryngol 84: 919-926.
464. Cobourne MT, Sharpe PT (2003). Tooth and jaw: molecular mechanisms of patterning in the first branchial arch. Arch Oral Biol 48: 1-14.
465. Cocke EW (1962). Benign Cartilaginous Tumors of the Larynx. Laryngoscope 1678-1730.
466. Coffin CM, Patel A, Perkins S, Elenitoba-Johnson KS, Perlman E, Griffin CA (2001). ALK1 and p80 expression and chromosomal rearrangements involving 2p23 in inflammatory myofibroblastic tumor. Mod Pathol 14: 569-576.
467. Coffin CM, Watterson J, Priest JR, Dehner LP (1995). Extrapulmonary inflammatory myofibroblastic tumor (inflammatory pseudotumor). A clinicopathologic and immunohistochemical study of 84 cases. Am J Surg Pathol 19: 859-872.
468. Cogliatti SB, Schmid U, Schumacher U, Eckert F, Hansmann ML, Hedderich J, Takahashi H, Lennert K (1991). Primary B-cell gastric lymphoma: a clinicopathological study of 145 patients. Gastroenterology 101: 1159-1170.
469. Cohen J, Guillamondegui OM, Batsakis JG, Medina JE (1985). Cancer of the minor salivary glands of the larynx. Am J Surg 150: 513-518.
470. Cohen MA, Batsakis JG (1968). Oncocytic tumors (oncocytomas) of minor salivary glands. Arch Otolaryngol 88: 71-73.
471. Cohen MMJr (1999). Nevoid basal cell carcinoma syndrome: molecular biology and new hypotheses. Int J Oral Maxillofac Surg 28: 216-223.
472. Cohen MMJr, Howell RE (1999). Etiology of fibrous dysplasia and McCune-Albright syndrome. Int J Oral Maxillofac Surg 28: 366-371.
473. Colby TV, Dorfman RF (1979). Malignant lymphomas involving the salivary glands. Pathol Annu 14 Pt 2: 307-324.
474. Colby TV, Koss MN, Travis WD (1995). Tumours of the Lower Respiratory Tract. 3rd ed. Armed Forces Institute of Pathology: Washington DC.
475. Coleman H, Altini M (1999). Intravascular tumour in intra-oral pleomorphic adenomas: a diagnostic and therapeutic dilemma. Histopathology 35: 439-444.
476. Coli A, Bigotti G, Bartolazzi A (1998). Malignant oncocytoma of major salivary glands. Report of a post-irradiation case. J Exp Clin Cancer Res 17: 65-70.
477. Collins BM, Jones AC (1995). Multiple granular cell tumors of the oral cavity: report of a case and review of the literature. J Oral Maxillofac Surg 53: 707-711.
478. Colmenero C, Patron M, Sierra I (1991). Acinic cell carcinoma of the salivary glands. A review of 20 new cases. J Craniomaxillofac Surg 19: 260-266.
479. Colombo F, Cursiefen C, Neukam FW, Holbach LM (2001). Orbital involvement in cherubism. Ophthalmology 108: 1884-1888.
480. Colreavy MP, Sigston E, Lacy PD, Balasubramaniam GS, Lyons BM (2001). Post-nasal space oncocytoma: a different approach to a rare tumour. J Laryngol Otol 115: 57-59.
481. Colwell AS, D'Cunha J, Maddaus MA (2001). Carney's triad paragangliomas. J Thorac Cardiovasc Surg 121: 1011-1012.
482. Compagno J, Hyams VJ (1976). Hemangiopericytoma-like intranasal tumors. A clinicopathologic study of 23 cases. Am J Clin Pathol 66: 672-683.
483. Compagno J, Wong RT (1977). Intranasal mixed tumors (pleomorphic adenomas): a clinicopathologic study of 40 cases. Am J Clin Pathol 68: 213-218.
484. Conley J, Pack GT (1974). Melanoma of the mucous membranes of the head and neck. Arch Otolaryngol 99: 315-319.
485. Conti JA, Kemeny N, Klimstra D, Minsky B, Rusch V (1994). Colon carcinoma metastatic to the trachea. Report of a case and a review of the literature. Am J Clin Oncol 17: 227-229.
486. Cook JR, Dehner LP, Collins MH, Ma Z, Morris SW, Coffin CM, Hill DA (2001). Anaplastic lymphoma kinase (ALK) expression in the inflammatory myofibroblastic tumor: a comparative immunohistochemical study. Am J Surg Pathol 25: 1364-1371.
487. Cook JR, Hill DA, Humphrey PA, Pfeifer JD, el Mofty SK (2000). Squamous cell carcinoma arising in recurrent respiratory papillomatosis with pulmonary involvement: emerging common pattern of clinical features and human papillomavirus serotype association. Mod Pathol 13: 914-918.
488. Cooper DS, Wenig BM (1996). Hyperthyroidism caused by an ectopic TSH-secreting pituitary tumor. Thyroid 6: 337-343.
489. Cooper JR, Hellquist HB, Michaels L (1992). Image analysis in the discrimination of verrucous carcinoma and squamous papilloma. J Pathol 166: 383-387.
490. Cooper JS, Cohen R, Stevens RE (1998). A comparison of staging systems for nasopharyngeal carcinoma. Cancer 83: 213-219.
491. Corenblum B, LeBlanc FE, Watanabe M (1980). Acromegaly with an adenomatous pharyngeal pituitary. JAMA 243: 1456-1457.
492. Corio RL, Goldblatt LI, Edwards PA, Hartman KS (1987). Ameloblastic carcinoma: a clinicopathologic study and assessment of eight cases. Oral Surg Oral Med Oral Pathol 64: 570-576.
493. Corio RL, Sciubba JJ, Brannon RB, Batsakis JG (1982). Epithelial-myoepithelial carcinoma of intercalated duct origin. A clinicopathologic and ultrastructural assessment of sixteen cases. Oral Surg Oral Med Oral Pathol 53: 280-287.
494. Corridan M (1956). Glycogen-rich clear-cell adenoma of the parotid gland. J Pathol Bacteriol 72: 623-626.
495. Costas A, Castro P, Martin-Granizo R, Monje F, Marron C, Amigo A (2000). Fine needle aspiration biopsy (FNAB) for lesions of the salivary glands. Br J Oral Maxillofac Surg 38: 539-542.
496. Coumbaras M, Pierot L, Felgeres AA, Boulin A, Gaillard S, Derome PJ (1999). Giant-cell tumour involving the cranial vault: imaging and treatment. Neuroradiology 41: 826-828.
497. Cox DP, Muller S, Carlson GW, Murray D (2000). Ameloblastic carcinoma ex ameloblastoma of the mandible with malignancy-associated hypercalcemia. Oral Surg Oral Med Oral Pathol Oral Radiol Endod 90: 716-722.
498. Cox SC, Walker DM (1996). Oral submucous fibrosis. A review. Aust Dent J 41: 294-299.
499. Coyas A, Eliadellis E, Anastassiades O (1983). Kaposi's Sarcoma of the larynx. J Laryngol Otol 97: 647-649.
500. Crawford RI, Tron VA, Ma R, Rivers JK (1995). Sinonasal malignant melanoma—a clinicopathologic analysis of 18 cases. Melanoma Res 5: 261-265.
501. Crissman JD, Kessis T, Shah KV, Fu YS, Stoler MH, Zarbo RJ, Weiss MA (1988). Squamous papillary neoplasia of the adult upper aerodigestive tract. Hum Pathol 19: 1387-1396.
502. Crissman JD, Sakr WA (2001). Squamous neoplasia of the upper aerodigestive tract. Intraepithelial and invasive squamous cell carcinoma. In: Head and Neck Surgical Pathology, Pilch BZ, ed., Lippincott Williams & Wilkins: Philadelphia , pp. 34-52.
503. Crissman JD, Visscher DW, Sakr W (1993). Premalignant lesions of the upper aerodigestive tract: pathologic classification. J Cell Biochem Suppl 17F: 49-56.
504. Crissman JD, Zarbo RJ (1989). Dysplasia, in situ carcinoma, and progression to invasive squamous cell carcinoma of the upper aerodigestive tract. Am J Surg Pathol 13 Suppl 1: 5-16.
505. Croitoru CM, Suarez PA, Luna MA (1999). Hybrid carcinomas of salivary glands. Report of 4 cases and review of the literature. Arch Pathol Lab Med 123: 698-702.
506. Crook T, Nicholls JM, Brooks L, O'Nions J, Allday MJ (2000). High level expression of deltaN-p63: a mechanism for the inactivation of p53 in undifferentiated nasopharyngeal carcinoma (NPC)? Oncogene 19: 3439-3444.
507. Cross JJ, Pilkington RJ, Antoun NM, Adlam DM (2000). Value of computed tomography and magnetic resonance imaging in the treatment of a calcifying epithelial odontogenic (Pindborg) tumour. Br J Oral Maxillofac Surg 38: 154-157.
508. Crotty PL, Nakhleh RE, Dehner LP (1993). Juvenile rhabdomyoma. An intermediate form of skeletal muscle tumor in children. Arch Pathol Lab Med 117: 43-47.
509. Crowell WT, Grizzle WE, Siegel AL (1982). Functional carotid paragangliomas. Biochemical, ultrastructural, and histochemical correlation with clinical symptoms. Arch Pathol Lab Med 106: 599-603.
510. Crowther JA, Colman BH (1987). Chemodectoma of the larynx. J Laryngol Otol 101: 1095-1098.
511. Cuadra-Garcia I, Proulx GM, Wu CL, Wang CC, Pilch BZ, Harris NL, Ferry JA (1999). Sinonasal lymphoma: a clinicopathologic analysis of 58 cases from the Massachusetts General Hospital. Am J Surg Pathol 23: 1356-1369.
512. Cummings BJ, Blend R, Keane T, Fitzpatrick P, Beale F, Clark R, Garrett P, Harwood A, Payne D, Rider W (1984). Primary radiation therapy for juvenile nasopharyngeal angiofibroma. Laryngoscope 94: 1599-1605.
513. Cunningham BA, Hemperly JJ, Murray BA, Prediger EA, Brackenbury R, Edelman GM (1987). Neural cell adhesion molecule: structure, immunoglobulin-like domains, cell surface modulation, and alternative RNA splicing. Science 236: 799-806.
514. Cupero TM, Thomas RW, Manning SC (2001). Desmoplastic fibroma of the maxillary sinus. Otolaryngol Head Neck Surg 125: 661-662.
515. Curtin HD, Rabinov JD (1998). Extension to the orbit from paraorbital disease. The sinuses. Radiol Clin North Am 36: 1201-13, xi.
516. Curtin HD, Williams R, Johnson J (1985). CT of perineural tumor extension: pterygopalatine fossa. AJR Am J Roentgenol 144: 163-169.
517. Cutler LS, Chaudhry AP, Topazian R (1981). Melanotic neuroectodermal tumor of infancy: an ultrastructural study, literature review, and reevaluation. Cancer 48: 257-270.
518. Da Mosto MC, Marchiori C, Rinaldo A, Ferlito A (1996). Laryngeal pleomorphic rhabdomyosarcoma. A critical review of the literature. Ann Otol Rhinol Laryngol 105: 289-294.
519. Dadas B, Alkan S, Turgut S, Basak T (2001). Primary papillary adenocarcinoma confined to the middle ear and mastoid. Eur Arch Otorhinolaryngol 258: 93-95.
520. Daffner RH, Kirks DR, Gehweiler JAJr, Heaston DK (1982). Computed tomography of fibrous dysplasia. AJR Am J Roentgenol 139: 943-948.
521. Dahiya S, Kumar R, Sarkar C, Ralte M, Sharma MC (2002). Clear cell odontogenic carcinoma: a diagnostic dilemma. Pathol Oncol Res 8: 283-285.
522. Dahl EC, Wolfson SH, Haugen JC (1981). Central odontogenic fibroma: review of literature and report of cases. J Oral Surg 39: 120-124.
523. Dahlin DC (1985). Caldwell Lecture. Giant cell tumor of bone: highlights of 407 cases. AJR Am J Roentgenol 144: 955-960.
524. Dahlkemper P, Wolcott JF, Pringle GA, Hicks ML (2000). Periapical central giant cell granuloma: a potential endodontic misdiagnosis. Oral Surg Oral Med Oral Pathol Oral Radiol Endod 90: 739-745.
525. Dahlqvist A, Carlsoo B, Hellstrom S (1986). Paraganglia of the human recurrent laryngeal nerve. Am J Otolaryngol 7: 366-369.
526. Dahm LJ, Schaefer SD, Carder HM, Vellios F (1978). Osteosarcoma of the soft tissue of the larynx: report of a case with light and electron microscopic studies. Cancer 42: 2343-2351.
527. Dal Cin P, Sciot R, Brys P, De Wever I, Dorfman H, Fletcher CD, Jonsson K, Mandahl N, Mertens F, Mitelman F, Rosai J, Rydholm A, Samson I, Tallini G, Van den Berghe H, Vanni R, Willen H (2000). Recurrent chromosome aberrations in fibrous dysplasia of the bone: a report of the CHAMP study group. CHromosomes And MorPhology. Cancer Genet Cytogenet 122: 30-32.
528. Dal Cin P, Sciot R, Fossion E, Van Damme B, Van den Berghe H (1993). Chromosome abnormalities in cementifying fibroma. Cancer Genet Cytogenet 71: 170-172.
529. Daley TD, Gardner DG, Smout MS (1984). Canalicular adenoma: not a basal cell adenoma. Oral Surg Oral Med Oral Pathol 57: 181-188.
530. Daley TD, Wysocki GP (1994). Peripheral odontogenic fibroma. Oral Surg Oral Med Oral Pathol 78: 329-336.
531. Daley TD, Wysocki GP, Pringle GA (1994). Relative incidence of odontogenic tumors and oral and jaw cysts in a Canadian population. Oral Surg Oral Med Oral Pathol 77: 276-280.
532. Dallera P, Bertoni F, Marchetti C, Bacchini P, Campobassi A (1994). Ameloblastic fibrosarcoma of the jaw: report of five cases. J Craniomaxillofac Surg 22: 349-354.
533. Damiani JM, Damiani KK, Hauck K, Hyams VJ (1981). Mucoepidermoid-adenosquamous carcinoma of the larynx and hypopharynx: a report of 21 cases and a review of the literature. Otolaryngol Head Neck Surg 89: 235-243.

534. Dammann F, Pereira P, Laniado M, Plinkert P, Lowenheim H, Claussen CD (1999). Inverted papilloma of the nasal cavity and the paranasal sinuses: using CT for primary diagnosis and follow-up. AJR Am J Roentgenol 172: 543-548.
535. Danford M, Eveson JW, Flood TR (1992). Papillary cystadenocarcinoma of the sublingual gland presenting as a ranula. Br J Oral Maxillofac Surg 30: 270-272.
536. Daou RA, Attia EL, Viloria JB (1983). Malignant fibrous histiocytomas of the head and neck. J Otolaryngol 12: 383-388.
537. Dardari R, Hinderer W, Lang D, Benider A, El Gueddari B, Joab I, Benslimane A, Khyatti M (2001). Antibody responses to recombinant Epstein-Barr virus antigens in nasopharyngeal carcinoma patients: complementary test of ZEBRA protein and early antigens p54 and p138. J Clin Microbiol 39: 3164-3170.
538. Dardick I (1995). Myoepithelioma: definitions and diagnostic criteria. Ultrastruct Pathol 19: 335-345.
539. Dardick I (1998). Mounting evidence against current histogenetic concepts for salivary gland tumorigenesis. Eur J Morphol 36 Suppl: 257-261.
540. Dardick I, Burford-Mason AP (1993). Current status of histogenetic and morphogenetic concepts of salivary gland tumorigenesis. Crit Rev Oral Biol Med 4: 639-677.
541. Dardick I, Cavell S, Boivin M, Hoppe D, Parks WR, Stinson J, Yamada S, Burns BF (1989). Salivary gland myoepithelioma variants. Histological, ultrastructural, and immunocytological features. Virchows Arch A Pathol Anat Histopathol 416: 25-42.
542. Dardick I, Daley TD, van Nostrand AW (1986). Basal cell adenoma with myoepithelial cell-derived "stroma": a new major salivary gland tumor entity. Head Neck Surg 8: 257-267.
543. Dardick I, George D, Jeans MT, Wittkuhn JF, Skimming L, Rippstein P, van Nostrand AW (1987). Ultrastructural morphology and cellular differentiation in acinic cell carcinoma. Oral Surg Oral Med Oral Pathol 63: 325-334.
544. Dardick I, Hammar SP, Scheithauer BW (1989). Ultrastructural spectrum of hemangiopericytoma: a comparative study of fetal, adult, and neoplastic pericytes. Ultrastruct Pathol 13: 111-154.
545. Dardick I, Ostrynski VL, Ekem JK, Leung R, Burford-Mason AP (1992). Immunohistochemical and ultrastructural correlates of muscle-actin expression in pleomorphic adenomas and myoepitheliomas based on comparison of formalin and methanol fixation. Virchows Arch A Pathol Anat Histopathol 421: 95-104.
546. Dardick I, Thomas MJ, van Nostrand AW (1989). Myoepithelioma—new concepts of histology and classification: a light and electron microscopic study. Ultrastruct Pathol 13: 187-224.
547. Darling MR, Schneider JW, Phillips VM (2002). Polymorphous low-grade adenocarcinoma and adenoid cystic carcinoma: a review and comparison of immunohistochemical markers. Oral Oncol 38: 641-645.
548. Datta R, Winston JS, Diaz-Reyes G, Loree TR, Myers L, Kuriakose MA, Rigual NR, Hicks WLJr (2003). Ameloblastic carcinoma: report of an aggressive case with multiple bony metastases. Am J Otolaryngol 24: 64-69.
549. Davis GL (1987). Tumours and inflammatory conditions of the ear. In: Pathology of the Head and Neck, Gnepp DR, ed., Churchill Livingstone: New York , pp. 547-583.
550. Davis G (2000). Ear - External, Middle and Temporal Bone. In: Diagnostic Surgical Pathology of the Head and Neck, Gnepp DR, ed., W.B. Saunders Ltd.: Philadelphia , pp. 681-714.
551. Davy CL, Dardick I, Hammond E, Thomas MJ (1994). Relationship of clear cell oncocytoma to mitochondrial-rich (typical) oncocytomas of parotid salivary gland. An ultrastructural study. Oral Surg Oral Med Oral Pathol 77: 469-479.
552. de Alava E, Kawai A, Healey JH, Fligman I, Meyers PA, Huvos AG, Gerald WL, Jhanwar SC, Argani P, Antonescu CR, Pardo-Mindan FJ, Ginsberg J, Womer R, Lawlor ER, Wunder J, Andrulis I, Sorensen PH, Barr FG, Ladanyi M (1998). EWS-FLI1 fusion transcript structure is an independent determinant of prognosis in Ewing's sarcoma. J Clin Oncol 16: 1248-1255.
553. de Araujo VC, de Sousa SO, Carvalho YR, de Araujo NS (2000). Application of immunohistochemistry to the diagnosis of salivary gland tumors. Appl Immunohistochem Mol Morphol 8: 195-202.
554. de Araujo VC, Martins MT, Leite KR, Gomez RS, de Araujo NS (2000). Immunohistochemical Mdm2 expression in minor salivary gland tumours and its relationship to p53 gene status. Oral Oncol 36: 67-69.
555. de Bree R, Scheeren RA, Kummer A, Tiwari RM (2002). Nasolacrimal duct obstruction caused by an oncocytoma. Rhinology 40: 165-167.
556. de Campora E, Calabrese V, Bianchi PM, Camaioni A, Corradini C (1983). Malignant hemangiopericytoma of the nasal cavity. Report of a case and review of the literature. J Laryngol Otol 97: 963-968.
557. de Graaf JH, Tamminga RY, Dam-Meiring A, Kamps WA, Timens W (1996). The presence of cytokines in Langerhans' cell histiocytosis. J Pathol 180: 400-406.
558. de Lange J, Rosenberg AJ, van den Akker HP, Koole R, Wirds JJ, van den Berg H (1999). Treatment of central giant cell granuloma of the jaw with calcitonin. Int J Oral Maxillofac Surg 28: 372-376.
559. de Lange J, van den Akker HP, Klip H (2004). Incidence and disease-free survival after surgical therapy of central giant cell granulomas of the jaw in The Netherlands: 1990-1995. Head Neck 26: 792-795.
560. De Meerleer GO, Vermeersch H, van Eijkeren M, Lemmerling M, Caemaert J, De Naeyer B, Delrue L, Moerman M, Huys J (1998). Primary sinonasal mucosal melanoma: three different therapeutic approaches to inoperable local disease or recurrence and a review of the literature. Melanoma Res 8: 449-457.
561. de Serres LM, Sie KC, Richardson MA (1995). Lymphatic malformations of the head and neck. A proposal for staging. Arch Otolaryngol Head Neck Surg 121: 577-582.
562. de Silva DC, Wright MF, Stevenson DA, Clark C, Gray ES, Holmes JD, Dean JC, Haites NE, Dunlop MG (1996). Cranial desmoid tumor associated with homozygous inactivation of the adenomatous polyposis coli gene in a 2-year-old girl with familial adenomatous polyposis. Cancer 77: 972-976.
563. de Sousa SO, Schwarzschild M, de Araujo NS, de Araujo VC (2000). Basal cell adenocarcinoma of the palate with squamous metaplasia. J Clin Pathol 53: 153-156.
564. de Souza CE, Sperling NM, da Costa SS, Yoon TH, Abdel Hamid M, de Souza RA (1989). Congenital cholesteatomas of the cerebellopontine angle. Am J Otol 10: 358-363.
565. De Stefani E, Correa P, Oreggia F, Leiva J, Rivero S, Fernandez G, Deneo-Pellegrini H, Zavala D, Fontham E (1987). Risk factors for laryngeal cancer. Cancer 60: 3087-3091.
566. De Stefani E, Oreggia F, Rivero S, Fierro L (1992). Hand-rolled cigarette smoking and risk of cancer of the mouth, pharynx, and larynx. Cancer 70: 679-682.
567. de Vathaire F, Sancho-Garnier H, de The H, Pieddeloup C, Schwaab G, Ho JH, Ellouz R, Micheau C, Cammoun M, Cachin Y, de The G (1988). Prognostic value of EBV markers in the clinical management of nasopharyngeal carcinoma (NPC): a multicenter follow-up study. Int J Cancer 42: 176-181.
568. Dehner LP (2003). Juvenile xanthogranulomas in the first two decades of life: a clinicopathologic study of 174 cases with cutaneous and extracutaneous manifestations. Am J Surg Pathol 27: 579-593.
569. Dehner LP, Chen KT (1980). Primary tumors of the external and middle ear. Benign and malignant glandular neoplasms. Arch Otolaryngol 106: 13-19.
570. Dehner LP, Mills A, Talerman A, Billman GF, Krous HF, Platz CE (1990). Germ cell neoplasms of head and neck soft tissues: a pathologic spectrum of teratomatous and endodermal sinus tumors. Hum Pathol 21: 309-318.
571. Dehner LP, Sibley RK, Sauk JJJr, Vickers RA, Nesbit ME, Leonard AS, Waite DE, Neeley JE, Ophoven J (1979). Malignant melanotic neuroectodermal tumor of infancy: a clinical, pathologic, ultrastructural and tissue culture study. Cancer 43: 1389-1410.
572. Dehner LP, Valbuena L, Perez-Atayde A, Reddick RL, Askin FB, Rosai J (1994). Salivary gland anlage tumor ("congenital pleomorphic adenoma"). A clinicopathologic, immunohistochemical and ultrastructural study of nine cases. Am J Surg Pathol 18: 25-36.
573. Dei Tos AP, Dal Cin P, Sciot R, Furlanetto A, Da Mosto MC, Giannini C, Rinaldo A, Ferlito A (1998). Synovial sarcoma of the larynx and hypopharynx. Ann Otol Rhinol Laryngol 107: 1080-1085.
574. Del Valle-Zapico A, Fernandez FF, Suarez AR, Angulo CM, Quintela JR (1998). Prognostic value of histopathologic parameters and DNA flow cytometry in squamous cell carcinoma of the pyriform sinus. Laryngoscope 108: 269-272.
575. Delattre O, Zucman J, Melot T, Garau XS, Zucker JM, Lenoir GM, Ambros PF, Sheer D, Turc-Carel C, Triche TJ, . (1994). The Ewing family of tumors—a subgroup of small-round-cell tumors defined by specific chimeric transcripts. N Engl J Med 331: 294-299.
576. Delecluse HJ, Anagnostopoulos I, Dallenbach F, Hummel M, Marafioti T, Schneider U, Huhn D, Schmidt-Westhausen A, Reichart PA, Gross U, Stein H (1997). Plasmablastic lymphomas of the oral cavity: a new entity associated with the human immunodeficiency virus infection. Blood 89: 1413-1420.
577. DeLellis RA, Lloyd RV, Heitz PU, Eng C (2004). World Health Organization Classification of Tumours. Pathology and Genetics of Tumours of Endocrine Organs. IARC Press: Lyon.
578. Delgado R, Klimstra D, Albores-Saavedra J (1996). Low grade salivary duct carcinoma. A distinctive variant with a low grade histology and a predominant intraductal growth pattern. Cancer 78: 958-967.
579. Delgado R, Vuitch F, Albores-Saavedra J (1993). Salivary duct carcinoma. Cancer 72: 1503-1512.
580. Della Torre G, Pilotti S, Donghi R, Pasquini G, Longoni A, Grandi C, Salvatori P, Pierotti MA, Rilke F (1994). Epstein-Barr virus genomes in undifferentiated and squamous cell nasopharyngeal carcinomas in Italian patients. Diagn Mol Pathol 3: 32-37.
581. DeMoura LF, Yook TS (1978). Malignant fibrous histiocytoma of the maxillary sinus. Otolaryngology 86: ORL-8.
582. Denoyelle F, Ducroz V, Roger G, Garabedian EN (1997). Nasal dermoid sinus cysts in children. Laryngoscope 107: 795-800.
583. Denton AB, Anderson DW, Berean KW (2000). Malignant epithelioid peripheral nerve sheath tumour of the pterygopalatine fossa. J Otolaryngol 29: 392-395.
584. DeRienzo DP, Greenberg SD, Fraire AE (1991). Carcinoma of the larynx. Changing incidence in women. Arch Otolaryngol Head Neck Surg 117: 681-684.
585. Derkay CS (1995). Task force on recurrent respiratory papillomas. A preliminary report. Arch Otolaryngol Head Neck Surg 121: 1386-1391.
586. Derkay CS (2001). Recurrent Papillary Fibromatosis. Laryngoscope 57-69.
587. Derkay CS, Darrow DH (2000). Recurrent respiratory papillomatosis of the larynx: current diagnosis and treatment. Otolaryngol Clin North Am 33: 1127-1142.
588. Derlacki EL, Barney PL (1976). Adenomatous tumors of the middle ear and mastoid. Laryngoscope 86: 1123-1135.
589. DeTomasi DC, Hann JR, Stewart HMJr (1985). Cherubism: report of a nonfamilial case. J Am Dent Assoc 111: 455-457.
590. Devaney KO, Ferlito A, Rinaldo A (1998). Giant cell tumor of the larynx. Ann Otol Rhinol Laryngol 107: 729-732.
591. Devaney KO, Ferlito A, Silver CE (1995). Cartilaginous tumors of the larynx. Ann Otol Rhinol Laryngol 104: 251-255.
592. Devlin J, Harrison CJ, Whitby DJ, David TJ (1990). Cartilaginous pseudocyst of the external auricle in children with atopic eczema. Br J Dermatol 122: 699-704.
593. Dhir K, Sciubba JJ, Tufano RP (2003). Ameloblastic carcinoma of the maxilla. Oral Oncol 39: 736-741.
594. Di Palma S, Corletto V, Lavarino C, Birindelli S, Pilotti S (1999). Unilateral aneuploid dedifferentiated acinic cell carcinoma associated with bilateral-low grade diploid acinic cell carcinoma of the parotid gland. Virchows Arch 434: 361-365.
595. Di Palma S, Guzzo M (1993). Malignant myoepithelioma of salivary glands: clinicopathological features of ten cases. Virchows Arch A Pathol Anat Histopathol 423: 389-396.
596. Di Palma S, Simpson RH, Skalova A, Michal M (1999). Metaplastic (infarcted) Warthin's tumour of the parotid gland: a possible consequence of fine needle aspiration biopsy. Histopathology 35: 432-438.
597. Di Sant'Agnese PA, Knowles DM (1980). Extracardiac rhabdomyoma: a clinicopathologic study and review of the literature. Cancer 46: 780-789.
598. DiCaprio MR, Murphy MJ, Camp RL (2000). Aneurysmal bone cyst of the spine with familial incidence. Spine 25: 1589-1592.

599. Dickens P, Srivastava G, Loke SL, Chan CW, Liu YT (1992). Epstein-Barr virus DNA in nasopharyngeal carcinomas from Chinese patients in Hong Kong. J Clin Pathol 45: 396-397.
600. Dickens P, Wei WI, Sham JS (1990). Osteosarcoma of the maxilla in Hong Kong Chinese postirradiation for nasopharyngeal carcinoma. A report of four cases. Cancer 66: 1924-1926.
601. Diebold J, Audouin J, Viry B, Ghandour C, Betti P, D'Ornano G (1990). Primary lymphoplasmacytic lymphoma of the larynx: a rare localization of MALT-type lymphoma. Ann Otol Rhinol Laryngol 99: 577-580.
602. Diedhiou A, Cazals-Hatem D, Rondini E, Sterkers O, Degott C, Wassef M (2001). [Sebaceous carcinoma of the submandibular gland: a case report]. Ann Pathol 21: 348-351.
603. Dietz A, Barme B, Gewelke U, Sennewald E, Heller WD, Maier H (1993). [The epidemiology of parotid tumors. A case control study]. HNO 41: 83-90.
604. DiGiuseppe JA, Corio RL, Westra WH (1996). Lymphoid infiltrates of the salivary glands: pathology, biology and clinical significance. Curr Opin Oncol 8: 232-237.
605. DiMaio SJ, DiMaio VJ, DiMaio TM, Nicastri AD, Chen CK (1980). Oncocytic carcinoma of the nasal cavity. South Med J 73: 803-806.
606. Dimery IW, Jones LA, Verjan RP, Raymond AK, Goepfert H, Hong WK (1987). Estrogen receptors in normal salivary gland and salivary gland carcinoma. Arch Otolaryngol Head Neck Surg 113: 1082-1085.
607. Dini M, Lo Russo G, Colafranceschi M (1998). So-called nasal glioma: case report with immunohistochemical study. Tumori 84: 398-402.
608. Diss TC, Wotherspoon AC, Speight P, Pan L, Isaacson PG (1995). B-cell monoclonality, Epstein Barr virus, and t(14;18) in myoepithelial sialadenitis and low-grade B-cell MALT lymphoma of the parotid gland. Am J Surg Pathol 19: 531-536.
609. Dixon WR, Ziskind J (1956). Odontogenic fibroma. Oral Surg Oral Med Oral Pathol 9: 813-816.
610. Doganay L, Bilgi S, Ozdil A, Yoruk Y, Altaner S, Kutlu K (2003). Epithelial-myoepithelial carcinoma of the lung. A case report and review of the literature. Arch Pathol Lab Med 127: e177-e180.
611. Dolcetti R, Menezes J (2003). Epstein-Barr virus and undifferentiated nasopharyngeal carcinoma: new immunobiological and molecular insights on a long-standing etiopathogenic association. Adv Cancer Res 87: 127-157.
612. Dolcetti R, Pelucchi S, Maestro R, Rizzo S, Pastore A, Boiocchi M (1991). Proto-oncogene allelic variations in human squamous cell carcinomas of the larynx. Eur Arch Otorhinolaryngol 248: 279-285.
613. Donaldson SS, Belli JA (1984). A rational clinical staging system for childhood rhabdomyosarcoma. J Clin Oncol 2: 135-139.
614. Donath K, Seifert G, Schmitz R (1972). [Diagnosis and ultrastructure of the tubular carcinoma of salivary gland ducts. Epithelial-myoepithelial carcinoma of the intercalated ducts]. Virchows Arch A Pathol Pathol Anat 356: 16-31.
615. Dong Y, Sui L, Sugimoto K, Tai Y, Tokuda M (2001). Cyclin D1-CDK4 complex, a possible critical factor for cell proliferation and prognosis in laryngeal squamous cell carcinomas. Int J Cancer 95: 209-215.
616. Dori S, Trougouboff P, David R, Buchner A (2000). Immunohistochemical evaluation of estrogen and progesterone receptors in adenoid cystic carcinoma of salivary gland origin. Oral Oncol 36: 450-453.
617. Doval DC, Rao CR, Saitha KS, Vigayakumar M, Misra S, Mani K, Bapsy PP, Kumaraswamy SV (1996). Magliant melanoma of the oral cavity: report of 14 cases from a regional cancer centre. Eur J Surg Oncol 22: 245-249.
618. Doyle DJ, Gianoli GJ, Espinola T, Miller RH (1994). Recurrent respiratory papillomatosis: juvenile versus adult forms. Laryngoscope 104: 523-527.
619. Doyle DJ, Henderson LA, LeJeune FEJr, Miller RH (1994). Changes in human papillomavirus typing of recurrent respiratory papillomatosis progressing to malignant neoplasm. Arch Otolaryngol Head Neck Surg 120: 1273-1276.
620. Doyle JL, Lamster IB, Baden E (1985). Odontogenic fibroma of the complex or WHO type. Report on six cases. J Oral Maxillofac Surg 43: 666-674.
621. Dray T, Vargas H, Weidner N, Sofferman RA (1998). Lymphoepitheliomas of the laryngohypopharynx. Am J Otolaryngol 19: 263-266.
622. Dreizen S, McCredie KB, Keating MJ, Luna MA (1983). Malignant gingival and skin "infiltrates" in adult leukemia. Oral Surg Oral Med Oral Pathol 55: 572-579.
623. Dubey P, Ha CS, Ang KK, El Naggar AK, Knapp C, Byers RM, Morrison WH (1998). Nonnasopharyngeal lymphoepithelioma of the head and neck. Cancer 82: 1556-1562.
624. Dubois J, Garel L, Grignon A, David M, Laberge L, Filiatrault D, Powell J (1998). Imaging of hemangiomas and vascular malformations in children. Acad Radiol 5: 390-400.
625. Dulguerov P, Allal AS, Calcaterra TC (2001). Esthesioneuroblastoma: a meta-analysis and review. Lancet Oncol 2: 683-690.
626. Dulguerov P, Calcaterra T (1992). Esthesioneuroblastoma: the UCLA experience 1970-1990. Laryngoscope 102: 843-849.
627. Dunkel IJ, Gerald WL, Rosenfield NS, Strong EW, Abramson DH, Ghavimi F (1998). Outcome of patients with a history of bilateral retinoblastoma treated for a second malignancy: the Memorial Sloan-Kettering experience. Med Pediatr Oncol 30: 59-62.
628. Dunlap CL (1999). Odontogenic fibroma. Semin Diagn Pathol 16: 293-296.
629. Dunlap CL, Barker BF (1984). Central odontogenic fibroma of the WHO type. Oral Surg Oral Med Oral Pathol 57: 390-394.
630. Dunphy CH, Grosso LE, Rodriquez JJ, Dunphy FR (1996). Bilateral mucosa-associated lymphoid tissue lymphomas of parotid glands: a 13-year interval. Mod Pathol 9: 560-565.
631. Duwel V, Michielssen P (1996). Primary malignant melanoma of the larynx. A case report. Acta Otorhinolaryngol Belg 50: 47-49.
632. Earl PD, Lowry JC, Sloan P (1993). Intraoral inflammatory pseudotumor. Oral Surg Oral Med Oral Pathol 76: 279-283.
633. Ebbs SR, Webb AJ (1986). Adenolymphoma of the parotid: aetiology, diagnosis and treatment. Br J Surg 73: 627-630.
634. Eden BV, Debo RF, Larner JM, Kelly MD, Levine PA, Stewart FM, Cantrell RW, Constable WC (1994). Esthesioneuroblastoma. Long-term outcome and patterns of failure—the University of Virginia experience. Cancer 73: 2556-2562.
635. Edmondson HD, Browne RM, Potts AJ (1982). Intra-oral basal cell carcinoma. Br J Oral Surg 20: 239-247.
636. Edwards PC, Bhuiya T, Kelsch RD (2003). C-kit expression in the salivary gland neoplasms adenoid cystic carcinoma, polymorphous low-grade adenocarcinoma, and monomorphic adenoma. Oral Surg Oral Med Oral Pathol Oral Radiol Endod 95: 586-593.
637. Eibling DE, Johnson JT, McCoy JPJr, Barnes EL, Syms CA, Wagner RL, Campbell J (1991). Flow cytometric evaluation of adenoid cystic carcinoma: correlation with histologic subtype and survival. Am J Surg 162: 367-372.
638. Eichhorn JH, Dickersin GR, Bhan AK, Goodman ML (1990). Sinonasal hemangiopericytoma. A reassessment with electron microscopy, immunohistochemistry, and long-term follow-up. Am J Surg Pathol 14: 856-866.
639. Eisenberg E (2000). Oral lichen planus: a benign lesion. J Oral Maxillofac Surg 58: 1278-1285.
640. El-Mofty SK, O'Leary TR, Swanson PE (1994). Malignant myoepithelioma of salivary glands: clinicopathologic and immunophenotypic features. Review of literature and report of two cases. Int J Surg Pathol 2: 133-140.
641. El Hakim IE, Uthman MA (1999). Squamous cell carcinoma and keratoacanthoma of the lower lip associated with "Goza" and "Shisha" smoking. Int J Dermatol 38: 108-110.
642. el Jabbour JN, Ferlito A (2003). Salivary gland neoplasms. In: Neoplasms of the Larynx, Ferlito A, ed., Churchill-Livingstone: Edinburgh , pp. 231-264.
643. El Labban NG, Lee KW (1983). Myofibroblasts in central giant cell granuloma of the jaws: an ultrastructural study. Histopathology 7: 907-918.
644. El Mofty S (2002). Psammomatoid and trabecular juvenile ossifying fibroma of the craniofacial skeleton: two distinct clinicopathologic entities. Oral Surg Oral Med Oral Pathol Oral Radiol Endod 93: 296-304.
645. el Mofty SK, Swanson PE, Wick MR, Miller AS (1993). Eosinophilic ulcer of the oral mucosa. Report of 38 new cases with immunohistochemical observations. Oral Surg Oral Med Oral Pathol 75: 716-722.
646. el Naggar A, Batsakis JG, Luna MA, Goepfert H, Tortoledo ME (1989). DNA content and proliferative activity of myoepitheliomas. J Laryngol Otol 103: 1192-1197.
647. El Naggar AK, Abdul-Karim FW, Hurr K, Callender D, Luna MA, Batsakis JG (1998). Genetic alterations in acinic cell carcinoma of the parotid gland determined by microsatellite analysis. Cancer Genet Cytogenet 102: 19-24.
648. El Naggar AK, Batsakis JG (1991). Carcinoid tumor of the larynx. A critical review of the literature. ORL J Otorhinolaryngol Relat Spec 53: 188-193.
649. El Naggar AK, Batsakis JG, Garcia GM, Luna ML, Goepfert H (1992). Sinonasal hemangiopericytomas. A clinicopathologic and DNA content study. Arch Otolaryngol Head Neck Surg 118: 134-137.
650. El Naggar AK, Batsakis JG, Luna MA, McLemore D, Byers RM (1990). DNA flow cytometry of acinic cell carcinomas of major salivary glands. J Laryngol Otol 104: 410-416.
651. El Naggar AK, Callender D, Coombes MM, Hurr K, Luna MA, Batsakis JG (2000). Molecular genetic alterations in carcinoma ex-pleomorphic adenoma: a putative progression model? Genes Chromosomes Cancer 27: 162-168.
652. El Naggar AK, Dinh M, Tucker S, Luna MA, Goepfert H, Hsu P, Batsakis JG (1996). Genotypic analysis of primary head and neck squamous carcinoma by combined fluorescence in situ hybridization and DNA flow cytometry. Am J Clin Pathol 105: 102-108.
653. El Naggar AK, Lovell M, Callender DL, Ordonez NG, Killary AM (1998). Concurrent cytogenetic, interphase fluorescence in situ hybridization and DNA flow cytometric analyses of a carcinoma ex-pleomorphic adenoma of parotid gland. Cancer Genet Cytogenet 107: 132-136.
654. El Naggar AK, Lovell M, Callender DL, Ordonez NG, Killary AM (1999). Cytogenetic analysis of a primary salivary gland myoepithelioma. Cancer Genet Cytogenet 113: 49-53.
655. El Naggar AK, Lovell M, Killary AM, Clayman GL, Batsakis JG (1996). A mucoepidermoid carcinoma of minor salivary gland with t(11;19)(q21;p13.1) as the only karyotypic abnormality. Cancer Genet Cytogenet 87: 29-33.
656. El Naggar AK, Lovell M, Ordonez NG, Killary AM (1998). Multiple unrelated translocations in a metastatic epimyoepithelial carcinoma of the parotid gland. Cancer Genet Cytogenet 100: 155-158.
657. El Rifai W, Rutherford S, Knuutila S, Frierson HFJr, Moskaluk CA (2001). Novel DNA copy number losses in chromosome 12q12—q13 in adenoid cystic carcinoma. Neoplasia 3: 173-178.
658. el Sayed Y, al Serhani A (1997). Lobular capillary haemangioma (pyogenic granuloma) of the nose. J Laryngol Otol 111: 941-945.
659. el Serafy S (1971). Rare benign tumors of the larynx. J Laryngol Otol 85: 837-851.
660. Elamin F, Steingrimsdottir H, Wanakulasuriya S, Johnson N, Tavassoli M (1998). Prevalence of human papillomavirus infection in premalignant and malignant lesions of the oral cavity in U.K. subjects: a novel method of detection. Oral Oncol 34: 191-197.
661. Elder EE, Xu D, Hoog A, Enberg U, Hou M, Pisa P, Gruber A, Larsson C, Backdahl M (2003). KI-67 AND hTERT Expression Can Aid in the Distinction between Malignant and Benign Pheochromocytoma and Paraganglioma. Mod Pathol 16: 246-255.
662. Elenitoba-Johnson KS, Zarate-Osorno A, Meneses A, Krenacs L, Kingma DW, Raffeld M, Jaffe ES (1998). Cytotoxic granular protein expression, Epstein-Barr virus strain type, and latent membrane protein-1 oncogene deletions in nasal T-lymphocyte/natural killer cell lymphomas from Mexico. Mod Pathol 11: 754-761.
663. Elkon D, Hightower SI, Lim ML, Cantrell RW, Constable WC (1979). Esthesioneuroblastoma. Cancer 44: 1087-1094.
664. Ellies M, Laskawi R, Arglebe C (1998). Extraglandular Warthin's tumours: clinical evaluation and long-term follow-up. Br J Oral Maxillofac Surg 36: 52-53.
665. Ellis GL (1988). "Clear cell" oncocytoma of salivary gland. Hum Pathol 19: 862-867.
666. Ellis GL (1998). Clear cell neoplasms in salivary glands: clearly a diagnostic chal-

lenge. Ann Diagn Pathol 2: 61-78.
667. Ellis GL (1999). Odontogenic ghost cell tumor. Semin Diagn Pathol 16: 288-292.
668. Ellis GL, Auclair PL (1996). Tumours of the salivary glands. 3rd ed. Armed Forces Institute of Pathology: Washington.
669. Ellis GL, Auclair PL, Gnepp DR (1991). Surgical Pathology of the Salivary Glands. WB Saunders: Philadelphia.
670. Ellis GL, Corio RL (1983). Acinic cell adenocarcinoma. A clinicopathologic analysis of 294 cases. Cancer 52: 542-549.
671. Ellis GL, Langloss JM, Heffner DK, Hyams VJ (1987). Spindle-cell carcinoma of the aerodigestive tract. An immunohistochemical analysis of 21 cases. Am J Surg Pathol 11: 335-342.
672. Ellis GL, Shmookler BM (1986). Aggressive (malignant?) epithelial odontogenic ghost cell tumor. Oral Surg Oral Med Oral Pathol 61: 471-478.
673. Ellis GL, Wiscovitch JG (1990). Basal cell adenocarcinomas of the major salivary glands. Oral Surg Oral Med Oral Pathol 69: 461-469.
674. Elzay RP (1983). Traumatic ulcerative granuloma with stromal eosinophilia (Riga-Fede's disease and traumatic eosinophilic granuloma). Oral Surg Oral Med Oral Pathol 55: 497-506.
675. Emile JF, Wechsler J, Brousse N, Boulland ML, Cologon R, Fraitag S, Voisin MC, Gaulard P, Boumsell L, Zafrani ES (1995). Langerhans' cell histiocytosis. Definitive diagnosis with the use of monoclonal antibody O10 on routinely paraffin-embedded samples. Am J Surg Pathol 19: 636-641.
676. Emley WE (1971). Giant cell tumor of the sphenoid bone. A case report and review of the literature. Arch Otolaryngol 94: 369-374.
677. Endo M, Kawabe R, Ito K, Ohmura S, Fujita K (1992). Plasma cell granuloma of the oral cavity. J Jpn Stomatol Soc 41: 136-140.
678. Eneroth CM (1964). Histological and clinical aspects of parotid tumors. Acta Otolaryngol (Stockh) Suppl 191: 1-99.
679. Eneroth CM (1971). Salivary gland tumors in the parotid gland, submandibular gland, and the palate region. Cancer 27: 1415-1418.
680. Enokihara H, Koike T, Arimura H, Aoyagi M, Watanabe K, Nakamura Y, Yamashiro K, Tsuruoka N, Tsujimoto M, Saito K, Furusawa S, Shishido H (1994). IL-5 mRNA expression in blood lymphocytes from patients with Kimura's disease and parasite infection. Am J Hematol 47: 69-73.
681. Enzinger FM, Smith BH (1976). Hemangiopericytoma. An analysis of 106 cases. Hum Pathol 7: 61-82.
682. Epivatianos A, Dimitrakopoulos J, Trigonidis G (1995). Intraoral salivary duct carcinoma: a clinicopathological study of four cases and review of the literature. Ann Dent 54: 36-40.
683. Epstein JB, Epstein JD, Le ND, Gorsky M (2001). Characteristics of oral and paraoral malignant lymphoma: a population-based review of 361 cases. Oral Surg Oral Med Oral Pathol Oral Radiol Endod 92: 519-525.
684. Erdamar B, Suoglu Y, Sirin M, Karatay C, Katircioglu S, Kiyak E (2000). Basaloid squamous cell carcinoma of the supraglottic larynx. Eur Arch Otorhinolaryngol 257: 154-157.
685. Erdheim J (1909). Über einen Hypophysentumor von ungewöhnlichem Sitz. Beitr Path Anat 46: 233-240.
686. Ereno C, Lopez JI, Grande J, Santaolalla F, Bilbao FJ (2001). Inflammatory myofibroblastic tumour of the larynx. J Laryngol Otol 115: 856-858.
687. Ereno C, Lopez JI, Sanchez JM, Bilbao FJ (2001). Papillary squamous cell carcinoma of the larynx. J Laryngol Otol 115: 164-166.
688. Ereno C, Lopez JI, Sanchez JM, Toledo JD (1994). Basaloid-squamous cell carcinoma of the larynx and hypopharynx. A clinicopathologic study of 7 cases. Pathol Res Pract 190: 186-193.
689. Eriksen C, Girdhar-Gopal H, Lowry LD (1991). Vagal paragangliomas: a report of nine cases. Am J Otolaryngol 12: 278-287.
690. Eriksson L, Hansson LG, Akesson L, Stahlberg F (2001). Simple bone cyst: a discrepancy between magnetic resonance imaging and surgical observations. Oral Surg Oral Med Oral Pathol Oral Radiol Endod 92: 694-698.
691. Ernster JA, Franquemont DW, Sweeney JP (2000). Initial report of a case of carcinosarcoma of the supraglottis. Ear Nose Throat J 79: 384-387.
692. Esmaeli B, Wang X, Youssef A, Gershenwald JE (2001). Patterns of regional and distant metastasis in patients with conjunctival melanoma: experience at a cancer center over four decades. Ophthalmology 108: 2101-2105.
693. Esnal Leal F, Garcia-Rostan y Perez GM, Garatea Crelgo J, Gorriaran Terreros M, Arzoz Sainz de Murieta E (1997). Sebaceous carcinoma of the salivary gland. Report of two cases of infrequent location. An Otorrinolaringol Ibero Am 24: 401-413.
694. Evans AT, Guthrie W (1991). Lymphoepithelioma-like carcinoma of the uvula and soft palate: a rare lesion in an unusual site. Histopathology 19: 184-186.
695. Evans HL (1984). Mucoepidermoid carcinoma of salivary glands: a study of 69 cases with special attention to histologic grading. Am J Clin Pathol 81: 696-701.
696. Evans HL, Batsakis JG (1984). Polymorphous low-grade adenocarcinoma of minor salivary glands. A study of 14 cases of a distinctive neoplasm. Cancer 53: 935-942.
697. Evans HL, Luna MA (2000). Polymorphous low-grade adenocarcinoma: a study of 40 cases with long-term follow up and an evaluation of the importance of papillary areas. Am J Surg Pathol 24: 1319-1328.
698. Evans RW, Cruickshank AH (1970). Epithelial tumours of the salivary glands. 1st ed. W.B. Saunders: Philadelphia.
699. Eversole LR, Belton CM, Hansen LS (1985). Clear cell odontogenic tumor: histochemical and ultrastructural features. J Oral Pathol 14: 603-614.
700. Eversole LR, Laipis PJ, Merrell P, Choi E (1987). Demonstration of human papillomavirus DNA in oral condyloma acuminatum. J Oral Pathol 16: 266-272.
701. Eversole LR, Leider AS, Jacobsen PL, Kidd PM (1985). Atypical histiocytic granuloma. Light microscopic, ultrastructural, and histochemical findings in an unusual pseudomalignant reactive lesion of the oral cavity. Cancer 55: 1722-1729.
702. Eversole LR, Leider AS, Strub D (1984). Radiographic characteristics of cystogenic ameloblastoma. Oral Surg Oral Med Oral Pathol 57: 572-577.
703. Eveson JW, Cawson RA (1985). Salivary gland tumours. A review of 2410 cases with particular reference to histological types, site, age and sex distribution. J Pathol 146: 51-58.
704. Eveson JW, Cawson RA (1985). Tumours of the minor (oropharyngeal) salivary glands: a demographic study of 336 cases. J Oral Pathol 14: 500-509.
705. Eveson JW, Cawson RA (1986). Warthin's tumor (cystadenolymphoma) of salivary glands. A clinicopathologic investigation of 278 cases. Oral Surg Oral Med Oral Pathol 61: 256-262.
706. Eveson JW, Cawson RA (1989). Infarcted ('infected') adenolymphomas. A clinicopathological study of 20 cases. Clin Otolaryngol 14: 205-210.
707. Eyden B (2003). Electron microscopy in the study of myofibroblastic lesions. Semin Diagn Pathol 20: 13-24.
708. Fagan JJ, Collins B, Barnes L, D'Amico F, Myers EN, Johnson JT (1998). Perineural invasion in squamous cell carcinoma of the head and neck. Arch Otolaryngol Head Neck Surg 124: 637-640.
709. Fagundes MA, Hug EB, Liebsch NJ, Daly W, Efird J, Munzenrider JE (1995). Radiation therapy for chordomas of the base of skull and cervical spine: patterns of failure and outcome after relapse. Int J Radiat Oncol Biol Phys 33: 579-584.
710. Falzon M, Isaacson PG (1991). The natural history of benign lymphoepithelial lesion of the salivary gland in which there is a monoclonal population of B cells. A report of two cases. Am J Surg Pathol 15: 59-65.
711. Fan CY, Melhem MF, Hosal AS, Grandis JR, Barnes EL (2001). Expression of androgen receptor, epidermal growth factor receptor, and transforming growth factor alpha in salivary duct carcinoma. Arch Otolaryngol Head Neck Surg 127: 1075-1079.
712. Fan CY, Wang J, Barnes EL (2000). Expression of androgen receptor and prostatic specific markers in salivary duct carcinoma: an immunohistochemical analysis of 13 cases and review of the literature. Am J Surg Pathol 24: 579-586.
713. Fanburg-Smith JC, Meis-Kindblom JM, Fante R, Kindblom LG (1998). Malignant granular cell tumor of soft tissue: diagnostic criteria and clinicopathologic correlation. Am J Surg Pathol 22: 779-794.
714. Fanburg-Smith JC, Spiro IJ, Katapuram SV, Mankin HJ, Rosenberg AE (1999). Infiltrative subcutaneous malignant fibrous histiocytoma: a comparative study with deep malignant fibrous histiocytoma and an observation of biologic behavior. Ann Diagn Pathol 3: 1-10.
715. Fang SY, Yan JJ, Ohyama M (1998). Immunohistochemistry of p53 in sinonasal inverted papilloma and associated squamous cell carcinoma. Am J Rhinol 12: 119-124.
716. Fang Y, Guan X, Guo Y, Sham J, Deng M, Liang Q, Li H, Zhang H, Zhou H, Trent J (2001). Analysis of genetic alterations in primary nasopharyngeal carcinoma by comparative genomic hybridization. Genes Chromosomes Cancer 30: 254-260.
717. Farag MM, Ghanimah SE, Ragaie A, Saleem TH (1987). Hormonal receptors in juvenile nasopharyngeal angiofibroma. Laryngoscope 97: 208-211.
718. Farchi G (1992). [Estimation of the impact of cigarette smoking reduction on mortality from tumors of the lung and larynx]. Ann Ist Super Sanita 28: 147-153.
719. Farman AG, van Wyk CW, Dreyer WP, Staz J, Thomas CJ, Louw JH, Bester D (1978). Central papillary atrophy of the tongue and denture stomatitis. J Prosthet Dent 40: 253-256.
720. Farndon PA, Del Mastro RG, Evans DG, Kilpatrick MW (1992). Location of gene for Gorlin syndrome. Lancet 339: 581-582.
721. Farr HW, Gray GFJr, Vrana M, Panio M (1973). Extracranial meningioma. J Surg Oncol 5: 411-420.
722. Fechner RE, Mills SE (1982). Verruca vulgaris of the larynx: a distinctive lesion of probable viral origin confused with verrucous carcinoma. Am J Surg Pathol 6: 357-362.
723. Fejerskov O, Krogh J (1972). The calcifying ghost cell odontogenic tumor - or the calcifying odontogenic cyst. J Oral Pathol 1: 273-287.
724. Feldman BA (1982). Rhabdomyosarcoma of the head and neck. Laryngoscope 92: 424-440.
725. Felix A, El Naggar AK, Press MF, Ordonez NG, Fonseca I, Tucker SL, Luna MA, Batsakis JG (1996). Prognostic significance of biomarkers (c-erbB-2, p53, proliferating cell nuclear antigen, and DNA content) in salivary duct carcinoma. Hum Pathol 27: 561-566.
726. Felix A, Rosa-Santos J, Mendonca ME, Torrinha F, Soares J (2002). Intracapsular carcinoma ex pleomorphic adenoma. Report of a case with unusual metastatic behaviour. Oral Oncol 38: 107-110.
727. Felix A, Rosa JC, Nunes JF, Fonseca I, Cidadao A, Soares J (2002). Hyalinizing clear cell carcinoma of salivary glands: a study of extracellular matrix. Oral Oncol 38: 364-368.
728. Felsberg GJ, Tien RD, McLendon RE (1995). Frontoethmoidal giant cell reparative granuloma. AJNR Am J Neuroradiol 16: 1551-1554.
729. Feng BJ, Huang W, Shugart YY, Lee MK, Zhang F, Xia JC, Wang HY, Huang TB, Jian SW, Huang P, Feng QS, Huang LX, Yu XJ, Li D, Chen LZ, Jia WH, Fang Y, Huang HM, Zhu JL, Liu XM, Zhao Y, Liu WQ, Deng MQ, Hu WH, Wu SX, Mo HY, Hong MF, King MC, Chen Z, Zeng YX (2002). Genome-wide scan for familial nasopharyngeal carcinoma reveals evidence of linkage to chromosome 4. Nat Genet 31: 395-399.
730. Ferlay J, Bray F, Pisani P, Parkin DM (2001). Globocan 2000: cancer incidence, mortality and prevalence worldwide. (1.0).
731. Ferlito A (1976). A pathologic and clinical study of adenosquamous carcinoma of the larynx. Report of four cases and review of the literature. Acta Otorhinolaryngol Belg 30: 379-389.
732. Ferlito A (1976). Histological classification of larynx and hypopharynx cancers and their clinical implications. Pathologic aspects of 2052 malignant neoplasms diagnosed at the ORL Department of Padua University from 1966 to 1976. Acta Otolaryngol Suppl 342: 1-88.
733. Ferlito A (1978). Primary pleomorphic liposarcoma of the larynx. J Otolaryngol 7: 161-166.
734. Ferlito A (1980). Acinic cell carcinoma of minor salivary glands. Histopathology 4: 331-343.
735. Ferlito A (1993). Neoplasms of the larynx. Churchill Livingstone: Edinburgh.
736. Ferlito A, Altavilla G, Rinaldo A, Doglioni C (1997). Basaloid squamous cell carcinoma of the larynx and hypopharynx. Ann Otol Rhinol Laryngol 106: 1024-1035.
737. Ferlito A, Antonutto G, Silvestri F (1976). Histological appearances and nuclear DNA content of verrucous squa-

mous cell carcinoma of the larynx. ORL J Otorhinolaryngol Relat Spec 38: 65-85.
738. Ferlito A, Barnes L, Rinaldo A, Gnepp DR, Milroy CM (1998). A review of neuroendocrine neoplasms of the larynx: update on diagnosis and treatment. J Laryngol Otol 112: 827-834.
739. Ferlito A, Barnes L, Wenig BM (1994). Identification, classification, treatment, and prognosis of laryngeal paraganglioma. Review of the literature and eight new cases. Ann Otol Rhinol Laryngol 103: 525-536.
740. Ferlito A, Caruso G (1991). Endolaryngeal synovial sarcoma. An update on diagnosis and treatment. ORL J Otorhinolaryngol Relat Spec 53: 116-119.
741. Ferlito A, Caruso G, Recher G (1988). Secondary laryngeal tumors. Report of seven cases with review of the literature. Arch Otolaryngol Head Neck Surg 114: 635-639.
742. Ferlito A, Devaney KO, Rinaldo A, Milroy CM, Carbone A (1996). Mucosal adenoid squamous cell carcinoma of the head and neck. Ann Otol Rhinol Laryngol 105: 409-413.
743. Ferlito A, Devaney KO, Rinaldo A, Putzi MJ (1999). Papillary squamous cell carcinoma versus verrucous squamous cell carcinoma of the head and neck. Ann Otol Rhinol Laryngol 108: 318-322.
744. Ferlito A, Friedmann J, Recher G (1985). Primary giant cell carcinoma of the larynx. A clinico-pathological study of four cases. ORL J Otorhinolaryngol Relat Spec 47: 105-112.
745. Ferlito A, Gale N, Hvala H (1981). Laryngeal salivary duct carcinoma: a light and electron microscopic study. J Laryngol Otol 95: 731-738.
746. Ferlito A, Recher G (1980). Ackerman's tumor (verrucous carcinoma) of the larynx: a clinicopathologic study of 77 cases. Cancer 46: 1617-1630.
747. Ferlito A, Recher G (1985). Chondrometaplasia of the larynx. ORL J Otorhinolaryngol Relat Spec 47: 174-177.
748. Ferlito A, Recher G (1986). Oncocytic lesions of the larynx. Arch Pathol Lab Med 245-247.
749. Ferlito A, Rinaldo A (2000). The pathology and management of subglottic cancer. Eur Arch Otorhinolaryngol 257: 168-173.
750. Ferlito A, Rinaldo A, Devaney KO, MacLennan K, Myers JN, Petruzzelli GJ, Shaha AR, Genden EM, Johnson JT, de Carvalho MB, Myers EN (2002). Prognostic significance of microscopic and macroscopic extracapsular spread from metastatic tumor in the cervical lymph nodes. Oral Oncol 38: 747-751.
751. Ferlito A, Rinaldo A, Mannara GM (1998). Is primary radiotherapy an appropriate option for the treatment of verrucous carcinoma of the head and neck? J Laryngol Otol 112: 132-139.
752. Ferlito A, Shaha AR, Rinaldo A (2002). Neuroendocrine neoplasms of the larynx: diagnosis, treatment and prognosis. ORL J Otorhinolaryngol Relat Spec 64: 108-113.
753. Ferlito A, Shaha AR, Rinaldo A (2002). The incidence of lymph node micrometastases in patients pathologically staged N0 in cancer of oral cavity and oropharynx. Oral Oncol 38: 3-5.
754. Ferlito A, Shaha AR, Silver CE, Rinaldo A, Mondin V (2001). Incidence and sites of distant metastases from head and neck cancer. ORL J Otorhinolaryngol Relat Spec 63: 202-207.
755. Fernandez PL, Cardesa A, Alos L, Pinto J, Traserra J (1995). Sinonasal teratocarcinosarcoma: an unusual neoplasm. Pathol Res Pract 191: 166-171.
756. Fernandez PL, Cardesa A, Bombi JA, Palacin A, Traserra J (1993). Malignant sinonasal epithelioid schwannoma. Virchows Arch A Pathol Anat Histopathol 423: 401-405.
757. Ferouz AS, Mohr RM, Paul P (1995). Juvenile nasopharyngeal angiofibroma and familial adenomatous polyposis: an association? Otolaryngol Head Neck Surg 113: 435-439.
758. Ferreiro JA (1994). Immunohistochemical analysis of salivary gland canalicular adenoma. Oral Surg Oral Med Oral Pathol 78: 761-765.
759. Fetsch JF, Weiss SW (1991). Observations concerning the pathogenesis of epithelioid hemangioma (angiolymphoid hyperplasia). Mod Pathol 4: 449-455.
760. Ficarra G, Prignano F, Romagnoli P (1997). Traumatic eosinophilic granuloma of the oral mucosa: a CD30+(Ki-1) lymphoproliferative disorder? Oral Oncol 33: 375-379.
761. Ficarra G, Silverman SJr, Quivey JM, Hansen LS, Giannotti K (1987). Granulocytic sarcoma (chloroma) of the oral cavity: a case with aleukemic presentation. Oral Surg Oral Med Oral Pathol 63: 709-714.
762. Fidias P, Wright C, Harris NL, Urba W, Grossbard ML (1996). Primary tracheal non-Hodgkin's lymphoma. A case report and review of the literature. Cancer 77: 2332-2338.
763. Filopoulos E, Angeli S, Daskalopoulou D, Kelessis N, Vassilopoulos P (1998). Preoperative evaluation of parotid tumours by fine needle biopsy. Eur J Surg Oncol 24: 180-183.
764. Fine SW, Li M (2003). Expression of calretinin and the alpha-subunit of inhibin in granular cell tumors. Am J Clin Pathol 119: 259-264.
765. Finkelstein SD, Tiffee JC, Bakker A, Swalsky P, Barnes L (1998). Malignant Transformation in Sinonasal Papillomas Is Closely Associated With Aberrant p53 Expression. Mol Diagn 3: 37-41.
766. Fiorella R, Di Nicola V, Resta L (1997). Epidemiological and clinical relief on hyperplastic lesions of the larynx. Acta Otolaryngol Suppl 527: 77-81.
767. Fisch U (1983). The infratemporal fossa approach for nasopharyngeal tumors. Laryngoscope 93: 36-44.
768. Fishback NF, Travis WD, Moran CA, Guinee DGJr, McCarthy WF, Koss MN (1994). Pleomorphic (spindle/giant cell) carcinoma of the lung. A clinicopathologic correlation of 78 cases. Cancer 73: 2936-2945.
769. Fisher EW, McManus TC (1994). Surgery for external auditory canal exostoses and osteomata. J Laryngol Otol 108: 106-110.
770. Fishleder A, Tubbs R, Hesse B, Levine H (1987). Uniform detection of immunoglobulin-gene rearrangement in benign lymphoepithelial lesions. N Engl J Med 316: 1118-1121.
771. Flanagan AM, Nui B, Tinkler SM, Horton MA, Williams DM, Chambers TJ (1988). The multinucleate cells in giant cell granulomas of the jaw are osteoclasts. Cancer 62: 1139-1145.
772. Flanders WD, Rothman KJ (1982). Interaction of alcohol and tobacco in laryngeal cancer. Am J Epidemiol 115: 371-379.
773. Fletcher CD (1994). Hemangiopericytoma - a dying breed? Reappraisal of an "entity" and its variants. A hypothesis. Curr Diagn Pathol 1: 19-23.
774. Fletcher CD (1995). Malignant peripheral nerve sheath tumours. Curr Top Pathol 89: 333-354.
775. Fletcher CDM, Unni K, Mertens F (2002). WHO Classification of Tumours. Pathology and Genetics of Tumours of Soft Tissue and Bone. IARC Press: Lyon.
776. Flezar M, Pogacnik A (2002). Warthin's tumour: unusual vs. common morphological findings in fine needle aspiration biopsies. Cytopathology 13: 232-241.
777. Fliss DM, Noble-Topham SE, McLachlin M, Freeman JL, Noyek AM, van Nostrand AW, Hartwick RW (1994). Laryngeal verrucous carcinoma: a clinicopathologic study and detection of human papillomavirus using polymerase chain reaction. Laryngoscope 104: 146-152.
778. Flores AD, Dickson RI, Riding K, Coy P (1986). Cancer of the nasopharynx in British Columbia. Am J Clin Oncol 9: 281-291.
779. Flynn MB, Maguire S, Martinez S, Tesmer T (1999). Primary squamous cell carcinoma of the parotid gland: the importance of correct histological diagnosis. Ann Surg Oncol 6: 768-770.
780. Folpe AL, Chand EM, Goldblum JR, Weiss SW (2001). Expression of Fli-1, a nuclear transcription factor, distinguishes vascular neoplasms from potential mimics. Am J Surg Pathol 25: 1061-1066.
781. Folpe AL, Veikkola T, Valtola R, Weiss SW (2000). Vascular endothelial growth factor receptor-3 (VEGFR-3): a marker of vascular tumors with presumed lymphatic differentiation, including Kaposi's sarcoma, kaposiform and Dabska-type hemangioendotheliomas, and a subset of angiosarcomas. Mod Pathol 13: 180-185.
782. Fonseca I, Felix A, Soares J (1997). Cell proliferation in salivary gland adenocarcinomas with myoepithelial participation. A study of 78 cases. Virchows Arch 430: 227-232.
783. Fonseca I, Felix A, Soares J (2000). Dedifferentiation in salivary gland carcinomas. Am J Surg Pathol 24: 469-471.
784. Fonseca I, Soares J (1993). Epithelial-myoepithelial carcinoma of the salivary glands. A study of 22 cases. Virchows Arch A Pathol Anat Histopathol 422: 389-396.
785. Fonseca I, Soares J (1996). Basal cell adenocarcinoma of minor salivary and seromucous glands of the head and neck region. Semin Diagn Pathol 13: 128-137.
786. Foote FW, Frazell EL (1953). Tumors of the major salivary glands. Cancer 6: 1065-1133.
787. Forastiere A, Koch W, Trotti A, Sidransky D (2001). Head and neck cancer. N Engl J Med 345: 1890-1900.
788. Fornelli A, Eusebi V, Pasquinelli G, Quattrone P, Rosai J (2001). Merkel cell carcinoma of the parotid gland associated with Warthin tumour: report of two cases. Histopathology 39: 342-346.
789. Forssell K, Forssell H, Happonen RP, Neva M (1988). Simple bone cyst. Review of the literature and analysis of 23 cases. Int J Oral Maxillofac Surg 17: 21-24.
790. Foss RD, Ellis GL, Auclair PL (1996). Salivary gland cystadenocarcinomas. A clinicopathologic study of 57 cases. Am J Surg Pathol 20: 1440-1447.
791. Foucar E, Rosai J, Dorfman R (1990). Sinus histiocytosis with massive lymphadenopathy (Rosai-Dorfman disease): review of the entity. Semin Diagn Pathol 7: 19-73.
792. Foulsham CK, Snyder GGI, Carpenter RJI (1981). Papillary cystadenoma lymphomatosum of the larynx. Otolaryngol Head Neck Surg 89: 960-964.
793. Fouret P, Dabit D, Sibony M, Alili D, Commo F, Saint-Guily JL, Callard P (1995). Expression of p53 protein related to the presence of human papillomavirus infection in precancer lesions of the larynx. Am J Pathol 146: 599-604.
794. Fracchiolla NS, Pignataro L, Capaccio P, Trecca D, Boletini A, Ottaviani A, Polli E, Maiolo AT, Neri A (1995). Multiple genetic lesions in laryngeal squamous cell carcinomas. Cancer 75: 1292-1301.
795. Fradis M, Rosenman D, Podoshin L, Ben-David Y, Misslevitch A (1988). Steroid therapy for plasma cell granuloma of the larynx. Ear Nose Throat J 67: 588-564.
796. Franceschi S, Bidoli E, Herrero R, Munoz N (2000). Comparison of cancers of the oral cavity and pharynx worldwide: etiological clues. Oral Oncol 36: 106-115.
797. Franceschi S, Talamini R, Barra S, Baron AE, Negri E, Bidoli E, Serraino D, La Vecchia C (1990). Smoking and drinking in relation to cancers of the oral cavity, pharynx, larynx, and esophagus in northern Italy. Cancer Res 50: 6502-6507.
798. Franchi A, Gallo O, Boddi V, Santucci M (1996). Prediction of occult neck metastases in laryngeal carcinoma: role of proliferating cell nuclear antigen, MIB-1, and E-cadherin immunohistochemical determination. Clin Cancer Res 2: 1801-1808.
799. Franchi A, Gallo O, Santucci M (1999). Clinical relevance of the histological classification of sinonasal intestinal-type adenocarcinomas. Hum Pathol 30: 1140-1145.
800. Franchi A, Massi D, Baroni G, Santucci M (2003). CDX-2 Homeobox Gene Expression. Am J Surg Pathol 27: 1390-1391.
801. Franchi A, Moroni M, Massi D, Paglierani M, Santucci M (2002). Sinonasal undifferentiated carcinoma, nasopharyngeal-type undifferentiated carcinoma, and keratinizing and nonkeratinizing squamous cell carcinoma express different cytokeratin patterns. Am J Surg Pathol 26: 1597-1604.
802. Francioso F, Carinci F, Tosi L, Scapoli L, Pezzetti F, Passerella E, Evangelisti R, Pastore A, Pelucchi S, Piattelli A, Rubini C, Fioroni M, Carinci P, Volinia S (2002). Identification of differentially expressed genes in human salivary gland tumors by DNA microarrays. Mol Cancer Ther 1: 533-538.
803. Franklin CD, Pindborg JJ (1976). The calcifying epithelial odontogenic tumor. A review and analysis of 113 cases. Oral Surg Oral Med Oral Pathol 42: 753-765.
804. Franquemont DW, Fechner RE, Mills SE (1991). Histologic classification of sinonasal intestinal-type adenocarcinoma. Am J Surg Pathol 15: 368-375.
805. Franquemont DW, Mills SE (1993). Plasmacytoid monomorphic adenoma of salivary glands. Absence of myogenous differentiation and comparison to spindle cell myoepithelioma. Am J Surg Pathol 17: 146-153.
806. Franzen A, Schmid S, Pfaltz M (1999). [Primary small cell carcinomas and metastatic disease in the head and neck]. HNO 47: 912-917.
807. Freedman HM, DeSanto LW, Devine KD, Weiland LH (1973). Malignant melanoma of the nasal cavity and paranasal sinuses. Arch Otolaryngol 97: 322-325.
808. Freedman PD, Lumerman H (1983).

Lobular carcinoma of intraoral minor salivary gland origin. Report of twelve cases. Oral Surg Oral Med Oral Pathol 56: 157-166.
809. Freeman C, Berg JW, Cutler SJ (1972). Occurrence and prognosis of extranodal lymphomas. Cancer 29: 252-260.
810. Fregnani ER, Pires FR, Falzoni R, Lopes MA, Vargas PA (2003). Lipomas of the oral cavity: clinical findings, histological classification and proliferative activity of 46 cases. Int J Oral Maxillofac Surg 32: 49-53.
811. Freier K, Joos S, Flechtenmacher C, Devens F, Benner A, Bosch FX, Lichter P, Hofele C (2003). Tissue microarray analysis reveals site-specific prevalence of oncogene amplifications in head and neck squamous cell carcinoma. Cancer Res 63: 1179-1182.
812. Freije JE, Beatty TW, Campbell BH, Woodson BT, Schultz CJ, Toohill RJ (1996). Carcinoma of the larynx in patients with gastroesophageal reflux. Am J Otolaryngol 17: 386-390.
813. Freimark B, Fantozzi R, Bone R, Bordin G, Fox R (1989). Detection of clonally expanded salivary gland lymphocytes in Sjogren's syndrome. Arthritis Rheum 32: 859-869.
814. Friedman CD, Costantino PD, Teitelbaum B, Berktold RE, Sisson GASr (1990). Primary extracranial meningiomas of the head and neck. Laryngoscope 100: 41-48.
815. Friedman M, Venkatesan TK, Caldarelli DD (1996). Intralesional vinblastine for treating AIDS-associated Kaposi's sarcoma of the oropharynx and larynx. Ann Otol Rhinol Laryngol 105: 272-274.
816. Friedrich RE, Bartel-Friedrich S, Lobeck H, Niedobitek G, Arps H (2000). Epstein-Barr virus DNA, intermediate filaments and epithelial membrane antigen in nasopharyngeal carcinoma. Anticancer Res 20: 4909-4916.
817. Friedrich RE, Giese M, Mautner VF, Schmelzle R, Scheuer HA (2002). [Abnormalities of the maxillary sinus in type 1 neurofibromatosis]. Mund Kiefer Gesichtschir 6: 363-367.
818. Frierson HFJr, El Naggar AK, Welsh JB, Sapinoso LM, Su AI, Cheng J, Saku T, Moskaluk CA, Hampton GM (2002). Large scale molecular analysis identifies genes with altered expression in salivary adenoid cystic carcinoma. Am J Pathol 161: 1315-1323.
819. Frierson HFJr, Mills SE, Fechner RE, Taxy JB, Levine PA (1986). Sinonasal undifferentiated carcinoma. An aggressive neoplasm derived from schneiderian epithelium and distinct from olfactory neuroblastoma. Am J Surg Pathol 10: 771-779.
820. Fries JW (1957). The roentgen features of fibrous dysplasia of the skull and facial bones: a critical analysis of thirty-nine pathologically proven cases. AJR Am J Roentgenol 77: 71-87.
821. Fritz A, Percy C, Jack A, Shanmugaratnam K, Sobin LH, Parkin DM, Whelan S (2000). International Classification of Diseases for Oncology. 3rd ed. World Health Organization: Geneva.
822. Frodel JL, Larrabee WF, Raisis J (1989). The nasal dermoid. Otolaryngol Head Neck Surg 101: 392-396.
823. Fu YS, Perzin KH (1974). Non-epithelial tumors of the nasal cavity, paranasal sinuses, and nasopharynx: A clinicopathologic study. I. General features and vascular tumors. Cancer 33: 1275-1288.
824. Fu YS, Perzin KH (1975). Nonepithelial tumors of the nasal cavity, paranasal sinuses, and nasopharynx: a clinicopathologic study. IV. Smooth muscle tumors (leiomyoma, leiomyosarcoma). Cancer 35: 1300-1308.
825. Fu YS, Perzin KH (1976). Nonepithelial tumors of the nasal cavity paranasal sinuses, and nasopharynx: a clinicopathologic study. V. Skeletal muscle tumors (rhabdomyoma and rhabdomyosarcoma). Cancer 37: 364-376.
826. Fu YS, Perzin KH (1976). Nonepithelial tumors of the nasal cavity, paranasal sinuses, and nasopharynx. A clinicopathologic study. VI. Fibrous tissue tumors (fibroma, fibromatosis, fibrosarcoma). Cancer 37: 2912-2928.
827. Fu YS, Perzin KH (1978). Nonepithelial tumors of the nasal cavity, paranasal sinuses and nasopharynx. A clinicopathologic study. IX. Plasmacytomas. Cancer 42: 2399-2406.
828. Fujieda S, Lee K, Sunaga H, Tsuzuki H, Ikawa H, Fan GK, Imanaka M, Takenaka H, Saito H (1999). Staining of interleukin-10 predicts clinical outcome in patients with nasopharyngeal carcinoma. Cancer 85: 1439-1445.
829. Fujii M, Kumanomidou H, Ohno Y, Kanzaki J (1995). Acinic cell carcinoma of maxillary sinus. Rhinology 33: 177-179.
830. Fujii M, Yamashita T, Ishiguro R, Tashiro M, Kameyama K (2002). Significance of epidermal growth factor receptor and tumor associated tissue eosinophilia in the prognosis of patients with nasopharyngeal carcinoma. Auris Nasus Larynx 29: 175-181.
831. Fujino K, Ito J, Kanaji M, Shiomi Y, Saiga T (1995). Adenosquamous carcinoma of the larynx. Am J Otolaryngol 16: 115-118.
832. Fujitani T, Takahara T, Hattori H, Imajo Y, Ogasawara H (1984). Radiochemotherapy for non-Hodgkin's lymphoma in palatine tonsil. Cancer 54: 1288-1292.
833. Fukunaga M, Miyazawa Y, Harada T, Ushigome S, Ishikawa E (1995). Yolk sac tumour of the ear. Histopathology 27: 563-567.
834. Fukunaga M, Ushigome S, Nomura K, Ishikawa E (1995). Solitary fibrous tumor of the nasal cavity and orbit. Pathol Int 45: 952-957.
835. Funasaka Y, Boulton T, Cobb M, Yarden Y, Fan B, Lyman SD, Williams DE, Anderson DM, Zakut R, Mishima Y, Halaban R (1992). c-Kit-kinase induces a cascade of protein tyrosine phosphorylation in normal human melanocytes in response to mast cell growth factor and stimulates mitogen-activated protein kinase but is down-regulated in melanomas. Mol Biol Cell 3: 197-209.
836. Furlong MA, Fanburg-Smith JC (2001). Pleomorphic rhabdomyosarcoma in children: four cases in the pediatric age group. Ann Diagn Pathol 5: 199-206.
837. Furlong MA, Mentzel T, Fanburg-Smith JC (2001). Pleomorphic rhabdomyosarcoma in adults: a clinicopathologic study of 38 cases with emphasis on morphologic variants and recent skeletal muscle-specific markers. Mod Pathol 14: 595-603.
838. Furukawa M, Suzuki H, Matsuura K, Takahashi E, Suzuki H, Tezuka F (2001). Carcinoma ex pleomorphic adenoma of the palatal minor salivary gland with extension into the nasopharynx. Auris Nasus Larynx 28: 279-281.
839. Furuta Y, Shinohara T, Sano K, Nagashima K, Inoue K, Tanaka K, Inuyama Y (1991). Molecular pathologic study of human papillomavirus infection in inverted papilloma and squamous cell carcinoma of the nasal cavities and paranasal sinuses. Laryngoscope 101: 79-85.
840. Fusconi M, Magliulo G, Della Rocca C, Marcotullio D, Suriano M, de Vincentiis M (2002). Leiomyosarcoma of the sinonasal tract: a case report and literature review. Am J Otolaryngol 23: 108-111.
841. Futrell JW, Bennett SH, Hoye RC, Roth JA, Ketcham AS (1971). Predicting survival in cancer of the larynx or hypopharynx. Am J Surg 122: 451-457.
842. Gaffey MJ, Frierson HF, Weiss LM, Barber CM, Baber GB, Stoler MH (1996). Human papillomavirus and Epstein-Barr virus in sinonasal Schneiderian papillomas. An in situ hybridization and polymerase chain reaction study. Am J Clin Pathol 106: 475-482.
843. Gaffey MJ, Mills SE, Boyd JC (1994). Aggressive papillary tumor of middle ear/temporal bone and adnexal papillary cystadenoma. Manifestations of von Hippel-Lindau disease. Am J Surg Pathol 18: 1254-1260.
844. Gaffey MJ, Mills SE, Fechner RE, Intemann SR, Wick MR (1988). Aggressive papillary middle-ear tumor. A clinicopathologic entity distinct from middle-ear adenoma. Am J Surg Pathol 12: 790-797.
845. Galanis E, Frytak S, Lloyd RV (1997). Extrapulmonary small cell carcinoma. Cancer 79: 1729-1736.
846. Gale N, Kambic V, Michaels L, Cardesa A, Hellquist H, Zidar N, Poljak M (2000). The Ljubljana classification: a practical strategy for the diagnosis of laryngeal precancerous lesions. Adv Anat Pathol 7: 240-251.
847. Gale N, Kambic V, Poljak M, Cor A, Velkavrh D, Mlacak B (2000). Chromosomes 7,17 polysomies and overexpression of epidermal growth factor receptor and p53 protein in epithelial hyperplastic laryngeal lesions. Oncology 58: 117-125.
848. Gale N, Poljak M, Kambic V, Ferluga D, Fischinger J (1994). Laryngeal papillomatosis: molecular, histopathological, and clinical evaluation. Virchows Arch 425: 291-295.
849. Galera-Ruiz H, Villar-Rodriguez JL, Sanchez-Calzado JA, Martin-Mora J, Ruiz-Carmona E (2001). Sinonasal neuroendocrine carcinoma presenting as a nasopharyngeal mass. Otolaryngol Head Neck Surg 124: 475-476.
850. Gallagher JC, Puzon BQ (1969). Oncocytic lesions of the larynx. Ann Otol Rhinol Laryngol 78: 307-318.
851. Gallivan MV, Chun B, Rowden G, Lack EE (1979). Laryngeal paraganglioma. Case report with ultrastructural analysis and literature review. Am J Surg Pathol 3: 85-92.
852. Gallo A, de Vincentiis M, Della Rocca C, Moi R, Simonelli M, Minni A, Shaha AR (2001). Evolution of precancerous laryngeal lesions: a clinicopathologic study with long-term follow-up on 259 patients. Head Neck 23: 42-47.
853. Gallo O, Bianchi S, Giannini A, Boccuzzi S, Calzolari A, Fini-Storchi O (1994). Lack of detection of human papillomavirus (HPV) in transformed laryngeal keratoses by in situ hybridization (ISH) technique. Acta Otolaryngol 114: 213-217.
854. Gallo O, Bianchi S, Giannini A, Gallina E, Libonati GA, Fini-Storchi O (1991). Correlations between histopathological and biological findings in nasopharyngeal carcinoma and its prognostic significance. Laryngoscope 101: 487-493.
855. Gallo O, Franchi A, Fini-Storchi I, Cilento G, Boddi V, Boccuzzi S, Urso C (1998). Prognostic significance of c-erbB-2 oncoprotein expression in intestinal-type adenocarcinoma of the sinonasal tract. Head Neck 20: 224-231.
856. Gallo O, Graziani P, Fini-Storchi O (1993). Undifferentiated carcinoma of the nose and paranasal sinuses. An immunohistochemical and clinical study. Ear Nose Throat J 72: 588-590, 593-5.
857. Gallo O, Santucci M, Calzolari A, Storchi OF (1994). Epstein-Barr virus (EBV) infection and undifferentiated carcinoma of the parotid gland in Caucasian patients. Acta Otolaryngol 114: 572-575.
858. Gangopadhyay K, Mahasin ZZ, Kfoury H, Ashraf Ali M (1997). Inflammatory myofibroblastic tumour of the tonsil. J Laryngol Otol 111: 880-882.
859. Gao Y, Di P, Peng X, Yu G, Sun K (2002). Mucinous adenocarcinoma of salivary glands. Zhonghua Kou Qiang Yi Xue Za Zhi 37: 356-358.
860. Garden AS, Weber RS, Morrison WH, Ang KK, Peters LJ (1995). The influence of positive margins and nerve invasion in adenoid cystic carcinoma of the head and neck treated with surgery and radiation. Int J Radiat Oncol Biol Phys 32: 619-626.
861. Gardner DG (1977). Peripheral ameloblastoma: a study of 21 cases, including 5 reported as basal cell carcinoma of the gingiva. Cancer 39: 1625-1633.
862. Gardner DG (1982). The peripheral odontogenic fibroma: an attempt at clarification. Oral Surg Oral Med Oral Pathol 54: 40-48.
863. Gardner DG (1996). Central odontogenic fibroma current concepts. J Oral Pathol Med 25: 556-561.
864. Gardner DG, Bell ME, Wesley RK, Wysocki GP (1980). Acinic cell tumors of minor salivary glands. Oral Surg Oral Med Oral Pathol 50: 545-551.
865. Gardner DG, Corio RL (1984). Plexiform unicystic ameloblastoma. A variant of ameloblastoma with a low-recurrence rate after enucleation. Cancer 53: 1730-1735.
866. Garlick JA, Taichman LB (1991). Human papillomavirus infection of the oral mucosa. Am J Dermatopathol 13: 386-395.
867. Garrido A, Humphrey G, Squire RS, Nishikawa H (2000). Sialoblastoma. Br J Plast Surg 53: 697-699.
868. Garrington GE, Scofield HH, Cornyn J, Hooker SP (1967). Osteosarcoma of the jaws. Analysis of 56 cases. Cancer 20: 377-391.
869. Gaughan RK, Olsen KD, Lewis JE (1992). Primary squamous cell carcinoma of the parotid gland. Arch Otolaryngol Head Neck Surg 118: 798-801.
870. Gebhart M, Vandeweyer E, Nemec E (1998). Paget's disease of bone complicated by giant cell tumor. Clin Orthop 187-193.
871. Gee MS, Kliewer KE, Hinton DR (1992). Nucleolar organizer regions in paragangliomas of the head and neck. Arch Otolaryngol Head Neck Surg 118: 380-383.
872. Genden EM, Ferlito A, Bradley PJ, Rinaldo A, Scully C (2003). Neck disease and distant metastases. Oral Oncol 39: 207-212.
873. Geoffray A, Lee YY, Jing BS, Wallace S (1984). Extracranial meningiomas of the head and neck. AJNR Am J Neuroradiol 5: 599-604.
874. George CD, Ng YY, Hall-Craggs MA, Jones BM (1991). Parotid haemangioma in infants: MR imaging at 1.5T. Pediatr Radiol 21: 483-485.

875. Germano A, Caruso G, Caffo M, Galatioto S, Belvedere M, Cardia E (1998). Temporal osteoclastoma: an exceptional lesion in infancy. Childs Nerv Syst 14: 213-217.

876. Gerughty RM, Hennigar GR, Brown FM (1968). Adenosquamous carcinoma of the nasal, oral and laryngeal cavities. A clinicopathologic survey of ten cases. Cancer 22: 1140-1155.

877. Gerughty RM, Scofield HH, Brown FM, Hennigar GR (1969). Malignant mixed tumors of salivary gland origin. Cancer 24: 471-486.

878. Geurts JM, Schoenmakers EF, Roijer E, Astrom AK, Stenman G, Van de Ven WJ (1998). Identification of NFIB as recurrent translocation partner gene of HMGIC in pleomorphic adenomas. Oncogene 16: 865-872.

879. Geurts JM, Schoenmakers EF, Roijer E, Stenman G, Van de Ven WJ (1997). Expression of reciprocal hybrid transcripts of HMGIC and FHIT in a pleomorphic adenoma of the parotid gland. Cancer Res 57: 13-17.

880. Ghadially FN (1985). Diagnostic Electron Microscopy of Tumours. 2nd ed. Butterworths: London.

881. Ghadially FN (2003). Keratoacanthoma. In: Fitzpatricks's Dermatology in General Medicine, Freedberg IM, Eisen AZ, Wolff K, Austen KF, Goldsmith LA, Katz SI, eds., McGraw-Hill: New York , pp. 766-772.

882. Ghandur-Mnaymneh L (1984). Multinodular oncocytoma of the parotid gland: a benign lesion simulating malignancy. Hum Pathol 15: 485-486.

883. Giannini A, Bianchi S, Messerini L, Gallo O, Gallina E, Asprella Libonati G, Olmi P, Zampi G (1991). Prognostic significance of accessory cells and lymphocytes in nasopharyngeal carcinoma. Pathol Res Pract 187: 496-502.

884. Giannoni C, El Naggar AK, Ordonez NG, Tu ZN, Austin J, Luna MA, Batsakis JG (1995). c-erbB-2/neu oncogene and Ki-67 analysis in the assessment of palatal salivary gland neoplasms. Otolaryngol Head Neck Surg 112: 391-398.

885. Giardiello FM, Hamilton SR, Krush AJ, Offerhaus JA, Booker SV, Petersen GM (1993). Nasopharyngeal angiofibroma in patients with familial adenomatous polyposis. Gastroenterology 105: 1550-1552.

886. Gibas Z, Miettinen M (1992). Recurrent parapharyngeal rhabdomyoma. Evidence of neoplastic nature of the tumor from cytogenetic study. Am J Surg Pathol 16: 721-728.

887. Gibbons MD, Manne U, Carroll WR, Peters GE, Weiss HL, Grizzle WE (2001). Molecular differences in mucoepidermoid carcinoma and adenoid cystic carcinoma of the major salivary glands. Laryngoscope 111: 1373-1378.

888. Gillison ML, Koch WM, Capone RB, Spafford M, Westra WH, Wu L, Zahurak ML, Daniel RW, Viglione M, Symer DE, Shah KV, Sidransky D (2000). Evidence for a causal association between human papillomavirus and a subset of head and neck cancers. J Natl Cancer Inst 92: 709-720.

889. Gimenez-Roqueplo AP, Favier J, Rustin P, Mourad JJ, Plouin PF, Corvol P, Rotig A, Jeunemaitre X (2001). The R22X mutation of the SDHD gene in hereditary paraganglioma abolishes the enzymatic activity of complex II in the mitochondrial respiratory chain and activates the hypoxia pathway. Am J Hum Genet 69: 1186-1197.

890. Ginsberg SS, Buzaid AC, Stern H,

Carter D (1992). Giant cell carcinoma of the lung. Cancer 70: 606-610.

891. Giunta JL, Kaplan MA (1990). Peripheral, soft tissue odontomas. Two case reports. Oral Surg Oral Med Oral Pathol 69: 406-411.

892. Glas AS, Hollema H, Nap RE, Plukker JT (2002). Expression of estrogen receptor, progesterone receptor, and insulin-like growth factor receptor-1 and of MIB-1 in patients with recurrent pleomorphic adenoma of the parotid gland. Cancer 94: 2211-2216.

893. Gleeson MJ, Bennett MH, Cawson RA (1986). Lymphomas of salivary glands. Cancer 58: 699-704.

894. Glenner GG, Grimley PM (1974). Tumors of the extra- adrenal paraganglion system (including chemoreceptors). 2nd ed. Armed Forces Institute of Pathology: Washington, DC.

895. Gloria-Cruz TI, Schachern PA, Paparella MM, Adams GL, Fulton SE (2000). Metastases to temporal bones from primary nonsystemic malignant neoplasms. Arch Otolaryngol Head Neck Surg 126: 209-214.

896. Gnepp DR (1983). Sebaceous neoplasms of salivary gland origin: a review. Pathol Annu 18 Pt 1: 71-102.

897. Gnepp DR (1991). Small cell neuroendocrine carcinoma of the larynx. A critical review of the literature. ORL J Otorhinolaryngol Relat Spec 53: 210-219.

898. Gnepp DR (1993). Malignant mixed tumors of the salivary glands: a review. Pathol Annu 28 Pt 1: 279-328.

899. Gnepp DR (2001). Diagnostic Surgical Pathology of the Head and Neck. W.B. Saunders: Philadelphia.

900. Gnepp DR, Brandwein MS, Henley JD (2001). Salivary and lacrymal glands. In: Diagnostic Surgical Pathology of the Head and Neck, Gnepp DR, Saunders WB, eds., New York , pp. 408-429.

901. Gnepp DR, Brannon R (1984). Sebaceous neoplasms of salivary gland origin. Report of 21 cases. Cancer 53: 2155-2170.

902. Gnepp DR, Corio RL, Brannon RB (1986). Small cell carcinoma of the major salivary glands. Cancer 58: 705-714.

903. Gnepp DR, Henley J, Weiss S, Heffner D (1996). Desmoid fibromatosis of the sinonasal tract and nasopharynx. A clinicopathologic study of 25 cases. Cancer 78: 2572-2579.

904. Gnepp DR, Rader WR, Cramer SF, Cook LL, Sciubba J (1987). Accuracy of frozen section diagnosis of the salivary gland. Otolaryngol Head Neck Surg 96: 325-330.

905. Gnepp DR, Schroeder W, Heffner D (1989). Synchronous tumors arising in a single major salivary gland. Cancer 63: 1219-1224.

906. Gnepp DR, Vogler C, Sotelo-Avila C, Kielmovitch IH (1990). Focal mucinosis of the upper aerodigestive tract in children. Hum Pathol 21: 856-858.

907. Gnepp DR, Wick MR (1990). Small cell carcinoma of the major salivary glands. An immunohistochemical study. Cancer 66: 185-192.

908. Go C, Schwartz MR, Donovan DT (2003). Molecular transformation of recurrent respiratory papillomatosis: viral typing and p53 overexpression. Ann Otol Rhinol Laryngol 112: 298-302.

909. Goedert JJ (2000). The epidemiology of acquired immunodeficiency syndrome malignancies. Semin Oncol 27: 390-401.

910. Goel MM, Agrawal SP, Srivastava AN (2003). Salivary duct carcinoma of the larynx: report of a rare case. Ear Nose Throat J 82: 371-373.

911. Gogas J, Markopoulos C, Karydakis V, Gogas G, Delladetsima J (1999). Carcinosarcoma of the submandibular salivary gland. Eur J Surg Oncol 25: 333-335.

912. Goldman JL, Lawson W, Zak FG, Roffman JD (1972). The presence of melanocytes in the human larynx. Laryngoscope 82: 824-835.

913. Goldman RL, Klein HZ (1972). Glycogen-rich adenoma of the parotid gland. An uncommon benign clear-cell tumor resembling certain clear-cell carcinomas of salivary origin. Cancer 30: 749-754.

914. Goldman RL, Perzik SL (1969). Infantile hemangioma of the parotid gland; a clinicopathological study of 15 cases. Arch Otolaryngol 90: 605-608.

915. Goldman RL, Weidner N (1993). Pure squamous cell carcinoma of the larynx with cervical nodal metastasis showing rhabdomyosarcomatous differentiation. Clinical, pathologic, and immunohistochemical study of a unique example of divergent differentiation. Am J Surg Pathol 17: 415-421.

916. Goldsmith DB, West TM, Morton R (2002). HLA associations with nasopharyngeal carcinoma in Southern Chinese: a meta-analysis. Clin Otolaryngol 27: 61-67.

917. Goldstein G, Parker FP, Hugh GS (1976). Ameloblastic sarcoma: pathogenesis and treatment with chemotherapy. Cancer 37: 1673-1678.

918. Golledge J, Fisher C, Rhys-Evans PH (1995). Head and neck liposarcoma. Cancer 76: 1051-1058.

919. Gollin SM, Storto PD, Malone PS, Barnes L, Washington JA, Chidambaram A, Janecka IP (1992). Cytogenetic abnormalities in an ossifying fibroma from a patient with bilateral retinoblastoma. Genes Chromosomes Cancer 4: 146-152.

920. Gomez-Roman JJ, Ocejo-Vinyals G, Sanchez-Velasco P, Nieto EH, Leyva-Cobian F, Val-Bernal JF (2000). Presence of human herpesvirus-8 DNA sequences and overexpression of human IL-6 and cyclin D1 in inflammatory myofibroblastic tumor (inflammatory pseudotumor). Lab Invest 80: 1121-1126.

921. Goode RK, Auclair PL, Ellis GL (1998). Mucoepidermoid carcinoma of the major salivary glands: clinical and histopathologic analysis of 234 cases with evaluation of grading criteria. Cancer 82: 1217-1224.

922. Goode RK, Corio RL (1988). Oncocytic adenocarcinoma of salivary glands. Oral Surg Oral Med Oral Pathol 65: 61-66.

923. Goodnight JW, Wang MB, Sercarz JA, Fu YS (1996). Extranodal Rosai-Dorfman disease of the head and neck. Laryngoscope 106: 253-256.

924. Goodstein ML, Eisele DW, Hyams VJ, Kashima HK (1990). Multiple synchronous granular cell tumors of the upper aerodigestive tract. Otolaryngol Head Neck Surg 103: 664-668.

925. Gordon A, McManus A, Anderson J, Fisher C, Abe S, Nojima T, Pritchard-Jones K, Shipley J (2003). Chromosomal imbalances in pleomorphic rhabdomyosarcomas and identification of the alveolar rhabdomyosarcoma-associated PAX3-FOXO1A fusion gene in one case. Cancer Genet Cytogenet 140: 73-77.

926. Gorenstein A, Neel HBI, Weiland LH, Devine KD (1980). Sarcomas of the larynx.

Arch Otolaryngol 106: 8-12.

927. Gorgoulis V, Rassidakis G, Karameris A, Giatromanolaki A, Barbatis C, Kittas C (1994). Expression of p53 protein in laryngeal squamous cell carcinoma and dysplasia: possible correlation with human papillomavirus infection and clinicopathological findings. Virchows Arch 425: 481-489.

928. Gorgoulis VG, Zacharatos P, Kotsinas A, Kyroudi A, Rassidakis AN, Ikonomopoulos JA, Barbatis C, Herrington CS, Kittas C (1999). Human papilloma virus (HPV) is possibly involved in laryngeal but not in lung carcinogenesis. Hum Pathol 30: 274-283.

929. Gorlin RJ (1995). Nevoid basal cell carcinoma syndrome. Dermatol Clin 13: 113-125.

930. Gorsky M, Epstein JB (1998). Melanoma arising from the mucosal surfaces of the head and neck. Oral Surg Oral Med Oral Pathol Oral Radiol Endod 86: 715-719.

931. Gorsky M, Raviv M, Taicher S (1993). Squamous cell carcinoma mimicking median rhomboid glossitis region: report of a case. J Oral Maxillofac Surg 51: 798-800.

932. Gotte K, Riedel F, Coy JF, Spahn V, Hormann K (2000). Salivary gland carcinosarcoma: immunohistochemical, molecular genetic and electron microscopic findings. Oral Oncol 36: 360-364.

933. Graeme-Cook F, Pilch BZ (1992). Hamartomas of the nose and nasopharynx. Head Neck 14: 321-327.

934. Graham CT, Roberts AH, Padel AF (1998). Pleomorphic lipoma of the parotid gland. J Laryngol Otol 112: 202-203.

935. Graham S, Blanchet M, Rohrer T (1977). Cancer in asbestos-mining and other areas of Quebec. J Natl Cancer Inst 59: 1139-1145.

936. Granter SR, Badizadegan K, Fletcher CD (1998). Myofibromatosis in adults, glomangiopericytoma, and myopericytoma: a spectrum of tumors showing perivascular myoid differentiation. Am J Surg Pathol 22: 513-525.

937. Grattan CE, Gentle TA, Basu MK (1992). Oral papillary plasmacytosis resembling candidosis without demonstrable fungus in lesional tissue. Clin Exp Dermatol 17: 112-116.

938. Gravanis MB, Giansanti JS (1970). Malignant histopathologic counterpart of the benign lymphoepithelial lesion. Cancer 26: 1332-1342.

939. Gray MH, Rosenberg AE, Dickersin GR, Bhan AK (1990). Cytokeratin expression in epithelioid vascular neoplasms. Hum Pathol 21: 212-217.

940. Gray SR, Cornog JLJr, Seo IS (1976). Oncocytic neoplasms of salivary glands: a report of fifteen cases including two malignant oncocytomas. Cancer 38: 1306-1317.

941. Graziadei PP (1973). Cell dynamics in the olfactory mucosa. Tissue Cell 5: 113-131.

942. Graziadei PP, Levine RR, Monti Graziadei GA (1979). Plasticity of connections of the olfactory sensory neuron: regeneration into the forebrain following bulbectomy in the neonatal mouse. Neuroscience 4: 713-727.

943. Greco F, De Palma L, Coletti V (1983). [A familial case of aneurysmal bone cyst]. Arch Putti Chir Organi Mov 33: 441-446.

944. Green GE, Bauman NM, Smith RJ (2000). Pathogenesis and treatment of juvenile onset recurrent respiratory papillomatosis. Otolaryngol Clin North Am 33: 187-207.

945. Green RS, Tunkel DE, Small D, Westra WH, Argani P (2000). Sialoblastoma: association with cutaneous hamartoma (organoid nevus)? Pediatr Dev Pathol 3: 504-505.

946. Greenberger JS, Crocker AC, Vawter G, Jaffe N, Cassady JR (1981). Results of treatment of 127 patients with systemic histiocytosis. Medicine (Baltimore) 60: 311-338.

947. Greene FL, Page DL, Fleming ID, Fritz AG, Balch CM, Haller DG, Morrow M (2002). American Joint Committee on Cancer. Cancer Staging Manual. Springer: New York.

948. Grenevicki LF, Barker BF, Fiorella RM, Mosby EL (2001). Clear cell carcinoma of the palate. Int J Oral Maxillofac Surg 30: 452-454.

949. Griffin CA, Hawkins AL, Dvorak C, Henkle C, Ellingham T, Perlman EJ (1999). Recurrent involvement of 2p23 in inflammatory myofibroblastic tumors. Cancer Res 59: 2776-2780.

950. Grinspan D, Abulafia J (1979). Oral florid papillomatosis (verrucous carcinoma). Int J Dermatol 18: 608-622.

951. Grufferman S, Gillman MW, Pasternak LR, Peterson CL, Young WGJr (1980). Familial carotid body tumors: case report and epidemiologic review. Cancer 46: 2116-2122.

952. Grulich AE, McCredie M, Coates M (1995). Cancer incidence in Asian migrants to New South Wales, Australia. Br J Cancer 71: 400-408.

953. Guarino M, Giordano F, Pallotti F, Ponzi S (1998). Solitary fibrous tumour of the submandibular gland. Histopathology 32: 571-573.

954. Guarino M, Tricomi P, Giordano F, Cristofori E (1996). Sarcomatoid carcinomas: pathological and histopathogenetic considerations. Pathology 28: 298-305.

955. Guarisco JL, Butcher RB (1990). Congenital cystic teratoma of the maxillary sinus. Otolaryngol Head Neck Surg 103: 1035-1038.

956. Guibaud L, Herbreteau D, Dubois J, Stempfle N, Berard J, Pracros JP, Merland JJ (1998). Aneurysmal bone cysts: percutaneous embolization with an alcoholic solution of zein—series of 18 cases. Radiology 208: 369-373.

957. Guild SR (1953). The glomus jugulare, a nonchromaffin paraganglion, in man. Ann Otol Rhinol Laryngol 62: 1045-1071.

958. Guillemot F, Lo LC, Johnson JE, Auerbach A, Anderson DJ, Joyner AL (1993). Mammalian achaete-scute homolog 1 is required for the early development of olfactory and autonomic neurons. Cell 75: 463-476.

959. Guillou L, Sahli R, Chaubert P, Monnier P, Cuttat JF, Costa J (1991). Squamous cell carcinoma of the lung in a nonsmoking, nonirradiated patient with juvenile laryngotracheal papillomatosis. Evidence of human papillomavirus-11 DNA in both carcinoma and papillomas. Am J Surg Pathol 15: 891-898.

960. Guimaraes DS, Amaral AP, Prado LF, Nascimento AG (1989). Acinic cell carcinoma of salivary glands: 16 cases with clinicopathologic correlation. J Oral Pathol Med 18: 396-399.

961. Gulley ML, Amin MB, Nicholls JM, Banks PM, Ayala AG, Srigley JR, Eagan PA, Ro JY (1995). Epstein-Barr virus is detected in undifferentiated nasopharyngeal carcinoma but not in lymphoepithelioma-like carcinoma of the urinary bladder. Hum Pathol 26: 1207-1214.

962. Gulley ML, Sargeant KP, Grider DJ, Eagan PA, Davey DD, Damm DD, Robinson RA, Vandersteen DP, McGuff HS, Banks PM (1995). Lymphomas of the oral soft tissues are not preferentially associated with latent or replicative Epstein-Barr virus. Oral Surg Oral Med Oral Pathol Oral Radiol Endod 80: 425-431.

963. Gunn A, Parrott NR (1988). Parotid tumours: a review of parotid tumour surgery in the Northern Regional Health Authority of the United Kingdom 1978-1982. Br J Surg 75: 1144-1146.

964. Guo X, Lui WO, Qian CN, Chen JD, Gray SG, Rhodes D, Haab B, Stanbridge E, Wang H, Hong MH, Min HQ, Larsson C, Teh BT (2002). Identifying cancer-related genes in nasopharyngeal carcinoma cell lines using DNA and mRNA expression profiling analyses. Int J Oncol 21: 1197-1204.

965. Guo X, Min HQ, Zeng MS, Qian CN, Huang XM, Shao JY, Hou JH (1998). nm23-H1 expression in nasopharyngeal carcinoma: correlation with clinical outcome. Int J Cancer 79: 596-600.

966. Gupta DS, Gupta MK (1986). Odontoameloblastoma. J Oral Maxillofac Surg 44: 146-148.

967. Gupta M, Kaste SC, Hopkins KP (2002). Radiologic appearance of primary jaw lesions in children. Pediatr Radiol 32: 153-168.

968. Gupta PC, Mehta HC (2000). Cohort study of all-cause mortality among tobacco users in Mumbai, India. Bull World Health Organ 78: 877-883.

969. Gupta PC, Murti PR, Bhonsle RB (1996). Epidemiology of cancer by tobacco products and the significance of TSNA. Crit Rev Toxicol 26: 183-198.

970. Gussen R (1971). Meniere's disease: new temporal bone findings in two cases. Laryngoscope 81: 1695-1707.

971. Gustafsson H, Carlsoo B, Henriksson R (1985). Ultrastructural morphometry and secretory behavior of acinic cell carcinoma. Cancer 55: 1706-1710.

972. Guzzo M, Andreola S, Sirizzotti G, Cantu G (2002). Mucoepidermoid carcinoma of the salivary glands: clinicopathologic review of 108 patients treated at the National Cancer Institute of Milan. Ann Surg Oncol 9: 688-695.

973. Habel G, O'Regan B, Eissing A, Khoury F, Donath K (1991). Intra-oral keratoacanthoma: an eruptive variant and review of the literature. Br Dent J 170: 336-339.

974. Haberman RS, Stanley DE (1989). Pleomorphic adenoma of the nasal septum. Otolaryngol Head Neck Surg 100: 610-612.

975. Hachisuga T, Hashimoto H, Enjoji M (1984). Angioleiomyoma. A clinicopathologic reappraisal of 562 cases. Cancer 54: 126-130.

976. Hadar T, Rahima M, Kahan E, Sidi J, Rakowsky E, Sarov B, Sarov I (1986). Significance of specific Epstein-Barr virus IgA and elevated IgG antibodies to viral capsid antigens in nasopharyngeal carcinoma patients. J Med Virol 20: 329-339.

977. Haddadin KJ, Soutar DS, Oliver RJ, Webster MH, Robertson AG, MacDonald DG (1999). Improved survival for patients with clinically T1/T2, N0 tongue tumors undergoing a prophylactic neck dissection. Head Neck 21: 517-525.

978. Hagen P, Lyons GD, Haindel C (1993). Verrucous carcinoma of the larynx: role of human papillomavirus, radiation, and surgery. Laryngoscope 103: 253-257.

979. Haghighat K, Kalmar JR, Mariotti AJ (2002). Squamous odontogenic tumor: diagnosis and management. J Periodontol 73: 653-656.

980. Hagiwara A, Inoue Y, Nakayama T, Yamato K, Nemoto Y, Shakudo M, Daikokuya H, Nakayama K, Yamada R (2001). The "botryoid sign": a characteristic feature of rhabdomyosarcomas in the head and neck. Neuroradiology 43: 331-335.

981. Hagiwara T, Yoshida H, Takeda Y (1995). Epithelial-myoepithelial carcinoma of a minor salivary gland of the palate. A case report. Int J Oral Maxillofac Surg 24: 160-161.

982. Hall-Jones J (1972). Giant cell tumour of the larynx. J Laryngol Otol 86: 371-381.

983. Halpin SF, Britton JA, Uttley D (1992). Giant cell tumour of the skull base: MRI appearances. Case report. Neuroradiology 34: 526-527.

984. Hamazaki S, Yoshida M, Yao M, Nagashima Y, Taguchi K, Nakashima H, Okada S (2001). Mutation of von Hippel-Lindau tumor suppressor gene in a sporadic endolymphatic sac tumor. Hum Pathol 32: 1272-1276.

985. Hamed G, Shmookler BM, Ellis GL, Punja U, Feldman D (1994). Oncocytic mucoepidermoid carcinoma of the parotid gland. Arch Pathol Lab Med 118: 313-314.

986. Hamilton-Dutoit SJ, Therkildsen MH, Neilsen NH, Jensen H, Hansen JP, Pallesen G (1991). Undifferentiated carcinoma of the salivary gland in Greenlandic Eskimos: demonstration of Epstein-Barr virus DNA by in situ nucleic acid hybridization. Hum Pathol 22: 811-815.

987. Hamilton AE, Rubinstein LJ, Poole GJ (1973). Primary intracranial esthesioneuroblastoma, (olfactory neuroblastoma). J Neurosurg 38: 548-556.

988. Hammad HM, Hammond HL, Kurago ZB, Frank JA (1998). Chondromyxoid fibroma of the jaws. Case report and review of the literature. Oral Surg Oral Med Oral Pathol Oral Radiol Endod 85: 293-300.

989. Hammar SP (1995). Common Neoplasms in Pulmonary Pathology - Tumors. Springer-Verlag: New York.

990. Hamner JEI (1969). The demonstration of perivascular collagen deposition in cherubism. Oral Surg Oral Med Oral Pathol 27: 129-141.

991. Hamoir M, Plouin-Gaudon I, Rombaux P, Francois G, Cornu AS, Desuter G, Clapuyt P, Debauche C, Verellen G, Beguin C (2001). Lymphatic malformations of the head and neck: a retrospective review and a support for staging. Head Neck 23: 326-337.

992. Hamper K, Brugmann M, Koppermann R, Caselitz J, Arps H, Askensten U, Auer G, Seifert G (1989). Epithelial-myoepithelial duct carcinoma of salivary glands: a follow-up and cytophotometric study of 21 cases. J Oral Pathol Med 18: 299-304.

993. Hamper K, Lazar F, Dietel M, Caselitz J, Berger J, Arps H, Falkmer U, Auer G, Seifert G (1990). Prognostic factors for adenoid cystic carcinoma of the head and neck: a retrospective evaluation of 96 cases. J Oral Pathol Med 19: 101-107.

994. Hamper K, Mausch HE, Caselitz J, Arps H, Berger J, Askensten U, Auer G, Seifert G (1990). Acinic cell carcinoma of the salivary glands: the prognostic relevance of DNA cytophotometry in a retrospective study of long duration (1965-1987). Oral Surg Oral Med Oral Pathol 69: 68-75.

995. Hamper K, Schmitz-Watjen W, Mausch HE, Caselitz J, Seifert G (1989). Multiple expression of tissue markers in mucoepidermoid carcinomas and acinic cell carcinomas of the salivary glands. Virchows Arch A Pathol Anat Histopathol 414: 407-413.

996. Hanada T, Moriyama I, Fukami K (1988). Acinic cell carcinoma originating in the nasal cavity. Arch Otorhinolaryngol 245: 344-347.

997. Hanau CA, Miettinen M (1995). Solitary fibrous tumor: histological and immunohistochemical spectrum of benign and malignant variants presenting at different sites. Hum Pathol 26: 440-449.

998. Handler SD, Ward PH (1979). Oncocytoma of the maxillary sinus. Laryngoscope 89: 372-376.

999. Handlers JP, Abrams AM, Melrose RJ, Danforth R (1991). Central odontogenic fibroma: clinicopathologic features of 19 cases and review of the literature. J Oral Maxillofac Surg 49: 46-54.

1000. Hanji D, Gohao L (1983). Malignant lymphoepithelial lesions of the salivary glands with anaplastic carcinomatous change. Report of nine cases and review of literature. Cancer 52: 2245-2252.

1001. Hanji D, Shujing S, Shuwei H, Gohao L (1983). The cytological diagnosis of nasopharyngeal carcinoma from exfoliated cells collected by suction method. An eight-year experience. J Laryngol Otol 97: 727-734.

1002. Hannon TS, Noonan K, Steinmetz R, Eugster EA, Levine MA, Pescovitz OH (2003). Is McCune-Albright syndrome overlooked in subjects with fibrous dysplasia of bone? J Pediatr 142: 532-538.

1003. Hansen LA, Prakash UB, Colby TV (1989). Pulmonary lymphoma in Sjogren's syndrome. Mayo Clin Proc 64: 920-931.

1004. Hansen LS, Eversole LR, Green TL, Powell NB (1985). Clear cell odontogenic tumor—a new histologic variant with aggressive potential. Head Neck Surg 8: 115-123.

1005. Hansen LS, Olson JA, Silverman SJr (1985). Proliferative verrucous leukoplakia. A long-term study of thirty patients. Oral Surg Oral Med Oral Pathol 60: 285-298.

1006. Hansen LS, Sapone J, Sproat RC (1974). Traumatic bone cysts of jaws. Oral Surg Oral Med Oral Pathol 37: 899-910.

1007. Har-El G, Zirkin HY, Tovi F, Sidi J (1985). Congenital pleomorphic adenoma of the nasopharynx (report of a case). J Laryngol Otol 99: 1281-1287.

1008. Hara H, Oyama T, Omori K, Misawa T, Kasai H, Kimura M, Ishii E, Inoue T, Takaso K, Suda K (1999). Fine needle aspiration cytology of an intraductal papilloma originating in a sublingual gland. A case report. Acta Cytol 43: 457-463.

1009. Harabuchi Y, Tsubota H, Ohguro S, Himi T, Asakura K, Kataura A, Ohuchi A, Hareyama M (1997). Prognostic factors and treatment outcome in non-Hodgkin's lymphoma of Waldeyer's ring. Acta Oncol 36: 413-420.

1010. Harada H (2000). Histomorphological investigation regarding to malignant transformation of pleomorphic adenoma (so-called malignant mixed tumor) of the salivary gland origin: special reference to carcinosarcoma. Kurume Med J 47: 307-323.

1011. Harada H, Kashiwagi SI, Fujiura H, Kusukawa J, Morimatsu M (1996). Epithelial-myoepithelial carcinoma—report of a case arising in the nasal cavity. J Laryngol Otol 110: 397-400.

1012. Haraf DJ, Nodzenski E, Brachman D, Mick R, Montag A, Graves D, Vokes EE,

Weichselbaum RR (1996). Human papilloma virus and p53 in head and neck cancer: clinical correlates and survival. Clin Cancer Res 2: 755-762.
1013. Harbo G, Grau C, Bundgaard T, Overgaard M, Elbrond O, Sogaard H, Overgaard J (1997). Cancer of the nasal cavity and paranasal sinuses. A clinico-pathological study of 277 patients. Acta Oncol 36: 45-50.
1014. Harris AM, van Wyk CW (1993). Heck's disease (focal epithelial hyperplasia): a longitudinal study. Community Dent Oral Epidemiol 21: 82-85.
1015. Harris M (1993). Central giant cell granulomas of the jaws regress with calcitonin therapy. Br J Oral Maxillofac Surg 31: 89-94.
1016. Harris MD, McKeever P, Robertson JM (1990). Congenital tumours of the salivary gland: a case report and review. Histopathology 17: 155-157.
1017. Harris NL (1999). Lymphoid proliferations of the salivary glands. Am J Clin Pathol 111: S94-103.
1018. Harris WH, Dudley HR, Barry RJ (1962). The natural history of fibrous dysplasia. J Bone Joint Surg AM 44: 207-233.
1019. Harrison MG, O'Neill ID, Chadwick BL (1997). Odontogenic myxoma in an adolescent with tuberous sclerosis. J Oral Pathol Med 26: 339-341.
1020. Hartman E (1960). Chemodectoma larynx. Acta Otolaryngol 51: 528-532.
1021. Hartman KS (1980). Histiocytosis X: a review of 114 cases with oral involvement. Oral Surg Oral Med Oral Pathol 49: 38-54.
1022. Hartwell LH, Kastan MB (1994). Cell cycle control and cancer. Science 266: 1821-1828.
1023. Hasegawa SL, Mentzel T, Fletcher CD (1997). Schwannomas of the sinonasal tract and nasopharynx. Mod Pathol 10: 777-784.
1024. Hashimoto M, Izumi J, Sakuma I, Iwama T, Watarai J (1998). Chondromyxoid fibroma of the ethmoid sinus. Neuroradiology 40: 577-579.
1025. Hashimoto N, Kurihara K, Yamasaki H, Ohba S, Sakai H, Yoshida S (1987). Pathological characteristics of metastatic carcinoma in the human mandible. J Oral Pathol 16: 362-367.
1026. Hassard AD, Boudreau SF, Cron CC (1984). Adenoma of the endolymphatic sac. J Otolaryngol 13: 213-216.
1027. Haughey BH, Gates GA, Arfken CL, Harvey J (1992). Meta-analysis of second malignant tumors in head and neck cancer: the case for an endoscopic screening protocol. Ann Otol Rhinol Laryngol 101: 105-112.
1028. Hayashi K, Ohtsuki Y, Sonobe H, Takahashi K, Iwata J, Nishioka E, Kawakami T (1988). Glycogen-rich clear cell carcinoma arising from minor salivary glands of the uvula. A case report. Acta Pathol Jpn 38: 1227-1234.
1029. Hayashi N, Iwata J, Masaoka N, Ueno H, Ohtsuki Y, Moriki T (1997). Ameloblastoma of the mandible metastasizing to the orbit with malignant transformation. A histopathological and immunohistochemical study. Virchows Arch 430: 501-507.
1030. Hayashi Y, Nagamine S, Yanagawa T, Yoshida H, Yura Y, Azuma M, Sato M (1987). Small cell undifferentiated carcinoma of the minor salivary gland containing exocrine, neuroendocrine, and squamous cells. Cancer 60: 1583-1588.
1031. Hayashi Y, Nishida T, Yoshida H, Yanagawa T, Yura Y, Sato M (1987). Immunoreactive vasoactive intestinal polypeptide in acinic cell carcinoma of the parotid gland. Cancer 60: 962-968.
1032. Hazarika P, Nayak RG, Balasundaram V (1985). Primary malignant fibrous histiocytoma of ethmoid sinus. Indian J Cancer 22: 76-84.
1033. Headington JT, Batsakis JG, Beals TF, Campbell TE, Simmons JL, Stone WD (1977). Membranous basal cell adenoma of parotid gland, dermal cylindromas, and trichoepitheliomas. Comparative histochemistry and ultrastructure. Cancer 39: 2460-2469.
1034. Heath D, Smith P (1985). The Pathology of the Carotid Body and Sinus. Edward Arnold: Baltimore.
1035. Hedberg K, Vaughan TL, White E, Davis S, Thomas DB (1994). Alcoholism and cancer of the larynx: a case-control study in western Washington (United States). Cancer Causes Control 5: 3-8.
1036. Heffner DK (1983). Problems in pediatric otorhinolaryngic pathology. I. Sinonasal and nasopharyngeal tumors and masses with myxoid features. Int J Pediatr Otorhinolaryngol 5: 77-91.
1037. Heffner DK (1983). Problems in pediatric otorhinolaryngic pathology. II. Vascular tumors and lesions of the sinonasal tract and nasopharynx. Int J Pediatr Otorhinolaryngol 5: 125-138.
1038. Heffner DK (1989). Low-grade adenocarcinoma of probable endolymphatic sac origin A clinicopathologic study of 20 cases. Cancer 64: 2292-2302.
1039. Heffner DK (1991). Sinonasal and laryngeal salivary gland lesions. In: Surgical Pathology of the Salivary Glands, Ellis GL, Auclair PL, Gnepp DR, eds., WB Saunders: Philadelphia , pp. 544-559.
1040. Heffner DK (2001). Diseases of the trachea. In: Surgical Pathology of the Head and Neck, Barnes L, ed., 2nd ed. Marcel Dekker: New York , pp. 602-631.
1041. Heffner DK, Gnepp DR (1992). Sinonasal fibrosarcomas, malignant schwannomas, and "Triton" tumors. A clinicopathologic study of 67 cases. Cancer 70: 1089-1101.
1042. Heffner DK, Hyams VJ (1984). Teratocarcinosarcoma (malignant teratoma?) of the nasal cavity and paranasal sinuses A clinicopathologic study of 20 cases. Cancer 53: 2140-2154.
1043. Heffner DK, Hyams VJ (1986). Cystic chondromalacia (endochondral pseudocyst) of the auricle. Arch Pathol Lab Med 110: 740-743.
1044. Heffner DK, Hyams VJ, Hauck KW, Lingeman C (1982). Low-grade adenocarcinoma of the nasal cavity and paranasal sinuses. Cancer 50: 312-322.
1045. Heffner DK, Thompson LD, Schall DG, Anderson V (1996). Pharyngeal dermoids ("hairy polyps") as accessory auricles. Ann Otol Rhinol Laryngol 105: 819-824.
1046. Hegarty DJ, Hopper C, Speight PM (1994). Inverted ductal papilloma of minor salivary glands. J Oral Pathol Med 23: 334-336.
1047. Heikinheimo K, Jee KJ, Morgan PR, Nagy B, Happonen RP, Knuutila S, Leivo I (2004). Gene expression profiling of odontogenic keratocyst. J Oral Pathol Med 33: 462.
1048. Heikinheimo K, Jee KJ, Niini T, Aalto Y, Happonen RP, Leivo I, Knuutila S (2002). Gene expression profiling of ameloblastoma and human tooth germ by means of a cDNA microarray. J Dent Res 81: 525-530.
1049. Heikinheimo KA, Laine MA, Ritvos OV, Voutilainen RJ, Hogan BL, Leivo IV, Heikinheimo AK (1999). Bone morphogenetic protein-6 is a marker of serous acinar cell differentiation in normal and neoplastic human salivary gland. Cancer Res 59: 5815-5821.
1050. Heinrich MC, Harris AE, Bell WR (1985). Metastatic intravagal paraganglioma. Case report and review of the literature. Am J Med 78: 1017-1024.
1051. Heitzmann A, Jan M, Lecomte P, Ruchoux MM, Lhuintre Y, Tillet Y (1989). Ectopic prolactinoma within the sphenoid sinus. Neurosurgery 24: 279-282.
1052. Helliwell TR (2001). Molecular markers of metastasis in squamous carcinomas. J Pathol 194: 289-293.
1053. Helliwell TR (2003). acp Best Practice No 169. Evidence based pathology: squamous carcinoma of the hypopharynx. J Clin Pathol 56: 81-85.
1054. Hellquist H, Cardesa A, Gale N, Kambic V, Michaels L (1999). Criteria for grading in the Ljubljana classification of epithelial hyperplastic laryngeal lesions. A study by members of the Working Group on Epithelial Hyperplastic Laryngeal Lesions of the European Society of Pathology. Histopathology 34: 226-233.
1055. Hellquist H, Lundgren J, Olofsson J (1982). Hyperplasia, keratosis, dysplasia and carcinoma in situ of the vocal cords—a follow-up study. Clin Otolaryngol 7: 11-27.
1056. Hellquist H, Olofsson J (1989). Spindle cell carcinoma of the larynx. APMIS 97: 1103-1113.
1057. Hellquist HB, Hellqvist H, Vejlens L, Lindholm CE (1994). Epithelioid leiomyoma of the larynx. Histopathology 24: 155-159.
1058. Hellquist HB, Karlsson MG, Nilsson C (1994). Salivary duct carcinoma—a highly aggressive salivary gland tumour with overexpression of c-erbB-2. J Pathol 172: 35-44.
1059. Hellquist HB, Lundgren J (1991). Neurogenic sarcoma of the sinonasal tract. J Laryngol Otol 105: 186-190.
1060. Hellquist HB, Sundelin K, Di Bacco A, Tytor M, Manzotti M, Viale G (1997). Tumour growth fraction and apoptosis in salivary gland acinic cell carcinomas. Prognostic implications of Ki-67 and bcl-2 expression and of in situ end labelling (TUNEL). J Pathol 181: 323-329.
1061. Heng DM, Wee J, Fong KW, Lian LG, Sethi VK, Chua ET, Yang TL, Khoo Tan HS, Lee KS, Lee KM, Tan T, Chua EJ (1999). Prognostic factors in 677 patients in Singapore with nondisseminated nasopharyngeal carcinoma. Cancer 86: 1912-1920.
1062. Henick DH, Feghali JG (1994). Bilateral cholesterol granuloma: an unusual presentation as an intradural mass. J Otolaryngol 23: 15-18.
1063. Henley JD, Geary WA, Jackson CL, Wu CD, Gnepp DR (1997). Dedifferentiated acinic cell carcinoma of the parotid gland: a distinct rarely described entity. Hum Pathol 28: 869-873.
1064. Henley JD, Seo IS, Dayan D, Gnepp DR (2000). Sarcomatoid salivary duct carcinoma of the parotid gland. Hum Pathol 31: 208-213.
1065. Henriksson G, Westrin KM, Carlsoo B, Silfversward C (1998). Recurrent primary pleomorphic adenomas of salivary gland origin: intrasurgical rupture, histopathologic features, and pseudopodia. Cancer 82: 617-620.
1066. Henry K (1992). Langerhans cell histiocytosis (Histiocytosis X). In: Thymus, Lymph Nodes, Spleen and Lymphatics, Henry K, Symmers WS, eds., Churchill Livingstone: Edinburg , pp. 297-308.
1067. Henry K (1992). Mast cells in lymph node medulla. In: Thymus, Lymph Nodes, Spleen and Lymphatics, Henry K, Symmers WS, eds., Churchill Livingstone: Edinburg , pp. 154-155.
1068. Henry K (1992). Origin of follicular dendritic cells. In: Thymus, Lymph Nodes, Spleen and Lymphatics, Henry K, Symmers WS, eds., Churchill Livingstone: Edinburg , pp. 156-157.
1069. Henry K (1997). Lymphoid tissue self assessment. Current Diag Pathol 4: 181-185.
1070. Herait P, Ganem G, Lipinski M, Carlu C, Micheau C, Schwaab G, de The G, Tursz T (1987). Lymphocyte subsets in tumour of patients with undifferentiated nasopharyngeal carcinoma: presence of lymphocytes with the phenotype of activated T cells. Br J Cancer 55: 135-139.
1071. Herait P, Tursz T, Guillard MY, Hanna K, Lipinski M, Micheau C, Sancho-Garnier H, Schwaab G, Cachin Y, Degos L, de The G (1983). HLA-A, -B, and -DR antigens in North African patients with nasopharyngeal carcinoma. Tissue Antigens 22: 335-341.
1072. Herens C, Thiry A, Dresse MF, Born J, Flagothier C, Vanstraelen G, Allington N, Bex V (2001). Translocation (16;17)(q22;p13) is a recurrent anomaly of aneurysmal bone cysts. Cancer Genet Cytogenet 127: 83-84.
1073. Hermanek P, Hutter RV, Sobin LH, Wittekind C (1999). International Union Against Cancer. Classification of isolated tumor cells and micrometastasis. Cancer 86: 2668-2673.
1074. Hermsen M, Guervos MA, Meijer G, Baak J, van Diest P, Marcos CA, Sampedro A (2001). New chromosomal regions with high-level amplifications in squamous cell carcinomas of the larynx and pharynx, identified by comparative genomic hybridization. J Pathol 194: 177-182.
1075. Hernandez G, Sanchez G, Caballero T, Moskow BS (1992). A rare case of a multicentric peripheral ameloblastoma of the gingiva. A light and electron microscopic study. J Clin Periodontol 19: 281-287.
1076. Hernberg S, Westerholm P, Schultz-Larsen K, Degerth R, Kuosma E, Englund A, Engzell U, Hansen HS, Mutanen P (1983). Nasal and sinonasal cancer. Connection with occupational exposures in Denmark, Finland and Sweden. Scand J Work Environ Health 9: 315-326.
1077. Herrero R, Castellsagué X, Pawlita M, Lissowska J, Kee F, Balaram P, Rajkumar T, Sridhar H, Rose B, Pintos J, Fernandez L, Idris A, Sanchez MJ, Nieto A, Talamini R, Tavani A, Snijders PJF, Meijer CJLM, Viscidi R, Muñoz N, International Agency for Research on Cancer (IARC) Multicentric Cervical Cancer Study Group (2003). The viral etiology of oral cancer: evidence from the IARC multi-centric study. J Natl Cancer Inst 47-51.
1078. Herrold KM (1964). Induction of olfactory neuroepithelial tumors in Syrian hamsters by diethylnitrosamine. Cancer 17: 114-121.
1079. Hertenstein JC (1986). Pathologic quiz case 1. Acantholytic squamous cell carcinoma. Arch Otolaryngol Head Neck Surg 112: 780-782.
1080. Heutink P, van der Mey AG, Sandkuijl LA, van Gils AP, Bardoel A, Breedveld GJ, van Vliet M, van Ommen GJ,

Cornelisse CJ, Oostra BA (1992). A gene subject to genomic imprinting and responsible for hereditary paragangliomas maps to chromosome 11q23-qter. Hum Mol Genet 1: 7-10.
1081. Hew WS, Carey FA, Kernohan NM, Heppleston AD, Jackson R, Jarrett RF (2002). Primary T cell lymphoma of salivary gland: a report of a case and review of the literature. J Clin Pathol 55: 61-63.
1082. Hewan-Lowe K, Dardick I (1995). Ultrastructural distinction of basaloid-squamous carcinoma and adenoid cystic carcinoma. Ultrastruct Pathol 19: 371-381.
1083. Hickman RE, Cawson RA, Duffy SW (1984). The prognosis of specific types of salivary gland tumors. Cancer 54: 1620-1624.
1084. Hicks J, Flaitz C (2002). Rhabdomyosarcoma of the head and neck in children. Oral Oncol 38: 450-459.
1085. Hicks MJ, Flaitz CM (2000). Oral mucosal melanoma: epidemiology and pathobiology. Oral Oncol 36: 152-169.
1086. Hicks MJ, Flaitz CM, Wong ME, McDaniel RK, Cagle PT (1994). Clear cell variant of calcifying epithelial odontogenic tumor: case report and review of the literature. Head Neck 16: 272-277.
1087. Hildes JA, Schaefer O (1984). The changing picture of neoplastic disease in the western and central Canadian Arctic (1950-1980). Can Med Assoc J 130: 25-32.
1088. Hildesheim A, Anderson LM, Chen CJ, Cheng YJ, Brinton LA, Daly AK, Reed CD, Chen IH, Caporaso NE, Hsu MM, Chen JY, Idle JR, Hoover RN, Yang CS, Chhabra SK (1997). CYP2E1 genetic polymorphisms and risk of nasopharyngeal carcinoma in Taiwan. J Natl Cancer Inst 89: 1207-1212.
1089. Hildesheim A, Apple RJ, Chen CJ, Wang SS, Cheng YJ, Klitz W, Mack SJ, Chen IH, Hsu MM, Yang CS, Brinton LA, Levine PH, Erlich HA (2002). Association of HLA class I and II alleles and extended haplotypes with nasopharyngeal carcinoma in Taiwan. J Natl Cancer Inst 94: 1780-1789.
1090. Hildesheim A, Dosemeci M, Chan CC, Chen CJ, Cheng YJ, Hsu MM, Chen IH, Mittl BF, Sun B, Levine PH, Chen JY, Brinton LA, Yang CS (2001). Occupational exposure to wood, formaldehyde, and solvents and risk of nasopharyngeal carcinoma. Cancer Epidemiol Biomarkers Prev 10: 1145-1153.
1091. Hillstrom RP, Zarbo RJ, Jacobs JR (1990). Nerve sheath tumors of the paranasal sinuses: electron microscopy and histopathologic diagnosis. Otolaryngol Head Neck Surg 102: 257-263.
1092. Hinni ML (2000). Giant cell tumor of the larynx. Ann Otol Rhinol Laryngol 109: 63-66.
1093. Hinni ML, Beatty CW (1996). Salivary gland choristoma of the middle ear: report of a case and review of the literature. Ear Nose Throat J 75: 422-424.
1094. Hirabayashi H, Koshii K, Uno K, Ohgaki H, Nakasone Y, Fujisawa T, Syouno N, Hinohara T, Hirabayashi K (1991). Extracapsular spread of squamous cell carcinoma in neck lymph nodes: prognostic factor of laryngeal cancer. Laryngoscope 101: 502-506.
1095. Hirao M, Gushiken T, Imokawa H, Kawai S, Inaba H, Tsukuda M (2001). Solitary neurofibroma of the nasal cavity: resection with endoscopic surgery. J Laryngol Otol 115: 1012-1014.
1096. Hirose T, Scheithauer BW, Lopes MB, Gerber HA, Altermatt HJ, Harner SG, VandenBerg SR (1995). Olfactory neuroblastoma. An immunohistochemical, ultrastructural, and flow cytometric study. Cancer 76: 4-19.
1097. Hirsch MS, Faquin WC, Krane JF (2004). Thyroid transcription factor-1, but not p53, is helpful in distinguishing moderately differentiated neuroendocrine carcinoma of the larynx from medullary carcinoma of the thyroid. Mod Pathol 17: 631-636.
1098. Hirshberg A, Buchner A (1995). Metastatic tumours to the oral region. An overview. Eur J Cancer B Oral Oncol 31B: 355-360.
1099. Hirshberg A, Kaplan I, Buchner A (1994). Calcifying odontogenic cyst associated with odontoma: a possible separate entity (odontocalcifying odontogenic cyst). J Oral Maxillofac Surg 52: 555-558.
1100. Hirshberg A, Leibovich P, Buchner A (1993). Metastases to the oral mucosa: analysis of 157 cases. J Oral Pathol Med 22: 385-390.
1101. Hirshberg A, Leibovich P, Horowitz I, Buchner A (1993). Metastatic tumors to postextraction sites. J Oral Maxillofac Surg 51: 1334-1337.
1102. Hirunsatit R, Kongruttanachok N, Shotelersuk K, Supiyaphun P, Voravud N, Sakuntabhai A, Mutirangura A (2003). Polymeric immunoglobulin receptor polymorphisms and risk of nasopharyngeal cancer. BMC Genet 4: 3.
1103. Hirvikoski P, Kumpulainen E, Virtaniemi J, Johansson R, Haapasalo H, Marin S, Halonen P, Helin H, Raitiola H, Pukander J, Kellokumpu-Lehtinen P, Kosma VM (1997). p53 expression and cell proliferation as prognostic factors in laryngeal squamous cell carcinoma. J Clin Oncol 15: 3111-3120.
1104. Hisatomi M, Asaumi JI, Konouchi H, Honda Y, Wakasa T, Kishi K (2002). A case of complex odontoma associated with an impacted lower deciduous second molar and analysis of the 107 odontomas. Oral Dis 8: 100-105.
1105. Hitomi G, Nishide N, Mitsui K (1996). Cherubism: diagnostic imaging and review of the literature in Japan. Oral Surg Oral Med Oral Pathol Oral Radiol Endod 81: 623-628.
1106. Hiyama T, Sato T, Yoshino K, Tsukuma H, Hanai A, Fujimoto I (1992). Second primary cancer following laryngeal cancer with special reference to smoking habits. Jpn J Cancer Res 83: 334-339.
1107. Ho FC, Srivastava G, Loke SL, Fu KH, Leung BP, Liang R, Choy D (1990). Presence of Epstein-Barr virus DNA in nasal lymphomas of B and 'T' cell type. Hematol Oncol 8: 271-281.
1108. Ho JH (1971). Genetic and envrionmental factors in nasopharyngeal carcinoma. In: Recent Advances in Human Tumor Virology and Immunology: Proceedings of the First International Cancer Symposium of the Princess Takamatsu Cancer Research Fund, Nakahara W, Hirayama T, Ito Y, eds., University of Tokyo Press: Tokyo .
1109. Ho KL (1980). Primary meningioma of the nasal cavity and paranasal sinuses. Cancer 46: 1442-1447.
1110. Hoang MP, Callender DL, Sola Gallego JJ, Huang Z, Sneige N, Luna MA, Batsakis JG, El Naggar AK (2001). Molecular and biomarker analyses of salivary duct carcinomas: comparison with mammary duct carcinoma. Int J Oncol 19: 865-871.
1111. Hoffman DA, McConahey WM, Fraumeni JFJr, Kurland LT (1982). Cancer incidence following treatment of hyperthyroidism. Int J Epidemiol 11: 218-224.
1112. Hoffman HT, Karnell LH, Robinson RA, Pinkston JA, Menck HR (1999). National Cancer Data Base report on cancer of the head and neck: acinic cell carcinoma. Head Neck 21: 297-309.
1113. Hogg RP, Ayshford C, Watkinson JC (1999). Parotid duct carcinoma arising in bilateral chronic sialadenitis. J Laryngol Otol 113: 686-688.
1114. Holland RS, Abaza N, Balsara G, Lesser R (1998). Granular cell tumor of the larynx in a six-year-old child: case report and review of the literature. Ear Nose Throat J 77: 652-4, 656, 658.
1115. Hollstein M, Sidransky D, Vogelstein B, Harris CC (1991). p53 mutations in human cancers. Science 253: 49-53.
1116. Holman RL (1956). Rhabdomyosarcoma of the middle-ear region; report of a case. J Laryngol Otol 7: 415-419.
1117. Holst VA, Marshall CE, Moskaluk CA, Frierson HFJr (1999). KIT protein expression and analysis of c-kit gene mutation in adenoid cystic carcinoma. Mod Pathol 12: 956-960.
1118. Honda K, Kashima K, Daa T, Yokoyama S, Nakayama I (2000). Clonal analysis of the epithelial component of Warthin's tumor. Hum Pathol 31: 1377-1380.
1119. Hong MH, Mai HQ, Min HQ, Ma J, Zhang EP, Cui NJ (2000). A comparison of the Chinese 1992 and fifth-edition International Union Against Cancer staging systems for staging nasopharyngeal carcinoma. Cancer 89: 242-247.
1120. Hong SM, Park YK, Ro JY (1999). Chondroblastoma of the temporal bone: a clinicopathologic study of five cases. J Korean Med Sci 14: 559-564.
1121. Hong SP, Ellis GL, Hartman KS (1991). Calcifying odontogenic cyst. A review of ninety-two cases with reevaluation of their nature as cysts or neoplasms, the nature of ghost cells, and subclassification. Oral Surg Oral Med Oral Pathol 72: 56-64.
1122. Hoppe RT, Williams J, Warnke R, Goffinet DR, Bagshaw MA (1978). Carcinoma of the nasopharynx—the significance of histology. Int J Radiat Oncol Biol Phys 4: 199-205.
1123. Hordijk GJ, Ruiter DJ, Bosman FT, Mauw BJ (1981). Chemodectoma (paraganglioma) of the larynx. Clin Otolaryngol 6: 249-254.
1124. Hording U, Nielsen HW, Albeck H, Daugaard S (1993). Nasopharyngeal carcinoma: histopathological types and association with Epstein-Barr Virus. Eur J Cancer B Oral Oncol 29B: 137-139.
1125. Hording U, Nielsen HW, Daugaard S, Albeck H (1994). Human papillomavirus types 11 and 16 detected in nasopharyngeal carcinomas by the polymerase chain reaction. Laryngoscope 104: 99-102.
1126. Horinouchi H, Ishihara T, Kawamura M, Kato R, Kikuchi K, Kobayashi K, Maenaka Y, Torikata C (1993). Epithelial myoepithelial tumour of the tracheal gland. J Clin Pathol 46: 185-187.
1127. Horn-Ross PL, Ljung BM, Morrow M (1997). Environmental factors and the risk of salivary gland cancer. Epidemiology 8: 414-419.
1128. Horn-Ross PL, Morrow M, Ljung BM (1997). Diet and the risk of salivary gland cancer. Am J Epidemiol 146: 171-176.
1129. Hornigold R, Morgan PR, Pearce A, Gleeson MJ (2005). Congenital sialolipoma of the parotid gland first reported case and review of the literature. Int J Pediatr Otorhinolaryngol 69: 429-434.
1130. Horsman DE, Berean K, Durham JS (1995). Translocation (11;19)(q21;p13.1) in mucoepidermoid carcinoma of salivary gland. Cancer Genet Cytogenet 80: 165-166.
1131. Hosaka N, Kitajiri S, Hiraumi H, Nogaki H, Toki J, Yang G, Hisha H, Ikehara S (2002). Ectopic pituitary adenoma with malignant transformation. Am J Surg Pathol 26: 1078-1082.
1132. Housholder MS, Zeligman I (1980). Sebaceous neoplasms associated with visceral carcinomas. Arch Dermatol 116: 61-64.
1133. Houston GD, Fowler CB (1997). Extraosseous calcifying epithelial odontogenic tumor: report of two cases and review of the literature. Oral Surg Oral Med Oral Pathol Oral Radiol Endod 83: 577-583.
1134. Hoving EW (2000). Nasal encephaloceles. Childs Nerv Syst 16: 702-706.
1135. Howell RM, Burkes EJJr (1977). Malignant transformation of ameloblastic fibro-odontoma to ameloblastic fibrosarcoma. Oral Surg Oral Med Oral Pathol 43: 391-401.
1136. Hrynchak M, White V, Berean K, Horsman D (1994). Cytogenetic findings in seven lacrimal gland neoplasms. Cancer Genet Cytogenet 75: 133-138.
1137. Hsiao JR, Jin YT, Tsai ST (1998). EBER1 in situ hybridization as an adjuvant for diagnosis of recurrent nasopharyngeal carcinoma. Anticancer Res 18: 4585-4589.
1138. Hsu DW, Efird JT, Hedley-Whyte ET (1997). Progesterone and estrogen receptors in meningiomas: prognostic considerations. J Neurosurg 86: 113-120.
1139. Hsu DW, Pardo FS, Efird JT, Linggood RM, Hedley-Whyte ET (1994). Prognostic significance of proliferative indices in menangiomas. J Neuropathol Exp Neurol 53: 247-255.
1140. Hsueh C, Hsueh S, Gonzalez-Crussi F, Lee T, Su J (2001). Nasal chondromesenchymal hamartoma in children: report of 2 cases with review of the literature. Arch Pathol Lab Med 125: 400-403.
1141. Huang DP, Ho JH, Chan WK, Lau WH, Lui M (1989). Cytogenetics of undifferentiated nasopharyngeal carcinoma xenografts from southern Chinese. Int J Cancer 43: 936-939.
1142. Huang DP, Ho JH, Saw D, Teoh TB (1978). Carcinoma of the nasal and paranasal regions in rats fed Cantonese salted marine fish. IARC Sci Publ 315-328.
1143. Huang DP, Ng HK, Ho YH, Chan KM (1988). Epstein-Barr virus (EBV)-associated undifferentiated carcinoma of the parotid gland. Histopathology 13: 509-517.
1144. Huang HY, Antonescu CR (2003). Sinonasal smooth muscle cell tumors: a clinicopathologic and immunohistochemical analysis of 12 cases with emphasis on the low-grade end of the spectrum. Arch Pathol Lab Med 127: 297-304.
1145. Huang Q, Yu GP, McCormick SA, Mo J, Datta B, Mahimkar M, Lazarus P, Schaffer AA, Desper R, Schantz SP (2002). Genetic differences detected by comparative genomic hybridization in head and neck squamous cell carcinomas from different tumor sites: construction of oncogenetic trees for tumor progression. Genes Chromosomes Cancer 34: 224-233.
1146. Hug EB, Muenter MW, Adams JA, de Vries A, Rosenberg AE, Munzenrider JE (2002). 3-D-conformal radiation therapy for

pediatric giant cell tumors of the skull base. Strahlenther Onkol 178: 239-244.

1147. Huh KH, Heo MS, Lee SS, Choi SC (2003). Three new cases of salivary duct carcinoma in the palate: A radiologic investigation and review of the literature. Oral Surg Oral Med Oral Pathol Oral Radiol Endod 95: 752-760.

1148. Hui AB, Lo KW, Leung SF, Teo P, Fung MK, To KF, Wong N, Choi PH, Lee JC, Huang DP (1999). Detection of recurrent chromosomal gains and losses in primary nasopharyngeal carcinoma by comparative genomic hybridisation. Int J Cancer 82: 498-503.

1149. Hui AB, Lo KW, Teo PM, To KF, Huang DP (2002). Genome wide detection of oncogene amplifications in nasopharyngeal carcinoma by array based comparative genomic hybridization. Int J Oncol 20: 467-473.

1150. Hui EP, Chan AT, Pezzella F, Turley H, To KF, Poon TC, Zee B, Mo F, Teo PM, Huang DP, Gatter KC, Johnson PJ, Harris AL (2002). Coexpression of hypoxia-inducible factors 1alpha and 2alpha, carbonic anhydrase IX, and vascular endothelial growth factor in nasopharyngeal carcinoma and relationship to survival. Clin Cancer Res 8: 2595-2604.

1151. Hui KK, Luna MA, Batsakis JG, Ordonez NG, Weber R (1990). Undifferentiated carcinomas of the major salivary glands. Oral Surg Oral Med Oral Pathol 69: 76-83.

1152. Huizenga C, Balogh K (1970). Cartilaginous tumors of the larynx. A clinicopathologic study of 10 new cases and a review of the literature. Cancer 26: 201-210.

1153. Hujala K, Martikainen P, Minn H, Grenman R (1993). Malignant nerve sheath tumors of the head and neck: four case studies and review of the literature. Eur Arch Otorhinolaryngol 250: 379-382.

1154. Hungermann D, Roeser K, Buerger H, Jakel T, Loning T, Herbst H (2002). Relative paucity of gross genetic alterations in myoepitheliomas and myoepithelial carcinomas of salivary glands. J Pathol 198: 487-494.

1155. Hurtado JF, Lopez JJ, Aranda FI, Talavera J (1994). Primary liposarcoma of the larynx. Case report and literature review. Ann Otol Rhinol Laryngol 103: 315-318.

1156. Hussong JW, Brown M, Perkins SL, Dehner LP, Coffin CM (1999). Comparison of DNA ploidy, histologic, and immunohistochemical findings with clinical outcome in inflammatory myofibroblastic tumors. Mod Pathol 12: 279-286.

1157. Hwang TZ, Jin YT, Tsai ST (1998). EBER in situ hybridization differentiates carcinomas originating from the sinonasal region and the nasopharynx. Anticancer Res 18: 4581-4584.

1158. Hyams VJ (1971). Papillomas of the nasal cavity and paranasal sinuses. A clinicopathological study of 315 cases. Ann Otol Rhinol Laryngol 80: 192-206.

1159. Hyams VJ, Batsakis JG, Michaels L (1988). Tumors of the upper respiratory tract and ear. 2nd series ed. Armed Forces Institute of Pathology: Washington.

1160. Hyams VJ, Michaels L (1976). Benign adenomatous neoplasm (adenoma) of the middle ear. Clin Otolaryngol 1: 17-26.

1161. Hyams VJ, Rabuzzi DD (1970). Cartilaginous tumors of the larynx. Laryngoscope 80: 755-767.

1162. Hyjek E, Smith WJ, Isaacson PG (1988). Primary B-cell lymphoma of salivary glands and its relationship to myoepithelial sialadenitis. Hum Pathol 19: 766-776.

1163. Hyman BA, Scheithauer BW, Weiland LH, Irons GB (1988). Membranous basal cell adenoma of the parotid gland. Malignant transformation in a patient with multiple dermal cylindromas. Arch Pathol Lab Med 112: 209-211.

1164. Hyman GA, Wolff M (1976). Malignant lymphomas of the salivary glands. Review of the literature and report of 33 new cases, including four cases associated with the lymphoepithelial lesion. Am J Clin Pathol 65: 421-438.

1165. Hytiroglou P, Brandwein MS, Strauchen JA, Mirante JP, Urken ML, Biller HF (1992). Inflammatory pseudotumor of the parapharyngeal space: case report and review of the literature. Head Neck 14: 230-234.

1166. IARC Working Group (1997). Epstein Barr Virus and Kaposi's Sarcoma Herpes Virus / Human Herpes 8.

1167. Ibrahim R, Bird DJ, Sieler MW (1991). Malignant myoepithelioma of the larynx with massive metastatic spread to the liver: an ultrastructural and immunocytochemical study. Ultrastruct Pathol 15: 69-76.

1168. Ibrahim SA, Abdalla HA, El Hassan AM (2003). Case report: congenital salivary gland analage tumor presenting with neonatal respiratory distress. Pediatr Pathol Mol Med 209-211.

1169. Ide F, Mishima K, Saito I (2003). Ectomesenchymal chondromyxoid tumor of the anterior tongue with myxoglobulosislike change. Virchows Arch 442: 302-303.

1170. Ide F, Shimoyama T, Horie N, Shimizu S (1999). Intraosseous squamous cell carcinoma arising in association with a squamous odontogenic tumour of the mandible. Oral Oncol 35: 431-434.

1171. Idris AM, Ahmed HM, Malik MO (1995). Toombak dipping and cancer of the oral cavity in the Sudan: a case-control study. Int J Cancer 63: 477-480.

1172. Iezzi G, Rubini C, Fioroni M, Piattelli A (2002). Clear cell odontogenic carcinoma. Oral Oncol 38: 209-213.

1173. Iezzoni JC, Gaffey MJ, Weiss LM (1995). The role of Epstein-Barr virus in lymphoepithelioma-like carcinomas. Am J Clin Pathol 103: 308-315.

1174. Imate Y, Yamashita H, Endo S, Okami K, Kamada T, Takahashi M, Kawano H (2000). Epithelial-myoepithelial carcinoma of the nasopharynx. ORL J Otorhinolaryngol Relat Spec 62: 282-285.

1175. Ingle R, Jennings TA, Goodman ML, Pilch BZ, Bergman S, Ross JS (1998). CD44 expression in sinonasal inverted papillomas and associated squamous cell carcinoma. Am J Clin Pathol 109: 309-314.

1176. Inoue H, Sato Y, Tsuchiya B, Nagai H, Takahashi H, Kameya T (2002). Expression of Epstein-Barr virus-encoded small nuclear RNA 1 in Japanese nasopharyngeal carcinomas. Acta Otolaryngol Suppl 113-117.

1177. Inoue Y, Nomura J, Hashimoto M, Tagawa T (2001). Epithelial-myoepithelial carcinoma of the palate: a case report. J Oral Maxillofac Surg 59: 1502-1505.

1178. Inui M, Tagawa T, Mori A, Yoneda J, Nomura J, Fukumori T (1993). Inflammatory pseudotumor in the submandibular region. Clinicopathologic study and review of the literature. Oral Surg Oral Med Oral Pathol 76: 333-337.

1179. Iqbal SM, Bhogoliwal SK, Nandi NB (1986). Laryngeal leiomyoma. J Laryngol Otol 100: 723-725.

1180. Ireland AJ, Eveson JW, Leopard PJ (1988). Malignant fibrous histiocytoma: a report of two cases arising in sites of previous irradiation. Br J Oral Maxillofac Surg 26: 221-227.

1181. Isaacson PG, Norton AJ (1994). Malignant lymphoma of the salivary gland. In: Extranodal lymphomas, Isaacson PG, Norton AJ, eds., Churchill Livingstone: New York .

1182. Isaacson PG, Wotherspoon AC, Diss T, Pan LX (1991). Follicular colonization in B-cell lymphoma of mucosa-associated lymphoid tissue. Am J Surg Pathol 15: 819-828.

1183. Isago H, Kimura T, Kataura A (1986). A case of Weber-Christian disease accompanied by a nasal symptom (a clinicopathologic case report). J Laryngol Otol 100: 221-227.

1184. Ishida M, Hasegawa S, Sato T, Tateishi R (1971). Glomus tumor (nonchromaffin-paraganglioma) of the larynx. Laryngoscope 81: 957-961.

1185. Ishikawa E, Tsuboi K, Onizawa K, Hara A, Kusakari J, Noguchi M, Nose T (2002). Chondroblastoma of the temporal base with high mitotic activity. Neurol Med Chir (Tokyo) 42: 516-520.

1186. Ishikawa T, Imada S, Ijuhin N (1993). Intraductal papilloma of the anterior lingual salivary gland. Case report and immunohistochemical study. Int J Oral Maxillofac Surg 22: 116-117.

1187. Ishiyama A, Eversole LR, Ross DA, Raz Y, Kerner MM, Fu YS, Blackwell KE, Feneberg R, Bell TS, Calcaterra TC (1994). Papillary squamous neoplasms of the head and neck. Laryngoscope 104: 1446-1452.

1188. Ito K, Tsukuda M, Kawabe R, Nakagawa C, Matsushita K, Kubota A, Furukawa M, Kameda Y, Ito T (2000). Benign and malignant oncocytoma of the salivary glands with an immunohistochemical evaluation of Ki-67. ORL J Otorhinolaryngol Relat Spec 62: 338-341.

1189. Iwata N, Hattori K, Nakagawa T, Tsujimura T (2002). Hemangioma of the nasal cavity: a clinicopathologic study. Auris Nasus Larynx 29: 335-339.

1190. Izumi K, Nakajima T, Maeda T, Cheng J, Saku T (1998). Adenosquamous carcinoma of the tongue: report of a case with histochemical, immunohistochemical, and ultrastructural study and review of the literature. Oral Surg Oral Med Oral Pathol Oral Radiol Endod 85: 178-184.

1191. Jaaskelainen K, Jee KJ, Leivo I, Saloniemi I, Knuutila S, Heikinheimo K (2002). Cell proliferation and chromosomal changes in human ameloblastoma. Cancer Genet Cytogenet 136: 31-37.

1192. Jacobson S, Shear M (1972). Verrucous carcinoma of the mouth. J Oral Pathol 1: 66-75.

1193. Jaehne M, Ussmuller J, Jakel KT, Zschaber R (2001). The clinical presentation of non-hodgkin lymphomas of the major salivary glands. Acta Otolaryngol 121: 647-651.

1194. Jaffe BF (1973). Unusual laryngeal problems in children. Ann Otol Rhinol Laryngol 82: 637-642.

1195. Jaffe ES (1995). Nasal and nasal-type T/NK cell lymphoma: a unique form of lymphoma associated with the Epstein-Barr virus. Histopathology 27: 581-583.

1196. Jaffe ES, Chan JK, Su IJ, Frizzera G, Mori S, Feller AC, Ho FC (1996). Report of the Workshop on Nasal and Related Extranodal Angiocentric T/Natural Killer Cell Lymphomas. Definitions, differential diagnosis, and epidemiology. Am J Surg Pathol 20: 103-111.

1197. Jaffe ES, Harris NL, Stein H, Vardiman JW (2001). World Health Organization Classification of Tumours. Pathology and Genetics of Tumours of Haematopoietic and Lymphoid Tissues. IARC Press: Lyon.

1198. Jahan-Parwar B, Huberman RM, Donovan DT, Schwartz MR, Ostrowski ML (1999). Oncocytic mucoepidermoid carcinoma of the salivary glands. Am J Surg Pathol 23: 523-529.

1199. Jahn AF, Walter JB, Farkashidy J (1980). Verrucous carcinoma of the nasopharynx—a clinicopathologic case report. J Otolaryngol 9: 84-89.

1200. Jain D, Parkash V, Li M, Gill J, Crouch J, Howe G, Tallini G (2000). Epstein-Barr virus RNA detection and glandular differentiation in nasopharyngeal carcinoma: report of 2 cases. Arch Pathol Lab Med 124: 1369-1372.

1201. Jaiswal VR, Hoang MP (2004). Primary combined squamous and small cell carcinoma of the larynx: a case report and review of the literature. Arch Pathol Lab Med 128: 1279-1282.

1202. Jamal MN (1994). Schwannoma of the larynx: case report, and review of the literature. J Laryngol Otol 108: 788-790.

1203. James M, Norton AJ, Akosa AB (1993). Primary T-cell lymphoma of submandibular salivary gland. Histopathology 22: 83-85.

1204. Janse van Rensburg L, Nortje CJ, Thompson I (1997). Correlating imaging and histopathology of an odontogenic keratocyst in the nevoid basal cell carcinoma syndrome. Dentomaxillofac Radiol 26: 195-199.

1205. Jansen JC, van den Berg R, Kuiper A, van der Mey AG, Zwinderman AH, Cornelisse CJ (2000). Estimation of growth rate in patients with head and neck paragangliomas influences the treatment proposal. Cancer 88: 2811-2816.

1206. Janssen JH, Blijdorp PA (1985). Central odontogenic fibroma. A case report. J Maxillofac Surg 13: 236-238.

1207. Jares P, Fernandez PL, Campo E, Nadal A, Bosch F, Aiza G, Nayach I, Traserra J, Cardesa A (1994). PRAD-1/cyclin D1 gene amplification correlates with messenger RNA overexpression and tumor progression in human laryngeal carcinomas. Cancer Res 54: 4813-4817.

1208. Jares P, Fernandez PL, Nadal A, Cazorla M, Hernandez L, Pinyol M, Hernandez S, Traserra J, Cardesa A, Campo E (1997). p16MTS1/CDK4I mutations and concomitant loss of heterozygosity at 9p21-23 are frequent events in squamous cell carcinoma of the larynx. Oncogene 15: 1445-1453.

1209. Jares P, Nadal A, Fernandez PL, Pinyol M, Hernandez L, Cazorla M, Hernandez S, Bea S, Cardesa A, Campo E (1999). Disregulation of p16MTS1/CDK4I protein and mRNA expression is associated with gene alterations in squamous-cell carcinoma of the larynx. Int J Cancer 81: 705-711.

1210. Jassar P, Stafford ND, MacDonald AW (1999). Pleomorphic adenoma of the nasal septum. J Laryngol Otol 113: 483-485.

1211. Jayakrishnan A, Elmalah I, Hussain K, Odell EW (2003). Basal cell adenocarcinoma in minor salivary glands. Histopathology 42: 610-614.

1212. Jeannel D, Ghnassia M, Hubert A,

Sancho-Garnier H, Eschwege F, Crognier E, de The G (1993). Increased risk of nasopharyngeal carcinoma among males of French origin born in Maghreb (north Africa). Int J Cancer 54: 536-539.

1213. Jeannel D, Hubert A, de Vathaire F, Ellouz R, Camoun M, Ben Salem M, Sancho-Garnier H, de The G (1990). Diet, living conditions and nasopharyngeal carcinoma in Tunisia—a case-control study. Int J Cancer 46: 421-425.

1214. Jeannon JP, Soames JV, Bell H, Wilson JA (1999). Immunohistochemical detection of oestrogen and progesterone receptors in salivary tumours. Clin Otolaryngol 24: 52-54.

1215. Jeng YM, Lin CY, Hsu HC (2000). Expression of the c-kit protein is associated with certain subtypes of salivary gland carcinoma. Cancer Lett 154: 107-111.

1216. Jeng YM, Sung MT, Fang CL, Huang HY, Mao TL, Cheng W, Hsiao CH (2002). Sinonasal undifferentiated carcinoma and nasopharyngeal-type undifferentiated carcinoma: two clinically, biologically, and histopathologically distinct entities. Am J Surg Pathol 26: 371-376.

1217. Jeremic B, Shibamoto Y, Acimovic L, Milisavljevic S (1996). Radiotherapy for primary squamous cell carcinoma of the trachea. Radiother Oncol 41: 135-138.

1218. Jin C, Jin Y, Hoglund M, Wennerberg J, Akervall J, Willen R, Dictor M, Mandahl N, Mitelman F, Mertens F (1998). Cytogenetic and molecular genetic demonstration of polyclonality in an acinic cell carcinoma. Br J Cancer 78: 292-295.

1219. Jin C, Jin Y, Wennerberg J, Dictor M, Mertens F (2000). Nonrandom pattern of cytogenetic abnormalities in squamous cell carcinoma of the larynx. Genes Chromosomes Cancer 28: 66-76.

1220. Jin C, Martins C, Jin Y, Wiegant J, Wennerberg J, Dictor M, Gisselsson D, Strombeck B, Fonseca I, Mitelman F, Tanke HJ, Hoglund M, Mertens F (2001). Characterization of chromosome aberrations in salivary gland tumors by FISH, including multicolor COBRA-FISH. Genes Chromosomes Cancer 30: 161-167.

1221. Jin XL, Ding CN, Chu Q (1999). Epithelial-myoepithelial carcinoma arising in the nasal cavity: a case report and review of literature. Pathology 31: 148-151.

1222. Jin Y, Mertens F, Mandahl N, Wennerberg J, Dictor M, Heim S, Mitelman F (1995). Tetraploidization and progressive loss of 6q in a squamous cell carcinoma of the parotid gland. Cancer Genet Cytogenet 79: 157-159.

1223. Jing J, Louie E, Henderson BE, Terasaki P (1977). Histocompatibility leukocyte antigen patterns in nasopharyngeal carcinoma cases from California. Natl Cancer Inst Monogr 47: 153-156.

1224. Johansen C, Boice JJr, McLaughlin J, Olsen J (2001). Cellular telephones and cancer—a nationwide cohort study in Denmark. J Natl Cancer Inst 93: 203-207.

1225. Johansen EC, Illum P (1995). Rhabdomyoma of the larynx: a review of the literature with a summary of previously described cases of rhabdomyoma of the larynx and a report of a new case. J Laryngol Otol 109: 147-153.

1226. Johns ME, Headington JT (1974). Squamous cell carcinoma of the external auditory canal. A clinicopathologic study of 20 cases. Arch Otolaryngol 100: 45-49.

1227. Johns ME, Regezi JA, Batsakis JG (1977). Oncocytic neoplasms of salivary glands: an ultrastructural study.

Laryngoscope 87: 862-871.

1228. Johns MMI, Westra WH, Califano JA, Eisele D, Koch WM, Sidransky D (1996). Allelotype of salivary gland tumors. Cancer Res 56: 1151-1154.

1229. Johnson LC, Yousefi M, Vinh TN, Heffner DK, Hyams VJ, Hartman KS (1991). Juvenile active ossifying fibroma. Its nature, dynamics and origin. Acta Otolaryngol Suppl 488: 1-40.

1230. Johnson N (2001). Tobacco use and oral cancer: a global perspective. J Dent Educ 65: 328-339.

1231. Johnson PJ, Lydiatt DD, Hollins RR, Rydlund KW, Degenhardt JA (1996). Malignant nerve sheath tumor of the nasal septum. Otolaryngol Head Neck Surg 115: 132-134.

1232. Johnson RE, Scheithauer BW, Dahlin DC (1983). Melanotic neuroectodermal tumor of infancy. A review of seven cases. Cancer 52: 661-666.

1233. Johnson TL, Plieth DA, Crissman JD, Sarkar FH (1991). HPV detection by polymerase chain reaction (PCR) in verrucous lesions of the upper aerodigestive tract. Mod Pathol 4: 461-465.

1234. Jones ME, Wackym PA, Said-Al-Naief N, Brandwein M, Shaari CM, Som PM, Zhang DY, King WA (1998). Clinical and molecular pathology of aggressive Schneiderian papilloma involving the temporal bone. Head Neck 20: 83-88.

1235. Jones SR, Myers EN, Barnes L (1984). Benign neoplasms of the larynx. Otolaryngol Clin North Am 17: 151-178.

1236. Jones WA (1933). Familial multilocular cystic disease of the jaws. Am J Cancer 17: 946-950.

1237. Jones WA, Gerrie J, Pritchard J (1950). Cherubism - A familial fibrous dysplasia of the jaws. J Bone & Joint Surg 32B: 334-347.

1238. Jordan R, Diss TC, Lench NJ, Isaacson PG, Speight PM (1995). Immunoglobulin gene rearrangements in lymphoplasmacytic infiltrates of labial salivary glands in Sjogren's syndrome. A possible predictor of lymphoma development. Oral Surg Oral Med Oral Pathol Oral Radiol Endod 79: 723-729.

1239. Jundt G, Prein J (2000). [Bone tumors and tumor-like lesions of the jaw. Findings from the Basel DOSAK reference registry]. Mund Kiefer Gesichtschir 4 Suppl 1: S196-S207.

1240. Justrabo E, Michiels R, Calmettes C, Cabanne F, Bastein H, Horiot JC, Guerrin J (1980). An uncommon apudoma: a functional chemodectoma of the larynx. Report of a case and review of the literature. Acta Otolaryngol 89: 135-143.

1241. Kaban LB, Troulis MJ, Ebb D, August M, Hornicek FJ, Dodson TB (2002). Antiangiogenic therapy with interferon alpha for giant cell lesions of the jaws. J Oral Maxillofac Surg 60: 1103-1111.

1242. Kaddour HS, Woodhead CJ (1992). Transitional papilloma of the middle ear. J Laryngol Otol 106: 628-629.

1243. Kadish S, Goodman M, Wang CC (1976). Olfactory neuroblastoma. A clinical analysis of 17 cases. Cancer 37: 1571-1576.

1244. Kaffe I, Ardekian L, Taicher S, Littner MM, Buchner A (1996). Radiologic features of central giant cell granuloma of the jaws. Oral Surg Oral Med Oral Pathol Oral Radiol Endod 81: 720-726.

1245. Kaffe I, Naor H, Buchner A (1997). Clinical and radiological features of odontogenic myxoma of the jaws. Dentomaxillofac Radiol 26: 299-303.

1246. Kaffe I, Naor H, Calderon S, Buchner A (1999). Radiological and clinical features of aneurysmal bone cyst of the jaws. Dentomaxillofac Radiol 28: 167-172.

1247. Kainuma K, Kikukawa M, Itoh T, Osawa M, Watanabe M (2001). Leiomyosarcoma of the larynx: emergency tracheostomy. J Laryngol Otol 115: 570-572.

1248. Kakagia D, Alexiadis G, Kiziridou A, Lambropoulou M (2004). Brooke-Spiegler syndrome with parotid gland involvement. Eur J Dermatol 14: 139-141.

1249. Kalantar Motamedi MH (1998). Aneurysmal bone cysts of the jaws: clinicopathological features, radiographic evaluation and treatment analysis of 17 cases. J Craniomaxillofac Surg 26: 56-62.

1250. Kallis S, Stevens DJ (1989). Acinous cell carcinoma of the larynx. J Laryngol Otol 103: 638-641.

1251. Kamath VV, Varma RR, Gadewar DR, Muralidhar M (1989). Oral verrucous carcinoma. An analysis of 37 cases. J Craniomaxillofac Surg 17: 309-314.

1252. Kamb A (1996). Human melanoma genetics. J Investig Dermatol Symp Proc 1: 177-182.

1253. Kambic V, Gale N (1995). Epithelial hyperplastic lesions of the larynx. Elsevier: Amsterdam.

1254. Kambic V, Lenart I (1971). [Our classification of hyperplasia of the laryngeal epithelium from the prognostic point of view]. J Fr Otorhinolaryngol Audiophonol Chir Maxillofac 20: 1145-1150.

1255. Kambic V, Radsel Z, Gale N (1989). Alterations in the laryngeal mucosa after exposure to asbestos. Br J Ind Med 46: 717-723.

1256. Kambic V, Radsel Z, Prezelj J, Zargi M (1984). The role of testosterone in laryngeal carcinogenesis. Am J Otolaryngol 5: 344-349.

1257. Kamerer DB, Caparosa RJ (1982). Temporal bone encephalocele—diagnosis and treatment. Laryngoscope 92: 878-882.

1258. Kamerer DB, Love GL, Riehl PA (1983). Intranasal encephalocele masking as nasal polyp in an adult patient. Arch Otolaryngol 109: 420-421.

1259. Kameya T, Shimosato Y, Adachi I, Abe K, Ebihara S, Ono I (1980). Neuroendocrine carcinoma of the paranasal sinus: a morphological and endocrinological study. Cancer 45: 330-339.

1260. Kamijo R, Miyaoka K, Tachikawa T, Nagumo M (1999). Odontogenic ghost cell carcinoma: report of a case. J Oral Maxillofac Surg 57: 1266-1270.

1261. Kammer H, George R (1981). Cushing's disease in a patient with an ectopic pituitary adenoma. JAMA 246: 2722-2724.

1262. Kanavaros P, Kouvidou C, Dai Y (1995). MDM-2 protein expression in nasopharyngeal carcinomas — comparative study with p53 expression. J Clin Pathol: Clin Mol Pathol 48: M322-M325.

1263. Kanavaros P, Lescs MC, Briere J, Divine M, Galateau F, Joab I, Bosq J, Farcet JP, Reyes F, Gaulard P (1993). Nasal T-cell lymphoma: a clinicopathologic entity associated with peculiar phenotype and with Epstein-Barr virus. Blood 81: 2688-2695.

1264. Kane WJ, McCaffrey TV, Olsen KD, Lewis JE (1991). Primary parotid malignancies. A clinical and pathologic review. Arch Otolaryngol Head Neck Surg 117: 307-315.

1265. Kapadia SB, Barnes L (1998). Expression of androgen receptor, gross cystic disease fluid protein, and CD44 in salivary duct carcinoma. Mod Pathol 11: 1033-1038.

1266. Kapadia SB, Barnes L, Pelzman K, Mirani N, Heffner DK, Bedetti C (1993). Carcinoma ex oncocytic Schneiderian (cylindrical cell) papilloma. Am J Otolaryngol 14: 332-338.

1267. Kapadia SB, Desai U, Cheng VS (1982). Extramedullary plasmacytoma of the head and neck. A clinicopathologic study of 20 cases. Medicine (Baltimore) 61: 317-329.

1268. Kapadia SB, Enzinger FM, Heffner DK, Hyams VJ, Frizzera G (1993). Crystal-storing histiocytosis associated with lymphoplasmacytic neoplasms. Report of three cases mimicking adult rhabdomyoma. Am J Surg Pathol 17: 461-467.

1269. Kapadia SB, Frisman DM, Hitchcock CL, Ellis GL, Popek EJ (1993). Melanotic neuroectodermal tumor of infancy. Clinicopathological, immunohistochemical, and flow cytometric study. Am J Surg Pathol 17: 566-573.

1270. Kapadia SB, Heffner DK (1992). Pitfalls in the histopathologic diagnosis of pyogenic granuloma. Eur Arch Otorhinolaryngol 249: 195-200.

1271. Kapadia SB, Meis JM, Frisman DM, Ellis GL, Heffner DK (1993). Fetal rhabdomyoma of the head and neck: a clinicopathologic and immunophenotypic study of 24 cases. Hum Pathol 24: 754-765.

1272. Kapadia SB, Meis JM, Frisman DM, Ellis GL, Heffner DK, Hyams VJ (1993). Adult rhabdomyoma of the head and neck: a clinicopathologic and immunophenotypic study. Hum Pathol 24: 608-617.

1273. Kapadia SB, Popek EJ, Barnes L (1994). Pediatric otorhinolaryngic pathology: diagnosis of selected lesions. Pathol Annu 29 Pt 1: 159-209.

1274. Kapadia SB, Roman LN, Kingma DW, Jaffe ES, Frizzera G (1995). Hodgkin's disease of Waldeyer's ring. Clinical and histoimmunophenotypic findings and association with Epstein-Barr virus in 16 cases. Am J Surg Pathol 19: 1431-1439.

1275. Kaplan MA, Pettit CL, Zukerberg LR, Harris NL (1992). Primary lymphoma of the trachea with morphologic and immunophenotypic characteristics of low-grade B-cell lymphoma of mucosa-associated lymphoid tissue. Am J Surg Pathol 16: 71-75.

1276. Kar DK, Gupta SK, Agarwal A, Mishra SK (2001). Brown tumor of the palate and mandible in association with primary hyperparathyroidism. J Oral Maxillofac Surg 59: 1352-1354.

1277. Karagiannidis K, Noussios G, Sakellariou T, Kontzoglou G, Mantziaris V, Preponis C (1998). Primary laryngeal melanoma. J Otolaryngol 27: 104-106.

1278. Karakok M, Ozer E, Sari I, Mumbuc S, Aydin A, Kanlikama M, Kervancioglu R (2002). Inflammatory myofibroblastic tumor (inflammatory pseudotumor) of the maxillary sinus mimicking malignancy: a case report of an unusual location (is that a true neoplasm?). Auris Nasus Larynx 29: 383-386.

1279. Kas K, Voz ML, Roijer E, Astrom AK, Meyen E, Stenman G, Van de Ven WJ (1997). Promoter swapping between the genes for a novel zinc finger protein and beta-catenin in pleiomorphic adenomas with t(3;8)(p21;q12) translocations. Nat Genet 15: 170-174.

1280. Kashima H, Mounts P, Leventhal B, Hruban RH (1993). Sites of predilection in recurrent respiratory papillomatosis. Ann Otol Rhinol Laryngol 102: 580-583.

1281. Kashima HK, Mounts P, Shah K (1996). Recurrent respiratory papillomatosis. Obstet Gynecol Clin North Am 23: 699-706.
1282. Kashima HK, Shah F, Lyles A, Glackin R, Muhammad N, Turner L, Van Zandt S, Whitt S, Shah K (1992). A comparison of risk factors in juvenile-onset and adult-onset recurrent respiratory papillomatosis. Laryngoscope 102: 9-13.
1283. Kasperbauer JL, O'Halloran GL, Espy MJ, Smith TF, Lewis JE (1993). Polymerase chain reaction (PCR) identification of human papillomavirus (HPV) DNA in verrucous carcinoma of the larynx. Laryngoscope 103: 416-420.
1284. Kato K, Ijiri R, Tanaka Y, Hara M, Sekido K (1999). Nasal chondromesenchymal hamartoma of infancy: the first Japanese case report. Pathol Int 49: 731-736.
1285. Kato S, Sakura M, Takooda S, Sakurai M, Izumo T (1997). Primary non-Hodgkin's lymphoma of the larynx. J Laryngol Otol 111: 571-574.
1286. Katz JO, Dunlap CL, Ennis RL (1992). Cherubism: report of a case showing regression without treatment. J Oral Maxillofac Surg 50: 301-303.
1287. Kaugars GE, Niamtu JI, Svirsky JA (1992). Cherubism: diagnosis, treatment, and comparison with central giant cell granulomas and giant cell tumors. Oral Surg Oral Med Oral Pathol 73: 369-374.
1288. Kaugars GE, Zussmann HW (1991). Ameloblastic odontoma (odontoameloblastoma). Oral Surg Oral Med Oral Pathol 71: 371-373.
1289. Kawauchi S, Hayatsu Y, Takahashi M, Furuya T, Oga A, Niwa S, Sasaki K (2003). Spindle-cell ameloblastic carcinoma: A case report with immunohistochemical, ultrastructural, and comparative genomic hybridization analyses. Oncol Rep 10: 31-34.
1290. Kaya S, Saydam L, Ruacan S (1990). Laryngeal leiomyoma. Int J Pediatr Otorhinolaryngol 19: 285-288.
1291. Kaznelson DJ, Schindel J (1979). Mucoepidermoid carcinoma of the air passages: report of three cases. Laryngoscope 89: 115-121.
1292. Kearsley JH, Thomas S (1993). Prognostic markers in cancers of the head and neck region. Anticancer Drugs 4: 419-429.
1293. Kedar A, Cantrel G, Rosen G (1988). Rhabdomyosarcoma of the trachea. J Laryngol Otol 102: 735-736.
1294. Keelawat S, Liu CZ, Roehm PC, Barnes L (2002). Adenosquamous carcinoma of the upper aerodigestive tract: a clinicopathologic study of 12 cases and review of the literature. Am J Otolaryngol 23: 160-168.
1295. Keller AZ (1969). Residence, age, race and related factors in the survival and associations with salivary tumors. Am J Epidemiol 90: 269-277.
1296. Kelly A, Bough IDJr, Luft JD, Conard K, Reilly JS, Tuttle D (1996). Hairy polyp of the oropharynx: case report and literature review. J Pediatr Surg 31: 704-706.
1297. Kelly JH, Joseph M, Carroll E, Goodman ML, Pilch BZ, Levinson RM, Strome M (1980). Inverted papilloma of the nasal septum. Arch Otolaryngol 106: 767-771.
1298. Kelly KM, Womer RB, Sorensen PH, Xiong QB, Barr FG (1997). Common and variant gene fusions predict distinct clinical phenotypes in rhabdomyosarcoma. J Clin Oncol 15: 1831-1836.
1299. Kemp BL, Batsakis JG, El Naggar AK, Kotliar SN, Luna MA (1995). Terminal duct adenocarcinomas of the parotid gland. J Laryngol Otol 109: 466-468.
1300. Kent SE, Majumdar B (1985). Metastatic tumours in the maxillary sinus. A report of two cases and a review of the literature. J Laryngol Otol 99: 459-462.
1301. Keogh PV, Fisher V, Flint SR (2002). Resolution of oral non-Hodgkin's lymphoma by reduction of immunosuppressive therapy in a renal allograft recipient: a case report and review of the literature. Oral Surg Oral Med Oral Pathol Oral Radiol Endod 94: 697-701.
1302. Kerpel SM, Freedman PD, Lumerman H (1978). The papillary cystadenoma of minor salivary gland origin. Oral Surg Oral Med Oral Pathol 46: 820-826.
1303. Kershisnik M, Batsakis JG (1994). Aneurysmal bone cysts of the jaws. Ann Otol Rhinol Laryngol 103: 164-165.
1304. Kessler A, Handler SD (1994). Salivary gland neoplasms in children: a 10-year survey at the Children's Hospital of Philadelphia. Int J Pediatr Otorhinolaryngol 29: 195-202.
1305. Keszler A, Piloni MJ (2002). Malignant transformation in odontogenic keratocysts. Case report. Med Oral 7: 331-335.
1306. Keukens F, Voorst Vader PC, Panders AK, Vinks S, Oosterhuis JW, Kleijer WJ (1989). Xeroderma pigmentosum: squamous cell carcinoma of the tongue. Acta Derm Venereol 69: 530-531.
1307. Khan MH, Jones AS, Haqqani MT (1994). Angioleiomyoma of the nasal cavity—report of a case and review of the literature. J Laryngol Otol 108: 244-246.
1308. Khullar SM, Best PV (1992). Adenomatosis of minor salivary glands. Report of a case. Oral Surg Oral Med Oral Pathol 74: 783-787.
1309. Khuri FR, Kim ES, Lee JJ, Winn RJ, Benner SE, Lippman SM, Fu KK, Cooper JS, Vokes EE, Chamberlain RM, Williams B, Pajak TF, Goepfert H, Hong WK (2001). The impact of smoking status, disease stage, and index tumor site on second primary tumor incidence and tumor recurrence in the head and neck retinoid chemoprevention trial. Cancer Epidemiol Biomarkers Prev 10: 823-829.
1310. Kieff DA, Curtin HD, Limb CJ, Nadol JB (1998). A hairy polyp presenting as a middle ear mass in a pediatric patient. Am J Otolaryngol 19: 228-231.
1311. Kim DW, Low W, Billman G, Wickersham J, Kearns D (1999). Chondroid hamartoma presenting as a neonatal nasal mass. Int J Pediatr Otorhinolaryngol 47: 253-259.
1312. Kim GE, Cho JH, Yang WI, Chung EJ, Suh CO, Park KR, Hong WP, Park IY, Hahn JS, Roh JK, Kim BS (2000). Angiocentric lymphoma of the head and neck: patterns of systemic failure after radiation treatment. J Clin Oncol 18: 54-63.
1313. Kim J, Ellis GL (1993). Dental follicular tissue: misinterpretation as odontogenic tumors. J Oral Maxillofac Surg 51: 762-767.
1314. Kim J, Lee EH, Yook JI, Han JY, Yoon JH, Ellis GL (2000). Odontogenic ghost cell carcinoma: a case report with reference to the relation between apoptosis and ghost cells. Oral Surg Oral Med Oral Pathol Oral Radiol Endod 90: 630-635.
1315. Kim J, Yook JI (1994). Immunohistochemical study on proliferating cell nuclear antigen expression in ameloblastomas. Eur J Cancer B Oral Oncol 30B: 126-131.
1316. Kim KI, Kim YS, Kim HK, Chae YS, Yoem BW, Kim I (1999). The detection of Epstein-Barr virus in the lesions of salivary glands. Pathol Res Pract 195: 407-412.
1317. Kim KI, Yoo SL (1996). Infantile fibrosarcoma in the nasal cavity. Otolaryngol Head Neck Surg 114: 98-102.
1318. Kim SS, Han MH, Kim JE, Lee CH, Chung HW, Lee JS, Chang KH (2000). Malignant melanoma of the sinonasal cavity: explanation of magnetic resonance signal intensities with histopathologic characteristics. Am J Otolaryngol 21: 366-378.
1319. Kim ST, Kim CW, Han GC, Park C, Jang IH, Cha HE, Choi G, Lee HM (2001). Malignant triton tumor of the nasal cavity. Head Neck 23: 1075-1078.
1320. Kim T, Yoon GS, Kim O, Gong G (1998). Fine needle aspiration diagnosis of malignant mixed tumor (carcinosarcoma) arising in pleomorphic adenoma of the salivary gland. A case report. Acta Cytol 42: 1027-1031.
1321. Kim YH, Chae SW, Jung HH (2003). Mucoepidermoid carcinoma arising from the eustachian tube and middle ear. J Laryngol Otol 117: 202-204.
1322. Kimura T, Ishikawa E, Yoshimura S (1948). On the unusual granulation combined with hyperplastic changes of lymphatic tissues. Trans Soc Pathol Jpn 37: 179-180.
1323. Kindblom LG, Angervall L, Haglid K (1984). An immunohistochemical analysis of S-100 protein and glial fibrillary acidic protein in nasal glioma. Acta Pathol Microbiol Immunol Scand [A] 92: 387-389.
1324. Kingdom TT, Kaplan MJ (1995). Mucosal melanoma of the nasal cavity and paranasal sinuses. Head Neck 17: 184-189.
1325. Kirita T, Okabe S, Izumo T, Sugimura M (1994). Risk factors for the postoperative local recurrence of tongue carcinoma. J Oral Maxillofac Surg 52: 149-154.
1326. Kishore A, O'Reilly BF (2000). A clinical study of vestibular schwannomas in type 2 neurofibromatosis. Clin Otolaryngol 25: 561-565.
1327. Kiyoshima T, Shima K, Kobayashi I, Matsuo K, Okamura K, Komatsu S, Rasul AM, Sakai H (2001). Expression of p53 tumor suppressor gene in adenoid cystic and mucoepidermoid carcinomas of the salivary glands. Oral Oncol 37: 315-322.
1328. Klap P, Reizine D, Monteil JP, Despreaux G, Hadjean E, Merland JJ, Tran Ba Huy P (1984). [Tumors and vascular malformations of the larynx. Angiographic aspects and therapeutic indications]. Ann Otolaryngol Chir Cervicofac 101: 579-583.
1329. Kleihues P, Cavenee WK (2000). Pathology and Genetics of Tumours of the Nervous System. IARC Press: Lyon.
1330. Klein EA, Anzil AP, Mezzacappa P, Borderon M, Ho V (1992). Sinonasal primitive neuroectodermal tumor arising in a long-term survivor of heritable unilateral retinoblastoma. Cancer 70: 423-431.
1331. Kleinsasser O (1964). Das Glomus Laryngieum inferior. Arch Ohrenheilk 184: 214-224.
1332. Kleinsasser O (1988). Tumors of the Larynx and Hypopharynx. Georg Thieme Pub: Stuttgart.
1333. Kleinsasser O, Schroeder HG (1988). Adenocarcinomas of the inner nose after exposure to wood dust. Morphological findings and relationships between histopathology and clinical behavior in 79 cases. Arch Otorhinolaryngol 245: 1-15.
1334. Klemi PJ, Joensuu H, Siivonen L, Virolainen E, Syrjanen S, Syrjanen K (1989). Association of DNA aneuploidy with human papillomavirus-induced malignant transformation of sinonasal transitional papillomas. Otolaryngol Head Neck Surg 100: 563-567.
1335. Kliewer KE, Cochran AJ (1989). A review of the histology, ultrastructure, immunohistology, and molecular biology of extra-adrenal paragangliomas. Arch Pathol Lab Med 113: 1209-1218.
1336. Kliewer KE, Wen DR, Cancilla PA, Cochran AJ (1989). Paragangliomas: assessment of prognosis by histologic, immunohistochemical, and ultrastructural techniques. Hum Pathol 20: 29-39.
1337. Klijanienko J, el Naggar A, Ponzio-Prion A, Marandas P, Micheau C, Caillaud JM (1993). Basaloid squamous carcinoma of the head and neck. Immunohistochemical comparison with adenoid cystic carcinoma and squamous cell carcinoma. Arch Otolaryngol Head Neck Surg 119: 887-890.
1338. Klijanienko J, El Naggar AK, Servois V, Rodriguez J, Validire P, Vielh P (1998). Mucoepidermoid carcinoma ex pleomorphic adenoma: nonspecific preoperative cytologic findings in six cases. Cancer 84: 231-234.
1339. Klijanienko J, Micheau C, Azli N, Cvitkovic E, Eschwege F, Marandas P, Armand JP, Casiraghi O, Schwaab G, de Vathaire F (1989). Undifferentiated carcinoma of nasopharyngeal type of tonsil. Arch Otolaryngol Head Neck Surg 115: 731-734.
1340. Klima M, Wolfe K, Johnson PE (1978). Basal cell tumors of the parotid gland. Arch Otolaryngol 104: 111-116.
1341. Klintenberg C, Olofsson J, Hellquist H, Sokjer H (1984). Adenocarcinoma of the ethmoid sinuses. A review of 28 cases with special reference to wood dust exposure. Cancer 54: 482-488.
1342. Knapp MJ (1971). Oral disease in 181,338 consecutive oral examinations. J Am Dent Assoc 83: 1288-1293.
1343. Knott PD, Gannon FH, Thompson LDR (2003). Mesenchymal chondrosarcoma of the sinonasal tract: a clinicopathologic study of 13 cases with a review of the literature. Laryngoscope 113: 783-790.
1344. Knudson AGJr (1971). Mutation and cancer: statistical study of retinoblastoma. Proc Natl Acad Sci U S A 68: 820-823.
1345. Ko JY, Chen CL, Lui LT, Hsu MM (1996). Radiation-induced malignant fibrous histiocytoma in patients with nasopharyngeal carcinoma. Arch Otolaryngol Head Neck Surg 122: 535-538.
1346. Ko YH, Choi KE, Han JH, Kim JM, Ree HJ (2001). Comparative genomic hybridization study of nasal-type NK/T-cell lymphoma. Cytometry 46: 85-91.
1347. Ko YH, Ree HJ, Kim WS, Choi WH, Moon WS, Kim SW (2000). Clinicopathologic and genotypic study of extranodal nasal-type natural killer/T-cell lymphoma and natural killer precursor lymphoma among Koreans. Cancer 89: 2106-2116.
1348. Koay CB, Freeland AP, Athanasou NA (1995). Chondromyxoid fibroma of the nasal bone with extension into the frontal and ethmoidal sinuses. J Laryngol Otol 109: 258-261.
1349. Kobayashi Y, Murakami R, Toba M, Ichikawa T, Kanazawa R, Sanno N, Shimura T, Sawada N, Hosone M, Kumazaki T (2001). Chondroblastoma of the temporal bone. Skeletal Radiol 30: 714-718.
1350. Koch BB, Trask DK, Hoffman HT,

Karnell LH, Robinson RA, Zhen W, Menck HR (2001). National survey of head and neck verrucous carcinoma: patterns of presentation, care, and outcome. Cancer 92: 110-120.
1351. Koch WM, Lango M, Sewell D, Zahurak M, Sidransky D (1999). Head and neck cancer in nonsmokers: a distinct clinical and molecular entity. Laryngoscope 109: 1544-1551.
1352. Koita H, Suzumiya J, Ohshima K, Takeshita M, Kimura N, Kikuchi M, Koono M (1997). Lymphoblastic lymphoma expressing natural killer cell phenotype with involvement of the mediastinum and nasal cavity. Am J Surg Pathol 21: 242-248.
1353. Koivunen P, Suutala L, Schorsch I, Jokinen K, Alho OP (2002). Malignant epithelial salivary gland tumors in northern Finland: incidence and clinical characteristics. Eur Arch Otorhinolaryngol 259: 146-149.
1354. Kojya S, Matsumura J, Ting L, Hongyo T, Inazawa J, Kirihata M, Aozasa K (2001). Familial nasal NK/T-cell lymphoma and pesticide use. Am J Hematol 66: 145-147.
1355. Kollur SM, El Hag IA (2003). Fine-needle aspiration cytology of metastatic nasopharyngeal carcinoma in cervical lymph nodes: comparison with metastatic squamous-cell carcinoma, and Hodgkin's and non-Hodgkin's lymphoma. Diagn Cytopathol 28: 18-22.
1356. Kondoh T, Hamada Y, Kamei K, Seto K (2002). Chondroblastoma of the mandibular condyle: report of a case. J Oral Maxillofac Surg 60: 198-203.
1357. Konowitz PM, Lawson W, Som PM, Urken ML, Breakstone BA, Biller HF (1988). Laryngeal paraganglioma: update on diagnosis and treatment. Laryngoscope 98: 40-49.
1358. Koss LG, Spiro RH, Hajdu S (1972). Small cell (oat cell) carcinoma of minor salivary gland origin. Cancer 30: 737-741.
1359. Kotsianti A, Costopoulos J, Morgello S, Papadimitriou C (1996). Undifferentiated carcinoma of the parotid gland in a white patient: detection of Epstein-Barr virus by in situ hybridization. Hum Pathol 27: 87-90.
1360. Kotwall CA (1992). Smoking as an etiologic factor in the development of Warthin's tumor of the parotid gland. Am J Surg 164: 646-647.
1361. Kourea HP, Orlow I, Scheithauer BW, Cordon-Cardo C, Woodruff JM (1999). Deletions of the INK4A gene occur in malignant peripheral nerve sheath tumors but not in neurofibromas. Am J Pathol 155: 1855-1860.
1362. Koury ME, Stella JP, Epker BN (1993). Vascular transformation in cherubism. Oral Surg Oral Med Oral Pathol 76: 20-27.
1363. Kovarik P, Pyle J, Chou PM (1998). Ploidy, proliferative activity, and p53 as biologic markers in inflammatory myofibroblastic tumors. Mod Pathol 11.
1364. Kowalski PJ, Paulino AF (2001). Proliferation index as a prognostic marker in hemangiopericytoma of the head and neck. Head Neck 23: 492-496.
1365. Koyi H, Branden E (2000). Intratracheal metastasis from malignant melanoma. J Eur Acad Dermatol Venereol 14: 407-408.
1366. Kragh LV, Dahlin DC, Erich JB (1958). Osteogenic sarcoma of the jaws and facial bones. Am J Surger 96: 496-505.
1367. Kragh LV, Dahlin DC, Erich JB (1960). Cartilaginous tumors of the jaws and facial regions. Am J Surg 99: 852-856.
1368. Kramer IR, Lucas RB, el Labban N, Lister L (1970). The use of discriminant analysis for examining the histological feathers of oral keratoses and lichen planus. Br J Cancer 24: 673-683.
1369. Kransdorf MJ, Sweet DE, Buetow PC, Giudici MA, Moser RPJr (1992). Giant cell tumor in skeletally immature patients. Radiology 184: 233-237.
1370. Kraus DH, Zelefsky MJ, Brock HA, Huo J, Harrison LB, Shah JP (1997). Combined surgery and radiation therapy for squamous cell carcinoma of the hypopharynx. Otolaryngol Head Neck Surg 116: 637-641.
1371. Krausen AS, Gall AM, Garza R, Spector GJ, Ansel DG (1977). Liposarcoma of the larynx: a multicentric or a metastatic malignancy. Laryngoscope 87: 1116-1124.
1372. Krecicki T, Jelen M, Zalesska-Krecicka M, Szkudlarek T (1998). Ki-67 immunostaining and prognosis in laryngeal cancer. Clin Otolaryngol 23: 539-542.
1373. Krishnamurthy S, Lanier AP, Dohan P, Lanier JF, Henle W (1987). Salivary gland cancer in Alaskan natives, 1966-1980. Hum Pathol 18: 986-996.
1374. Krogdahl AS, Schou C (1997). Mucinous adenocarcinoma of the sublingual gland. J Oral Pathol Med 26: 198-200.
1375. Krogdahl AS, Svane-Knudsen V (2002). Intraductal papilloma of the parotid gland in a child. Histopathology 41: 83-85.
1376. Kroll AJ, Alexander B, Cochios F, Pechet L (1964). Hereditary deficiencies of clotting factors VII and X associated with carotid-body tumors. N Engl J Med 270: 6-13.
1377. Kronenberg J, Ben Shoshan J, Modan M, Leventon G (1988). Blast injury and cholesteatoma. Am J Otol 9: 127-130.
1378. Ku PK, Tong MC, Leung CY, Pak MW, van Hasselt CA (1999). Nasal manifestation of extranodal Rosai-Dorfman disease—diagnosis and management. J Laryngol Otol 113: 275-280.
1379. Kuhn JJ, Schoem SR, Warnock GR (1996). Squamous cell carcinoma arising in a benign teratoma of the maxilla. Otolaryngol Head Neck Surg 114: 447-452.
1380. Kui LL, Xiu HZ, Ning LY (2003). Condyloma acuminatum and human papilloma virus infection in the oral mucosa of children. Pediatr Dent 25: 149-153.
1381. Kujawski M, Sarlomo-Rikala M, Gabriel A, Szyfter K, Knuutila S (1999). Recurrent DNA copy number losses associated with metastasis of larynx carcinoma. Genes Chromosomes Cancer 26: 253-257.
1382. Kumaki N, Kajiwara H, Kameyama K, DeLellis RA, Asa SL, Osamura RY, Takami H (2002). Prediction of malignant behavior of pheochromocytomas and paragangliomas using immunohistochemical techniques. Endocr Pathol 13: 149-156.
1383. Kumar RV, Kini L, Bhargava AK, Mukherjee G, Hazarika D, Shenoy AM, Anantha N (1993). Salivary duct carcinoma. J Surg Oncol 54: 193-198.
1384. Kumar S, Perlman E, Pack S, Davis M, Zhang H, Meltzer P, Tsokos M (1999). Absence of EWS/FLI1 fusion in olfactory neuroblastomas indicates these tumors do not belong to the Ewing's sarcoma family. Hum Pathol 30: 1356-1360.
1385. Kung IT, Gibson JB, Bannatyne PM (1984). Kimura's disease: a clinico-pathological study of 21 cases and its distinction from angiolymphoid hyperplasia with eosinophilia. Pathology 16: 39-44.
1386. Kunze E, Donath K, Luhr HG, Engelhardt W, De Vivie R (1985). Biology of metastasizing ameloblastoma. Pathol Res Pract 180: 526-535.
1387. Kuo T, Hsueh C (1997). Lymphoepithelioma-like salivary gland carcinoma in Taiwan: a clinicopathological study of nine cases demonstrating a strong association with Epstein-Barr virus. Histopathology 31: 75-82.
1388. Kuo T, Sayers CP, Rosai J (1976). Masson's "vegetant intravascular hemangioendothelioma:" a lesion often mistaken for angiosarcoma: study of seventeen cases located in the skin and soft tissues. Cancer 38: 1227-1236.
1389. Kuo T, Tsang NM (2001). Salivary gland type nasopharyngeal carcinoma: a histologic, immunohistochemical, and Epstein-Barr virus study of 15 cases including a psammomatous mucoepidermoid carcinoma. Am J Surg Pathol 25: 80-86.
1390. Kuo TT, Shih LY, Chan HL (1988). Kimura's disease; involvement of regional lymph nodes and distinction from angiolymphoid hyperplasia with eosinophilia. Am J Surg Pathol 12: 843-854.
1391. Kuratomi Y, Kumamoto Y, Sakai Y, Komiyama S (1994). Carotid body tumor associated with differentiated thyroid carcinoma. Eur Arch Otorhinolaryngol 251 Suppl 1: S91-S94.
1392. Kuroi M (1980). Simple bone cyst of the jaw: review of the literature and report of case. J Oral Surg 38: 456-459.
1393. Kurokawa H, Murata T, Fukuyama H, Kajiyama M (1999). Sebaceous lymphadenoma in the midline of the maxilla: report of case. J Oral Maxillofac Surg 57: 1461-1463.
1394. Kurtz M, Mesa M, Alberto P (2001). Treatment of a central giant cell lesion of the mandible with intralesional glucocorticosteroids. Oral Surg Oral Med Oral Pathol Oral Radiol Endod 91: 636-637.
1395. Kuruvilla A, Wenig BM, Humphrey DM, Heffner DK (1990). Leiomyosarcoma of the sinonasal tract. A clinicopathologic study of nine cases. Arch Otolaryngol Head Neck Surg 116: 1278-1286.
1396. Kusafuka K, Hiraki Y, Shukunami C, Yamaguchi A, Kayano T, Takemura T (2001). Cartilage-specific matrix protein chondromodulin-I is associated with chondroid formation in salivary pleomorphic adenomas: immunohistochemical analysis. Am J Pathol 158: 1465-1472.
1397. Kusafuka K, Yamaguchi A, Kayano T, Takemura T (1999). Immunohistochemical localization of the bone morphogenetic protein-6 in salivary pleomorphic adenomas. Pathol Int 49: 1023-1027.
1398. Kwekkeboom DJ, van Urk H, Pauw BK, Lamberts SW, Kooij PP, Hoogma RP, Krenning EP (1993). Octreotide scintigraphy for the detection of paragangliomas. J Nucl Med 34: 873-878.
1399. Kwon GY, Kim EJ, Go JH (2002). Lymphadenoma arising in the parotid gland: a case report. Yonsei Med J 43: 536-538.
1400. Kwon MY, Gu M (2001). True malignant mixed tumor (carcinosarcoma) of parotid gland with unusual mesenchymal component: a case report and review of the literature. Arch Pathol Lab Med 125: 812-815.
1401. Kwong DL, Nicholls J, Wei WI, Chua DT, Sham JS, Yuen PW, Cheng AC, Wan KY, Kwong PW, Choy DT (1999). The time course of histologic remission after treatment of patients with nasopharyngeal carcinoma. Cancer 85: 1446-1453.
1402. Kwong DL, Nicholls J, Wei WI, Chua DT, Sham JS, Yuen PW, Cheng AC, Yau CC, Kwong PW, Choy DT (2001). Correlation of endoscopic and histologic findings before and after treatment for nasopharyngeal carcinoma. Head Neck 23: 34-41.
1403. Kwong J, Lo KW, To KF, Teo PM, Johnson PJ, Huang DP (2002). Promoter hypermethylation of multiple genes in nasopharyngeal carcinoma. Clin Cancer Res 8: 131-137.
1404. La Vecchia C, Franceschi S, Favero A, Talamini R, Negri E (1999). Alcohol intake and cancer of the upper digestive tract. Pattern of risk in Italy is different from that in Denmark. BMJ 318: 1289-1290.
1405. La Vecchia C, Negri E, D'Avanzo B, Franceschi S, Decarli A, Boyle P (1990). Dietary indicators of laryngeal cancer risk. Cancer Res 50: 4497-4500.
1406. La Vecchia C, Talamini R, Bosetti C, Negri E, Franceschi S (1999). RESPONSE: re: cancer of the oral cavity and pharynx in nonsmokers who drink alcohol and in nondrinkers who smoke tobacco. J Natl Cancer Inst 91: 1337-1338.
1407. Laane CJ, Murr AH, Mhatre AN, Jones KD, Lalwani AK (2002). Role of Epstein-Barr virus and cytomegalovirus in the etiology of benign parotid tumors. Head Neck 24: 443-450.
1408. Lack EE (1985). Extragonadal germ cell tumors of the head and neck region: review of 16 cases. Hum Pathol 16: 56-64.
1409. Lack EE (1994). Pathology of Adrenal & Extra-Adrenal Paraganglia. WB Saunders: Philidelphia.
1410. Lack EE, Cubilla AL, Woodruff JM (1979). Paragangliomas of the head and neck region. A pathologic study of tumors from 71 patients. Hum Pathol 10: 191-218.
1411. Lack EE, Cubilla AL, Woodruff JM, Farr HW (1977). Paragangliomas of the head and neck region: a clinical study of 69 patients. Cancer 39: 397-409.
1412. Lack EE, Lloyd RV, Carney JA, Woodruff JW (2003). Recommendations for the reporting of extra-adrenal paragangliomas. The Association of Directors of Anatomic and Surgical Pathology. Hum Pathol 34: 112-113.
1413. Lack EE, Upton MP (1988). Histopathologic review of salivary gland tumors in childhood. Arch Otolaryngol Head Neck Surg 114: 898-906.
1414. LaGuette J, Matias-Guiu X, Rosai J (1997). Thyroid paraganglioma: a clinicopathologic and immunohistochemical study of three cases. Am J Surg Pathol 21: 748-753.
1415. Lai JP, Tong CL, Hong C, Xiao JY, Tao ZD, Zhang Z, Tong WM, Betz CS (2002). Association between high initial tissue levels of cyclin d1 and recurrence of nasopharyngeal carcinoma. Laryngoscope 112: 402-408.
1416. Lalwani AK, Kaplan MJ (1990). Paranasal sinus leiomyosarcoma after cyclophosphamide and irradiation. Otolaryngol Head Neck Surg 103: 1039-1042.
1417. Lam KH, Ho HC, Ho CM, Wei WI (1994). Multifocal nature of adenolymphoma of the parotid. Br J Surg 81: 1612-1614.
1418. Lam KH, Wei WI, Ho HC, Ho CM (1990). Whole organ sectioning of mixed parotid tumors. Am J Surg 160: 377-381.
1419. Lam PW, Chan JK, Sin VC (1997). Nasal pleomorphic adenoma with skeletal

muscle differentiation: potential misdiagnosis as rhabdomyosarcoma. Hum Pathol 28: 1299-1302.
1420. Lambert PR, Ward PH, Berci G (1980). Pseudosarcoma of the larynx: a comprehensive analysis. Arch Otolaryngol 106: 700-708.
1421. Lamelas J, Terry JHJr, Alfonso AE (1987). Warthin's tumor: multicentricity and increasing incidence in women. Am J Surg 154: 347-351.
1422. Lamovec J, Frkovic-Grazio S, Bracko M (1998). Nonsporadic cases and unusual morphological features in pheochromocytoma and paraganglioma. Arch Pathol Lab Med 122: 63-68.
1423. Lampertico P, Russel WO, MacComb WS (1963). Squamous papilloma of the upper respiratory epithelium. Arch Pathol 75: 293-302.
1424. Lane S, Ironside JW (1990). Extraskeletal Ewing's sarcoma of the nasal fossa. J Laryngol Otol 104: 570-573.
1425. Langford L, Batsakis JG (1995). Pituitary gland involvement of the sinonasal tract. Ann Otol Rhinol Laryngol 104: 167-169.
1426. Langford LA (1996). Pathology of meningiomas. J Neurooncol 29: 217-221.
1427. Lanier A, Bender T, Talbot M, Wilmeth S, Tschopp C, Henle W, Henle G, Ritter D, Terasaki P (1980). Nasopharyngeal carcinoma in Alaskan Eskimos Indians, and Aleuts: a review of cases and study of Epstein-Barr virus, HLA, and environmental risk factors. Cancer 46: 2100-2106.
1428. Lanier AP, Clift SR, Bornkamm G, Henle W, Goepfert H, Raab-Traub N (1991). Epstein-Barr virus and malignant lymphoepithelial lesions of the salivary gland. Arctic Med Res 50: 55-61.
1429. Laramore GE, Scott CB, al Sarraf M, Haselow RE, Ervin TJ, Wheeler R, Jacobs JR, Schuller DE, Gahbauer RA, Schwade JG, Campbell BH (1992). Adjuvant chemotherapy for resectable squamous cell carcinomas of the head and neck: report on Intergroup Study 0034. Int J Radiat Oncol Biol Phys 23: 705-713.
1430. Larraza-Hernandez O, Alberes-Saavedra J, Benavides G, Krause LG, Perez-Merizaldi JC, Ginzo A (1982). Multiple endocrine neoplasia. Pituitary adenoma, multicentric papillary thyroid carcinoma, bilateral carotid body paraganglioma, parathyroid hyperplasia, gastric leiomyoma, and systemic amyloidosis. Am J Clin Pathol 78: 527-532.
1431. Larsson Å, Almeren H (1978). Ameloblastoma of the jaws. An analysis of a consecutive series of all cases reported to the Swedish Cancer Registry during 1958—1971. Acta Pathol Microbiol Scand [A] 86A: 337-349.
1432. Larsson LG, Donner LR (1999). Large cell neuroendocrine carcinoma of the parotid gland: fine needle aspiration, and light microscopic and ultrastructural study. Acta Cytol 43: 534-536.
1433. Larsson LG, Sandstrom A, Westling P (1975). Relationship of Plummer-Vinson disease to cancer of the upper alimentary tract in Sweden. Cancer Res 35: 3308-3316.
1434. Lasjaunias P, Picard L, Manelfe C, Moret J, Doyon D (1980). Angiofibroma of the nasopharynx. A review of 53 cases treated by embolisation. The role of pretherapeutic angiography. Pathophysiological hypotheses. J Neuroradiol 7: 73-95.
1435. Laskawi R, Rodel R, Zirk A, Arglebe C (1998). Retrospective analysis of 35 patients with acinic cell carcinoma of the parotid gland. J Oral Maxillofac Surg 56: 440-443.
1436. Laskawi R, Schott T, Schroder M (1998). Recurrent pleomorphic adenomas of the parotid gland: clinical evaluation and long-term follow-up. Br J Oral Maxillofac Surg 36: 48-51.
1437. Laskin WB, Weiss SW, Bratthauer GL (1991). Epithelioid variant of malignant peripheral nerve sheath tumor (malignant epithelioid schwannoma). Am J Surg Pathol 15: 1136-1145.
1438. Laudio P (1971). Chemodectoma (paraganglioma non chromaffine) del laringeo superiore. Otorhinolaringol Ital 39.
1439. Laughlin EH (1989). Metastasizing ameloblastoma. Cancer 64: 776-780.
1440. Lawrence B, Perez-Atayde A, Hibbard MK, Rubin BP, Dal Cin P, Pinkus JL, Pinkus GS, Xiao S, Yi ES, Fletcher CD, Fletcher JA (2000). TPM3-ALK and TPM4-ALK oncogenes in inflammatory myofibroblastic tumors. Am J Pathol 157: 377-384.
1441. Lawrence WJr, Hays DM, Heyn R, Tefft M, Crist W, Beltangady M, Newton WJr, Wharam M (1987). Lymphatic metastases with childhood rhabdomyosarcoma. A report from the Intergroup Rhabdomyosarcoma Study. Cancer 60: 910-915.
1442. Lawson W, Ho BT, Shaari CM, Biller HF (1995). Inverted papilloma: a report of 112 cases. Laryngoscope 105: 282-288.
1443. Leclerc A, Luce D, Demers PA, Boffetta P, Kogevinas M, Belli S, Bolm-Audorff U, Brinton LA, Colin D, Comba P, Gerin M, Hardell L, Hayes RB, Magnani C, Merler E, Morcet JF, Preston-Martin S, Vaughan TL, Zheng W (1997). Sinonasal cancer and occupation. Results from the reanalysis of twelve case-control studies. Am J Ind Med 31: 153-165.
1444. Lee AW, Foo W, Law SC, Poon YF, SK O, Tung SY, Sze WM, Chappell R, Lau WH, Ho JH (1999). Staging of nasopharyngeal carcinoma: from Ho's to the new UICC system. Int J Cancer 84: 179-187.
1445. Lee AW, Foo W, Law SC, Poon YF, Sze WM, SK O, Tung SY, Chappell R, Lau WH, Ho JH (1999). Recurrent nasopharyngeal carcinoma: the puzzles of long latency. Int J Radiat Oncol Biol Phys 44: 149-156.
1446. Lee AW, Foo W, Mang O, Sze WM, Chappell R, Lau WH, Ko WM (2003). Changing epidemiology of nasopharyngeal carcinoma in Hong Kong over a 20-year period (1980-99): an encouraging reduction in both incidence and mortality. Int J Cancer 103: 680-685.
1447. Lee AW, Sze WM, Yau TK, Yeung RM, Chappell R, Fowler JF (2001). Retrospective analysis on treating nasopharyngeal carcinoma with accelerated fractionation (6 fractions per week) in comparison with conventional fractionation (5 fractions per week): report on 3-year tumor control and normal tissue toxicity. Radiother Oncol 58: 121-130.
1448. Lee AWM, Sze WM, Au JSK (2005). Treatment results for nasopharyngeal carcinoma in the modern era: The Hong Kong experience. Int J Radiat Oncol Biol Phys 61: 1107-1116.
1449. Lee DJ, Smith RR, Spaziani JT, Rostock R, Holliday M, Moses H (1985). Adenoid cystic carcinoma of the nasopharynx. Case reports and literature review. Ann Otol Rhinol Laryngol 94: 269-272.
1450. Lee HM, Kim AR, Lee SH (2000). Epithelial-myoepithelial carcinoma of the nasal cavity. Eur Arch Otorhinolaryngol 257: 376-378.
1451. Lee JH, Barich F, Karnell LH, Robinson RA, Zhen WK, Gantz BJ, Hoffman HT (2002). National Cancer Data Base report on malignant paragangliomas of the head and neck. Cancer 94: 730-737.
1452. Lee JH, Lee HK, Choi CG, Suh DC, Lee KS, Khang SK (2001). Malignant peripheral nerve sheath tumor in the parapharyngeal space: tumor spread through the eustachian tube. AJNR Am J Neuroradiol 22: 748-750.
1453. Lee JH, Lee MS, Lee BH, Choe DH, Do YS, Kim KH, Chin SY, Shim YS, Cho KJ (1996). Rhabdomyosarcoma of the head and neck in adults: MR and CT findings. AJNR Am J Neuroradiol 17: 1923-1928.
1454. Lee N, Xia P, Quivey JM, Sultanem K, Poon I, Akazawa C, Akazawa P, Weinberg V, Fu KK (2002). Intensity-modulated radiotherapy in the treatment of nasopharyngeal carcinoma: an update of the UCSF experience. Int J Radiat Oncol Biol Phys 53: 12-22.
1455. Lee PS, Sabbath-Solitare M, Redondo TC, Ongcapin EH (2000). Molecular evidence that the stromal and epithelial cells in pleomorphic adenomas of salivary gland arise from the same origin: clonal analysis using human androgen receptor gene (HUMARA) assay. Hum Pathol 31: 498-503.
1456. Lee S, Kim GE, Park CS, Choi EC, Yang WI, Lee CG, Keum KC, Kim YB, Suh CO (2001). Primary squamous cell carcinoma of the parotid gland. Am J Otolaryngol 22: 400-406.
1457. Lee YY, Van Tassel P, Nauert C, Raymond AK, Ediken J (1988). Craniofacial osteosarcomas: Plain film, CT, and MR findings in 46 cases. Am J Neuroradiol 9: 379-385.
1458. Lefor AT, Ord RA (1993). Multiple synchronous bilateral Warthin's tumors of the parotid glands with pleomorphic adenoma. Case report and review of the literature. Oral Surg Oral Med Oral Pathol 76: 319-324.
1459. Legius E, Dierick H, Wu R, Hall BK, Marynen P, Cassiman JJ, Glover TW (1994). TP53 mutations are frequent in malignant NF1 tumors. Genes Chromosomes Cancer 10: 250-255.
1460. Lei A, Wang S, Su Q (1998). [A study of histopathology and cell proliferation in calcifying odontogenic cyst]. Zhonghua Kou Qiang Yi Xue Za Zhi 33: 207-209.
1461. Leider AS, Eversole LR, Barkin ME (1985). Cystic ameloblastoma. A clinicopathologic analysis. Oral Surg Oral Med Oral Pathol 60: 624-630.
1462. Leider AS, Nelson JF, Trodahl JN (1972). Ameloblastic fibrosarcoma of the jaws. Oral Surg Oral Med Oral Pathol 33: 559-569.
1463. Leighton SE, Teo JG, Leung SF, Cheung AY, Lee JC, van Hasselt CA (1996). Prevalence and prognostic significance of tumor-associated tissue eosinophilia in nasopharyngeal carcinoma. Cancer 77: 436-440.
1464. Leithner A, Windhager R, Lang S, Haas OA, Kainberger F, Kotz R (1999). Aneurysmal bone cyst. A population based epidemiologic study and literature review. Clin Orthop 176-179.
1465. Lele SM, Pou AM, Ventura K, Gatalica Z, Payne D (2002). Molecular events in the progression of recurrent respiratory papillomatosis to carcinoma. Arch Pathol Lab Med 126: 1184-1188.
1466. LeMay DR, Sun JK, Mendel E, Hinton DR, Giannotta SL (1997). Chondromyxoid fibroma of the temporal bone. Surg Neurol 48: 148-152.
1467. Lench NJ, High AS, Markham AF, Hume WJ, Robinson PA (1996). Investigation of chromosome 9q22.3-q31 DNA marker loss in odontogenic keratocysts. Eur J Cancer B Oral Oncol 32B: 202-206.
1468. Lench NJ, Telford EA, High AS, Markham AF, Wicking C, Wainwright BJ (1997). Characterisation of human patched germ line mutations in naevoid basal cell carcinoma syndrome. Hum Genet 100: 497-502.
1469. Lengyel E, Somogyi A, Godeny M, Szerdahelyi A, Nemeth G (2000). Polymorphous low-grade adenocarcinoma of the nasopharynx. Case report and review of the literature. Strahlenther Onkol 176: 40-42.
1470. Lennert K, Kaiserling E, Mazzanti T (1978). Diagnosis and differential diagnosis of lymphoepithelial carcinoma in lymph nodes: histological, cytological and electron-microscopic findings. IARC Sci Publ 51-64.
1471. Lennox B, Clarke JA, Drake F, Ewen SW (1978). Incidence of salivary gland tumours in Scotland: accuracy of national records. Br Med J 1: 687-689.
1472. Lentsch EJ, Myers JN (2001). Melanoma of the head and neck: current concepts in diagnosis and management. Laryngoscope 111: 1209-1222.
1473. Leon X, Quer M, Diez S, Orus C, Lopez-Pousa A, Burgues J (1999). Second neoplasm in patients with head and neck cancer. Head Neck 21: 204-210.
1474. Leonard J, Gokden M, Kyriakos M, Derdeyn CP, Rich KM (2001). Malignant giant-cell tumor of the parietal bone: case report and review of the literature. Neurosurgery 48: 424-429.
1475. Leonard JR, Talbot ML (1970). Asymptomatic acoustic neurilemoma. Arch Otolaryngol 91: 117-124.
1476. Leong IT, Fernandes BJ, Mock D (2001). Epstein-Barr virus detection in non-Hodgkin's lymphoma of the oral cavity: an immunocytochemical and in situ hybridization study. Oral Surg Oral Med Oral Pathol Oral Radiol Endod 92: 184-193.
1477. Lesperance MM, Esclamado RM (1995). Squamous cell carcinoma arising in inverted papilloma. Laryngoscope 105: 178-183.
1478. Lesser RW, Spector GJ, Devineni VR (1987). Malignant tumors of the middle ear and external auditory canal: a 20-year review. Otolaryngol Head Neck Surg 96: 43-47.
1479. Leung SY, Chung LP, Yuen ST, Ho CM, Wong MP, Chan SY (1995). Lymphoepithelial carcinoma of the salivary gland: in situ detection of Epstein-Barr virus. J Clin Pathol 48: 1022-1027.
1480. Leung SY, Yuen ST, Chung LP, Kwong WK, Wong MP, Chan SY (1995). Epstein-Barr virus is present in a wide histological spectrum of sinonasal carcinomas. Am J Surg Pathol 19: 994-1001.
1481. Levanat S, Gorlin RJ, Fallet S, Johnson DR, Fantasia JE, Bale AE (1996). A two-hit model for developmental defects in Gorlin syndrome. Nat Genet 12: 85-87.
1482. Leventon GS, Evans HL (1981). Sarcomatoid squamous cell carcinoma of the mucous membranes of the head and neck: a clinicopathologic study of 20 cases. Cancer 48: 994-1003.
1483. Levi F, Lucchini F, Negri E, Boyle P, La Vecchia C (2004). Cancer mortality in

Europe, 1995-1999, and an overview of trends since 1960. Int J Cancer 110: 155-169.
1484. Levi JE, Delcelo R, Alberti VN, Torloni H, Villa LL (1989). Human papillomavirus DNA in respiratory papillomatosis detected by in situ hybridization and the polymerase chain reaction. Am J Pathol 135: 1179-1184.
1485. Levine AJ, Momand J, Finlay CA (1991). The p53 tumour suppressor gene. Nature 351: 453-456.
1486. Levine PH, Pearson GR, Armstrong M, Bengali Z, Berenberg J, Easton J, Goepfert H, Henle G, Henle W, Heffner D, Huang A, Hyams VJ, Lanier A, Neel HB, Pilch B, Pointek N, Taylor W, Terebelo H, Weiland L (1981). The reliability of IgA antibody to Epstein-Barr virus (EBV) capsid antigen as a test for the diagnosis of nasopharyngeal carcinoma (NPC). Cancer Detect Prev 4: 307-312.
1487. Levy FE, Tansek KM (1990). AIDS-associated Kaposi's sarcoma of the larynx. Ear Nose Throat J 69: 177, 182-177, 184.
1488. Lewis JE, McKinney BC, Weiland LH, Ferreiro JA, Olsen KD (1996). Salivary duct carcinoma. Clinicopathologic and immunohistochemical review of 26 cases. Cancer 77: 223-230.
1489. Lewis JE, Olsen KD, Inwards CY (1997). Cartilaginous tumors of the larynx: clinicopathologic review of 47 cases. Ann Otol Rhinol Laryngol 106: 94-100.
1490. Lewis JE, Olsen KD, Sebo TJ (1997). Spindle cell carcinoma of the larynx: review of 26 cases including DNA content and immunohistochemistry. Hum Pathol 28: 664-673.
1491. Lewis JE, Olsen KD, Sebo TJ (2001). Carcinoma ex pleomorphic adenoma: pathologic analysis of 73 cases. Hum Pathol 32: 596-604.
1492. Lewis JE, Olsen KD, Weiland LH (1991). Acinic cell carcinoma. Clinicopathologic review. Cancer 67: 172-179.
1493. Lewis JS, Castro EB (1972). Cancer of the nasal cavity and paranasal sinuses. J Laryngol Otol 86: 255-262.
1494. Lewis PD, Baxter P, Paul Griffiths A, Parry JM, Skibinski DO (2000). Detection of damage to the mitochondrial genome in the oncocytic cells of Warthin's tumour. J Pathol 191: 274-281.
1495. Li S, Baloch ZW, Tomaszewski JE, LiVolsi VA (2000). Worrisome histologic alterations following fine-needle aspiration of benign parotid lesions. Arch Pathol Lab Med 124: 87-91.
1496. Li T, Hongyo T, Syaifudin M, Nomura T, Dong Z, Shingu N, Kojya S, Nakatsuka S, Aozasa K (2000). Mutations of the p53 gene in nasal NK/T-cell lymphoma. Lab Invest 80: 493-499.
1497. Li TJ, Chen XM, Wang SZ, Fan MW, Semba I, Kitano M (1996). Kimura's disease: a clinicopathologic study of 54 Chinese patients. Oral Surg Oral Med Oral Pathol Oral Radiol Endod 82: 549-555.
1498. Li TJ, Yu SF (2003). Clinicopathologic spectrum of the so-called calcifying odontogenic cysts: a study of 21 intraosseous cases with reconsideration of the terminology and classification. Am J Surg Pathol 27: 372-384.
1499. Li TJ, Yu SF, Gao Y, Wang EB (2001). Clear cell odontogenic carcinoma: a clinicopathologic and immunocytochemical study of 5 cases. Arch Pathol Lab Med 125: 1566-1571.
1500. Li YX, Coucke PA, Li JY, Gu DZ, Liu XF, Zhou LQ, Mirimanoff RO, Yu ZH, Huang YR (1998). Primary non-Hodgkin's lymphoma of the nasal cavity: prognostic significance of paranasal extension and the role of radiotherapy and chemotherapy. Cancer 83: 449-456.
1501. Li ZQ, Pan QC, Chen JJ (1983). Epidemiology of nasopharyngeal carcinoma. In: Nasopharyngeal Carcinoma Clinical and Laboratory Researches, Li ZQ, Pan QC, Chen JJ, eds., Guangdong Science and Technology Press: Guangzhou, China , pp. 42-56.
1502. Liang A, Michaels L, Wright A (2003). Immunohistochemical characterizationof the epidermoid formation in the human middle ear. Laryngoscope 113: 1007-1014.
1503. Liang J, Yi Z, Lianq P (2000). The nature of juvenile nasopharyngeal angiofibroma. Otolaryngol Head Neck Surg 123: 475-481.
1504. Liang PC, Chen CC, Chu CC, Hu YF, Chu HM, Tsung YS (1961). The histologic classification, biological characteristics and histogenesis of nasopharyngeal carcinomas. Chin Med J 81: 629-658.
1505. Liang R, Todd D, Chan TK, Chiu E, Lie A, Kwong YL, Choy D, Ho FC (1995). Treatment outcome and prognostic factors for primary nasal lymphoma. J Clin Oncol 13: 666-670.
1506. Liao BS, Hilsinger RLJr, Chong E (1993). Septal pleomorphic adenoma masquerading as squamous cell carcinoma. Ear Nose Throat J 72: 781-782.
1507. Liao Z, Ha CS, McLaughlin P, Manning JT, Hess M, Cabanillas F, Cox JD (2000). Mucosa-associated lymphoid tissue lymphoma with initial supradiaphragmatic presentation: natural history and patterns of disease progression. Int J Radiat Oncol Biol Phys 48: 399-403.
1508. Libera DD, Falconieri G, Zanella M (1999). Embryonal "Botryoid" rhabdomyosarcoma of the larynx: a clinicopathologic and immunohistochemical study of two cases. Ann Diagn Pathol 3: 341-349.
1509. Lichtenstein L, Jaffee HL (1943). Chondrosarcoma of Bone. Am J Pathol 553-589.
1510. Lie ES, Karlsen F, Holm R (1996). Presence of human papillomavirus in squamous cell laryngeal carcinomas. A study of thirty-nine cases using polymerase chain reaction and in situ hybridization. Acta Otolaryngol 116: 900-905.
1511. Lieberman PH, Jones CR, Steinman RM, Erlandson RA, Smith J, Gee T, Huvos A, Garin-Chesa P, Filippa DA, Urmacher C, Gangi MD, Sperber M (1996). Langerhans cell (eosinophilic) granulomatosis. A clinicopathologic study encompassing 50 years. Am J Surg Pathol 20: 519-552.
1512. Liew SH, Leong AS, Tang HM (1981). Tracheal paraganglioma: a case report with review of the literature. Cancer 47: 1387-1393.
1513. Lin HS, Lin CS, Yeh S, Tu SM (1969). Fine structure of nasopharyngeal carcinoma with special reference to the anaplastic type. Cancer 23: 390-405.
1514. Lin JC, Chen KY, Wang WY, Jan JS, Liang WM, Tsai CS, Wei YH (2001). Detection of Epstein-Barr virus DNA the peripheral-blood cells of patients with nasopharyngeal carcinoma: relationship to distant metastasis and survival. J Clin Oncol 19: 2607-2615.
1515. Lin JC, Jan JS, Hsu CY, Liang WM, Jiang RS, Wang WY (2003). Phase III study of concurrent chemoradiotherapy versus radiotherapy alone for advanced nasopharyngeal carcinoma: positive effect on overall and progression-free survival. J Clin Oncol 21: 631-637.
1516. Lin SY, Hsu CY, Jan YJ (2001). Primary laryngeal melanoma. Otolaryngol Head Neck Surg 125: 569-570.
1517. Lind PO (1987). Malignant transformation in oral leukoplakia. Scand J Dent Res 95: 449-455.
1518. Lindberg R (1966). Unusual malignant tumors of the head and neck. Radiology 86: 1090-1095.
1519. Lindeberg H, Elbrond O (1989). Laryngeal papillomas: clinical aspects in a series of 231 patients. Clin Otolaryngol 14: 333-342.
1520. Lindeberg H, Elbrond O (1990). Laryngeal papillomas: the epidemiology in a Danish subpopulation 1965-1984. Clin Otolaryngol 15: 125-131.
1521. Lindeberg H, Elbrond O (1991). Malignant tumours in patients with a history of multiple laryngeal papillomas: the significance of irradiation. Clin Otolaryngol 149-151.
1522. Lindeberg H, Krogdahl A (1997). Laryngeal dysplasia and the human papillomavirus. Clin Otolaryngol 22: 382-386.
1523. Lindeberg H, Krogdahl A (1999). Laryngeal cancer and human papillomavirus: HPV is absent in the majority of laryngeal carcinomas. Cancer Lett 146: 9-13.
1524. Lindeberg H, Oster S, Oxlund I, Elbrond O (1986). Laryngeal papillomas: classification and course. Clin Otolaryngol 11: 423-429.
1525. Linhartova A (1974). Sebaceous glands in salivary gland tissue. Arch Pathol 98: 320-324.
1526. Linnoila RI, Lack EE, Steinberg SM, Keiser HR (1988). Decreased expression of neuropeptides in malignant paragangliomas: an immunohistochemical study. Hum Pathol 19: 41-50.
1527. Lins JE, Gnepp DR (1986). Myoepithelioma of the palate in a child. Int J Pediatr Otorhinolaryngol 11: 5-13.
1528. Lippert BM, Eggers S, Schluter E, Rudert H, Werner JA (2002). Lipoma of the larynx. Report of 2 cases and review of the literature. Otolaryngol Pol 56: 669-674.
1529. Lippert BM, Godbersen GS, Luttges J, Werner JA (1996). Leiomyosarcoma of the nasal cavity. Case report and literature review. ORL J Otorhinolaryngol Relat Spec 58: 115-120.
1530. Lippert BM, Schluter E, Claassen H, Werner JA (1997). Leiomyosarcoma of the larynx. Eur Arch Otorhinolaryngol 254: 466-469.
1531. Liston SL, Dehner LP, Jarvis CW, Pitzele C, Huseby TL (1981). Inflammatory pseudotumors in the buccal tissues of children. Oral Surg Oral Med Oral Pathol 51: 287-291.
1532. Liu Q, Ohshima K, Sumie A, Suzushima H, Iwasaki H, Kikuchi M (2001). Nasal CD56 positive small round cell tumors. Differential diagnosis of hematological, neurogenic, and myogenic neoplasms. Virchows Arch 438: 271-279.
1533. LiVolsi VA, Perzin KH (1977). Malignant mixed tumors arising in salivary glands. I. Carcinomas arising in benign mixed tumors: a clinicopathologic study. Cancer 39: 2209-2230.
1534. Llewellyn CD, Linklater K, Bell J, Johnson NW, Warnakulasuriya KA (2003). Squamous cell carcinoma of the oral cavity in patients aged 45 years and under: a descriptive analysis of 116 cases diagnosed in the South East of England from 1990 to 1997. Oral Oncol 39: 106-114.
1535. Llorente JL, Suarez C, Seco M, Garcia A (1996). Leiomyoma of the nasal septum: report of a case and review of the literature. J Laryngol Otol 110: 65-68.
1536. Lloreta J, Serrano S, Corominas JM, Ferres-Padro E (1995). Polymorphous low-grade adenocarcinoma arising in the nasal cavities with an associated undifferentiated carcinoma. Ultrastruct Pathol 19: 365-370.
1537. Lloyd G, Lund VJ, Howard D, Savy L (2000). Optimum imaging for sinonasal malignancy. J Laryngol Otol 114: 557-562.
1538. Lloyd RV, Chandler WF, Kovacs K, Ryan N (1986). Ectopic pituitary adenomas with normal anterior pituitary glands. Am J Surg Pathol 10: 546-552.
1539. Lo Muzio L, Staibano S, Pannone G, Bucci P, Nocini PF, Bucci E, De Rosa G (1999). Expression of cell cycle and apoptosis-related proteins in sporadic odontogenic keratocysts and odontogenic keratocysts associated with the nevoid basal cell carcinoma syndrome. J Dent Res 78: 1345-1353.
1540. Lo AK, Topf JS, Jackson IT, Silberberg B (1992). Minor salivary gland basal cell adenocarcinoma of the palate. J Oral Maxillofac Surg 50: 531-534.
1541. Lo KW, Cheung ST, Leung SF, van Hasselt A, Tsang YS, Mak KF, Chung YF, Woo JK, Lee JC, Huang DP (1996). Hypermethylation of the p16 gene in nasopharyngeal carcinoma. Cancer Res 56: 2721-2725.
1542. Lo KW, Huang DP (2002). Genetic and epigenetic changes in nasopharyngeal carcinoma. Semin Cancer Biol 12: 451-462.
1543. Lo KW, Huang DP, Lau KM (1995). p16 gene alterations in nasopharyngeal carcinoma. Cancer Res 55: 2039-2043.
1544. Lo KW, Kwong J, Hui AB, Chan SY, To KF, Chan AS, Chow LS, Teo PM, Johnson PJ, Huang DP (2001). High frequency of promoter hypermethylation of RASSF1A in nasopharyngeal carcinoma. Cancer Res 61: 3877-3881.
1545. Lo KW, Teo PM, Hui AB, To KF, Tsang YS, Chan SY, Mak KF, Lee JC, Huang DP (2000). High resolution allelotype of microdissected primary nasopharyngeal carcinoma. Cancer Res 60: 3348-3353.
1546. Lo KW, Tsang YS, Kwong J, To KF, Teo PM, Huang DP (2002). Promoter hypermethylation of the EDNRB gene in nasopharyngeal carcinoma. Int J Cancer 98: 651-655.
1547. Lo YM, Chan AT, Chan LY, Leung SF, Lam CW, Huang DP, Johnson PJ (2000). Molecular prognostication of nasopharyngeal carcinoma by quantitative analysis of circulating Epstein-Barr virus DNA. Cancer Res 60: 6878-6881.
1548. Lo YM, Chan LY, Chan AT, Leung SF, Lo KW, Zhang J, Lee JC, Hjelm NM, Johnson PJ, Huang DP (1999). Quantitative and temporal correlation between circulating cell-free Epstein-Barr virus DNA and tumor recurrence in nasopharyngeal carcinoma. Cancer Res 59: 5452-5455.
1549. Lo YM, Chan LY, Lo KW, Leung SF, Zhang J, Chan AT, Lee JC, Hjelm NM, Johnson PJ, Huang DP (1999). Quantitative analysis of cell-free Epstein-Barr virus DNA in plasma of patients with nasopharyngeal carcinoma. Cancer Res 59: 1188-1191.
1550. Logsdon MD, Ha CS, Kavadi VS, Cabanillas F, Hess MA, Cox JD (1997).

Lymphoma of the nasal cavity and paranasal sinuses: improved outcome and altered prognostic factors with combined modality therapy. Cancer 80: 477-488.
1551. Loke YW (1967). Salivary gland tumours in Malaya. Br J Cancer 21: 665-674.
1552. Lomax-Smith JD, Azzopardi JG (1978). The hyaline cell: a distinctive feature of "mixed" salivary tumours. Histopathology 2: 77-92.
1553. Lombardi T, Kuffer R, Di Felice R, Samson J (1999). Epithelial odontogenic ghost cell tumour of the mandibular gingiva. Oral Oncol 35: 439-442.
1554. London SD, Schlosser RJ, Gross CW (2002). Endoscopic management of benign sinonasal tumors: a decade of experience. Am J Rhinol 16: 221-227.
1555. Looi LM (1987). Tumor-associated tissue eosinophilia in nasopharyngeal carcinoma. A pathologic study of 422 primary and 138 metastatic tumors. Cancer 59: 466-470.
1556. Loos BM, Wieneke JA, Thompson LD (2001). Laryngeal angiosarcoma: a clinicopathologic study of five cases with a review of the literature. Laryngoscope 111: 1197-1202.
1557. Looser KG, Shah JP, Strong EW (1978). The significance of "positive" margins in surgically resected epidermoid carcinomas. Head Neck Surg 1: 107-111.
1558. Lopategui JR, Gaffey MJ, Frierson HFJr, Chan JK, Mills SE, Chang KL, Chen YY, Weiss LM (1994). Detection of Epstein-Barr viral RNA in sinonasal undifferentiated carcinoma from Western and Asian patients. Am J Surg Pathol 18: 391-398.
1559. Lopes MA, de Abreu Alves F, Levy BA, de Almeida OP, Kowalski LP (2001). Intraoral salivary duct carcinoma: case report with immunohistochemical observations. Oral Surg Oral Med Oral Pathol Oral Radiol Endod 91: 689-692.
1560. Lopes MA, Kowalski LP, da Cunha Santos G, Paes de Almeida O (1999). A clinicopathologic study of 196 intraoral minor salivary gland tumours. J Oral Pathol Med 28: 264-267.
1561. Lopes MA, Nikitakis NG, Reynolds MA, Ord RA, Sauk JJr (2002). Biomarkers predictive of lymph node metastases in oral squamous cell carcinoma. J Oral Maxillofac Surg 60: 142-147.
1562. Loree TR, North JHJr, Werness BA, Nangia R, Mullins AP, Hicks WLJr (2000). Malignant peripheral nerve sheath tumors of the head and neck: analysis of prognostic factors. Otolaryngol Head Neck Surg 122: 667-672.
1563. Lovin JD, Talarico CL, Wegert SL, Gaynor LF, Sutley SS (1991). Gorlin's syndrome with associated odontogenic cysts. Pediatr Radiol 21: 584-587.
1564. Loyola AM, Gatti AF, Pinto DSJr, Mesquita RA (1997). Alveolar and extra-alveolar granular cell lesions of the newborn: report of case and review of literature. Oral Surg Oral Med Oral Pathol Oral Radiol Endod 84: 668-671.
1565. Lu CC, Chen JC, Jin YT, Yang HB, Chan SH, Tsai ST (2003). Genetic susceptibility to nasopharyngeal carcinoma within the HLA-A locus in Taiwanese. Int J Cancer 103: 745-751.
1566. Lu QL, Elia G, Lucas S, Thomas JA (1993). Bcl-2 proto-oncogene expression in Epstein-Barr-virus-associated nasopharyngeal carcinoma. Int J Cancer 53: 29-35.
1567. Lu SJ, Day NE, Degos L, Lepage V, Wang PC, Chan SH, Simons M, McKnight B, Easton D, Zeng Y, de The G (1990). Linkage of a nasopharyngeal carcinoma susceptibility locus to the HLA region. Nature 346: 470-471.
1568. Lu Y, Mock D, Takata T, Jordan RC (1999). Odontogenic ghost cell carcinoma: report of four new cases and review of the literature. J Oral Pathol Med 28: 323-329.
1569. Lu Y, Xuan M, Takata T, Wang C, He Z, Zhou Z, Mock D, Nikai H (1998). Odontogenic tumors. A demographic study of 759 cases in a Chinese population. Oral Surg Oral Med Oral Pathol Oral Radiol Endod 86: 707-714.
1570. Lucas DR, Unni KK, McLeod RA, O'Connor MI, Sim FH (1994). Osteoblastoma: clinicopathologic study of 306 cases. Hum Pathol 25: 117-134.
1571. Luce D, Gerin M, Leclerc A, Morcet JF, Brugere J, Goldberg M (1993). Sinonasal cancer and occupational exposure to formaldehyde and other substances. Int J Cancer 53: 224-231.
1572. Ludvikova M, Ryska A, Korabecna M, Rydlova M, Michal M (2001). Oncocytic papillary carcinoma with lymphoid stroma (Warthin-like tumour) of the thyroid: a distinct entity with favourable prognosis. Histopathology 39: 17-24.
1573. Luna MA (1996). Salivary gland neoplasms. In: Surgical Pathology of Laryngeal Neoplasms, Ferlito A, ed., Chapman and Hall: London , pp. 257-294.
1574. Luna MA (1999). Sialoblastoma and epithelial tumors in children: their morphologic spectrum and distribution by age. Adv Anat Pathol 6: 287-292.
1575. Luna MA (2000). Salivary Glands. In: Head and Neck Surgical Pathology, Pilch BZ, ed., Lippincott Williams & Wilkins: Philadelphia , pp. 284-349.
1576. Luna MA, Batsakis JG, Tortoledo ME, del Junco GW (1989). Carcinomas ex monomorphic adenoma of salivary glands. J Laryngol Otol 103: 756-759.
1577. Luna MA, el Naggar A, Batsakis JG, Weber RS, Garnsey LA, Goepfert H (1990). Flow cytometric DNA content of adenoid cystic carcinoma of submandibular gland. Correlation of histologic features and prognosis. Arch Otolaryngol Head Neck Surg 116: 1291-1296.
1578. Luna MA, el Naggar A, Parichatikanond P, Weber RS, Batsakis JG (1990). Basaloid squamous carcinoma of the upper aerodigestive tract. Clinicopathologic and DNA flow cytometric analysis. Cancer 66: 537-542.
1579. Luna MA, Mackay B, Gamez-Araujo J (1973). Myoepithelioma of the palate. Report of a case with histochemical and electron microscopic observations. Cancer 32: 1429-1435.
1580. Luna MA, Ordonez NG, Mackay B, Batsakis JG, Guillamondegui O (1985). Salivary epithelial-myoepithelial carcinomas of intercalated ducts: a clinical, electron microscopic, and immunocytochemical study. Oral Surg Oral Med Oral Pathol 59: 482-490.
1581. Luna MA, Pineda-Daboin K (2001). Upper aerodigestive tract. In: Pathology of Incipient Neoplasia, Henson D, Albores-Saavedra J, eds., Oxford University Press: New York , pp. 57-85.
1582. Luna MA, Tortoledo ME, Allen M (1987). Salivary dermal analogue tumors arising in lymph nodes. Cancer 59: 1165-1169.
1583. Luna MA, Tortoledo ME, Ordonez NG, Frankenthaler RA, Batsakis JG (1991). Primary sarcomas of the major salivary glands. Arch Otolaryngol Head Neck Surg 117: 302-306.
1584. Lundgren J, Olofsson J, Hellquist H (1982). Oncocytic lesions of the larynx. Acta Otolaryngol 94: 335-344.
1585. Lussier C, Klijanienko J, Vielh P (2000). Fine-needle aspiration of metastatic nonlymphomatous tumors to the major salivary glands: a clinicopathologic study of 40 cases cytologically diagnosed and histologically correlated. Cancer 90: 350-356.
1586. Lustig LR, Holliday MJ, McCarthy EF, Nager GT (2001). Fibrous dysplasia involving the skull base and temporal bone. Arch Otolaryngol Head Neck Surg 127: 1239-1247.
1587. Lustrin ES, Palestro C, Vaheesan K (2001). Radiographic evaluation and assessment of paragangliomas. Otolaryngol Clin North Am 34: 881-906, vi.
1588. Luzar B, Poljak M, Marin IJ, Fischinger J, Gale N (2001). Quantitative measurement of telomerase catalytic subunit (hTERT) mRNA in laryngeal squamous cell carcinomas. Anticancer Res 21: 4011-4015.
1589. Lynde CW, McLean DI, Wood WS (1984). Tumors of ceruminous glands. J Am Acad Dermatol 11: 841-847.
1590. Ma B, Corry J, Rischin D, Leong T, Peters LJ (2001). Combined modality treatment for locally advanced squamous-cell carcinoma of the oropharynx in a woman with Bloom's syndrome: a case report and review of the literature. Ann Oncol 12: 1015-1017.
1591. Ma J, Chan JK, Chow CW, Orell SR (2002). Lymphadenoma: a report of three cases of an uncommon salivary gland neoplasm. Histopathology 41: 342-350.
1592. Ma J, Mai HQ, Hong MH, Cui NJ, Lu TX, Lu LX, Mo HY, Min HQ (2001). Is the 1997 AJCC staging system for nasopharyngeal carcinoma prognostically useful for Chinese patient populations? Int J Radiat Oncol Biol Phys 50: 1181-1189.
1593. Ma Z, Hill DA, Collins MH, Morris SW, Sumegi J, Zhou M, Zuppan C, Bridge JA (2003). Fusion of ALK to the Ran-binding protein 2 (RANBP2) gene in inflammatory myofibroblastic tumor. Genes Chromosomes Cancer 37: 98-105.
1594. Macbeth R (1965). Malignant disease of the paranasal sinuses. J Laryngol 79: 592-612.
1595. MacCollin MM (2003). www.genetests.org. Genereviews
1596. Macdonald MR, Le KT, Freeman J, Hui MF, Cheung RK, Dosch HM (1995). A majority of inverted sinonasal papillomas carries Epstein-Barr virus genomes. Cancer 75: 2307-2312.
1597. Macfarlane GJ, Macfarlane TV, Lowenfels AB (1996). The influence of alcohol consumption on worldwide trends in mortality from upper aerodigestive tract cancers in men. J Epidemiol Community Health 50: 636-639.
1598. Machado de Sousa SO, Soares de Araujo N, Correa L, Pires Soubhia AM, Cavalcanti de Araujo V (2001). Immunohistochemical aspects of basal cell adenoma and canalicular adenoma of salivary glands. Oral Oncol 37: 365-368.
1599. Mackenzie IJ, Morgan JM, Mitchell JF (1981). Secondary tracheal carcinoma. J Laryngol Otol 95: 973-978.
1600. MacLeod RI, Soames JV (1988). Squamous cell carcinoma arising in an odontogenic keratocyst. Br J Oral Maxillofac Surg 26: 52-57.
1601. MacMillan C, Kapadia SB, Finkelstein SD, Nalesnik MA, Barnes L (1996). Lymphoepithelial carcinoma of the larynx and hypopharynx: study of eight cases with relationship to Epstein-Barr virus and p53 gene alterations, and review of the literature. Hum Pathol 27: 1172-1179.
1602. MacNaughton DM, Tewfik TL, Bernstein ML (1990). Hodgkin's disease in the nasopharynx. J Otolaryngol 19: 282-284.
1603. Maddox JC, Evans HL (1981). Angiosarcoma of skin and soft tissue: a study of forty-four cases. Cancer 48: 1907-1921.
1604. Madrigal FM, Godoy LM, Daboin KP, Casiraghi O, Garcia AM, Luna MA (2002). Laryngeal osteosarcoma: a clinicopathologic analysis of four cases and comparison with a carcinosarcoma. Ann Diagn Pathol 6: 1-9.
1605. Magnano M, Cavalot AL, Gervasio CF, Lerda W, Gabriele P, Orecchia R, Ruo-Redda MG, Beltramo G, Ragona R, Cortesina G (1999). Surgery or radiotherapy for early stages carcinomas of the glottic larynx. Tumori 85: 188-193.
1606. Mahlstedt K, Ussmuller J, Donath K (2002). Malignant sialogenic tumours of the larynx. J Laryngol Otol 116: 119-122.
1607. Maier H, Dietz A, Gewelke U, Heller WD, Weidauer H (1992). Tobacco and alcohol and the risk of head and neck cancer. Clin Investig 70: 320-327.
1608. Maier H, Tisch M (1997). Epidemiology of laryngeal cancer: results of the Heidelberg case-control study. Acta Otolaryngol Suppl 527: 160-164.
1609. Maier HC (1985). Craniopharyngioma with erosion and drainage into the nasopharynx. An autobiographical case report. J Neurosurg 62: 132-134.
1610. Maiorano E, Lo Muzio L, Favia G, Piattelli A (2002). Warthin's tumour: a study of 78 cases with emphasis on bilaterality, multifocality and association with other malignancies. Oral Oncol 38: 35-40.
1611. Maitra A, Baskin LB, Lee EL (2001). Malignancies arising in oncocytic schneiderian papillomas: a report of 2 cases and review of the literature. Arch Pathol Lab Med 125: 1365-1367.
1612. Maiuri F, Corriero G, Elefante R, Cirillo S, Giamundo A (1987). Craniopharyngioma of the cranial base and nasopharynx. Surg Neurol 27: 191-194.
1613. Majumdar S, Raghavan U, Jones NS (2002). Solitary plasmacytoma and extramedullary plasmacytoma of the paranasal sinuses and soft palate. J Laryngol Otol 116: 962-965.
1614. Makepeace AR, Fermont DC, Bennett MH (1987). Non-Hodgkin's lymphoma of the tonsil. Experience of treatment over a 27-year period. J Laryngol Otol 101: 1151-1158.
1615. Makowski GJ, McGuff S, Van Sickels JE (2001). Squamous cell carcinoma in a maxillary odontogenic keratocyst. J Oral Maxillofac Surg 59: 76-80.
1616. Maldjian JA, Norton KI, Groisman GM, Som PM (1994). Inflammatory pseudotumor of the maxillary sinus in a 15-year-old boy. AJNR Am J Neuroradiol 15: 784-786.
1617. Mallofre C, Cardesa A, Campo E, Condom E, Palacin A, Garin-Chesa P, Traserra J (1993). Expression of cytokeratins in squamous cell carcinomas of the larynx: immunohistochemical analysis and correlation with prognostic factors. Pathol Res Pract 189: 275-282.
1618. Mallow RD, Spatz SS, Zubrow HJ, Kline SN (1966). Odontogenic fibroma with

calcification. Report of a case with a review of the literature. Oral Surg Oral Med Oral Pathol 22: 564-568.
1619. Malpica A, Luna MA, Lyos AT, Silva EG (1995). Sinonasal Teratocarcinosarcoma: a clinocopathologic study of 9 cases. Lab Invest 72: 103.
1620. Mancuso TF, Brennan MJ (1970). Epidemiological considerations of cancer of the gallbladder, bile ducts and salivary glands in the rubber industry. J Occup Med 12: 333-341.
1621. Mangion J, Rahman N, Edkins S, Barfoot R, Nguyen T, Sigurdsson A, Townend JV, Fitzpatrick DR, Flanagan AM, Stratton MR (1999). The gene for cherubism maps to chromosome 4p16.3. Am J Hum Genet 65: 151-157.
1622. Mani NJ (1974). Odontoma syndrome: report of an unusual case with multiple multiform odontomas of both jaws. J Dent 2: 149-152.
1623. Manivel C, Wick MR, Dehner LP (1986). Transitional (cylindric) cell carcinoma with endodermal sinus tumor-like features of the nasopharynx and paranasal sinuses. Clinicopathologic and immunohistochemical study of two cases. Arch Pathol Lab Med 110: 198-202.
1624. Manolidis S, Donald PJ (1997). Malignant mucosal melanoma of the head and neck: review of the literature and report of 14 patients. Cancer 80: 1373-1386.
1625. Mantravadi J, Roth LM, Kafrawy AH (1993). Vascular neoplasms of the parotid gland. Parotid vascular tumors. Oral Surg Oral Med Oral Pathol 75: 70-75.
1626. Mao L, El Naggar AK, Papadimitrakopoulou V, Shin DM, Shin HC, Fan Y, Zhou X, Clayman G, Lee JJ, Lee JS, Hittelman WN, Lippman SM, Hong WK (1998). Phenotype and genotype of advanced premalignant head and neck lesions after chemopreventive therapy. J Natl Cancer Inst 90: 1545-1551.
1627. Mao L, Lee JS, Fan YH, Ro JY, Batsakis JG, Lippman S, Hittelman W, Hong WK (1996). Frequent microsatellite alterations at chromosomes 9p21 and 3p14 in oral premalignant lesions and their value in cancer risk assessment. Nat Med 2: 682-685.
1628. Marchioni DL, Fisberg RM, do Rosario M, Latorre DO, Wunsch V (2002). Diet and cancer of oral cavity and pharynx: a case-control study in Sao Paulo, Brazil. IARC Sci Publ 156: 559-561.
1629. Margiotta V, Franco V, Rizzo A, Porter S, Scully C, Di Alberti L (1999). Gastric and gingival localization of mucosa-associated lymphoid tissue (MALT) lymphoma. An immunohistochemical, virological and clinical case report. J Periodontol 70: 914-918.
1630. Margolis FL (1972). A brain protein unique to the olfactory bulb. Proc Natl Acad Sci U S A 69: 1221-1224.
1631. Margolis FL, Verhaagen J, Biffo S, Huang FL, Grillo M (1991). Regulation of gene expression in the olfactory neuroepithelium: a neurogenetic matrix. Prog Brain Res 89: 97-122.
1632. Marianowski R, Wassef M, Amanou L, Herman P, Tran-Ba-Huy P (1998). Primary T-cell non-Hodgkin lymphoma of the larynx with subsequent cutaneous involvement. Arch Otolaryngol Head Neck Surg 124: 1037-1040.
1633. Marie PJ, de Pollak C, Chanson P, Lomri A (1997). Increased proliferation of osteoblastic cells expressing the activating Gs alpha mutation in monostotic and polyostotic fibrous dysplasia. Am J Pathol 150: 1059-1069.
1634. Mariman EC, van Beersum SE, Cremers CW, Struycken PM, Ropers HH (1995). Fine mapping of a putatively imprinted gene for familial non-chromaffin paragangliomas to chromosome 11q13.1: evidence for genetic heterogeneity. Hum Genet 95: 56-62.
1635. Marioni G, Bertino G, Mariuzzi L, Bergamin-Bracale AM, Lombardo M, Beltrami CA (2000). Laryngeal leiomyosarcoma. J Laryngol Otol 114: 398-401.
1636. Marioni G, Bottin R, Staffieri A, Altavilla G (2003). Spindle-cell tumours of the larynx: diagnostic pitfalls. A case report and review of the literature. Acta Otolaryngol 123: 86-90.
1637. Marioni G, Mariuzzi L, Gaio E, Portaleone S, Pertoldi B, Staffieri A (2002). Lymphoepithelial carcinoma of the larynx. Acta Otolaryngol 122: 429-434.
1638. Mark J, Dahlenfors R, Stenman G, Nordquist A (1989). A human adenolymphoma showing the chromosomal aberrations del (7)(p12p14-15) and t(11;19)(q21;p12-13). Anticancer Res 9: 1565-1566.
1639. Mark J, Dahlenfors R, Wedell B (1997). Impact of the in vitro technique used on the cytogenetic patterns in pleomorphic adenomas. Cancer Genet Cytogenet 95: 9-15.
1640. Mark RJ, Tran LM, Sercarz J, Fu YS, Calcaterra TC, Juillard GF (1993). Angiosarcoma of the head and neck. The UCLA experience 1955 through 1990. Arch Otolaryngol Head Neck Surg 119: 973-978.
1641. Martin-Hirsch DP, Lannigan FJ, Irani B, Batman P (1992). Oncocytic papillary cystadenomatosis of the larynx. J Laryngol Otol 106: 656-658.
1642. Martin PC, Hoda SA, Pigman HT, Pulitzer DR (1994). Giant cell tumor of the larynx. Case report and review of the literature. Arch Pathol Lab Med 118: 834-837.
1643. Martinelli M, Martini F, Rinaldi E, Caramanico L, Magri E, Grandi E, Carinci F, Pastore A, Tognon M (2002). Simian virus 40 sequences and expression of the viral large T antigen oncoprotein in human pleomorphic adenomas of parotid glands. Am J Pathol 161: 1127-1133.
1644. Martinez-Barba E, Cortes-Guardiola JA, Minguela-Puras A, Torroba-Caron A, Mendez-Trujillo S, Bermejo-Lopez J (1997). Salivary duct carcinoma: clinicopathological and immunohistochemical studies. J Craniomaxillofac Surg 25: 328-334.
1645. Martinez-Gavidia EM, Bagan JV, Milian-Masanet MA, Lloria de Miguel E, Perez-Valles A (2000). Highly aggressive brown tumour of the maxilla as first manifestation of primary hyperparathyroidism. Int J Oral Maxillofac Surg 29: 447-449.
1646. Martinez-Madrigal F, Baden E, Casiraghi O, Micheau C (1991). Oral and pharyngeal adenosquamous carcinoma. A report of four cases with immunohistochemical studies. Eur Arch Otorhinolaryngol 248: 255-258.
1647. Martinez-Madrigal F, Santiago Payan H, Meneses A, Dominguez Malagon H, Rojas ME (1995). Plasmacytoid myoepithelioma of the laryngeal region: a case report. Hum Pathol 26: 802-804.
1648. Martinez S, Bosch R, Pardo J, Salvado MT, Alvaro T (2001). Inflammatory myofibroblastic tumour of larynx. J Laryngol Otol 115: 140-142.
1649. Martins C, Carvalho YR, do Carmo MA (2001). Argyrophilic nucleolar organizer regions (AgNORs) in odontogenic myxoma (OM) and ameloblastic fibroma (AF). J Oral Pathol Med 30: 489-493.
1650. Martins C, Fonseca I, Roque L, Pinto AE, Soares J (1996). Malignant salivary gland neoplasms: a cytogenetic study of 19 cases. Eur J Cancer B Oral Oncol 32B: 128-132.
1651. Martins C, Fonseca I, Roque L, Ribeiro C, Soares J (2001). Cytogenetic similarities between two types of salivary gland carcinomas: adenoid cystic carcinoma and polymorphous low-grade adenocarcinoma. Cancer Genet Cytogenet 128: 130-136.
1652. Maruya S, Kim HW, Weber RS, Lee JJ, Kies M, Luna MA, Batsakis JG, El Naggar AK (2004). Gene expression screening of salivary gland neoplasms: molecular markers of potential histogenetic and clinical significance. J Mol Diagn 6: 180-190.
1653. Maruya S, Kurotaki H, Shimoyama N, Kaimori M, Shinkawa H, Yagihashi S (2003). Expression of p16 protein and hypermethylation status of its promoter gene in adenoid cystic carcinoma of the head and neck. ORL J Otorhinolaryngol Relat Spec 65: 26-32.
1654. Maruyama S, Cheng J, Inoue T, Takagi R, Saku T (2002). Sebaceous lymphadenoma of the lip: report of a case of minor salivary gland origin. J Oral Pathol Med 31: 242-243.
1655. Mashberg A, Samit A (1995). Early diagnosis of asymptomatic oral and oropharyngeal squamous cancers. CA Cancer J Clin 45: 328-351.
1656. Massey V, Wallner K (1992). Treatment of metastatic chemodectoma. Cancer 69: 790-792.
1657. Mast BA, Kapadia SB, Yunis E, Bentz M (1999). Subtotal maxillectomy for melanotic neuroectodermal tumor of infancy. Plast Reconstr Surg 103: 1961-1963.
1658. Masuda M, Shinokuma A, Hirakawa N, Nakashima T, Komiyama S (1998). Expression of bcl-2-, p53, and Ki-67 and outcome of patients with primary nasopharyngeal carcinomas following DNA-damaging treatment. Head Neck 20: 640-644.
1659. Mathews FR, Appleton SS, Wear DJ (1989). Intraoral Hodgkin's disease. J Oral Maxillofac Surg 47: 502-504.
1660. Mathisen DJ, Grillo HC (1996). Tumors of the cervical trachea. In: Cancer of the Head and Neck, Myers EN, Suen JY, eds., 3rd ed. WB Saunders: Philadelphia , pp. 439-461.
1661. Matias C, Corde J, Soares J (1988). Primary malignant melanoma of the nasal cavity: a clinicopathologic study of nine cases. J Surg Oncol 39: 29-32.
1662. Matsuba HM, Mauney M, Simpson JR, Thawley SE, Pikul FJ (1988). Adenocarcinomas of major and minor salivary gland origin: a histopathologic review of treatment failure patterns. Laryngoscope 98: 784-788.
1663. Matsuba HM, Thawley SE, Simpson JR, Levine LA, Mauney M (1984). Adenoid cystic carcinoma of major and minor salivary gland origin. Laryngoscope 94: 1316-1318.
1664. Matsumoto Y, Yanagihara N (1982). Renal clear cell carcinoma metastatic to the nose and paranasal sinuses. Laryngoscope 92: 1190-1193.
1665. Matsumura S, Murakami S, Kakimoto N, Furukawa S, Kishino M, Ishida T, Fuchihata H (1998). Histopathologic and radiographic findings of the simple bone cyst. Oral Surg Oral Med Oral Pathol Oral Radiol Endod 85: 619-625.
1666. Matsuno A, Nagashima T, Matsuura R, Tanaka H, Hirakawa M, Murakami M, Tamura A, Kirino T (1996). Correlation between MIB-1 staining index and the immunoreactivity of p53 protein in recurrent and non-recurrent meningiomas. Am J Clin Pathol 106: 776-781.
1667. Matsushita H, Matsuya S, Endo Y, Hara M, Shishiba Y, Yamaguchi H, Kameya T (1984). A prolactin producing tumor originated in the sphenoid sinus. Acta Pathol Jpn 34: 103-109.
1668. Mattavelli F, Di Palma S, Guzzo M (1995). Primary mucosal malignant melanoma of the larynx: case report and review of the literature. Tumori 81: 460-463.
1669. Mazzoni A, Pareschi R, Calabrese V (1988). Intratemporal vascular tumours. J Laryngol Otol 102: 353-356.
1670. McCaffrey TV, Meyer FB, Michels VV, Piepgras DG, Marion MS (1994). Familial paragangliomas of the head and neck. Arch Otolaryngol Head Neck Surg 120: 1211-1216.
1671. McCaffrey TV, Witte M, Ferguson MT (1998). Verrucous carcinoma of the larynx. Ann Otol Rhinol Laryngol 107: 391-395.
1672. McClain K, Jin H, Gresik V, Favara B (1994). Langerhans cell histiocytosis: lack of a viral etiology. Am J Hematol 47: 16-20.
1673. McClatchey KD (1987). Tumors of the dental lamina: a selective review. Semin Diagn Pathol 4: 200-204.
1674. McClatchey KD, Sullivan MJ, Paugh DR (1989). Peripheral ameloblastic carcinoma: a case report of a rare neoplasm. J Otolaryngol 18: 109-111.
1675. McCluggage WG, Cameron CH, Brooker D, O'Hara MD (1996). Paraganglioma: an unusual tumour of the parathyroid gland. J Laryngol Otol 110: 196-199.
1676. McCluggage WG, Napier SS, Primrose WJ, Adair RA, Toner PG (1995). Sinonasal neuroendocrine carcinoma exhibiting amphicrine differentiation. Histopathology 27: 79-82.
1677. McCoy JM, Waldron CA (1981). Verrucous carcinoma of the oral cavity. A review of forty-nine cases. Oral Surg Oral Med Oral Pathol 52: 623-629.
1678. McDermott MB, Ponder TB, Dehner LP (1998). Nasal chondromesenchymal hamartoma: an upper respiratory tract analogue of the chest wall mesenchymal hamartoma. Am J Surg Pathol 22: 425-433.
1679. McGavran MH, Bauer WC, Ogura JH (1961). The incidence of cervical lymph node metastases from epidermoid carcinoma of the larynx and their relationship to certain characteristics of the primary tumor: A study based on the clinical and pathological findings for 96 patients treated by primary en bloc laryngectomy and radical neck dissection. Cancer 14: 55-66.
1680. McGill T (1984). Congenital diseases of the larynx. Otolaryngol Clin North Am 17: 57-62.
1681. McGregor AD, Burgoyne M, Tan KC (1988). Recurrent pleomorphic salivary adenoma—the relevance of age at first presentation. Br J Plast Surg 41: 177-181.
1682. McGregor AD, MacDonald DG (1988). Routes of entry of squamous cell carcinoma to the mandible. Head Neck Surg 10: 294-301.
1683. McGregor AD, MacDonald DG (1989). Patterns of spread of squamous cell carcinoma within the mandible. Head Neck 11: 457-461.
1684. McGuirt WF, Ray M (1999). Second laryngeal cancers in previously treated

larynges. Laryngoscope 109: 1406-1408.

1685. McKay MJ, Carr PJ, Jaworski R, Kalnins I (1989). Cancer of distant primary site relapsing in the nasopharynx: a report of two cases and review of the literature. Head Neck 11: 534-537.

1686. McKiernan DC, Watters GW (1995). Smooth muscle tumours of the larynx. J Laryngol Otol 109: 77-79.

1687. McKinney CD, Mills SE, Franquemont DW (1995). Sinonasal intestinal-type adenocarcinoma: immunohistochemical profile and comparison with colonic adenocarcinoma. Mod Pathol 8: 421-426.

1688. McKnight HA (1939). Malignant parotid tumor in the newborn. Am J Surg 130.

1689. McLaren KM, Burnett RA, Goodlad JR, Howatson SR, Lang S, Lee FD, Lessells AM, Ogston S, Robertson AJ, Simpson JG, Smith GD, Tavadia HB, Walker F (2000). Consistency of histopathological reporting of laryngeal dysplasia. The Scottish Pathology Consistency Group. Histopathology 37: 460-463.

1690. McMenamin ME, Fletcher CD (2001). Expanding the spectrum of malignant change in schwannomas: epithelioid malignant change, epithelioid malignant peripheral nerve sheath tumor, and epithelioid angiosarcoma: a study of 17 cases. Am J Surg Pathol 25: 13-25.

1691. McNeil C (2000). HPV in oropharyngeal cancers: new data inspire hope for vaccines. J Natl Cancer Inst 92: 680-681.

1692. McRae RD, Gatland DJ, McNab Jones RF, Khan S (1990). Malignant transformation in a laryngeal hemangioma. Ann Otol Rhinol Laryngol 99: 562-565.

1693. Medeiros LJ, Peiper SC, Elwood L, Yano T, Raffeld M, Jaffe ES (1991). Angiocentric immunoproliferative lesions: a molecular analysis of eight cases. Hum Pathol 22: 1150-1157.

1694. Medeiros LJ, Rizzi R, Lardelli P, Jaffe ES (1990). Malignant lymphoma involving a Warthin's tumor: a case with immunophenotypic and gene rearrangement analysis. Hum Pathol 21: 974-977.

1695. Medina JE, Dichtel W, Luna MA (1984). Verrucous-squamous carcinomas of the oral cavity. A clinicopathologic study of 104 cases. Arch Otolaryngol 110: 437-440.

1696. Megerian CA, Haynes DS, Poe DS, Choo DI, Keriakas TJ, Glasscock MEI (2002). Hearing preservation surgery for small endolymphatic sac tumors in patients with von Hippel-Lindau syndrome. Otol Neurotol 23: 378-387.

1697. Megerian CA, Maniglia AJ (1994). Parotidectomy: a ten year experience with fine needle aspiration and frozen section biopsy correlation. Ear Nose Throat J 73: 377-380.

1698. Megerian CA, Sofferman RA, McKenna MJ, Eavy RD, Nadol JBJ (1982). Fibrous dysplasia of the temporal bone. Ann Otol Rhinol Laryngol 91 Suppl.92.

1699. Mehta FS, Shroff BC, Gupta PC, Daftary DK (1972). Oral leukoplakia in relation to tobacco habits. A ten-year follow-up study of Bombay policemen. Oral Surg Oral Med Oral Pathol 34: 426-433.

1700. Meijer JW, Ramaekers FC, Manni JJ, Slooff JJ, Aldeweireldt J, Vooys GP (1988). Intermediate filament proteins in spindle cell carcinoma of the larynx and tongue. Acta Otolaryngol 106: 306-313.

1701. Meis JM, Butler JJ, Osborne BM, Manning JT (1986). Granulocytic sarcoma

in nonleukemic patients. Cancer 58: 2697-2709.

1702. Melato M, Falconieri G, Fanin R, Baccarani M (1986). Hodgkin's disease occurring in a Warthin's tumor: first case report. Pathol Res Pract 181: 615-620.

1703. Melrose RJ (1999). Desmoplastic ameloblastoma. Pathol Rev 4: 21-27.

1704. Menarguez J, Mollejo M, Carrion R, Oliva H, Bellas C, Forteza J, Martin C, Ruiz-Marcellan C, Morente M, Romagosa V, Cuena R, Piris MA (1994). Waldeyer ring lymphomas. A clinicopathological study of 79 cases. Histopathology 24: 13-22.

1705. Menck HR, Henderson BE (1982). Cancer incidence patterns in the Pacific Basin. Natl Cancer Inst Monogr 62: 101-109.

1706. Mentzel T, Bainbridge TC, Katenkamp D (1997). Solitary fibrous tumour: clinicopathological, immunohistochemical, and ultrastructural analysis of 12 cases arising in soft tissues, nasal cavity and nasopharynx, urinary bladder and prostate. Virchows Arch 430: 445-453.

1707. Merrick RE, Rhone DP, Chilis TJ (1980). Malignant fibrous histiocytoma of the maxillary sinus. Case report and literature review. Arch Otolaryngol 106: 365-367.

1708. Merrick Y, Albeck H, Nielsen NH, Hansen HS (1986). Familial clustering of salivary gland carcinoma in Greenland. Cancer 57: 2097-2102.

1709. Mezzelani A, Tornielli S, Minoletti F, Pierotti MA, Sozzi G, Pilotti S (1999). Esthesioneuroblastoma is not a member of the primitive peripheral neuroectodermal tumour-Ewing's group. Br J Cancer 81: 586-591.

1710. Michaels L (1996). Benign mucosal tumors of the nose and paranasal sinuses. Semin Diagn Pathol 13: 113-117.

1711. Michaels L, Hellquist H (2001). Ear, Nose and Throat Histopathology. 2nd ed. Springer Verlag: Berlin.

1712. Michaels L, Lee K, Manuja SL, Soucek SO (1999). Family with low-grade neuroendocrine carcinoma of salivary glands, severe sensorineural hearing loss, and enamel hypoplasia. Am J Med Genet 83: 183-186.

1713. Michaels L, Wells M (1980). Squamous cell carcinoma of the middle ear. Clin Otolaryngol 5: 235-248.

1714. Michaels L, Young M (1995). Histogenesis of papillomas of the nose and paranasal sinuses. Arch Pathol Lab Med 119: 821-826.

1715. Michal M, Hrabal P, Skalova A (1998). Oncocytic cystadenoma of the parotid gland with prominent signet-ring cell features. Pathol Int 48: 629-633.

1716. Michal M, Skalova A, Mukensnabl P (2000). Micropapillary carcinoma of the parotid gland arising in mucinous cystadenoma. Virchows Arch 437: 465-468.

1717. Michal M, Skalova A, Simpson RH, Leivo I, Ryska A, Starek I (1997). Well-differentiated acinic cell carcinoma of salivary glands associated with lymphoid stroma. Hum Pathol 28: 595-600.

1718. Michal M, Skalova A, Simpson RH, Raslan WF, Curik R, Leivo I, Mukensnabl P (1999). Cribriform adenocarcinoma of the tongue: a hitherto unrecognized type of adenocarcinoma characteristically occurring in the tongue. Histopathology 35: 495-501.

1719. Michal M, Skalova A, Simpson RH, Rychterova V, Leivo I (1996). Clear cell malignant myoepithelioma of the salivary glands. Histopathology 28: 309-315.

1720. Michal M, Sokol L, Mukensnabl P (1996). Salivary gland anlage tumor. A case with widespread necrosis and large cyst formation. Pathology 28: 128-130.

1721. Michalek AM, Mahoney MC, McLaughlin CC, Murphy D, Metzger BB (1994). Historical and contemporary correlates of syphilis and cancer. Int J Epidemiol 23: 381-385.

1722. Micheau C, Luboinski B, Schwaab G, Richard J, Cachin Y (1979). Lymphoepitheliomas of the larynx (undifferentiated carcinomas of nasopharyngeal type). Clin Otolaryngol 4: 43-48.

1723. Miettinen M (1988). Antibody specific to muscle actins in the diagnosis and classification of soft tissue tumors. Am J Pathol 130: 205-215.

1724. Miettinen M, Paal E, Lasota J, Sobin LH (2002). Gastrointestinal glomus tumors: a clinicopathologic, immunohistochemical, and molecular genetic study of 32 cases. Am J Surg Pathol 26: 301-311.

1725. Mihailescu D, Shore-Freedman E, Mukani S, Lubin J, Ron E, Schneider AB (2002). Multiple neoplasms in an irradiated cohort: pattern of occurrence and relationship to thyroid cancer outcome. J Clin Endocrinol Metab 87: 3236-3241.

1726. Mikaelian DO, Contrucci RB, Batsakis JG (1986). Epithelial-myoepithelial carcinoma of the subglottic region: a case presentation and review of the literature. Otolaryngol Head Neck Surg 95: 104-106.

1727. Milasin J, Pujic N, Dedovic N, Gavric M, Vranic V, Petrovic V, Minic A (1993). H-ras gene mutations in salivary gland pleomorphic adenomas. Int J Oral Maxillofac Surg 22: 359-361.

1728. Milchgrub S, Gnepp DR, Vuitch F, Delgado R, Albores-Saavedra J (1994). Hyalinizing clear cell carcinoma of salivary gland. Am J Surg Pathol 18: 74-82.

1729. Milford CA, Mugliston TA, O'Flynn P, McCarthy K (1989). Carcinoma arising in a pleomorphic adenoma of the epiglottis. J Laryngol Otol 103: 324-327.

1730. Milham SJr (1976). Cancer mortality pattern associated with exposure to metals. Ann N Y Acad Sci 271: 243-249.

1731. Milian MA, Bagan JV, Jimenez Y, Perez A, Scully C, Antoniades D (2001). Langerhans' cell histiocytosis restricted to the oral mucosa. Oral Surg Oral Med Oral Pathol Oral Radiol Endod 91: 76-79.

1732. Miller AS, Hartman GG, Chen SY, Edmonds PR, Brightman SA, Harwick RD (1994). Estrogen receptor assay in polymorphous low-grade adenocarcinoma and adenoid cystic carcinoma of salivary gland origin. An immunohistochemical study. Oral Surg Oral Med Oral Pathol 77: 36-40.

1733. Miller AS, Harwick RD, Alfaro-Miranda M, Sundararajan M (1993). Search for correlation of radon levels and incidence of salivary gland tumors. Oral Surg Oral Med Oral Pathol 75: 58-63.

1734. Miller DC, Goodman ML, Pilch BZ, Shi SR, Dickersin GR, Halpern H, Norris CMJr (1984). Mixed olfactory neuroblastoma and carcinoma. A report of two cases. Cancer 54: 2019-2028.

1735. Miller LH, Santaella-Latimer L, Miller T (1975). Synovial sarcoma of the larynx. Trans Am Acad Ophthalmol Otolaryngol 80: 448-451.

1736. Miller RB, Boon MS, Atkins JP, Lowry LD (2000). Vagal paraganglioma: the Jefferson experience. Otolaryngol Head Neck Surg 122: 482-487.

1737. Mills RP, Hussain SS (1984). Teratomas of the head and neck in infancy

and childhood. Int J Pediatr Otorhinolaryngol 8: 177-180.

1738. Mills SE, Cooper PH, Fechner RE (1980). Lobular capillary hemangioma: the underlying lesion of pyogenic granuloma. A study of 73 cases from the oral and nasal mucous membranes. Am J Surg Pathol 4: 470-479.

1739. Mills SE, Fechner RE, Cantrell RW (1982). Aggressive sinonasal lesion resembling normal intestinal mucosa. Am J Surg Pathol 6: 803-809.

1740. Mills SE, Frierson HFJr (1985). Olfactory neuroblastoma. A clinicopathologic study of 21 cases. Am J Surg Pathol 9: 317-327.

1741. Mills SE, Gaffey MJ, Frierson HFJr (2000). Tumors of the Upper Aerodigestive Tract and Ear. 3 ed. Armed Forces Institute of Pathology: Washington.

1742. Mills SE, Garland TA, Allen MSJr (1984). Low-grade papillary adenocarcinoma of palatal salivary gland origin. Am J Surg Pathol 8: 367-374.

1743. Min KW (1995). Usefulness of electron microscopy in the diagnosis of "small" round cell tumors of the sinonasal region. Ultrastruct Pathol 19: 347-363.

1744. Minami M, Kaneda T, Ozawa K, Yamamoto H, Itai Y, Ozawa M, Yoshikawa K, Sasaki Y (1996). Cystic lesions of the maxillomandibular region: MR imaging distinction of odontogenic keratocysts and ameloblastomas from other cysts. AJR Am J Roentgenol 166: 943-949.

1745. Mindell RS, Calcaterra TC, Ward PH (1975). Leiomyosarcoma of the head and neck: a review of the literature and report of two cases. Laryngoscope 85: 904-910.

1746. Mineta H, Miura K, Takebayashi S, Araki K, Ueda Y, Harada H, Misawa K (2001). Immunohistochemical analysis of small cell carcinoma of the head and neck: a report of four patients and a review of sixteen patients in the literature with ectopic hormone production. Ann Otol Rhinol Laryngol 110: 76-82.

1747. Miragall F, Kadmon G, Husmann M, Schachner M (1988). Expression of cell adhesion molecules in the olfactory system of the adult mouse: presence of the embryonic form of N-CAM. Dev Biol 129: 516-531.

1748. Miro Castillo N, Roca-Ribas Serda F, Barnadas Molins A, Prades Marti J, Casamitjana Claramunt F, Perello Scherdel E (2000). [Facial paralysis of metastatic origin. Review of metastatic lesions of the temporal bone]. An Otorrinolaringol Ibero Am 27: 255-263.

1749. Mirza S, Dutt SN, Irving RM, Jones EL (2000). Intraductal papilloma of the submandibular gland. J Laryngol Otol 114: 481-483.

1750. Mitchell DB, Humphreys S, Kearns DB (1988). Mucoepidermoid carcinoma of the larynx in a child. Int J Pediatr Otorhinolaryngol 15: 211-215.

1751. Mitleman F, Johansson B, Mertens F (2003). Mitelman Database of Chromosome Aberrations in Cancer (2003. http://cgap nci nih/gov/Chromosomes/ Mitelman http://cgap.nci.nih.gov/Chromosomes/ Mitelman.

1752. Miyauchi M, Ogawa I, Takata T, Ito H, Nikai H, Ijuhin N, Tanimoto K (1995). Florid cemento-osseous dysplasia with concomitant simple bone cysts: a case in a Japanese woman. J Oral Pathol Med 24: 285-287.

1753. Mochloulis G, Irving RM, Grant HR, Miller RF (1996). Laryngeal Kaposi's sarcoma in patients with AIDS. J Laryngol Otol

110: 1034-1037.
1754. Modan B, Chetrit A, Alfandary E, Tamir A, Lusky A, Wolf M, Shpilberg O (1998). Increased risk of salivary gland tumors after low-dose irradiation. Laryngoscope 108: 1095-1097.
1755. Moench HC, Phillips TL (1972). Carcinoma of the nasopharynx. Review of 146 patients with emphasis on radiation dose and time factors. Am J Surg 124: 515-518.
1756. Moghe GM, Borges AM, Soman CS, Naresh KN (2001). Hodgkin's disease involving Waldeyer's ring: a study of four cases. Leuk Lymphoma 41: 151-156.
1757. Moh'd Hadi U, Kahwaji GJ, Mufarrij AA, Tawil A, Noureddine B (2002). Low grade primary clear cell carcinoma of the sinonasal tract. Rhinology 40: 44-47.
1758. Mohamed AH, Cherrick HM (1975). Glycogen-rich adenocarcinoma of minor salivary glands. A light and electron microscopic study. Cancer 36: 1057-1066.
1759. Mohammadi-Araghi H, Haery C (1993). Fibro-osseous lesions of craniofacial bones. The role of imaging. Radiol Clin North Am 31: 121-134.
1760. Mohanty SK, Dey P, Ghoshal S, Saikia UN (2002). Cytologic features of metastatic nasopharyngeal carcinoma. Diagn Cytopathol 27: 340-342.
1761. Mok JS, Pak MW, Chan KF, Chow J, Hasselt CA (2001). Unusual T- and T/NK-cell non-Hodgkin's lymphoma of the larynx: a diagnostic challenge for clinicians and pathologists. Head Neck 23: 625-628.
1762. Mokni-Baizig N, Ayed K, Ayed FB, Ayed S, Sassi F, Ladgham A, Bel Hadj O, El May A (2001). Association between HLA-A/-B antigens and -DRB1 alleles and nasopharyngeal carcinoma in Tunisia. Oncology 61: 55-58.
1763. Molony NC, Stewart A, Ah-See K, McLaren M (1998). Hodgkin's lymphoma of the nasopharynx. J Laryngol Otol 112: 103-105.
1764. Molteni A, Warpeha RL, Brizio-Molteni L, Fors EM (1981). Estradiol receptor-binding protein in head and neck neoplastic and normal tissue. Arch Surg 116: 207-210.
1765. Monk JSJr, Church JS (1992). Warthin's tumor. A high incidence and no sex predominance in central Pennsylvania. Arch Otolaryngol Head Neck Surg 118: 477-478.
1766. Monoo K, Sageshima M, Ito E, Nishihira S, Ishikawa K (2003). [Histopathological grading and clinical features of patients with mucoepidermoid carcinoma of the salivary glands]. Nippon Jibiinkoka Gakkai Kaiho 106: 192-198.
1767. Moore C, Catlin D (1967). Anatomic origins and locations of oral cancer. Am J Surg 114: 510-513.
1768. Moore JG, Bocklage T (1998). Fine-needle aspiration biopsy of large-cell undifferentiated carcinoma of the salivary glands: presentation of two cases, literature review, and differential cytodiagnosis of high-grade salivary gland malignancies. Diagn Cytopathol 19: 44-50.
1769. Moore SB, Pearson GR, Neel HBI, Weiland LH (1983). HLA and nasopharyngeal carcinoma in North American Caucasoids. Tissue Antigens 22: 72-75.
1770. Moretti JA, Miller D (1973). Laryngeal involvement in benign symmetric lipomatosis. Arch Otolaryngol 97: 495-496.
1771. Morgan K, MacLennan KA, Narula A, Bradley PJ, Morgan DA (1989). Non-Hodgkin's lymphoma of the larynx (stage IE). Cancer 64: 1123-1127.
1772. Morgan MN, Mackenzie DH (1968). Tumours of salivary glands. A review of 204 cases with 5-year follow-up. Br J Surg 55: 284-288.
1773. Mori N, Yatabe Y, Oka K, Kinoshita T, Kobayashi T, Ono T, Asai J (1996). Expression of perforin in nasal lymphoma. Additional evidence of its natural killer cell derivation. Am J Pathol 149: 699-705.
1774. Morice WG, Ferreiro JA (1998). Distinction of basaloid squamous cell carcinoma from adenoid cystic and small cell undifferentiated carcinoma by immunohistochemistry. Hum Pathol 29: 609-612.
1775. Morinaga S, Hashimoto S, Tezuka F (1992). Epithelial-myoepithelial carcinoma of the parotid gland in a child. Acta Pathol Jpn 42: 358-363.
1776. Morinaga S, Nakajima T, Shimosato Y (1987). Normal and neoplastic myoepithelial cells in salivary glands: an immunohistochemical study. Hum Pathol 18: 1218-1226.
1777. Morita A, Ebersold MJ, Olsen KD, Foote RL, Lewis JE, Quast LM (1993). Esthesioneuroblastoma: prognosis and management. Neurosurgery 32: 706-714.
1778. Morita T, Fujiki N, Sudo M, Miyata K, Kurata K (2000). Neonatal mature teratoma of the sphenoidal sinus: a case report. Am J Otolaryngol 21: 398-401.
1779. Moriya S, Tei K, Notani K, Shindoh M (2001). Malignant hemangiopericytoma of the head and neck: a report of 3 cases. J Oral Maxillofac Surg 59: 340-345.
1780. Morland B, Cox G, Randall C, Ramsay A, Radford M (1994). Synovial sarcoma of the larynx in a child: case report and histological appearances. Med Pediatr Oncol 23: 64-68.
1781. Morris KM, Campbell D, Stell PM, MacKenzie I, Miles JB (1990). Meningiomas presenting with paranasal sinus involvement. Br J Neurosurg 4: 511-515.
1782. Morrison MD (1988). Is chronic gastroesophageal reflux a causative factor in glottic carcinoma? Otolaryngol Head Neck Surg 99: 370-373.
1783. Mosqueda-Taylor A, Carlos-Bregni R, Ramirez-Amador V, Palma-Guzman JM, Esquivel-Bonilla D, Hernandez-Rojase LA (2002). Odontoameloblastoma. Clinicopathologic study of three cases and critical review of the literature. Oral Oncol 38: 800-805.
1784. Mosqueda-Taylor A, Meneses-Garcia A, Ruiz-Godoy Rivera LM, Lourdes Suarez-Roa M (2002). Clear cell odontogenic carcinoma of the mandible. J Oral Pathol Med 31: 439-441.
1785. Moss WT (1965). Therapeutic Radiology. 2nd ed. Mosby: St Louis.
1786. Mostafapour SP, Folz B, Barlow D, Manning S (2000). Sialoblastoma of the submandibular gland: report of a case and review of the literature. Int J Pediatr Otorhinolaryngol 53: 157-161.
1787. Motamedi MH (2002). Destructive aneurysmal bone cyst of the mandibular condyle: report of a case and review of the literature. J Oral Maxillofac Surg 60: 1357-1361.
1788. Mounts P, Shah KV, Kashima H (1982). Viral etiology of juvenile- and adult-onset squamous papilloma of the larynx. Proc Natl Acad Sci U S A 79: 5425-5429.
1789. Mukherji SK, Armao D, Joshi VM (2001). Cervical nodal metastases in squamous cell carcinoma of the head and neck: what to expect. Head Neck 23: 995-1005.
1790. Muller E, Beleites E (2000). The basaloid squamous cell carcinoma of the nasopharynx. Rhinology 38: 208-211.
1791. Muller S, Barnes L (1995). Basaloid squamous cell carcinoma of the head and neck with a spindle cell component. An unusual histologic variant. Arch Pathol Lab Med 119: 181-182.
1792. Muller S, Barnes L (1996). Basal cell adenocarcinoma of the salivary glands. Report of seven cases and review of the literature. Cancer 78: 2471-2477.
1793. Muller S, DeRose PB, Cohen C (1993). DNA ploidy of ameloblastoma and ameloblastic carcinoma of the jaws. Analysis by image and flow cytometry. Arch Pathol Lab Med 117: 1126-1131.
1794. Muller S, Parker DC, Kapadia SB, Budnick SD, Barnes EL (1995). Ameloblastic fibrosarcoma of the jaws. A clinicopathologic and DNA analysis of five cases and review of the literature with discussion of its relationship to ameloblastic fibroma. Oral Surg Oral Med Oral Pathol Oral Radiol Endod 79: 469-477.
1795. Muraki Y, Tateishi A, Tominaga K, Fukuda J, Haneji T, Iwata Y (1999). Malignant peripheral nerve sheath tumour in the maxilla associated with von Recklinghausen's disease. Oral Dis 5: 250-252.
1796. Murono S, Ohmura T, Sugimori S, Furukawa M (1998). Vascular leiomyoma with abundant adipose cells of the nasal cavity. Am J Otolaryngol 19: 50-53.
1797. Murrah VA, Batsakis JG (1994). Proliferative verrucous leukoplakia and verrucous hyperplasia. Ann Otol Rhinol Laryngol 103: 660-663.
1798. Murti PR, Bhonsle RB, Pindborg JJ, Daftary DK, Gupta PC, Mehta FS (1985). Malignant transformation rate in oral submucous fibrosis over a 17-year period. Community Dent Oral Epidemiol 13: 340-341.
1799. Murty GE, Welch AR, Soames JV (1990). Basal cell adenocarcinoma of the parotid gland. J Laryngol Otol 104: 150-151.
1800. Muscat JE, Wynder EL (1992). Tobacco, alcohol, asbestos, and occupational risk factors for laryngeal cancer. Cancer 69: 2244-2251.
1801. Muscat JE, Wynder EL (1998). A case/control study of risk factors for major salivary gland cancer. Otolaryngol Head Neck Surg 118: 195-198.
1802. Musy PY, Reibel JF, Levine PA (2002). Sinonasal undifferentiated carcinoma: the search for a better outcome. Laryngoscope 112: 1450-1455.
1803. Mutoh H, Nagata H, Ohno K, Numata T, Nagao T, Nagao K, Konno A (2001). Analysis of the p53 gene in parotid gland cancers: a relatively high frequency of mutations in low-grade mucoepidermoid carcinomas. Int J Oncol 18: 781-786.
1804. Muzumdar DP, Goel A, Pakhmode CK (2002). Multicystic acoustic neurinoma: report of two cases. J Clin Neurosci 9: 453-455.
1805. Mwang'ombe NJ, Kirongo G, Byakika W (2002). Fronto-ethmoidal teratoma: case report. East Afr Med J 79: 106-107.
1806. Myssiorek D, Halaas Y, Silver C (2001). Laryngeal and sinonasal paragangliomas. Otolaryngol Clin North Am 34: 971-82, vii.
1807. Myssiorek D, Patel M, Wasserman P, Rofeim O (1998). Osteosarcoma of the larynx. Ann Otol Rhinol Laryngol 107: 70-74.
1808. Myssiorek D, Vambutas A, Abramson AL (1994). Carcinoma in situ of the glottic larynx. Laryngoscope 104: 463-467.
1809. Nadal A, Campo E, Pinto J, Mallofre C, Palacin A, Arias C, Traserra J, Cardesa A (1995). p53 expression in normal, dysplastic, and neoplastic laryngeal epithelium. Absence of a correlation with prognostic factors. J Pathol 175: 181-188.
1810. Nadal A, Cardesa A (2003). Molecular biology of laryngeal squamous cell carcinoma. Virchows Arch 442: 1-7.
1811. Nadal A, Jares P, Cazorla M, Fernandez PL, Sanjuan X, Hernandez L, Pinyol M, Aldea M, Mallofre C, Muntane J, Traserra J, Campo E, Cardesa A (1997). p21WAF1/Cip1 expression is associated with cell differentiation but not with p53 mutations in squamous cell carcinomas of the larynx. J Pathol 183: 156-163.
1812. Nagai MA, Butugan O, Logullo A, Brentani MM (1996). Expression of growth factors, proto-oncogenes, and p53 in nasopharyngeal angiofibromas. Laryngoscope 106: 190-195.
1813. Nagai N, Takeshita N, Nagatsuka H, Inoue M, Nishijima K, Nojima T, Yamasaki M, Hoh C (1991). Ameloblastic carcinoma: case report and review. J Oral Pathol Med 20: 460-463.
1814. Nagao K, Matsuzaki O, Saiga H, Sugano I, Kaneko T, Katoh T, Kitamura T (1980). Histopathological studies on parotid gland tumors in Japanese children. Virchows Arch A Pathol Anat Histol 388: 263-272.
1815. Nagao K, Matsuzaki O, Saiga H, Sugano I, Kaneko T, Katoh T, Kitamura T, Shigematsu H, Maruyama N (1986). Histopathologic studies on adenocarcinoma of the parotid gland. Acta Pathol Jpn 36: 337-347.
1816. Nagao K, Matsuzaki O, Saiga H, Sugano I, Shigematsu H, Kaneko T, Katoh T, Kitamura T (1982). Histopathologic studies of undifferentiated carcinoma of the parotid gland. Cancer 50: 1572-1579.
1817. Nagao K, Matsuzaki O, Shigematsu H, Kaneko T, Katoh T, Kitamura T (1980). Histopathologic studies of benign infantile hemangioendothelioma of the parotid gland. Cancer 46: 2250-2256.
1818. Nagao T, Gaffey TA, Olsen KD, Serizawa H, Lewis JE (2004). Small cell carcinoma of the major salivary glands: clinicopathologic study with emphasis on cytokeratin 20 immunoreactivity and clinical outcome. Am J Surg Pathol 28: 762-770.
1819. Nagao T, Gaffey TA, Serizawa H, Iwaya K, Watanabe A, Yoshida T, Yamazaki K, Sageshima M, Lewis JE (2004). Sarcomatoid variant of salivary duct carcinoma: clinicopathologic and immunohistochemical study of eight cases with review of the literature. Am J Clin Pathol 122: 222-231.
1820. Nagao T, Gaffey TA, Visscher DW, Kay PA, Minato H, Serizawa H, Lewis JE (2004). Invasive micropapillary salivary duct carcinoma: a distinct histologic variant with biologic significance. Am J Surg Pathol 28: 319-326.
1821. Nagao T, Ishida Y, Sugano I, Tajima Y, Matsuzaki O, Hino T, Konno A, Kondo Y, Nagao K (1996). Epstein-Barr virus-associated undifferentiated carcinoma with lymphoid stroma of the salivary gland in Japanese patients. Comparison with benign lymphoepithelial lesion. Cancer 78: 695-703.
1822. Nagao T, Serizawa H, Iwaya K, Shimizu T, Sugano I, Ishida Y, Yamazaki K, Shimizu M, Itoh T, Konno A, Ebihara Y

(2002). Keratocystoma of the parotid gland: a report of two cases of an unusual pathologic entity. Mod Pathol 15: 1005-1010.
1823. Nagao T, Sugano I, Ishida Y, Asoh A, Munakata S, Yamazaki K, Konno A, Iwaya K, Shimizu T, Serizawa H, Ebihara Y (2002). Hybrid carcinomas of the salivary glands: report of nine cases with a clinicopathologic, immunohistochemical, and p53 gene alteration analysis. Mod Pathol 15: 724-733.
1824. Nagao T, Sugano I, Ishida Y, Asoh A, Munakata S, Yamazaki K, Konno A, Kondo Y, Nagao K (2001). Sialolipoma: a report of seven cases of a new variant of salivary gland lipoma. Histopathology 38: 30-36.
1825. Nagao T, Sugano I, Ishida Y, Matsuzaki O, Konno A, Kondo Y, Nagao K (1997). Carcinoma in basal cell adenoma of the parotid gland. Pathol Res Pract 193: 171-178.
1826. Nagao T, Sugano I, Ishida Y, Tajima Y, Furuya N, Kondo Y, Nagao K (1998). Mucoepidermoid carcinoma arising in Warthin's tumour of the parotid gland: report of two cases with histopathological, ultrastructural and immunohistochemical studies. Histopathology 33: 379-386.
1827. Nagao T, Sugano I, Ishida Y, Tajima Y, Matsuzaki O, Konno A, Kondo Y, Nagao K (1998). Salivary gland malignant myoepithelioma: a clinicopathologic and immunohistochemical study of ten cases. Cancer 83: 1292-1299.
1828. Nagao T, Sugano I, Ishida Y, Tajima Y, Munakata S, Asoh A, Yamazaki K, Muto H, Konno A, Kondo Y, Nagao K (2000). Primary large-cell neuroendocrine carcinoma of the parotid gland: immunohistochemical and molecular analysis of two cases. Mod Pathol 13: 554-561.
1829. Nagao T, Sugano I, Matsuzaki O, Hara H, Kondo Y, Nagao K (2000). Intraductal papillary tumors of the major salivary glands: case reports of benign and malignant variants. Arch Pathol Lab Med 124: 291-295.
1830. Nager GT (1964). Meningiomas Involving the Temporal Bone. Charles C.Thomas: Springfield, IL.
1831. Nageris B, Elidan J, Sherman Y (1994). Fibrosarcoma of the vocal fold: a late complication of radiotherapy. J Laryngol Otol 108: 993-994.
1832. Nagler RM, Laufer D (1997). Tumors of the major and minor salivary glands: review of 25 years of experience. Anticancer Res 17: 701-707.
1833. Nakada M, Nishizaki K, Akagi H, Masuda Y, Yoshino T (1998). Oncocytic carcinoma of the submandibular gland: a case report and literature review. J Oral Pathol Med 27: 225-228.
1834. Nakagawa T, Hattori K, Iwata N, Tsujimura T (2002). Papillary cystadenocarcinoma arising from minor salivary glands in the anterior portion of the tongue: a case report. Auris Nasus Larynx 29: 87-90.
1835. Nakajima T, Watanabe S, Sato Y, Shimosato Y, Motoi M, Lennert K (1982). S-100 protein in Langerhans cells, interdigitating reticulum cells and histiocytosis X cells. Gann 73: 429-432.
1836. Nakamura K, Uehara S, Omagari J, Kunitake N, Jingu K, Masuda K (1997). Primary non-Hodgkin's lymphoma of the maxillary sinus. Am J Clin Oncol 20: 272-275.
1837. Nakamura K, Uehara S, Omagari J, Kunitake N, Kimura M, Makino Y, Murakami J, Jingu K, Masuda K (1997). Primary non-Hodgkin lymphoma of the sinonasal cavities: correlation of CT evaluation with clinical outcome. Radiology 204: 431-435.
1838. Nakamura S, Katoh E, Koshikawa T, Yatabe Y, Nagasaka T, Ishida H, Tokoro Y, Koike K, Kagami Y, Ogura M, Kojima M, Nara Y, Mizoguchi Y, Hara K, Kurita S, Seto M, Suchi T (1997). Clinicopathologic study of nasal T/NK-cell lymphoma among the Japanese. Pathol Int 47: 38-53.
1839. Nakata M, Anno K, Matsumori LT, Sumie M, Sase M, Nakano T, Hara H, Imate Y, Nakamura Y, Kato H (2002). Prenatal diagnosis of congenital epulis: a case report. Ultrasound Obstet Gynecol 20: 627-629.
1840. Nakayama M, Wenig BM, Heffner DK (1995). Atypical stromal cells in inflammatory nasal polyps: immunohistochemical and ultrastructural analysis in defining histogenesis. Laryngoscope 105: 127-134.
1841. Nakhleh RE, Swanson PE, Dehner LP (1991). Juvenile (embryonal and alveolar) rhabdomyosarcoma of the head and neck in adults. A clinical, pathologic, and immunohistochemical study of 12 cases. Cancer 67: 1019-1024.
1842. Nall AV, Stringer SP, Baughman RA (1997). Vascular leiomyoma of the superior turbinate: first reported case. Head Neck 19: 63-67.
1843. Nandapalan V, Roland NJ, Helliwell TR, Williams EM, Hamilton JW, Jones AS (1998). Mucosal melanoma of the head and neck. Clin Otolaryngol 23: 107-116.
1844. Napier SS, Gormely JS, Newlands C, Ramsay-Baggs P (1995). Adenosquamous carcinoma. A rare neoplasm with an aggressive course. Oral Surg Oral Med Oral Pathol Oral Radiol Endod 79: 607-611.
1845. Napier SS, Herron BT, Herron BM (1995). Acinic cell carcinoma in Northern Ireland: a 10-year review. Br J Oral Maxillofac Surg 33: 145-148.
1846. Nappi O, Ritter JH, Pettinato G, Wick MR (1995). Hemangiopericytoma: histopathological pattern or clinicopathologic entity? Semin Diagn Pathol 12: 221-232.
1847. Nappi O, Wick MR, Pettinato G, Ghiselli RW, Swanson PE (1992). Pseudovascular adenoid squamous cell carcinoma of the skin. A neoplasm that may be mistaken for angiosarcoma. Am J Surg Pathol 16: 429-438.
1848. Narula AA, Vallis MP, el Silimy OE, Dowling F, Bradley PJ (1986). Radiation induced angiosarcomas of the nasopharynx. Eur J Surg Oncol 12: 147-152.
1849. Nascimento AG, Amaral AL, Prado LA, Kligerman J, Silveira TR (1986). Adenoid cystic carcinoma of salivary glands. A study of 61 cases with clinicopathologic correlation. Cancer 57: 312-319.
1850. Nascimento AG, Amaral LP, Prado LA, Kligerman J, Silveira TR (1986). Mucoepidermoid carcinoma of salivary glands: a clinicopathologic study of 46 cases. Head Neck Surg 8: 409-417.
1851. Nasser SM, Faquin WC, Dayal Y (2003). Expression of androgen, estrogen, and progesterone receptors in salivary gland tumors. Frequent expression of androgen receptor in a subset of malignant salivary gland tumors. Am J Clin Pathol 119: 801-806.
1852. Nauta JM, Panders AK, Schoots CJ, Vermey A, Roodenburg JL (1992). Peripheral ameloblastoma. A case report and review of the literature. Int J Oral Maxillofac Surg 21: 40-44.
1853. Nawroz H, Koch W, Anker P, Stroun M, Sidransky D (1996). Microsatellite alterations in serum DNA of head and neck cancer patients. Nat Med 2: 1035-1037.
1854. Nawshad AI, Savage NW, Young WG, Smyth I, Wicking C (2000). Allelic losses in chromosome 9q22.3-31q in odontogenic keratocysts. J Oral Pathol Med 29: 353 only.
1855. Nayak DR, Balakrishnan R, Rao RV, Hazarika P (2001). Clear cell carcinoma of the larynx—a case report. Int J Pediatr Otorhinolaryngol 57: 149-153.
1856. Nayar RC, Prudhomme F, Parise OJr, Gandia D, Luboinski B, Schwaab G (1993). Rhabdomyosarcoma of the head and neck in adults: a study of 26 patients. Laryngoscope 103: 1362-1366.
1857. Nazar-Stewart V, Vaughan TL, Burt RD, Chen C, Berwick M, Swanson GM (1999). Glutathione S-transferase M1 and susceptibility to nasopharyngeal carcinoma. Cancer Epidemiol Biomarkers Prev 8: 547-551.
1858. Nazeer T, Ro JY, Varma DG, de la Hermosa JR, Ayala AG (1996). Chondromyxoid fibroma of paranasal sinuses: report of two cases presenting with nasal obstruction. Skeletal Radiol 25: 779-782.
1859. Neel HBI (1985). Nasopharyngeal carcinoma. Clinical presentation, diagnosis, treatment, and prognosis. Otolaryngol Clin North Am 18: 479-490.
1860. Neel HBI, Pearson GR, Taylor WF (1984). Antibodies to Epstein-Barr virus in patients with nasopharyngeal carcinoma and in comparison groups. Ann Otol Rhinol Laryngol 93: 477-482.
1861. Neel HBI, Whicker JH, Devine KD, Weiland LH (1973). Juvenile angiofibroma. Review of 120 cases. Am J Surg 126: 547-556.
1862. Negri E, La Vecchia C, Franceschi S, Tavani A (1993). Attributable risk for oral cancer in northern Italy. Cancer Epidemiol Biomarkers Prev 2: 189-193.
1863. Nelson EG, Hinojosa R (1991). Histopathology of metastatic temporal bone tumors. Arch Otolaryngol Head Neck Surg 117: 189-193.
1864. Nelson JF, Jacoway JR (1973). Monomorphic adenoma (canalicular type). Report of 29 cases. Cancer 31: 1511-1513.
1865. Nelson RS, Perlman EJ, Askin FB (1995). Is esthesioneuroblastoma a peripheral neuroectodermal tumor? Hum Pathol 26: 639-641.
1866. Nelson ZL, Newman L, Loukota RA, Williams DM (1995). Bilateral multifocal canalicular adenomas of buccal minor salivary glands: a case report. Br J Oral Maxillofac Surg 33: 299-301.
1867. Nemoto Y, Inoue Y, Tashiro T, Mochizuki T, Katsuyama J, Hakuba A, Onoyama Y (1995). Central giant cell granuloma of the temporal bone. AJNR Am J Neuroradiol 16: 982-985.
1868. Netterville JL, Jackson CG, Miller FR, Wanamaker JR, Glasscock ME (1998). Vagal paraganglioma: a review of 46 patients treated during a 20-year period. Arch Otolaryngol Head Neck Surg 124: 1133-1140.
1869. Netterville JL, Reilly KM, Robertson D, Reiber ME, Armstrong WB, Childs P (1995). Carotid body tumors: a review of 30 patients with 46 tumors. Laryngoscope 105: 115-126.
1870. Neville BW, Damm DD, Allen CM, Bouquot JE (2002). Oral and Maxillofacial Pathology. 2 nd ed. W.B. Saunders: Philadelphia.
1871. Neville BW, Damm DD, Weir JC, Fantasia JE (1988). Labial salivary gland tumors. Cancer 61: 2113-2116.
1872. Newman AN, Colman M, Jayich SA (1983). Verrucous carcinoma of the frontal sinus: a case report and review of the literature. J Surg Oncol 24: 298-303.
1873. Newman J, Antonakopoulos GN, Darnton SJ, Matthews HR (1992). The ultrastructure of oesophageal carcinomas: multidirectional differentiation. A transmission electron microscopic study of 43 cases. J Pathol 167: 193-198.
1874. Newman JP, Funkhouser WK (1993). Pathologic quiz case 1. Clear cell carcinoma of the nasal cavity. Arch Otolaryngol Head Neck Surg 119: 1046-1049.
1875. Newman L, Howells GL, Coghlan KM, DiBiase A, Williams DM (1995). Malignant ameloblastoma revisited. Br J Oral Maxillofac Surg 33: 47-50.
1876. Newman L, Loukota RA, Bradley PF (1993). An infarcted Warthin's tumour presenting with facial weakness. Br J Oral Maxillofac Surg 31: 311-312.
1877. Ng CS, Lo ST, Chan JK (1999). Peripheral T and putative natural killer cell lymphomas commonly coexpress CD95 and CD95 ligand. Hum Pathol 30: 48-53.
1878. Ng CS, Lo ST, Chan JK, Chan WC (1997). CD56+ putative natural killer cell lymphomas: production of cytolytic effectors and related proteins mediating tumor cell apoptosis? Hum Pathol 28: 1276-1282.
1879. Ng KH, Siar CH (1990). Peripheral ameloblastoma with clear cell differentiation. Oral Surg Oral Med Oral Pathol 70: 210-213.
1880. Ng SH, Chang TC, Ko SF, Yen PS, Wan YL, Tang LM, Tsai MH (1997). Nasopharyngeal carcinoma: MRI and CT assessment. Neuroradiology 39: 741-746.
1881. Ng WK, Ma L (1995). Pleomorphic adenoma with extensive lipometaplasia. Histopathology 27: 285-288.
1882. Ngan RK, Lau WH, Yip TT, Cho WC, Cheng WW, Lim CK, Wan KK, Chu E, Joab I, Grunewald V, Poon YF, Ho JH (2001). Remarkable application of serum EBV EBER-1 in monitoring response of nasopharyngeal cancer patients to salvage chemotherapy. Ann N Y Acad Sci 945: 73-79.
1883. Nguyen-Tan PF, Le QT, Quivey JM, Singer M, Terris DJ, Goffinet DR, Fu KK (2001). Treatment results and prognostic factors of advanced T3—4 laryngeal carcinoma: the University of California, San Francisco (UCSF) and Stanford University Hospital (SUH) experience. Int J Radiat Oncol Biol Phys 50: 1172-1180.
1884. Nibu K, Li G, Zhang X, Rawson NE, Restrepo D, Kaga K, Lowry LD, Keane WM, Rothstein JL (1999). Olfactory neuron-specific expression of NeuroD in mouse and human nasal mucosa. Cell Tissue Res 298: 405-414.
1885. Nicholls JM, Agathanggelou A, Fung K, Zeng X, Niedobitek G (1997). The association of squamous cell carcinomas of the nasopharynx with Epstein-Barr virus shows geographical variation reminiscent of Burkitt's lymphoma. J Pathol 183: 164-168.
1886. Nicholls JM, Sham J, Chan CW, Choy D (1992). Radiation therapy for nasopharyngeal carcinoma: histologic appearances and patterns of tumor regression. Hum Pathol 23: 742-747.
1887. Nicholson HS, Egeler RM, Nesbit ME (1998). The epidemiology of Langerhans cell histiocytosis. Hematol Oncol Clin North Am 12: 379-384.

1888. Nicolai P, Ferlito A, Sasaki CT, Kirchner JA (1990). Laryngeal chondrosarcoma: incidence, pathology, biological behavior, and treatment. Ann Otol Rhinol Laryngol 99: 515-523.
1889. Nicolai P, Peretti G, Cappiello J, Renaldini G, Cavaliere S, Morassi ML (1991). [Melanoma metastatic to the trachea and nasal cavity: description of a case and review of the literature]. Acta Otorhinolaryngol Ital 11: 85-92.
1890. Nicolai P, Redaelli de Zinis LO, Tomenzoli D, Maroldi R, Antonelli AR (1991). Sphenoid mucocele with intracranial invasion secondary to nasopharyngeal acinic cell carcinoma. Head Neck 13: 540-544.
1891. Nicolai P, Tomenzoli D, Berlucchi M, Facchetti F, Morassi L, Maroldi R (2000). Malignant triton tumor of the ethmoid sinus and nasal cavity. Ann Otol Rhinol Laryngol 109: 880-886.
1892. Niedobitek G, Hansmann ML, Herbst H, Young LS, Dienemann D, Hartmann CA, Finn T, Pitteroff S, Welt A, Anagnostopoulos I, Friedrich RE, Lobeck H, Sam CK, Araujo I, Rickinson AB, Stein H (1991). Epstein-Barr virus and carcinomas: undifferentiated carcinomas but not squamous cell carcinomas of the nasopharynx are regularly associated with the virus. J Pathol 165: 17-24.
1893. Niedobitek G, Herbst H, Young LS (1993). Epstein-Barr virus and carcinomas. Int J Clin Lab Res 23: 17-24.
1894. Nielsen GP, Fletcher CD, Smith MA, Rybak L, Rosenberg AE (2002). Soft tissue aneurysmal bone cyst: a clinicopathologic study of five cases. Am J Surg Pathol 26: 64-69.
1895. Nielsen GP, Stemmer-Rachamimov AO, Ino Y, Moller MB, Rosenberg AE, Louis DN (1999). Malignant transformation of neurofibromas in neurofibromatosis 1 is associated with CDKN2A/p16 inactivation. Am J Pathol 155: 1879-1884.
1896. Nielsen TO, Sejean G, Onerheim RM (2000). Paraganglioma of the tongue. Arch Pathol Lab Med 124: 877-879.
1897. Niemann S, Steinberger D, Muller U (1999). PGL3, a third, not maternally imprinted locus in autosomal dominant paraganglioma. Neurogenetics 2: 167-170.
1898. Nikolaou AC, Markou CD, Petridis DG, Daniilidis IC (2000). Second primary neoplasms in patients with laryngeal carcinoma. Laryngoscope 110: 58-64.
1899. Nilles R, Lenarz T, Kaiserling E (1993). [Myoepithelial carcinoma of the nasopharynx. Case report and review of the literature]. HNO 41: 396-400.
1900. Ning JP, Yu MC, Wang QS, Henderson BE (1990). Consumption of salted fish and other risk factors for nasopharyngeal carcinoma (NPC) in Tianjin, a low-risk region for NPC in the People's Republic of China. J Natl Cancer Inst 82: 291-296.
1901. Noguchi K, Urade M, Sakurai K, Nishimura N, Hashitani S, Kishimoto H (2002). Small cell neuroendocrine carcinoma of the maxillary sinus—a case report and nude mouse transplantable model. Head Neck 24: 491-496.
1902. Nojeg MM, Jalaludin MA, Jayalakshmi P (1998). Papillary adenocarcinoma of the nasopharynx—case report and review of the literature. Med J Malaysia 53: 104-106.
1903. Nomori H, Watanabe S, Nakajima T, Shimosato Y, Kameya T (1986). Histiocytes in nasopharyngeal carcinoma in relation to prognosis. Cancer 57: 100-105.
1904. Nordkvist A, Gustafsson H, Juberg-Ode M, Stenman G (1994). Recurrent rearrangements of 11q14-22 in mucoepidermoid carcinoma. Cancer Genet Cytogenet 74: 77-83.
1905. Nordkvist A, Mark J, Dahlenfors R, Bende M, Stenman G (1994). Cytogenetic observations in 13 cystadenolymphomas (Warthin's tumors). Cancer Genet Cytogenet 76: 129-135.
1906. Nordkvist A, Mark J, Gustafsson H, Bang G, Stenman G (1994). Non-random chromosome rearrangements in adenoid cystic carcinoma of the salivary glands. Genes Chromosomes Cancer 10: 115-121.
1907. Nordkvist A, Roijer E, Bang G, Gustafsson H, Behrendt M, Ryd W, Thoresen S, Donath K, Stenman G (2000). Expression and mutation patterns of p53 in benign and malignant salivary gland tumors. Int J Oncol 16: 477-483.
1908. Norris HJ (1962). Papillary lesions of the nasal cavity and paranasal sinuses. Part I. Exophytic (squamous) papillomas. A study of 28 cases. Laryngoscope 72: 1797.
1909. Notani K, Iizuka T, Yamazaki Y, Henmi T, Sugiura C, Kohgo T, Fukuda H (2002). Mucinous adenocarcinoma of probable minor salivary gland origin. Oral Surg Oral Med Oral Pathol Oral Radiol Endod 94: 738-740.
1910. Notani PN, Jayant K (1987). Role of diet in upper aerodigestive tract cancers. Nutr Cancer 10: 103-113.
1911. Nunes JF, Fonseca I, Soares J (1996). Helioid inclusions in dedifferentiated acinic cell carcinoma of the parotid gland. Ultrastruct Pathol 20: 443-449.
1912. Nunez DA, Astley SM, Lewis FA, Wells M (1994). Human papilloma viruses: a study of their prevalence in the normal larynx. J Laryngol Otol 108: 319-320.
1913. Nuutinen J, Syrjanen K (1983). Angioleiomyoma of the larynx. Report of a case and review of the literature. Laryngoscope 93: 941-943.
1914. Nylander K, Dabelsteen E, Hall PA (2000). The p53 molecule and its prognostic role in squamous cell carcinomas of the head and neck. J Oral Pathol Med 29: 413-425.
1915. Nyrop M, Grontved A (2002). Cancer of the external auditory canal. Arch Otolaryngol Head Neck Surg 128: 834-837.
1916. O'Brien CJ, Malka VB, Mijailovic M (1993). Evaluation of 242 consecutive parotidectomies performed for benign and malignant disease. Aust N Z J Surg 63: 870-877.
1917. O'Brien CJ, McNeil EB, McMahon JD, Pathak I, Lauer CS, Jackson MA (2002). Significance of clinical stage, extent of surgery, and pathologic findings in metastatic cutaneous squamous carcinoma of the parotid gland. Head Neck 24: 417-422.
1918. O'Brien CJ, Soong SJ, Herrera GA, Urist MM, Maddox WA (1986). Malignant salivary tumors—analysis of prognostic factors and survival. Head Neck Surg 9: 82-92.
1919. O'Conor GTJr, Drake CR, Johns ME, Cail WS, Winn HR, Niskanen E (1985). Treatment of advanced esthesioneuroblastoma with high-dose chemotherapy and autologous bone marrow transplantation. A case report. Cancer 55: 347-349.
1920. O'Malley M, Pogrel MA, Stewart JC, Silva RG, Regezi JA (1997). Central giant cell granulomas of the jaws: phenotype and proliferation-associated markers. J Oral Pathol Med 26: 159-163.
1921. O'Regan EM, Gibb DH, Odell EW (2001). Rapid growth of giant cell granuloma in pregnancy treated with calcitonin. Oral Surg Oral Med Oral Pathol Oral Radiol Endod 92: 532-538.
1922. O'Reilly BJ, Kershaw JB (1987). Hodgkin's disease of the nasopharynx. J Laryngol Otol 101: 506-507.
1923. O'Reilly BJ, Ryan J, Reynard J, Chevretton E (1989). Malignant fibrous histiocytoma of the nasopharynx. J Laryngol Otol 103: 1076-1079.
1924. O'Reilly BJ, Zuk R (1989). Transitional type papilloma of the nasopharynx. J Laryngol Otol 103: 528-530.
1925. Ochsenius G, Ortega A, Godoy L, Penafiel C, Escobar E (2002). Odontogenic tumors in Chile: a study of 362 cases. J Oral Pathol Med 31: 415-420.
1926. Oda D, Persson GR, Haigh WG, Sabath DE, Penn I, Aziz S (1996). Oral presentation of posttransplantation lymphoproliferative disorders. An unusual manifestation. Transplantation 61: 435-440.
1927. Odell EW, Jani P, Sherriff M, Ahluwalia SM, Hibbert J, Levison DA, Morgan PR (1994). The prognostic value of individual histologic grading parameters in small lingual squamous cell carcinomas. The importance of the pattern of invasion. Cancer 74: 789-794.
1928. Odell EW, Lombardi T, Barrett AW, Morgan PR, Speight PM (1997). Hybrid central giant cell granuloma and central odontogenic fibroma-like lesions of the jaws. Histopathology 30: 165-171.
1929. Odell EW, Morgan PR (1998). Biopsy Pathology of the Oral Tissues. Chapman and Hall Medical: London.
1930. Odukoya O (1995). Odontogenic tumors: analysis of 289 Nigerian cases. J Oral Pathol Med 24: 454-457.
1931. Ogawa I, Nikai H, Takata T, Ijuhin N, Miyauchi M, Ito H, Vuhahula E (1991). Clear cell tumors of minor salivary gland origin. An immunohistochemical and ultrastructural analysis. Oral Surg Oral Med Oral Pathol 72: 200-207.
1932. Ogus HD, Bennett MH (1978). Carcinoma of the dorsum of the tongue: a rarity or misdiagnosis. Br J Oral Surg 16: 115-124.
1933. Ohashi Y, Nakai Y, Muraoka M, Takano H (1984). Asymptomatic leiomyosarcoma of maxillary sinus accompanied by primary mucocele. Arch Otorhinolaryngol 240: 73-78.
1934. Ohlms LA, McGill T, Healy GB (1994). Malignant laryngeal tumors in children: a 15-year experience with four patients. Ann Otol Rhinol Laryngol 103: 686-692.
1935. Ohshima K, Suzumiya J, Shimazaki K, Kato A, Tanaka T, Kanda M, Kikuchi M (1997). Nasal T/NK cell lymphomas commonly express perforin and Fas ligand: important mediators of tissue damage. Histopathology 31: 444-450.
1936. Okada H, Murai M, Yamamoto H (1994). Malignant fibrous histiocytoma of the maxillary sinus: a case study of proliferative activity, immunohistochemistry, and electron microscopy. J Oral Maxillofac Surg 52: 1193-1197.
1937. Okinaka Y, Sekitani T (1984). Mucoepidermoid carcinoma of the vocal cord. Report of a case. ORL J Otorhinolaryngol Relat Spec 46: 139-146.
1938. Oliveira P, Fonseca I, Soares J (1992). Acinic cell carcinoma of the salivary glands. A long term follow-up study of 15 cases. Eur J Surg Oncol 18: 7-15.
1939. Olivier M, Eeles R, Hollstein M, Khan MA, Harris CC, Hainaut P (2002). The IARC TP53 database: new online mutation analysis and recommendations to users. Hum Mutat 19: 607-614.
1940. Olofsson J, Grontoft O, Sokjer H, Risberg B (1984). Paraganglioma involving the larynx. ORL J Otorhinolaryngol Relat Spec 46: 57-65.
1941. Olofsson J, van Nostrand AW (1973). Growth and spread of laryngeal and hypopharyngeal carcinoma with reflections on the effect of preoperative irradiation. 139 cases studied by whole organ serial sectioning. Acta Otolaryngol Suppl 308: 1-84.
1942. Olofsson J, van Nostrand AW (1977). Adenoid cystic carcinoma of the larynx: a report of four cases and a review of the literature. Cancer 40: 1307-1313.
1943. Olsen J, Sabreo S, Fasting U (1985). Interaction of alcohol and tobacco as risk factors in cancer of the laryngeal region. J Epidemiol Community Health 39: 165-168.
1944. Olsen KD, Lewis JE, Suman VJ (1997). Spindle cell carcinoma of the larynx and hypopharynx. Otolaryngol Head Neck Surg 116: 47-52.
1945. Olsen TG, Helwig EB (1985). Angiolymphoid hyperplasia with eosinophilia. A clinicopathologic study of 116 patients. J Am Acad Dermatol 12: 781-796.
1946. Onitsuka T (1994). Sex hormones in papillary carcinoma of thyroid gland and pleomorphic adenoma of parotid gland. Acta Otolaryngol 114: 218-222.
1947. Ooi EE, Ren EC, Chan SH (1997). Association between microsatellites within the human MHC and nasopharyngeal carcinoma. Int J Cancer 74: 229-232.
1948. Ooi GC, Chim CS, Liang R, Tsang KW, Kwong YL (2000). Nasal T-cell/natural killer cell lymphoma: CT and MR imaging features of a new clinicopathologic entity. AJR Am J Roentgenol 174: 1141-1145.
1949. Ophir D (1991). Familial multicentric paragangliomas in a child. J Laryngol Otol 105: 376-380.
1949A. Or S, Yucetas S. (1987). Compound and complex odonotomas. Int J Oral Maxillofac Surg 16: 596-599
1950. Ordonez NG, Batsakis JG (1986). Acinic cell carcinoma of the nasal cavity: electron-optic and immunohistochemical observations. J Laryngol Otol 100: 345-349.
1951. Oreggia F, De Stefani E, Boffetta P, Brennan P, Deneo-Pellegrini H, Ronco AL (2001). Meat, fat and risk of laryngeal cancer: a case-control study in Uruguay. Oral Oncol 37: 141-145.
1952. Ortiz-Hidalgo C, de Leon-Bojorge B, Fernandez-Sobrino G, Sanchez Marle JF, Martin del Campo N (2001). Sialoblastoma: report of a congenital case with dysembryogenic alterations of the adjacent parotid gland. Histopathology 38: 79-80.
1953. Orvidas LJ, Kasperbauer JL (2000). Pediatric lymphangiomas of the head and neck. Ann Otol Rhinol Laryngol 109: 411-421.
1954. Orvidas LJ, Kasperbauer JL, Lewis JE, Olsen KD, Lesnick TG (2000). Pediatric parotid masses. Arch Otolaryngol Head Neck Surg 126: 177-184.
1955. Orvidas LJ, Lewis JE, Olsen KD, Weiner JS (1999). Intranasal verrucous carcinoma: relationship to inverting papilloma and human papillomavirus. Laryngoscope 109: 371-375.
1956. Orvidas LJ, Olsen KD, Lewis JE, Suman VJ (1998). Verrucous carcinoma of the larynx: a review of 53 patients. Head Neck 20: 197-203.

1957. Osaki T, Hirota J, Ohno A, Tatemoto Y (1990). Mucinous adenocarcinoma of the submandibular gland. Cancer 66: 1796-1801.
1958. Osaki T, Yoneda K, Yamamoto T, Kimura T, Matuoka H, Sakai H, Ryoke K (2000). Clinical investigation on pulmonary metastasis of head and neck carcinomas. Oncology 59: 196-203.
1959. Osmond DH, Buchbinder S, Cheng A, Graves A, Vittinghoff E, Cossen CK, Forghani B, Martin JN (2002). Prevalence of Kaposi sarcoma-associated herpesvirus infection in homosexual men at beginning of and during the HIV epidemic. JAMA 287: 221-225.
1960. Ostman J, Anneroth G, Gustafsson H, Tavelin B (1997). Malignant salivary gland tumours in Sweden 1960-1989—an epidemiological study. Oral Oncol 33: 169-176.
1961. Ott G, Katzenberger T, Greiner A, Kalla J, Rosenwald A, Heinrich U, Ott MM, Muller-Hermelink HK (1997). The t(11;18)(q21;q21) chromosome translocation is a frequent and specific aberration in low-grade but not high-grade malignant non-Hodgkin's lymphomas of the mucosa-associated lymphoid tissue (MALT-) type. Cancer Res 57: 3944-3948.
1962. Oudejans JJ, Harijadi H, Kummer JA, Tan IB, Bloemena E, Middeldorp JM, Bladergroen B, Dukers DF, Vos W, Meijer CJ (2002). High numbers of granzyme B/CD8-positive tumour-infiltrating lymphocytes in nasopharyngeal carcinoma biopsies predict rapid fatal outcome in patients treated with curative intent. J Pathol 198: 468-475.
1963. Owens OT, Calcaterra TC (1982). Salivary gland tumors of the lip. Arch Otolaryngol 108: 45-47.
1964. Oysu C, Aslan I, Bilgic B, Yazicioglu E (2001). Malignant triton tumour of the parapharyngeal space. J Laryngol Otol 115: 573-575.
1965. Ozono S, Onozuka M, Sato K, Ito Y (1992). Immunohistochemical localization of estradiol, progesterone, and progesterone receptor in human salivary glands and salivary adenoid cystic carcinomas. Cell Struct Funct 17: 169-175.
1966. Ozyar E, Yildiz F, Akyol FH, Atahan IL (1999). Comparison of AJCC 1988 and 1997 classifications for nasopharyngeal carcinoma. American Joint Committee on Cancer. Int J Radiat Oncol Biol Phys 44: 1079-1087.
1967. Pacheco-Ojeda L (2001). Malignant carotid body tumors: report of three cases. Ann Otol Rhinol Laryngol 110: 36-40.
1968. Packeisen J, Nowak M, Kruger A (2002). [Epulis in a newborn. histogenetic comparison with a granular cell tumor in adults]. Pathologe 23: 145-148.
Paczona R, Jori J, Tiszlavicz L, Czigner J (1999). Leiomyosarcoma of the larynx. Review of the literature and report of two cases. Ann Otol Rhinol Laryngol 108: 677-682.
1969 A. Pahl S, Henn W, Binger T, Stein U, Remberger K (2000). Malignant odontogenic myxoma of the maxilla: case with cytogenetic confirmation. J Laryngol Otol 114: 533-535.
1970. Pai SA, Naresh KN, Masih K, Ramarao C, Borges AM (1998). Teratocarcinosarcoma of the paranasal sinuses: a clinicopathologic and immunohistochemical study. Hum Pathol 29: 718-722.
1971. Pak MW, To KF, Lo YM, Chan LY, Tong JH, Lo KW, van Hasselt CA (2002). Nasopharyngeal carcinoma in situ (NPCIS)—pathologic and clinical perspectives. Head Neck 24: 989-995.
1972. Palacios E, Restrepo S, Rojas R (2002). Extramedullary plasmacytoma in the nasal cavity. Ear Nose Throat J 81: 499-500.
1973. Palmer TJ, Gleeson MJ, Eveson JW, Cawson RA (1990). Oncocytic adenomas and oncocytic hyperplasia of salivary glands: a clinicopathological study of 26 cases. Histopathology 16: 487-493.
1974. Palva T, Jokinen K, Karja J (1975). Neurilemmoma (schwannoma) of the larynx. J Laryngol Otol 89: 203-207.
1975. Panici PB, Scambia G, Perrone L, Battaglia F, Cattani P, Rabitti C, Dettori G, Capelli A, Sedlis A, Mancuso S (1992). Oral condyloma lesions in patients with extensive genital human papillomavirus infection. Am J Obstet Gynecol 167: 451-458.
1976. Panje WR, Moran WJ, Bostwick DG, Kitt VV (1986). Angiosarcoma of the head and neck: review of 11 cases. Laryngoscope 96: 1381-1384.
1977. Panoutsakopoulos G, Pandis N, Kyriazoglou I, Gustafson P, Mertens F, Mandahl N (1999). Recurrent t(16;17)(q22;p13) in aneurysmal bone cysts. Genes Chromosomes Cancer 26: 265-266.
1978. Pappo AS, Meza JL, Donaldson SS, Wharam MD, Wiener ES, Qualman SJ, Maurer HM, Crist WM (2003). Treatment of localized nonorbital, nonparameningeal head and neck rhabdomyosarcoma: lessons learned from intergroup rhabdomyosarcoma studies III and IV. J Clin Oncol 21: 638-645.
1979. Parkin DM, Muir CS, Whelan SL, Gao YT, Ferlay J, Powell J (1992). Cancer Incidence in Five Continents, Vol. VI. International Agency for Research on Cancer: Lyon.
1980. Parkin DM, Pisani P, Ferlay J (1999). Estimates of the worldwide incidence of 25 major cancers in 1990. Int J Cancer 80: 827-841.
1981. Parkin DM, Whelan SL, Ferlay J, Teppo L, Thomas DB (2003). Cancer Incidence in Five Continents, Vol. VIII. IARC Press: Lyon.
1982. Parnes SM (1990). Asbestos and cancer of the larynx: is there a relationship? Laryngoscope 100: 254-261.
1983. Partridge M, Li SR, Pateromichelakis S, Francis R, Phillips E, Huang XH, Tesfa-Selase F, Langdon JD (2000). Detection of minimal residual cancer to investigate why oral tumors recur despite seemingly adequate treatment. Clin Cancer Res 6: 2718-2725.
1984. Parwani AV, Ali SZ (2003). Diagnostic accuracy and pitfalls in fine-needle aspiration interpretation of Warthin tumor. Cancer 99: 166-171.
1985. Pastore A, Grandi E, Targa L, Marchese Ragona R (2001). [Malignant fibrous histiocytoma of the larynx. Presentation of a clinical case and review of the literature]. Acta Otorhinolaryngol Ital 21: 361-364.
1986. Patey DH, Thackray AC (1958). The treatment of parotid tumours in the light of a pathological study of parotidectomy material. Br J Surg 45: 477-487.
1987. Pathak I, O'Brien CJ, Petersen-Schaeffer K, McNeil EB, McMahon J, Quinn MJ, Thompson JF, McCarthy WH (2001). Do nodal metastases from cutaneous melanoma of the head and neck follow a clinically predictable pattern? Head Neck 23: 785-790.
1988. Pathmanathan R, Prasad U, Chandrika G, Sadler R, Flynn K, Raab-Traub N (1995). Undifferentiated, nonkeratinizing, and squamous cell carcinoma of the nasopharynx. Variants of Epstein-Barr virus-infected neoplasia. Am J Pathol 146: 1355-1367.
1989. Pathmanathan R, Prasad U, Sadler R, Flynn K, Raab-Traub N (1995). Clonal proliferations of cells infected with Epstein-Barr virus in preinvasive lesions related to nasopharyngeal carcinoma. N Engl J Med 333: 693-698.
1990. Patrikiou A, Sepheriadou-Mavropoulou T, Zambelis G (1981). Bilateral traumatic bone cyst of the mandible. A case report. Oral Surg Oral Med Oral Pathol 51: 131-133.
1991. Patternson K, Kapur S, Chandra RS (1986). "Nasal gliomas" and related brain heteropias: a pathologist's perspective. Pediatr Pathol 5: 353-362.
1992. Patterson GA, Campbell DB (2000). Clinical-pathologic conference in thoracic surgery: basaloid squamous carcinoma of the trachea. J Thorac Cardiovasc Surg 120: 187-193.
1993. Patton LL, McKaig R, Strauss R, Rogers D, Eron JJJr (2000). Changing prevalence of oral manifestations of human immuno-deficiency virus in the era of protease inhibitor therapy. Oral Surg Oral Med Oral Pathol Oral Radiol Endod 89: 299-304.
1994. Patton LL, Valdez IH (1991). Xeroderma pigmentosum: review and report of a case. Oral Surg Oral Med Oral Pathol 71: 297-300.
1995. Pauk J, Huang ML, Brodie SJ, Wald A, Koelle DM, Schacker T, Celum C, Selke S, Corey L (2000). Mucosal shedding of human herpesvirus 8 in men. N Engl J Med 343: 1369-1377.
1996. Paulino AF, Huvos AG (1999). Oncocytic and oncocytoid tumors of the salivary glands. Semin Diagn Pathol 16: 98-104.
1997. Paulino AF, Singh B, Shah JP, Huvos AG (2000). Basaloid squamous cell carcinoma of the head and neck. Laryngoscope 110: 1479-1482.
1998. Paulsen J, Lennert K (1994). Low-grade B-cell lymphoma of mucosa-associated lymphoid tissue type in Waldeyer's ring. Histopathology 24: 1-11.
1999. Paz IB, Cook N, Odom-Maryon T, Xie Y, Wilczynski SP (1997). Human papillomavirus (HPV) in head and neck cancer. An association of HPV 16 with squamous cell carcinoma of Waldeyer's tonsillar ring. Cancer 79: 595-604.
2000. Pellicano M, Zullo F, Catizone C, Guida F, Catizone F, Nappi C (1998). Prenatal diagnosis of congenital granular cell epulis. Ultrasound Obstet Gynecol 11: 144-146.
2001. Pellin A, Boix J, Blesa JR, Noguera R, Carda C, Llombart-Bosch A (1994). EWS/FLI-1 rearrangement in small round cell sarcomas of bone and soft tissue detected by reverse transcriptase polymerase chain reaction amplification. Eur J Cancer 30A: 827-831.
2002. Pelosi G, Fraggetta F (2002). Epithelial-myoepithelial carcinomas of the bronchus. Am J Surg Pathol 26: 950-951.
2003. Pelucchi C, Talamini R, Levi F, Bosetti C, La Vecchia C, Negri E, Parpinel M, Franceschi S (2003). Fibre intake and laryngeal cancer risk. Ann Oncol 14: 162-167.
2004. Penaloza-Plascencia M, Montoya-Fuentes H, Flores-Martinez SE, Fierro-Velasco FJ, Penaloza-Gonzalez JM, Sanchez-Corona J (2000). Molecular identification of 7 human papillomavirus types in recurrent respiratory papillomatosis. Arch Otolaryngol Head Neck Surg 126: 1119-1123.
2005. Peng JC, Sheen TS, Hsu MM (1995). Nasopharyngeal carcinoma with dermatomyositis. Analysis of 12 cases. Arch Otolaryngol Head Neck Surg 121: 1298-1301.
2006. Penner CR, Folpe AL, Budnick SD (2002). C-kit expression distinguishes salivary gland adenoid cystic carcinoma from polymorphous low-grade adenocarcinoma. Mod Pathol 15: 687-691.
2007. Perdigou JB, Pages M, Le Bodic MF, Pages A (1981). [Oncocytoma with neuro-secretory granules of nasal mucous membrane (author's transl)]. Arch Anat Cytol Pathol 29: 75-78.
2008. Perez-Ayala M, Ruiz-Cabello F, Esteban F, Concha A, Redondo M, Oliva MR, Cabrera T, Garrido F (1990). Presence of HPV 16 sequences in laryngeal carcinomas. Int J Cancer 46: 8-11.
2009. Perez-Ordonez B, Caruana SM, Huvos AG, Shah JP (1998). Small cell neuroendocrine carcinoma of the nasal cavity and paranasal sinuses. Hum Pathol 29: 826-832.
2010. Perez-Ordonez B, Erlandson RA, Rosai J (1996). Follicular dendritic cell tumor: report of 13 additional cases of a distinctive entity. Am J Surg Pathol 20: 944-955.
2011. Perez-Ordonez B, Linkov I, Huvos AG (1998). Polymorphous low-grade adenocarcinoma of minor salivary glands: a study of 17 cases with emphasis on cell differentiation. Histopathology 32: 521-529.
2012. Perez P, Dominguez O, Gonzalez S, Gonzalez S, Trivino A, Suarez C (1999). ras gene mutations in ethmoid sinus adenocarcinoma: prognostic implications. Cancer 86: 255-264.
2013. Perrone F, Oggionni M, Birindelli S, Suardi S, Tabano S, Romano R, Moiraghi ML, Bimbi G, Quattrone P, Cantu G, Pierotti MA, Licitra L, Pilotti S (2003). TP53, p14ARF, p16INK4a and H-ras gene molecular analysis in intestinal-type adenocarcinoma of the nasal cavity and paranasal sinuses. Int J Cancer 105: 196-203.
2014. Perzin KH, Cantor JO, Johannessen JV (1981). Acinic cell carcinoma arising in nasal cavity: report of a case with ultrastructural observations. Cancer 47: 1818-1822.
2015. Perzin KH, Fu YS (1980). Non-epithelial tumors of the nasal cavity, paranasal sinuses and nasopharynx: a clinico-pathologic study XI. fibrous histiocytomas. Cancer 45: 2616-2626.
2016. Perzin KH, Gullane P, Clairmont AC (1978). Adenoid cystic carcinomas arising in salivary glands: a correlation of histologic features and clinical course. Cancer 42: 265-282.
2017. Perzin KH, LiVolsi VA (1979). Acinic cell carcinomas arising in salivary glands: a clinicopathologic study. Cancer 44: 1434-1457.
2018. Perzin KH, Panyu H, Wechter S (1982). Nonepithelial tumors of the nasal cavity, paranasal sinuses and nasopharynx. A clinicopathologic study. XII: Schwann cell tumors (neurilemoma, neurofibroma, malignant schwannoma). Cancer 50: 2193-2202.
2019. Perzin KH, Pushparaj N (1984). Nonepithelial tumors of the nasal cavity,

paranasal sinuses, and nasopharynx. A clinicopathologic study. XIII: Meningiomas. Cancer 54: 1860-1869.
2020. Pesavento G, Ferlito A, Recher G (1980). Primary clear cell carcinoma of the larynx. J Clin Pathol 33: 1160-1164.
2021. Pesce C, Colacino R, Buffa P (1986). Duct carcinoma of the minor salivary glands: a case report. J Laryngol Otol 100: 611-613.
2022. Pesce C, Tobia-Gallelli F, Toncini C (1984). APUD cells of the larynx. Acta Otolaryngol 98: 158-162.
2023. Peters WJ (1979). Cherubism: a study of twenty cases from one family. Oral Surg Oral Med Oral Pathol 47: 307-311.
2024. Petrikowski CG, Pharoah MJ, Lee L, Grace MG (1995). Radiographic differentiation of osteogenic sarcoma, osteomyelitis, and fibrous dysplasia of the jaws. Oral Surg Oral Med Oral Pathol Oral Radiol Endod 80: 744-750.
2025. Petropoulos AE, Luetje CM, Camarata PJ, Whittaker CK, Lee G, Baysal BE (2000). Genetic analysis in the diagnosis of familial paragangliomas. Laryngoscope 110: 1225-1229.
2026. Pettinato G, Manivel JC, D'Amore ES, Jaszcz W, Gorlin RJ (1991). Melanotic neuroectodermal tumor of infancy. A reexamination of a histogenetic problem based on immunohistochemical, flow cytometric, and ultrastructural study of 10 cases. Am J Surg Pathol 15: 233-245.
2027. Pfeifer GP, Denissenko MF, Olivier M, Tretyakova N, Hecht SS, Hainaut P (2002). Tobacco smoke carcinogens, DNA damage and p53 mutations in smoking-associated cancers. Oncogene 21: 7435-7451.
2028. Philipsen HP, Birn H (1969). The adenomatoid odontogenic tumour. Ameloblastic adenomatoid tumour or adeno-ameloblastoma. Acta Pathol Microbiol Scand 75: 375-398.
2029. Philipsen HP, Reichart PA (1996). Squamous odontogenic tumor (SOT): a benign neoplasm of the periodontium. A review of 36 reported cases. J Clin Periodontol 23: 922-926.
2030. Philipsen HP, Reichart PA (1998). Unicystic ameloblastoma. A review of 193 cases from the literature. Oral Oncol 34: 317-325.
2031. Philipsen HP, Reichart PA (2000). Calcifying epithelial odontogenic tumour: biological profile based on 181 cases from the literature. Oral Oncol 36: 17-26.
2032. Philipsen HP, Reichart PA, Nikai H (1998). The adenomatoid odontogenic tumour (AOT): An update. Oral Med Pathol 2: 55-60.
2033. Philipsen HP, Reichart PA, Nikai H, Takata T, Kudo Y (2001). Peripheral ameloblastoma: biological profile based on 160 cases from the literature. Oral Oncol 37: 17-27.
2034. Philipsen HP, Reichart PA, Praetorius F (1997). Mixed odontogenic tumours and odontomas. Considerations on interrelationship. Review of the literature and presentation of 134 new cases of odontomas. Oral Oncol 33: 86-99.
2035. Philipsen HP, Reichart PA, Takata T (2001). Desmoplastic ameloblastoma (including "hybrid" lesion of ameloblastoma). Biological profile based on 100 cases from the literature and own files. Oral Oncol 37: 455-460.
2036. Philipsen HP, Samman N, Ormiston IW, Wu PC, Reichart PA (1992). Variants of the adenomatoid odontogenic tumor with a note on tumor origin. J Oral Pathol Med 21: 348-352.
2037. Philipsen HP, Thosaporn W, Reichart P, Grundt G (1992). Odontogenic lesions in opercula of permanent molars delayed in eruption. J Oral Pathol Med 21: 38-41.
2038. Phillips CD, Futterer SF, Lipper MH, Levine PA (1997). Sinonasal undifferentiated carcinoma: CT and MR imaging of an uncommon neoplasm of the nasal cavity. Radiology 202: 477-480.
2039. Piattelli A, Lezzi G, Rubini C, Fioroni M (2002). Intraduct papilloma of the palate. Report of a case. Oral Oncol 38: 398-400.
2040. Piattelli A, Sesenna E, Trisi P (1994). Clear cell odontogenic carcinoma. Report of a case with lymph node and pulmonary metastases. Eur J Cancer B Oral Oncol 30B: 278-280.
2040A. Piattelli A, Trisi P (1992). Morphodifferentiation and histodifferentiation of the dental hard tissues in compound odontoma: a study of undemineralized material. J Oral Pathol Med 21, 340-342.
2041. Piccirillo JF, Lacy PD, Basu A, Spitznagel EL (2002). Development of a new head and neck cancer-specific comorbidity index. Arch Otolaryngol Head Neck Surg 128: 1172-1179.
2042. Pierce ST, Cibull ML, Metcalfe MS, Sloan D (1994). Bone marrow metastases from small cell cancer of the head and neck. Head Neck 16: 266-271.
2043. Pileri SA, Grogan TM, Harris NL, Banks P, Campo E, Chan JK, Favera RD, Delsol G, Wolf-Peeters C, Falini B, Gascoyne RD, Gaulard P, Gatter KC, Isaacson PG, Jaffe ES, Kluin P, Knowles DM, Mason DY, Mori S, Muller-Hermelink HK, Piris MA, Ralfkiaer E, Stein H, Su IJ, Warnke RA, Weiss LM (2002). Tumours of histiocytes and accessory dendritic cells: an immunohistochemical approach to classification from the International Lymphoma Study Group based on 61 cases. Histopathology 41: 1-29.
2044. Pillsbury HC, Jones K (1989). Vascular tumors of the head and neck: presentation, prognosis, and treatment dilemmas. Oncology (Huntingt) 3: 23-29.
2045. Pincock LD, Bruce KW (1954). Odontogenic fibroma. Oral Surg Oral Med Oral Pathol 7: 307-311.
2046. Pindborg JJ (1955). Calcifying epithelial odontogenic tumors. Acta Pathol Microbiol Scand 111: 71.
2047. Pindborg JJ (1958). A calcifying epithelial odontogenic tumor. Cancer 11: 838-843.
2048. Pindborg JJ, Clausen F (1958). Classification of odontogenic tumors. A suggestion. Acta Odontol Scand 16: 293-301.
2049. Pindborg JJ, Jolst O, Renstrup G, Roed-Petersen B (1968). Studies in oral leukoplakia: a preliminary report on the period pervalence of malignant transformation in leukoplakia based on a follow-up study of 248 patients. J Am Dent Assoc 76: 767-771.
2050. Pindborg JJ, Kramer IRH (1971). Histological typing of odontogenic tumours, jaw cysts and allied lesions. 1st ed. World Health Organization: Geneva.
2051. Pindborg JJ, Shear M, Kramer IRH (1992). Histological Typing of Odontogenic Tumours. 2 ed. Springer Verlag: Berlin.
2052. Pinkston JA, Cole P (1996). Cigarette smoking and Warthin's tumor. Am J Epidemiol 144: 183-187.
2053. Pinkston JA, Cole P (1999). Incidence rates of salivary gland tumors: results from a population-based study. Otolaryngol Head Neck Surg 120: 834-840.
2054. Pinsolle J, LeCluse I, Demeaux H, Laur P, Rivel J, Siberchicot F (1990). Osteosarcoma of the soft tissue of the larynx: report of a case with electron microscopic studies. Otolaryngol Head Neck Surg 102: 276-280.
2055. Pisani P, Krengli M, Ramponi A, Olina M, Pia F (1994). Angiosarcoma of the hypopharynx. J Laryngol Otol 108: 905-908.
2056. Pitanguy I, Machado BH, Radwanski HN, Amorim NF (1996). Surgical treatment of hemangiomas of the nose. Ann Plast Surg 36: 586-592.
2057. Pitman KT, Ferlito A, Devaney KO, Shaha AR, Rinaldo A (2003). Sentinel lymph node biopsy in head and neck cancer. Oral Oncol 39: 343-349.
2058. Pivnick EK, Walter AW, Lawrence MD, Smith ME (1996). Gorlin syndrome associated with midline nasal dermoid cyst. J Med Genet 33: 704-706.
2059. Plath T, Dallenbach F (1998). [Basal cell adenocarcinoma of the minor salivary glands of the palate. Case report and review of the literature]. Mund Kiefer Gesichtschir 2: 275-278.
2060. Platz H, Fries R, Hudec M (1985). Retrospective DOSAK Study on carcinomas of the oral cavity: results and consequences. J Maxillofac Surg 13: 147-153.
2061. Plaza G, Manzanal AI, Fogue L, Santon A, Martinez-Montero JC, Bellas C (2002). Association of Epstein-Barr virus and nasopharyngeal carcinoma in Caucasian patients. Ann Otol Rhinol Laryngol 111: 210-216.
2062. Podoshin L, Rolan L, Altman MM, Peyser E (1970). 'Pharyngeal' craniopharyngioma. J Laryngol Otol 84: 93-99.
2063. Poirier S, Ohshima H, de The G, Hubert A, Bourgade MC, Bartsch H (1987). Volatile nitrosamine levels in common foods from Tunisia, south China and Greenland, high-risk areas for nasopharyngeal carcinoma (NPC). Int J Cancer 39: 293-296.
2064. Polin RS, Sheehan JP, Chenelle AG, Munoz E, Larner J, Phillips CD, Cantrell RW, Laws ERJr, Newman SA, Levine PA, Jane JA (1998). The role of preoperative adjuvant treatment in the management of esthesioneuroblastoma: the University of Virginia experience. Neurosurgery 42: 1029-1037.
2065. Poljak M, Gale N, Kambic V (1997). Human papillomaviruses: a study of their prevalence in the epithelial hyperplastic lesions of the larynx. Acta Otolaryngol Suppl 527: 66-69.
2066. Poljak M, Seme K, Gale N (1998). Detection of human papillomaviruses in tissue specimens. Adv Anat Pathol 5: 216-234.
2067. Pollandt K, Engels C, Werner M, Delling G (2002). [Fibrous dysplasia]. Pathologe 23: 351-356.
2068. Pomilla PV, Morris AB, Jaworek A (1995). Sinonasal non-Hodgkin's lymphoma in patients infected with human immunodeficiency virus: report of three cases and review. Clin Infect Dis 21: 137-149.
2069. Pontius KI, Sebek BA (1981). Extraskeletal Ewing's sarcoma arising in the nasal fossa. Light- and electron-microscopic observations. Am J Clin Pathol 75: 410-415.
2070. Porter PL, Bigler SA, McNutt M, Gown AM (1991). The immunophenotype of hemangiopericytomas and glomus tumors, with special reference to muscle protein expression: an immunohistochemical study and review of the literature. Mod Pathol 4: 46-52.
2071. Porter WM, Sidwell RU, Catovsky D, Bunker CB (2001). Cutaneous presentation of chronic lymphatic leukaemia and response to ultraviolet B phototherapy. Br J Dermatol 144: 1092-1094.
2072. Portugal LG, Goldenberg JD, Wenig BL, Ferrer KT, Nodzenski E, Sabnani JB, Javier C, Weichselbaum RR, Vokes EE (1997). Human papillomavirus expression and p53 gene mutations in squamous cell carcinoma. Arch Otolaryngol Head Neck Surg 123: 1230-1234.
2073. Potter AJJr, Khatib G, Peppard SB (1984). Intranasal glomus tumor. Arch Otolaryngol 110: 755-756.
2074. Pou AM, Rimell FL, Jordan JA, Shoemaker DL, Johnson JT, Barua P, Post JC, Ehrlich GD (1995). Adult respiratory papillomatosis: human papillomavirus type and viral coinfections as predictors of prognosis. Ann Otol Rhinol Laryngol 104: 758-762.
2075. Poulsen P, Jorgensen K, Grontved A (1987). Benign and malignant neoplasms of the parotid gland: incidence and histology in the Danish County of Funen. Laryngoscope 97: 102-104.
2076. Praetorius F (1997). HPV-associated diseases of oral mucosa. Clin Dermatol 15: 399-413.
2077. Praetorius F, Hjorting-Hansen E, Gorlin RJ, Vickers RA (1981). Calcifying odontogenic cyst. Range, variations and neoplastic potential. Acta Odontol Scand 39: 227-240.
2078. Prasad ML, Busam KJ, Patel SG, Hoshaw-Woodard S, Shah JP, Huvos AG (2003). Clinicopathologic differences in malignant melanoma arising in oral squamous and sinonasal respiratory mucosa of the upper aerodigestive tract. Arch Pathol Lab Med ?: ?
2079. Prasad ML, Jungbluth AA, Iversen K, Huvos AG, Busam KJ (2001). Expression of melanocytic differentiation markers in malignant melanomas of the oral and sinonasal mucosa. Am J Surg Pathol 25: 782-787.
2080. Prasad ML, Patel S, Hoshaw-Woodard S, Escrig M, Shah JP, Huvos AG, Busam KJ (2002). Prognostic factors for malignant melanoma of the squamous mucosa of the head and neck. Am J Surg Pathol 26: 883-892.
2081. Prasad ML, Patel SG, Huvos AG, Shah JP, Busam KJ (2004). Primary mucosal melanoma of the head and neck: a proposal for microstaging localized, Stage I (lymph node-negative) tumors. Cancer 100: 1657-1664.
2082. Prasad U (1974). Cells of origin of nasopharyngeal carcinoma: an electron microscopic study. J Laryngol Otol 88: 1087-1094.
2083. Prasad U, Kwi NK (1975). Nasopharyngeal craniopharyngioma. J Laryngol Otol 89: 445-452.
2084. Prathap K, Looi LM, Prasad U (1984). Localized amyloidosis in nasopharyngeal carcinoma. Histopathology 8: 27-34.
2085. Prescher A, Brors D (2001). [Metastases to the paranasal sinuses: case report and review of the literature]. Laryngorhinootologie 80: 583-594.
2086. Press MF, Pike MC, Hung G, Zhou JY, Ma Y, George J, Dietz-Band J, James W, Slamon DJ, Batsakis JG, El Naggar AK (1994). Amplification and overexpression of HER-2/neu in carcinomas of the salivary

gland: correlation with poor prognosis. Cancer Res 54: 5675-5682.

2087. Pressman J, Dowdy A, Libby R, Fields M (1956). Further studies upon the submucosal compartments and lymphatics of the larynx by the injection of dyes and radioisotopes. Ann Otol Rhinol Laryngol 65: 766-980.

2088. Preston-Martin S, Thomas DC, White SC, Cohen D (1988). Prior exposure to medical and dental x-rays related to tumors of the parotid gland. J Natl Cancer Inst 80: 943-949.

2089. Preston-Martin S, White SC (1990). Brain and salivary gland tumors related to prior dental radiography: implications for current practice. J Am Dent Assoc 120: 151-158.

2090. Prime SS, Thakker NS, Pring M, Guest PG, Paterson IC (2001). A review of inherited cancer syndromes and their relevance to oral squamous cell carcinoma. Oral Oncol 37: 1-16.

2091. Proulx GM, Caudra-Garcia I, Ferry J, Harris N, Greco WR, Kaya U, Chan A, Wang CC (2003). Lymphoma of the nasal cavity and paranasal sinuses: treatment and outcome of early-stage disease. Am J Clin Oncol 26: 6-11.

2092. Puchalski R, Shah UK, Carpentieri D, McLaughlin R, Handler SD (2000). Melanotic neuroectodermal tumor of infancy (MNTI) of the hard palate: presentation and management. Int J Pediatr Otorhinolaryngol 53: 163-168.

2093. Pugnale N, Waridel F, Bouzourene H, Boubaker A, Pugnale M, Gaillard RC, Gomez F (2003). Pharyngeal pituitary nonfunctioning adenoma with normal intra-sellar gland: massive tumor shrinkage on octreotide therapy. Eur J Endocrinol 148: 357-364.

2094. Qian CN, Guo X, Cao B, Kort EJ, Lee CC, Chen J, Wang LM, Mai WY, Min HQ, Hong MH, Vande Woude GF, Resau JH, Teh BT (2002). Met protein expression level correlates with survival in patients with late-stage nasopharyngeal carcinoma. Cancer Res 62: 589-596.

2095. Qian CN, Zhang CQ, Guo X, Hong MH, Cao SM, Mai WY, Min HQ, Zeng YX (2000). Elevation of serum vascular endothelial growth factor in male patients with metastatic nasopharyngeal carcinoma. Cancer 88: 255-261.

2096. Qin DX, Hu YH, Yan JH, Xu GZ, Cai WM, Wu XL, Cao DX, Gu XZ (1988). Analysis of 1379 patients with nasopharyngeal carcinoma treated by radiation. Cancer 61: 1117-1124.

2097. Quddus MR, Henley JD, Affify AM, Dardick I, Gnepp DR (1999). Basal cell adenocarcinoma of the salivary gland: an ultrastructural and immunohistochemical study. Oral Surg Oral Med Oral Pathol Oral Radiol Endod 87: 485-492.

2098. Queimado L, Reis A, Fonseca I, Martins C, Lovett M, Soares J, Parreira L (1998). A refined localization of two deleted regions in chromosome 6q associated with salivary gland carcinomas. Oncogene 16: 83-88.

2099. Quesada P, Navarrete ML, Perello E (1990). Eosinophilic granuloma of the temporal bone. Eur Arch Otorhinolaryngol 247: 194-196.

2100. Quick CA, Foucar E, Dehner LP (1979). Frequency and significance of epithelial atypia in laryngeal papillomatosis. Laryngoscope 89: 550-560.

2101. Quiney RE, Wells M, Lewis FA, Terry RM, Michaels L, Croft CB (1989). Laryngeal

papillomatosis: correlation between severity of disease and presence of HPV 6 and 11 detected by in situ DNA hybridisation. J Clin Pathol 42: 694-698.

2102. Quinn HJJr (1984). Synovial sarcoma of the larynx treated by partial laryngectomy. Laryngoscope 94: 1158-1161.

2103. Quintana PG, Kapadia SB, Bahler DW, Johnson JT, Swerdlow SH (1997). Salivary gland lymphoid infiltrates associated with lymphoepithelial lesions: a clinicopathologic, immunophenotypic, and genotypic study. Hum Pathol 28: 850-861.

2104. Quintanilla-Martinez L, Franklin JL, Guerrero I, Krenacs L, Naresh KN, Rama-Rao C, Bhatia K, Raffeld M, Magrath IT (1999). Histological and immunophenotypic profile of nasal NK/T cell lymphomas from Peru: high prevalence of p53 overexpression. Hum Pathol 30: 849-855.

2105. Quintanilla-Martinez L, Kremer M, Keller G, Nathrath M, Gamboa-Dominguez A, Meneses A, Luna-Contreras L, Cabras A, Hoefler H, Mohar A, Fend F (2001). p53 Mutations in nasal natural killer/T-cell lymphoma from Mexico: association with large cell morphology and advanced disease. Am J Pathol 159: 2095-2105.

2106. Quon H, Liu FF, Cummings BJ (2001). Potential molecular prognostic markers in head and neck squamous cell carcinomas. Head Neck 23: 147-159.

2107. Raab-Traub N (2002). Epstein-Barr virus in the pathogenesis of NPC. Semin Cancer Biol 12: 431-441.

2108. Raab-Traub N, Flynn K, Pearson G, Huang A, Levine P, Lanier A, Pagano J (1987). The differentiated form of nasopharyngeal carcinoma contains Epstein-Barr virus DNA. Int J Cancer 39: 25-29.

2109. Raab SS, Sigman JD, Hoffman HT (1998). The utility of parotid gland and level I and II neck fine-needle aspiration. Arch Pathol Lab Med 122: 823-827.

2110. Rabah R, Sakr W, Thomas R, Lancaster WD, Gregoire L (2000). Human papillomavirus type, proliferative activity, and p53: potential markers of aggressive papillomatosis. Arch Pathol Lab Med 124: 721-724.

2110A. Rachanis CC, Shear M (1978). Age-standardized incidence rates of primordial cyst (keratocyst) on the Witwatersrand. Community Dent Oral Epidemiol 6: 296-299.

2111. Radkowski D, McGill T, Healy GB, Ohlms L, Jones DT (1996). Angiofibroma. Changes in staging and treatment. Arch Otolaryngol Head Neck Surg 122: 122-129.

2112. Rady PL, Schnadig VJ, Weiss RL, Hughes TK, Tyring SK (1998). Malignant transformation of recurrent respiratory papillomatosis associated with integrated human papillomavirus type 11 DNA and mutation of p53. Laryngoscope 108: 735-740.

2113. Rafferty MA, Fenton JE, Jones AS (2001). The history, aetiology and epidemiology of laryngeal carcinoma. Clin Otolaryngol 26: 442-446.

2114. Ragbeer MS, Stone J (1990). Vascular leiomyoma of the nasal cavity: report of a case and review of literature. J Oral Maxillofac Surg 48: 1113-1117.

2115. Rajendran R (1994). Oral submucous fibrosis: etiology, pathogenesis, and future research. Bull World Health Organ 72: 985-996.

2116. Rajentheran R, McLean NR, Kelly CG, Reed MF, Nolan A (1999). Malignant transformation of oral lichen planus. Eur J Surg Oncol 25: 520-523.

2117. Raji A, Essaadi M, Mahtar M, Roubal M, Chekkoury IA, Benchakroun Y (2002). [Cervicofacial lymphangioma in adults (10 case reports)]. Rev Laryngol Otol Rhinol (Bord) 123: 27-32.

2118. Ram B, Saleh HA, Baird AR, Mountain RE (1998). Verrucous carcinoma of the maxillary antrum. J Laryngol Otol 112: 399-402.

2119. Ramanathan RC, Thomas JM (1999). Malignant peripheral nerve sheath tumours associated with von Recklinghausen's neurofibromatosis. Eur J Surg Oncol 25: 190-193.

2120. Ramirez-Amador V, Esquivel-Pedraza L, Sierra-Madero J, Anaya-Saavedra G, Gonzalez-Ramirez I, Ponce-de-Leon S (2003). The Changing Clinical Spectrum of Human Immunodeficiency Virus (HIV)-Related Oral Lesions in 1,000 Consecutive Patients: A 12-Year Study in a Referral Center in Mexico. Medicine (Baltimore) 82: 39-50.

2121. Ramirez-Camacho R, Vincente J, Berrocal JRG, Ramon y Cajal S (1999). Fibro-osseous lesions of the external auditory canal. Laryngoscope 109: 488-491.

2122. Raney RB, Asmar L, Newton WAJr, Bagwell C, Breneman JC, Crist W, Gehan EA, Webber B, Wharam M, Wiener ES, Anderson JR, Maurer HM (1997). Ewing's sarcoma of soft tissues in childhood: a report from the Intergroup Rhabdomyosarcoma Study, 1972 to 1991. J Clin Oncol 15: 574-582.

2123. Raney RB, Asmar L, Vassilopoulou-Sellin R, Klein MJ, Donaldson SS, Green J, Heyn R, Wharam M, Glicksman AS, Gehan EA, Anderson J, Maurer HM (1999). Late complications of therapy in 213 children with localized, nonorbital soft-tissue sarcoma of the head and neck: A descriptive report from the Intergroup Rhabdomyosarcoma Studies (IRS)-II and -III. IRS Group of the Children's Cancer Group and the Pediatric Oncology Group. Med Pediatr Oncol 33: 362-371.

2124. Rao AB, Koeller KK, Adair CF (1999). From the archives of the AFIP. Paragangliomas of the head and neck: radiologic-pathologic correlation. Armed Forces Institute of Pathology. Radiographics 19: 1605-1632.

2125. Rao PH, Murty VV, Louie DC, Chaganti RS (1998). Nonsyntenic amplification of MYC with CDK4 and MDM2 in a malignant mixed tumor of salivary gland. Cancer Genet Cytogenet 105: 160-163.

2126. Rao VK, Weiss SW (1992). Angiomatosis of soft tissue. An analysis of the histologic features and clinical outcome in 51 cases. Am J Surg Pathol 16: 764-771.

2127. Rapini RP, Golitz LE, Greer ROJr, Krekorian EA, Poulson T (1985). Primary malignant melanoma of the oral cavity. A review of 177 cases. Cancer 55: 1543-1551.

2128. Raslan WF, Barnes L, Krause JR, Contis L, Killeen R, Kapadia SB (1994). Basaloid squamous cell carcinoma of the head and neck: a clinicopathologic and flow cytometric study of 10 new cases with review of the English literature. Am J Otolaryngol 15: 204-211.

2129. Rasmussen P, Lindholm J (1979). Ectopic pituitary adenomas. Clin Endocrinol (Oxf) 11: 69-74.

2130. Rassekh CH, Nuss DW, Kapadia SB, Curtin HD, Weissman JL, Janecka IP (1996). Chondrosarcoma of the nasal septum: skull base imaging and clinicopathologic correlation. Otolaryngol Head Neck

Surg 115: 29-37.

2131. Raut A, Huryn J, Pollack A, Zlotolow I (2000). Unusual gingival presentation of post-transplantation lymphoproliferative disorder: a case report and review of the literature. Oral Surg Oral Med Oral Pathol Oral Radiol Endod 90: 436-441.

2132. Ravasz LA, Hordijk GJ, Slootweg PJ, Smit F, Van der Tweel I (1993). Uni- and multivariate analysis of eight indications for post-operative radiotherapy and their significance for local-regional cure in advanced head and neck cancer. J Laryngol Otol 107: 437-440.

2133. Rawson AJ, Howard.J.M., Royster HP, Horn RCJr (1950). Tumors of the salivary glands: a clinicopathologic study of 160 cases. Cancer 3: 445-458.

2134. Raychowdhuri RN (1965). Oat-cell carcinoma and paranasal sinuses. J Laryngol Otol 79: 253-255.

2135. Raymond MR, Yoo JH, Heathcote JG, McLachlin CM, Lampe HB (2002). Accuracy of fine-needle aspiration biopsy for Warthin's tumours. J Otolaryngol 31: 263-270.

2136. Reddy SP, Raslan WF, Gooneratne S, Kathuria S, Marks JE (1995). Prognostic significance of keratinization in nasopharyngeal carcinoma. Am J Otolaryngol 16: 103-108.

2137. Redman RS, Keegan BP, Spector CJ, Patterson RH (1994). Peripheral ameloblastoma with unusual mitotic activity and conflicting evidence regarding histogenesis. J Oral Maxillofac Surg 52: 192-197.

2138. Ree HJ, Kikuchi M, Lee SS, Ohshima K, Yang WI, Ko YH, Cho EY, Rhee JC (2002). Focal follicular features in tonsillar diffuse large B-cell lymphomas: follicular lymphoma with diffuse areas or follicular colonization. Hum Pathol 33: 732-740.

2139. Ree HJ, Rege VB, Knisley RE, Thayer WR, D'Amico RP, Song JY, Crowley JP (1980). Malignant lymphoma of Waldeyer's ring following gastrointestinal lymphoma. Cancer 46: 1528-1535.

2140. Regezi JA, Kerr DA, Courtney RM (1978). Odontogenic tumors: analysis of 706 cases. J Oral Surg 36: 771-778.

2141. Regezi JA, McMillan A, Dekker N, Daniels TE, Silverman SJr, Schoelch M, Ziober BL (1998). Apoptosis-associated proteins in oral lymphomas from HIV-positive patients. Oral Surg Oral Med Oral Pathol Oral Radiol Endod 86: 196-202.

2142. Regezi JA, Zarbo RJ, Stewart JC (1991). Extranodal oral lymphomas: histologic subtypes and immunophenotypes (in routinely processed tissue). Oral Surg Oral Med Oral Pathol 72: 702-708.

2143. Regnard JF, Fourquier P, Levasseur P (1996). Results and prognostic factors in resections of primary tracheal tumors: a multicenter retrospective study. The French Society of Cardiovascular Surgery. J Thorac Cardiovasc Surg 111: 808-813.

2144. Rehberg E, Kleinsasser O (1999). Malignant transformation in non-irradiated juvenile laryngeal papillomatosis. Eur Arch Otorhinolaryngol 256: 450-454.

2145. Reibel J (2003). Prognosis of oral pre-malignant lesions: significance of clinical, histopathological, and molecular biological characteristics. Crit Rev Oral Biol Med 14: 47-62.

2146. Reibel JF, McLean WC, Cantrell RW (1981). Laryngeal acinic cell carcinoma following thyroid irradiation. Otolaryngol Head Neck Surg 89: 398-401.

2147. Reich DS, Palmer CA, Peters GE

(1995). Ethmoid sinus leiomyosarcoma after cyclophosphamide treatment. Otolaryngol Head Neck Surg 113: 495-498.
2148. Reichart PA, Philipsen HP (2004). Odontogenic Tumours and Allied Lesions. Quintessence Publishing: London.
2149. Reichart PA, Philipsen HP, Sonner S (1995). Ameloblastoma: biological profile of 3677 cases. Eur J Cancer B Oral Oncol 31B: 86-99.
2150. Reichart PA, Schmidt-Westhausen A, Samaranayake LP, Philipsen HP (1994). Candida-associated palatal papillary hyperplasia in HIV infection. J Oral Pathol Med 23: 403-405.
2151. Reid BC, Winn DM, Morse DE, Pendrys DG (2000). Head and neck in situ carcinoma: incidence, trends, and survival. Oral Oncol 36: 414-420.
2152. Reinshagen K, Wessel LM, Roth H, Waag KL (2002). Congenital epulis: a rare diagnosis in paediatric surgery. Eur J Pediatr Surg 12: 124-126.
2153. Rejowski JE, Campanella RS, Block LJ (1982). Small cell carcinoma of the nose and paranasal sinuses. Otolaryngol Head Neck Surg 90: 516-517.
2154. Remagen W, Lohr J, von Westernhagen B (1983). [Osteosarcoma of the larynx]. HNO 31: 366-368.
2155. Remine WH, Weiland LH, Remine SG (1978). Carotid body tumors. Curr Prob Cancer 11: 3-27.
2156. Renan MJ (1993). How many mutations are required for tumorigenesis? Implications from human cancer data. Mol Carcinog 7: 139-146.
2157. Renehan A, Gleave EN, Hancock BD, Smith P, McGurk M (1996). Long-term follow-up of over 1000 patients with salivary gland tumours treated in a single centre. Br J Surg 83: 1750-1754.
2158. Requena L, Sangueza OP (1997). Cutaneous vascular proliferation. Part II. Hyperplasias and benign neoplasms. J Am Acad Dermatol 37: 887-919.
2159. Reuter VE, Woodruff JM (1986). Melanoma of the larynx. Laryngoscope 96: 389-393.
2160. Revel MP, Vanel D, Sigal R, Luboinski B, Michel G, Legrand I, Masselot J (1992). Aneurysmal bone cysts of the jaws: CT and MR findings. J Comput Assist Tomogr 16: 84-86.
2161. Rhea JT, Weber AL (1983). Giant-cell granuloma of the sinuses. Radiology 147: 135-137.
2162. Riazimand SH, Brieger J, Jacob R, Welkoborsky HJ, Mann WJ (2002). Analysis of cytogenetic aberrations in esthesioneuroblastomas by comparative genomic hybridization. Cancer Genet Cytogenet 136: 53-57.
2163. Ribari O, Elemr G, Balint A (1975). Laryngeal giant cell tumour. J Laryngol Otol 89: 857-861.
2164. Ribe A, Fernandez PL, Ostertarg H, Claros P, Bombi JA, Palacin A, Cardesa A (1997). Middle-ear adenoma (MEA): a report of two cases, one with predominant "plasmacytoid' features. Histopathology 30: 359-364.
2165. Ribeiro AC, Joshi VM, Funkhouser WK, Mukherji SK (2001). Inflammatory myofibroblastic tumor involving the pterygopalatine fossa. AJNR Am J Neuroradiol 22: 518-520.
2166. Richkind KE, Mortimer E, Mowery-Rushton P, Fraire A (2002). Translocation (16;20)(p11.2;q13). sole cytogenetic abnormality in a unicameral bone cyst. Cancer Genet Cytogenet 137: 153-155.
2167. Ries LAG, Hankey BF, Miller BA, Hartman AM, Edwards BK (1991). Cancer Statistics Review, 1973- 88. National Cancer Institute: Bethesda.
2167A. Riddett SA (2004) A composite odontoma at a very early age. Br Dent J 77: 129-131
2168. Riese U, Dahse R, Fiedler W, Theuer C, Koscielny S, Ernst G, Beleites E, Claussen U, von Eggeling F (1999). Tumor suppressor gene p16 (CDKN2A) mutation status and promoter inactivation in head and neck cancer. Int J Mol Med 4: 61-65.
2169. Righi PD, Li YQ, Deutsch M, McDonald JS, Wilson KM, Bejarano P, Stambrook PJ, Osterhage D, Nguyen C, Gluckman JL, Pavelic ZP (1994). The role of the p53 gene in the malignant transformation of pleomorphic adenomas of the parotid gland. Anticancer Res 14: 2253-2257.
2170. Rigual NR, Milley P, Lore JMJr, Kaufman S (1986). Accuracy of frozen-section diagnosis in salivary gland neoplasms. Head Neck Surg 8: 442-446.
2171. Rihkanen H, Aaltonen LM, Syrjanen SM (1993). Human papillomavirus in laryngeal papillomas and in adjacent normal epithelium. Clin Otolaryngol 18: 470-474.
2172. Rihkanen H, Peltomaa J, Syrjanen S (1994). Prevalence of human papillomavirus (HPV) DNA in vocal cords without laryngeal papillomas. Acta Otolaryngol 114: 348-351.
2173. Rimell F, Maisel R, Dayton V (1992). In situ hybridization and laryngeal papillomas. Ann Otol Rhinol Laryngol 101: 119-126.
2174. Rimell FL, Shoemaker DL, Pou AM, Jordan JA, Post JC, Ehrlich GD (1997). Pediatric respiratory papillomatosis: prognostic role of viral typing and cofactors. Laryngoscope 107: 915-918.
2175. Riminucci M, Fisher LW, Shenker A, Spiegel AM, Bianco P, Gehron Robey P (1997). Fibrous dysplasia of bone in the McCune-Albright syndrome: abnormalities in bone formation. Am J Pathol 151: 1587-1600.
2176. Riminucci M, Liu B, Corsi A, Shenker A, Spiegel AM, Robey PG, Bianco P (1999). The histopathology of fibrous dysplasia of bone in patients with activating mutations of the Gs alpha gene: site-specific patterns and recurrent histological hallmarks. J Pathol 187: 249-258.
2177. Rimmelin A, Roth T, George B, Dias P, Clouet PL, Dietemann JL (1996). Giant-cell tumour of the sphenoid bone: case report. Neuroradiology 38: 650-653.
2178. Rinaldo A, Howard DJ, Ferlito A (2000). Laryngeal chondrosarcoma: a 24-year experience at the Royal National Throat, Nose and Ear Hospital. Acta Otolaryngol 120: 680-688.
2179. Rinaldo A, McLaren KM, Boccato P, Maran AG (1999). Hyalinizing clear cell carcinoma of the oral cavity and of the parotid gland. ORL J Otorhinolaryngol Relat Spec 61: 48-51.
2180. Rischin D, Corry J, Smith J, Stewart J, Hughes P, Peters L (2002). Excellent disease control and survival in patients with advanced nasopharyngeal cancer treated with chemoradiation. J Clin Oncol 20: 1845-1852.
2181. Risdall RJ, Dehner LP, Duray P, Kobrinsky N, Robison L, Nesbit MEJr (1983). Histiocytosis X (Langerhans' cell histiocytosis). Prognostic role of histopathology. Arch Pathol Lab Med 107: 59-63.
2182. Roa RA, Atkins JPJr, Cunnane MF, Keane WM (1988). Papillary adenocarcinoma of the larynx: a case report. Otolaryngol Head Neck Surg 99: 601-603.
2183. Robbins KT, Clayman G, Levine PA, Medina J, Sessions R, Shaha A, Som P, Wolf GT (2002). Neck dissection classification update: revisions proposed by the American Head and Neck Society and the American Academy of Otolaryngology-Head and Neck Surgery. Arch Otolaryngol Head Neck Surg 128: 751-758.
2184. Roberts WH, Dinges DL, Hanly MG (1993). Inverted papilloma of the middle ear. Ann Otol Rhinol Laryngol 102: 890-892.
2185. Robertson JS, Wiegand DA, Schaitkin BM (1991). Life-threatening hemangioma arising from the parotid gland. Otolaryngol Head Neck Surg 104: 858-862.
2186. Robin PE, Powell DJ, Stansbie JM (1979). Carcinoma of the nasal cavity and paranasal sinuses: incidence and presentation of different histological types. Clin Otolaryngol 4: 431-456.
2187. Rodrigo JP, Fernandez JA, Suarez C, Gomez J, Llorente JL, Herrero A (2000). Malignant fibrous histiocytoma of the nasal cavity and paranasal sinuses. Am J Rhinol 14: 427-431.
2188. Rodriguez-Cuevas S, Lopez-Garza J, Labastida-Almendaro S (1998). Carotid body tumors in inhabitants of altitudes higher than 2000 meters above sea level. Head Neck 20: 374-378.
2189. Rodriguez JC, Arranz JS, Forcelledo MF (1990). Isolated granulocytic sarcoma: report of a case in the oral cavity. J Oral Maxillofac Surg 48: 748-752.
2190. Roessner A, von Bassewitz DB, Schlake W, Thorwesten G, Grundmann E (1984). Biologic characterization of human bone tumors. III. Giant cell tumor of bone. A combined electron microscopical, histochemical, and autoradiographical study. Pathol Res Pract 178: 431-440.
2191. Rohn GN, Close LG, Vuitch F, Merkel MA (1994). Fibrous neoplasms of the adult larynx. Head Neck 16: 227-231.
2192. Rohrmus B, Thoma-Greber EM, Bogner JR, Rocken M (2000). Outlook in oral and cutaneous Kaposi's sarcoma. Lancet 356: 2160.
2193. Roijer E, Kas K, Behrendt M, Van de Ven W, Stenman G (1999). Fluorescence in situ hybridization mapping of breakpoints in pleomorphic adenomas with 8q12-13 abnormalities identifies a subgroup of tumors without PLAG1 involvement. Genes Chromosomes Cancer 24: 78-82.
2194. Roijer E, Nordkvist A, Strom AK, Ryd W, Behrendt M, Bullerdiek J, Mark J, Stenman G (2002). Translocation, deletion/amplification, and expression of HMGIC and MDM2 in a carcinoma ex pleomorphic adenoma. Am J Pathol 160: 433-440.
2195. Roland NJ, Caslin AW, Nash J, Stell PM (1992). Value of grading squamous cell carcinoma of the head and neck. Head Neck 14: 224-229.
2196. Rollins CE, Yost BA, Costa MJ, Vogt PJ (1995). Squamous differentiation in small-cell carcinoma of the parotid gland. Arch Pathol Lab Med 119: 183-185.
2197. Ron E, Saftlas AF (1996). Head and neck radiation carcinogenesis: epidemiologic evidence. Otolaryngol Head Neck Surg 115: 403-408.
2198. Rosa JC, Felix A, Fonseca I, Soares J (1997). Immunoexpression of c-erbB-2 and p53 in benign and malignant salivary neoplasms with myoepithelial differentiation. J Clin Pathol 50: 661-663.
2199. Rosai J, Suster S (2001). Warthin's tumors. Hum Pathol 32: 352.
2200. Rosenberg A, Biesma DH, Sie-Go DM, Slootweg PJ (1996). Primary extranodal CD30-positive T-cell non-Hodgkins lymphoma of the oral mucosa. Report of two cases. Int J Oral Maxillofac Surg 25: 57-59.
2201. Rosin MP, Cheng X, Poh C, Lam WL, Huang Y, Lovas J, Berean K, Epstein JB, Priddy R, Le ND, Zhang L (2000). Use of allelic loss to predict malignant risk for low-grade oral epithelial dysplasia. Clin Cancer Res 6: 357-362.
2202. Ross G, Shoaib T, Soutar DS, Camilleri IG, Gray HW, Bessent RG, Robertson AG, MacDonald DG (2002). The use of sentinel node biopsy to upstage the clinically N0 neck in head and neck cancer. Arch Otolaryngol Head Neck Surg 128: 1287-1291.
2203. Rossi RM, Landas SK, Kelly DR, Marsh WL (1998). Osteosarcoma of the larynx. Otolaryngol Head Neck Surg 118: 385-388.
2204. Roth MJ, Medeiros LJ, Elenitoba-Johnson K, Kuchnio M, Jaffe ES, Stetler-Stevenson M (1995). Extramedullary myeloid cell tumors. An immunohistochemical study of 29 cases using routinely fixed and processed paraffin-embedded tissue sections. Arch Pathol Lab Med 119: 790-798.
2205. Roush GC (1979). Epidemiology of cancer of the nose and paranasal sinuses: current concepts. Head Neck Surg 2: 3-11.
2206. Rousseau A, Mock D, Dover DG, Jordan RC (1999). Multiple canalicular adenomas: a case report and review of the literature. Oral Surg Oral Med Oral Pathol Oral Radiol Endod 87: 346-350.
2207. Roux S, Amazit L, Meduri G, Guiochon-Mantel A, Milgrom E, Mariette X (2002). RANK (receptor activator of nuclear factor kappa B) and RANK ligand are expressed in giant cell tumors of bone. Am J Clin Pathol 117: 210-216.
2208. Rowe-Jones JM, Solomons NB, Ratcliffe NA (1994). Leiomyosarcoma of the larynx. J Laryngol Otol 108: 359-362.
2209. Roychowdhury DF, Tseng AJr, Fu KK, Weinburg V, Weidner N (1996). New prognostic factors in nasopharyngeal carcinoma. Tumor angiogenesis and C-erbB2 expression. Cancer 77: 1419-1426.
2210. Royer B, Cazals-Hatem D, Sibilia J, Agbalika F, Cayuela JM, Soussi T, Maloisel F, Clauvel JP, Brouet JC, Mariette X (1997). Lymphomas in patients with Sjogren's syndrome are marginal zone B-cell neoplasms, arise in diverse extranodal and nodal sites, and are not associated with viruses. Blood 90: 766-775.
2211. Rud NP, Reiman HM, Pritchard DJ, Frassica FJ, Smithson WA (1989). Extraosseous Ewing's sarcoma. A study of 42 cases. Cancer 64: 1548-1553.
2212. Rufenacht H, Mihatsch MJ, Jundt K, Gachter A, Tanner K, Heitz PU (1985). Gastric epitheloid leiomyomas, pulmonary chondroma, non-functioning metastasizing extra-adrenal paraganglioma and myxoma: a variant of Carney's triad. Report of a patient. Klin Wochenschr 63: 282-284.
2213. Ruggieri P, Sim FH, Bond JR, Unni KK (1994). Malignancies in fibrous dysplasia. Cancer 73: 1411-1424.
2214. Rulon DB, Helwig EB (1973). Multiple sebaceous neoplasms of the skin: an association with multiple visceral carcinomas, especially of the colon. Am J Clin

Pathol 60: 745-752.
2215. Ruske DR, Glassford N, Costello S, Stewart IA (1998). Laryngeal rhabdomyosarcoma in adults. J Laryngol Otol 112: 670-672.
2216. Ruszczak Z, Mayer da Silva A, Orfanos CE (1987). Angioproliferative changes in clinically noninvolved, perilesional skin in AIDS-associated Kaposi's sarcoma. Dermatologica 175: 270-279.
2217. Ryan SJ, Font RL (1973). Primary epithelial neoplasms of the lacrimal sac. Am J Ophthalmol 76: 73-88.
2218. Saber AT, Nielsen LR, Dictor M, Hagmar L, Mikoczy Z, Wallin H (1998). K-ras mutations in sinonasal adenocarcinomas in patients occupationally exposed to wood or leather dust. Cancer Lett 126: 59-65.
2219. Sabo R, Sela M, Sabo G, Herskovitz P, Feinmesser R (2001). Metastatic hypernephroma to the head and neck: unusual case reports and review of the literature. J Otolaryngol 30: 140-144.
2220. Sabri JA, Hajjar MA (1967). Malignant mixed tumor of the vocal cord. Report of a case. Arch Otolaryngol 85: 332-334.
2221. Sadar ES, Conomy JP, Benjamin SP, Levine HL (1979). Meningiomas of the paranasal sinuses, benign and malignant. Neurosurgery 4: 227-232.
2222. Said-Al-Naief N, Ivanov K, Jones M, Som P, Urken M, Brandwein M (1999). Granular cell tumor of the parotid. Ann Diagn Pathol 3: 35-38.
2223. Saito K, Unni KK, Wollan PC, Lund BA (1995). Chondrosarcoma of the jaw and facial bones. Cancer 76: 1550-1558.
2224. Saito Y, Hoshina Y, Nagamine T, Nakajima T, Suzuki M, Hayashi T (1992). Simple bone cyst. A clinical and histopathologic study of fifteen cases. Oral Surg Oral Med Oral Pathol 74: 487-491.
2225. Sakabe H, Bamba M, Nomura K, Kitamura S, Segawa H, Yasui H, Inoue T, Taniwaki M, Fujiyama Y, Bamba T (2003). MALT lymphoma at the base of the tongue developing without any background of immunodeficiency or autoimmune disease. Leuk Lymphoma 44: 875-878.
2226. Sakakura A, Yamamoto Y, Takasaki T, Makimoto K, Nakamura M, Takahashi H (1996). Recurrent laryngeal papillomatosis developing into laryngeal carcinoma with human papilloma virus (HPV) type 18: a case report. J Laryngol Otol 110: 75-77.
2227. Sakakura Y, Ohi M, Yamada S, Miyoshi Y (1980). A case of subglottic hemangioma: a new technique of surgical removal. Auris Nasus Larynx 7: 81-88.
2228. Saksela E, Tarkkanen J, Wartiovaara J (1972). Parotid clear-cell adenoma of possible myoepithelial origin. Cancer 30: 742-748.
2229. Saku T, Hayashi Y, Takahara O, Matsuura H, Tokunaga M, Tokunaga M, Tokuoka S, Soda M, Mabuchi K, Land CE (1997). Salivary gland tumors among atomic bomb survivors, 1950-1987. Cancer 79: 1465-1475.
2230. Sakurai K, Urade M, Noguchi K, Kishimoto H, Ishibashi M, Yasoshima H, Yamamoto T, Kubota A (2001). Increased expression of cyclooxygenase-2 in human salivary gland tumors. Pathol Int 51: 762-769.
2231. Saldana MJ, Salem LE, Travezan R (1973). High altitude hypoxia and chemodectomas. Hum Pathol 4: 251-263.
2232. Saltarelli MG, Fleming MV, Wenig BM, Gal AA, Mansour KA, Travis WD (1995). Primary basaloid squamous cell carcinoma of the trachea. Am J Clin Pathol 104: 594-598.
2233. Sam CK, Brooks LA, Niedobitek G, Young LS, Prasad U, Rickinson AB (1993). Analysis of Epstein-Barr virus infection in nasopharyngeal biopsies from a group at high risk of nasopharyngeal carcinoma. Int J Cancer 53: 957-962.
2234. Sanchez-Casis G, Devine KD, Weiland LH (1971). Nasal adenocarcinomas that closely simulate colonic carcinomas. Cancer 28: 714-720.
2235. Sancho-Garnier H, Theobald S (1993). Black (air-cured) and blond (flue-cured) tobacco and cancer risk II: Pharynx and larynx cancer. Eur J Cancer 29A: 273-276.
2236. Sanders KW, Abreo F, Rivera E, Stucker FJ, Nathan CA (2001). A diagnostic and therapeutic approach to paragangliomas of the larynx. Arch Otolaryngol Head Neck Surg 127: 565-569.
2237. Sanderson RJ, Rivron RP, Wallace WA (1991). Adenosquamous carcinoma of the hypopharynx. J Laryngol Otol 105: 678-680.
2238. Sandros J, Mark J, Happonen RP, Stenman G (1988). Specificity of 6q- markers and other recurrent deviations in human malignant salivary gland tumors. Anticancer Res 8: 637-643.
2239. Sandros J, Stenman G, Mark J (1990). Cytogenetic and molecular observations in human and experimental salivary gland tumors. Cancer Genet Cytogenet 44: 153-167.
2240. Sankary S, Sherwin RN, Malone PS, Janecka I, Barnes L, Storto PD, Gollin SM (1993). Clonal chromosomal aberrations in a leiomyosarcoma of the sinonasal tract. Cancer Genet Cytogenet 65: 21-26.
2241. Sans A, Bartolami S, Fraysse B (1996). Histopathology of the peripheral vestibular system in small vestibular schwannomas. Am J Otol 17: 326-24.
2242. Santon Roldan A, De San Jose S, Gomez Sanz E, Fernandez Munoz R, Herrera P, Bellas Menendez C (2002). [Human herpesvirus-8 detection in Kaposi's sarcoma, multiple myeloma, and lymphoproliferative syndromes occurring in immunocompetent and immunocompromised patients]. Med Clin (Barc) 119: 241-244.
2243. Santos-Briz A, Lobato RD, Ramos A, Millan JM, Ricoy JR, Martinez-Tello FJ (2003). Giant cell reparative granuloma of the occipital bone. Skeletal Radiol 32: 151-155.
2244. Sapci T, Yildirim G, Peker K, Karavus A, Akbulut UG (2000). Acinic cell carcinoma originating in the nasal septum. Rhinology 38: 140-143.
2245. Saravanappa N, Rashid AM, Thebe PR, Davis JP (2000). Juvenile xanthogranuloma of the nasal cavity. J Laryngol Otol 114: 460-461.
2246. Sarkar FH, Visscher DW, Kintanar EB, Zarbo RJ, Crissman JD (1992). Sinonasal Schneiderian papillomas: human papillomavirus typing by polymerase chain reaction. Mod Pathol 5: 329-332.
2247. Sataloff RT, Ressue JC, Portell M, Harris RM, Ossoff R, Merati AL, Zeitels S (2000). Granular cell tumors of the larynx. J Voice 14: 119-134.
2248. Sato J, Asakura K, Yokoyama Y, Satoh M (1998). Solitary fibrous tumor of the parotid gland extending to the parapharyngeal space. Eur Arch Otorhinolaryngol 255: 18-21.
2249. Satoh K, Hibi G, Yamamoto Y, Urano M, Kuroda M, Nakamura S (2003). Follicular dendritic cell tumor in the oro-pharyngeal region: report of a case and a review of the literature. Oral Oncol 39: 415-419.
2250. Saul SH, Kapadia SB (1985). Primary lymphoma of Waldeyer's ring. Clinicopathologic study of 68 cases. Cancer 56: 157-166.
2251. Savera AT, Sloman A, Huvos AG, Klimstra DS (2000). Myoepithelial carcinoma of the salivary glands: a clinicopathologic study of 25 patients. Am J Surg Pathol 24: 761-774.
2252. Saw D, Ho JH, Lau WH, Chan J (1986). Parotid swelling as the first manifestation of nasopharyngeal carcinoma: a report of two cases. Eur J Surg Oncol 12: 71-75.
2253. Saw D, Lau WH, Ho JH, Chan JK, Ng CS (1986). Malignant lymphoepithelial lesion of the salivary gland. Hum Pathol 17: 914-923.
2254. Sawyer JR, Tryka AF, Bell JM, Boop FA (1995). Nonrandom chromosome breakpoints at Xq26 and 2q33 characterize cemento-ossifying fibromas of the orbit. Cancer 76: 1853-1859.
2255. Schaefer O, Hildes JA, Medd LM, Cameron DG (1975). The changing pattern of neoplastic disease in Canadian Eskimos. Can Med Assoc J 112: 1399-1404.
2256. Schaefer SD, Denton RA, Blend BL, Carder HM (1980). Malignant fibrous histiocytoma of the frontal sinus. Laryngoscope 90: 2021-2026.
2257. Schafer DR, Thompson LD, Smith BC, Wenig BM (1998). Primary ameloblastoma of the sinonasal tract: a clinicopathologic study of 24 cases. Cancer 82: 667-674.
2258. Schantz SP, Byers RM, Goepfert H, Shallenberger RC, Beddingfield N (1988). The implication of tobacco use in the young adult with head and neck cancer. Cancer 62: 1374-1380.
2259. Schantz SP, Yu GP (2002). Head and neck cancer incidence trends in young Americans, 1973-1997, with a special analysis for tongue cancer. Arch Otolaryngol Head Neck Surg 128: 268-274.
2260. Schenk P, Handisurya A, Steurer M (2002). Ultrastructural morphology of a middle ear ceruminoma. ORL J Otorhinolaryngol Relat Spec 64: 358-363.
2261. Schepman KP, van der Meij EH, Smeele LE, van der Waal I (1998). Malignant transformation of oral leukoplakia: a follow-up study of a hospital-based population of 166 patients with oral leukoplakia from The Netherlands. Oral Oncol 34: 270-275.
2262. Schiff NF, Annino DJ, Woo P, Shapshay SM (1997). Kaposi's sarcoma of the larynx. Ann Otol Rhinol Laryngol 106: 563-567.
2263. Schimpf A, Musebeck K, Mootz W (1969). [Histologic report No 222. Nevus cell nevus (compound nevus) in the larynx region (Plica ventricularis)]. Z Haut Geschlechtskr 44: 137-144.
2264. Schiodt M (1984). Oral manifestations of lupus erythematosus. Int J Oral Surg 13: 101-147.
2265. Schmid-Wendtner MH, Sander C, Volkenandt M, Wendtner CM (1999). Unusual manifestations of B-cell disorders. Case 2: chronic lymphocytic leukemia presenting with cutaneous lesions. J Clin Oncol 17: 1084-1085.
2266. Schmid U, Helbron D, Lennert K (1982). Development of malignant lymphoma in myoepithelial sialadenitis (Sjogren's syndrome). Virchows Arch A Pathol Anat Histol 395: 11-43.
2267. Schmid U, Helbron D, Lennert K (1982). Primary malignant lymphomas localized in salivary glands. Histopathology 6: 673-687.
2267A. Schmidseder R, HausamenJE (1975). Multiple odontogenic tumors and other anomalies. An autosomal dominantly inherited syndrome. Oral Surg Oral Med Oral Pathol 39: 249-258.
2268. Schneider AB, Favus MJ, Stachura ME, Arnold MJ, Frohman LA (1977). Salivary gland neoplasms as a late consequence of head and neck irradiation. Ann Intern Med 87: 160-164.
2269. Schoenmakers EF, Wanschura S, Mols R, Bullerdiek J, Van den Berghe H, Van de Ven WJ (1995). Recurrent rearrangements in the high mobility group protein gene, HMGI-C, in benign mesenchymal tumours. Nat Genet 10: 436-444.
2270. Schofield ID (1981). Central odontogenic fibroma: report of case. J Oral Surg 39: 218-220.
2271. Scholes AG, Woolgar JA, Boyle MA, Brown JS, Vaughan ED, Hart CA, Jones AS, Field JK (1998). Synchronous oral carcinomas: independent or common clonal origin? Cancer Res 58: 2003-2006.
2272. Scholl RJ, Kellett HM, Neumann DP, Lurie AG (1999). Cysts and cystic lesions of the mandible: clinical and radiologic-histopathologic review. Radiographics 19: 1107-1124.
2273. Schramm VLJr, Imola MJ (2001). Management of nasopharyngeal salivary gland malignancy. Laryngoscope 111: 1533-1544.
2274. Schteingart DE, Chandler WF, Lloyd RV, Ibarra-Perez G (1987). Cushing's syndrome caused by an ectopic pituitary adenoma. Neurosurgery 21: 223-227.
2275. Schuknecht HF (1993). Pathology of the Ear. 2nd ed. Lea & Febiger: Philadelphia.
2276. Schurch W, Skalli O, Lagace R, Seemayer TA, Gabbiani G (1990). Intermediate filament proteins and actin isoforms as markers for soft-tissue tumor differentiation and origin. III. Hemangiopericytomas and glomus tumors. Am J Pathol 136: 771-786.
2277. Schwaber MK, Glasscock ME, Nissen AJ, Jackson CG, Smith PG (1984). Diagnosis and management of catecholamine secreting glomus tumors. Laryngoscope 94: 1008-1015.
2278. Schwartz RA (1995). Verrucous carcinoma of the skin and mucosa. J Am Acad Dermatol 32: 1-21.
2279. Schwerer MJ, Kraft K, Baczako K, Maier H (2001). Cytokeratin expression and epithelial differentiation in Warthin's tumour and its metaplastic (infarcted) variant. Histopathology 39: 347-352.
2280. Sciot R, Delaere P, Van Damme B, Desmet V (1995). Angiosarcoma of the larynx. Histopathology 26: 177-180.
2281. Sciot R, Dorfman H, Brys P, Dal Cin P, De Wever I, Fletcher CD, Jonson K, Mandahl N, Mertens F, Mitelman F, Rosai J, Rydholm A, Samson I, Tallini G, Van den Berghe H, Vanni R, Willen H (2000). Cytogenetic-morphologic correlations in aneurysmal bone cyst, giant cell tumor of bone and combined lesions. A report from the CHAMP study group. Mod Pathol 13: 1206-1210.
2282. Sciubba JJ, Brannon RB (1982). Myoepithelioma of salivary glands: report of 23 cases. Cancer 49: 562-572.

2283. Scott KM, Carter CS (1995). Malignant fibrous histiocytoma of the larynx: case report and literature review. J Otolaryngol 24: 198-200.
2284. Scully C (2002). Oral squamous cell carcinoma; from an hypothesis about a virus, to concern about possible sexual transmission. Oral Oncol 38: 227-234.
2285. Scully C, Porter SR, Speight PM, Eveson JW, Gale D (1999). Adenosquamous carcinoma of the mouth: a rare variant of squamous cell carcinoma. Int J Oral Maxillofac Surg 28: 125-128.
2286. Scully C, Sudbo J, Speight PM (2003). Progress in determining the malignant potential of oral lesions. J Oral Pathol Med 32: 251-256.
2287. Seals JL, Shenefelt RE, Babin RW (1986). Intralaryngeal nevus in a child. A case report. Int J Pediatr Otorhinolaryngol 12: 55-58.
2288. Sedano HO, Gorlin RJ (1989). Epidermolysis bullosa. Oral Surg Oral Med Oral Pathol 67: 555-563.
2288A. Sedano HO, Pindborg JJ (2003) Ghost cell eepithelium in odontomas. J Oral Pathol 4: 27-30
2289. Seibert RW, Seibert JJ, Jimenez JF, Angtuaco EJ (1984). Nasopharyngeal brain heterotopia—a cause of upper airway obstruction in infancy. Laryngoscope 94: 818-819.
2290. Seifert G (1992). Histopathology of malignant salivary gland tumours. Eur J Cancer B Oral Oncol 28B: 49-56.
2291. Seifert G (1996). Classification and differential diagnosis of clear and basal cell tumors of the salivary glands. Semin Diagn Pathol 13: 95-103.
2292. Seifert G (1996). Mucoepidermoid carcinoma in a salivary duct cyst of the parotid gland. Contribution to the development of tumours in salivary gland cysts. Pathol Res Pract 192: 1211-1217.
2293. Seifert G (1996). Oralpathologie I. Pathologie der Speicheldrusen. Springer Verlag: Berlin.
2294. Seifert G (1997). Bilateral mucoepidermoid carcinomas arising in bilateral pre-existing Warthin's tumours of the parotid gland. Oral Oncol 33: 284-287.
2295. Seifert G, Bull HG, Donath K (1980). Histologic subclassification of the cystadenolymphoma of the parotid gland. Analysis of 275 cases. Virchows Arch A Pathol Anat Histol 388: 13-38.
2296. Seifert G, Caselitz J (1983). Tumor markers in parotid gland carcinomas: immunohistochemical investigations. Cancer Detect Prev 6: 119-130.
2297. Seifert G, Donath K (1996). Hybrid tumours of salivary glands. Definition and classification of five rare cases. Eur J Cancer B Oral Oncol 32B: 251-259.
2298. Seifert G, Donath K (1996). Multiple tumours of the salivary glands—terminology and nomenclature. Eur J Cancer B Oral Oncol 32B: 3-7.
2299. Seifert G, Donath K, Schafer R (1999). Lipomatous pleomorphic adenoma of the parotid gland. Classification of lipomatous tissue in salivary glands. Pathol Res Pract 195: 247-252.
2300. Seifert G, Hennings K, Caselitz J (1986). Metastatic tumors to the parotid and submandibular glands—analysis and differential diagnosis of 108 cases. Pathol Res Pract 181: 684-692.
2301. Seifert G, Miehlke A, Haubrich J, Chilla R (1986). Diseases of the Salivary Glands: Pathology - Diagnosis - Treatment - Facial Nerve Surgery. Thieme Publishing Group: Stuttgart.
2302. Seifert G, Okabe H, Caselitz J (1986). Epithelial salivary gland tumors in children and adolescents. Analysis of 80 cases (Salivary Gland Register 1965-1984). ORL J Otorhinolaryngol Relat Spec 48: 137-149.
2303. Seifert G, Schulz CP (1979). [The monomorphic salivary duct adenoma. Classification and analysis of 79 cases]. Virchows Arch A Pathol Anat Histol 383: 77-99.
2304. Seifert G, Sobin LH (1991). Histological Typing of Salivary Gland Tumours. 2nd ed. Springer-Verlag: Berlin.
2305. Seikaly H, Cuyler JP (1994). Infantile subglottic hemangioma. J Otolaryngol 23: 135-137.
2306. Seo IS, Tomich CE, Warfel KA, Hull MT (1980). Clear cell carcinoma of the larynx A variant of mucoepidermoid carcinoma. Ann Otol Rhinol Laryngol 89: 168-172.
2307. Servenius B, Vernachio J, Price J, Andersson LC, Peterson PA (1994). Metastasizing neuroblastomas in mice transgenic for simian virus 40 large T (SV40T) under the olfactory marker protein gene promoter. Cancer Res 54: 5198-5205.
2308. Seshul MJ, Eby TL, Crowe DR, Peters GE (1995). Nasal inverted papilloma with involvement of middle ear and mastoid. Arch Otolaryngol Head Neck Surg 121: 1045-1048.
2309. Sessions RB, Bryan RN, Naclerio RM, Alford BR (1981). Radiographic staging of juvenile angiofibroma. Head Neck Surg 3: 279-283.
2310. Shah JP, Huvos AG, Strong EW (1977). Mucosal melanomas of the head and neck. Am J Surg 134: 531-535.
2311. Shah KV, Stern WF, Shah FK, Bishai D, Kashima HK (1998). Risk factors for juvenile onset recurrent respiratory papillomatosis. Pediatr Infect Dis J 17: 372-376.
2312. Shaheen KW, Cohen SR, Muraszko K, Newman MH (1991). Massive teratoma of the sphenoid sinus in a premature infant. J Craniofac Surg 2: 140-145.
2313. Shaida AM, McFerran DJ, da Cruz M, Hardy DG, Moffat DA (2000). Cavernous haemangioma of the internal auditory canal. J Laryngol Otol 114: 453-455.
2314. Sham JS, Choy D, Wei WI (1990). Nasopharyngeal carcinoma: orderly neck node spread. Int J Radiat Oncol Biol Phys 19: 929-933.
2315. Shamaskin RG, Svirsky JA, Kaugars GE (1989). Intraosseous and extraosseous calcifying odontogenic cyst (Gorlin cyst). J Oral Maxillofac Surg 47: 562-565.
2316. Shanmugaratnam K (1978). Histological typing of nasopharyngeal carcinoma. IARC Sci Publ 3-12.
2317. Shanmugaratnam K (1991). Histological Typing of Tumours of the Upper Respiratory Tract and Ear. 2nd ed. Springer-Verlag: Berlin.
2318. Shanmugaratnam K, Chan SH, de The G, Goh JE, Khor TH, Simons MJ, Tye CY (1979). Histopathology of nasopharyngeal carcinoma: correlations with epidemiology, survival rates and other biological characteristics. Cancer 44: 1029-1044.
2319. Shanmugaratnam K, Kunaratnam N, Chia KB, Chiang GS, Sinniah R (1983). Teratoid carcinosarcoma of the paranasal sinuses. Pathology 15: 413-419.
2320. Shanmugaratnam K, Sobin LH (1978). Histological typing of upper respiratory tract tumours. WHO: Geneva.
2321. Shapeero LG, Vanel D, Ackerman LV, Terrier-Lacombe MJ, Housin D, Schwaab G, Sigal R, Masselot J (1993). Aggressive fibrous dysplasia of the maxillary sinus. Skeletal Radiol 22: 563-568.
2322. Sharma RR, Verma A, Pawar SJ, Dev E, Devadas RV, Shiv VK, Musa MM (2002). Pediatric giant cell granuloma of the temporal bone: a case report and brief review of the literature. J Clin Neurosci 9: 459-462.
2323. Shear M (1992). Ondotogenic keratocyst (primordial cyst). In: Cysts of the Oral Regions, Cysts of the Oral Regions, 3rd ed. Butterworth Heinemann: Oxford , pp. 27-32.
2324. Shear M (1994). Developmental odontogenic cysts. An update. J Oral Pathol Med 23: 1-11.
2325. Shear M, Singh S (1978). Age-standardized incidence rates of ameloblastoma and dentigerous cyst on the Witwatersrand, South Africa. Community Dent Oral Epidemiol 6: 195-199.
2326. Sheen TS, Tsai CC, Ko JY, Chang YL, Hsu MM (1997). Undifferentiated carcinoma of the major salivary glands. Cancer 80: 357-363.
2327. Sheen TS, Wu CT, Hsieh T, Hsu MM (1997). Postirradiation laryngeal osteosarcoma: case report and literature review. Head Neck 19: 57-62.
2328. Sheikh M, Chisti FA, Sinan T (1999). Giant cell tumour of the temporal bone: case report and review of the literature. Australas Radiol 43: 113-115.
2329. Shemen LJ, Huvos AG, Spiro RH (1987). Squamous cell carcinoma of salivary gland origin. Head Neck Surg 9: 235-240.
2330. Shen J, Tate JE, Crum CP, Goodman ML (1996). Prevalence of human papillomaviruses (HPV) in benign and malignant tumors of the upper respiratory tract. Mod Pathol 9: 15-20.
2331. Shen L, Liang AC, Lu L, Au WY, Kwong YL, Liang RH, Srivastava G (2002). Frequent deletion of Fas gene sequences encoding death and transmembrane domains in nasal natural killer/T-cell lymphoma. Am J Pathol 161: 2123-2131.
2332. Sheng WQ, Hashimoto H, Okamoto S, Ishida T, Meis-Kindblom JM, Kindblom LG, Hisaoka M (2001). Expression of COL1A1-PDGFB fusion transcripts in superficial adult fibrosarcoma suggests a close relationship to dermatofibrosarcoma protuberans. J Pathol 194: 88-94.
2333. Sheppard LM, Mickelson SA (1990). Hemangiomas of the nasal septum and paranasal sinuses. Henry Ford Hosp Med J 38: 25-27.
2334. Shibata K, Komune S (1980). Laryngeal angiomyoma (vascular leiomyoma): clinicopathological findings. Laryngoscope 90: 1880-1886.
2335. Shick PC, Riordan GP, Foss RD (1995). Estrogen and progesterone receptors in salivary gland adenoid cystic carcinoma. Oral Surg Oral Med Oral Pathol Oral Radiol Endod 80: 440-444.
2336. Shiffman NJ (1975). Squamous cell carcinomas of the skin of the pinna. Can J Surg 18: 279-283.
2337. Shikhani AH, Johns ME (1988). Tumors of the major salivary glands in children. Head Neck Surg 10: 257-263.
2338. Shikhani AH, Shikhani LT, Kuhajda FP, Allam CK (1993). Warthin's tumor-associated neoplasms: report of two cases and review of the literature. Ear Nose Throat J 72: 264-3.
2339. Shimazaki H, Aida S, Tamai S, Miyazawa T, Nakanobou M (2000). Sinonasal teratocarcinosarcoma: ultrastructural and immunohistochemical evidence of neuroectodermal origin. Ultrastruct Pathol 24: 115-122.
2340. Shimm DS, Dosoretz DE, Harris NL, Pilch BZ, Linggood RM, Wang CC (1984). Radiation therapy of Waldeyer's ring lymphoma. Cancer 54: 426-431.
2341. Shimoyama T, Horie N, Nasu D, Kaneko T, Kato T, Tojo T, Suzuki T, Ide F (1999). So-called simple bone cyst of the jaw: a family of pseudocysts of diverse nature and etiology. J Oral Sci 41: 93-98.
2342. Shingaki S, Suzuki I, Nakajima T, Kawasaki T (1988). Evaluation of histopathologic parameters in predicting cervical lymph node metastasis of oral and oropharyngeal carcinomas. Oral Surg Oral Med Oral Pathol 66: 683-688.
2343. Shintaku M, Honda T (1997). Identification of oncocytic lesions of salivary glands by anti-mitochondrial immunohistochemistry. Histopathology 31: 408-411.
2344. Shirasuna K, Watatani K, Miyazaki T (1984). Ultrastructure of a sialadenoma papilliferum. Cancer 53: 468-474.
2345. Shoaib T, Soutar DS, MacDonald DG, Camilleri IG, Dunaway DJ, Gray HW, McCurrach GM, Bessent RG, MacLeod TI, Robertson AG (2001). The accuracy of head and neck carcinoma sentinel lymph node biopsy in the clinically N0 neck. Cancer 91: 2077-2083.
2346. Shotelersuk K, Khorprasert C, Sakdikul S, Pornthanakasem W, Voravud N, Mutirangura A (2000). Epstein-Barr virus DNA in serum/plasma as a tumor marker for nasopharyngeal cancer. Clin Cancer Res 6: 1046-1051.
2347. Shreif JA, Goumas PD, Mastronikolis N, Naxakis SS (2001). Extramedullary plasmacytoma of the nasal cavity. Otolaryngol Head Neck Surg 124: 119-120.
2348. Shrestha P, Yang LT, Liu BL, Namba M, Qin CL, Isono K, Tsukitani K, Mori M (1994). Clear cell carcinoma of salivary glands: immunohistochemical evaluation of clear tumor cells. Anticancer Res 14: 825-836.
2349. Shroyer KR, Greer RO, Fankhouser CA, McGuirt WF, Marshall R (1993). Detection of human papillomavirus DNA in oral verrucous carcinoma by polymerase chain reaction. Mod Pathol 6: 669-672.
2350. Shteyer A, Fundoianu-Dayan D (1986). Papillary cystic adenocarcinoma of minor salivary glands. Int J Oral Maxillofac Surg 15: 361-364.
2351. Shugar JM, Som PM, Biller HF, Som ML, Krespi YP (1981). Peripheral nerve sheath tumors of the paranasal sinuses. Head Neck Surg 4: 72-76.
2352. Siar CH, Ng KH (1993). Patterns of expression of intermediate filaments and S-100 protein in desmoplastic ameloblastoma. J Nihon Univ Sch Dent 35: 104-108.
2353. Siddiqi SH, Solomon MP, Haller JO (2000). Sialoblastoma and hepatoblastoma in a neonate. Pediatr Radiol 30: 349-351.
2354. Sidek D, Michaels L, Wright A (1996). Changes in the inner ear in vestibular schwannoma. In: Progress in Human Auditory and Vestibular Histopatholog, Iurato S, Veldman JE, eds., Kugler publications: Amsterdam .
2355. Siedentop KH, Jeantet C (1961). Primary adenocarcinoma of the middle ear. Report of three cases. Ann Otol Rhinol Laryngol 70: 719-733.
2356. Siegel SE, Cohen SR, Isaacs HJr, Stanley P (1979). Malignant transformation of tracheobronchial juvenile papillomatosis without prior radiotherapy. Ann Otol Rhinol

Laryngol 88: 192-197.
2357. Silverberg MJ, Thorsen P, Lindeberg H, Grant LA, Shah KV (2003). Condyloma in pregnancy is strongly predictive of juvenile-onset recurrent respiratory papillomatosis. Obstet Gynecol 101: 645-652.
2358. Silverman S, Bhargava K, Smith LW, Malaowalla AM (1976). Malignant transformation and natural history of oral leukoplakia in 57,518 industrial workers of Gujarat, India. Cancer 38: 1790-1795.
2359. Silverman SJr (2000). Oral lichen planus: a potentially premalignant lesion. J Oral Maxillofac Surg 58: 1286-1288.
2360. Silverman SJr, Gorsky M (1997). Proliferative verrucous leukoplakia: a follow-up study of 54 cases. Oral Surg Oral Med Oral Pathol Oral Radiol Endod 84: 154-157.
2361. Silverman SJr, Gorsky M, Lozada F (1984). Oral leukoplakia and malignant transformation. A follow-up study of 257 patients. Cancer 53: 563-568.
2362. Silverman SJr, Rosen RD (1968). Observations on the clinical characteristics and natural history of oral leukoplakia. J Am Dent Assoc 76: 772-777.
2363. Simko EJ, Brannon RB, Eibling DE (1998). Ameloblastic carcinoma of the mandible. Head Neck 20: 654-659.
2364. Simons MJ, Wee GB, Day NE, Morris PJ, Shanmugaratnam K, De The GB (1974). Immunogenetic aspects of nasopharyngeal carcinoma: I. Differences in HL-A antigen profiles between patients and control groups. Int J Cancer 13: 122-134.
2365. Simons MJ, Wee GB, Goh EH, Chan SH, Shanmugaratnam K, Day NE, de The G (1976). Immunogenetic aspects of nasopharyngeal carcinoma. IV. Increased risk in Chinese of nasopharyngeal carcinoma associated with a Chinese-related HLA profile (A2, Singapore 2). J Natl Cancer Inst 57: 977-980.
2366. Simons MJ, Wee GB, Singh D, Dharmalingham S, Yong NK, Chau JC, Ho JH, Day NE, de The G (1977). Immunogenetic aspects of nasopharyngeal carcinoma. V. Confirmation of a Chinese-related HLA profile (A2, Singapore 2) associated with an increased risk in Chinese for nasopharyngeal carcinoma. Natl Cancer Inst Monogr 47: 147-151.
2367. Simpson RH, Jones H, Beasley P (1995). Benign myoepithelioma of the salivary glands: a true entity? Histopathology 27: 1-9.
2368. Simpson RH, Pereira EM, Ribeiro AC, Abdulkadir A, Reis-Filho JS (2002). Polymorphous low-grade adenocarcinoma of the salivary glands with transformation to high-grade carcinoma. Histopathology 41: 250-259.
2369. Simpson RH, Sarsfield PT, Clarke T, Babajews AV (1990). Clear cell carcinoma of minor salivary glands. Histopathology 17: 433-438.
2370. Simpson RH, Skalova A (1997). Metastatic carcinoma of the prostate presenting as parotid tumour. Histopathology 30: 70-74.
2371. Simpson RHW, Prasad AR, Lewis JE, Skalova A, David L (2003). Mucin-rich variant of salivary duct carcinoma: a clinicopathologic and immunohistochemical study of four cases. Am J Surg Pathol 27: 1070-1079.
2372. Simpson RHW, Sarsfield PTL (1997). Benign and malignant lymphoid lesions of the salivary glands. Curr Diagn Pathol 4: 91-99.
2373. Sindwani R, Matthews TW, Thomas J, Venkatesan VM (1998). Epithelioid leiomyosarcoma of the larynx. Head Neck 20: 563-567.
2374. Singh B, Alfonso A, Sabin S, Poluri A, Shaha AR, Sundaram K, Lucente FE (2000). Outcome differences in younger and older patients with laryngeal cancer: a retrospective case-control study. Am J Otolaryngol 21: 92-97.
2375. Singh SP, Cottingham SL, Slone W, Boesel CP, Welling DB, Yates AJ (1996). Lipomas of the internal auditory canal. Arch Pathol Lab Med 120: 681-683.
2376. Sinkre P, Lindberg G, Albores-Saavedra J (2001). Nasopharyngeal gangliocytic paraganglioma. Arch Pathol Lab Med 125: 1098-1100.
2377. Sironi M, Isimbaldi G, Claren R, Delpiano C, Di Nuovo F, Spinelli M (2000). Carcinosarcoma of the parotid gland: cytological, clinicopathological and immunohistochemical study of a case. Pathol Res Pract 196: 511-517.
2378. Sisson GA, Beck SP (1981). Cancer of the nasal and paranasal sinuses. In: Cancer of the Head and Neck, Suen JY, Myers EN, eds., Churchill Livingstone: New York , pp. 242-279.
2379. Sissons HA, Malcolm AJ (1997). Fibrous dysplasia of bone: case report with autopsy study 80 years after the original clinical recognition of the bone lesions. Skeletal Radiol 26: 177-183.
2380. Siu LL, Chan JK, Wong KF, Choy C, Kwong YL (2003). Aberrant promoter CpG methylation as a molecular marker for disease monitoring in natural killer cell lymphomas. Br J Haematol 122: 70-77.
2381. Siu LL, Chan JK, Wong KF, Kwong YL (2002). Specific patterns of gene methylation in natural killer cell lymphomas : p73 is consistently involved. Am J Pathol 160: 59-66.
2382. Siu LL, Chan V, Chan JK, Wong KF, Liang R, Kwong YL (2000). Consistent patterns of allelic loss in natural killer cell lymphoma. Am J Pathol 157: 1803-1809.
2383. Siu LL, Wong KF, Chan JK, Kwong YL (1999). Comparative genomic hybridization analysis of natural killer cell lymphoma/leukemia. Recognition of consistent patterns of genetic alterations. Am J Pathol 155: 1419-1425.
2384. Siwersson U, Kindblom LG (1984). Oncocytic carcinoid of the nasal cavity and carcinoid of the lung in a child. Pathol Res Pract 178: 562-569.
2385. Sjogren H, Dahlenfors R, Stenman G, Mark J (2003). Observations by G-banding and multicolor spectral karyotyping in a salivary gland basal cell adenoma. Virchows Arch 442: 86-87.
2386. Skalli O, Pelte MF, Peclet MC, Gabbiani G, Gugliotta P, Bussolati G, Ravazzola M, Orci L (1989). Alpha-smooth muscle actin, a differentiation marker of smooth muscle cells, is present in microfilamentous bundles of pericytes. J Histochem Cytochem 37: 315-321.
2387. Skalova A, Lehtonen H, Von Boguslawsky K, Leivo I (1994). Prognostic significance of cell proliferation in mucoepidermoid carcinomas of the salivary gland: clinicopathological study using MIB 1 antibody in paraffin sections. Hum Pathol 25: 929-935.
2388. Skalova A, Leivo I, Von Boguslawsky K, Saksela E (1994). Cell proliferation correlates with prognosis in acinic cell carcinomas of salivary gland origin. Immunohistochemical study of 30 cases using the MIB 1 antibody in formalin-fixed paraffin sections. J Pathol 173: 13-21.
2389. Skalova A, Leivo I, Wolf H, Fakan F (2000). Oncocytic cystadenoma of the parotid gland with tyrosine-rich crystals. Pathol Res Pract 196: 849-851.
2390. Skalova A, Michal M, Nathansky Z (1994). Epidermoid carcinoma arising in Warthin's tumour: a case study. J Oral Pathol Med 23: 330-333.
2391. Skalova A, Simpson RH, Lehtonen H, Leivo I (1997). Assessment of proliferative activity using the MIB1 antibody help to distinguish polymorphous low grade adenocarcinoma from adenoid cystic carcinoma of salivary glands. Pathol Res Pract 193: 695-703.
2392. Skalova A, Starek, Kucerova V, Szepe P, Plank L (2001). Salivary duct carcinoma—a highly aggressive salivary gland tumor with HER-2/neu oncoprotein overexpression. Pathol Res Pract 197: 621-626.
2393. Skalova A, Starek I, Vanecek T, Kucerova V, Plank L, Szepe P, DiPalma S, Leivo I (2003). Expression of HER-2/neu gene and protein in salivary duct carcinoma of parotid gland as revealed by fluorescence in situ hybridization and immunohistochemistry. Histopathology 42: 1-9.
2394. Slater LJ (1999). Odontogenic sarcoma and carcinosarcoma. Semin Diagn Pathol 16: 325-332.
2395. Slavin JL, Woodford NW, Busmanis I (1995). Synchronous parotid myoepithelioma and Warthin's tumor. Pathology 27: 199-200.
2396. Slonim SM, Haykal HA, Cushing GW, Freidberg SR, Lee AK (1993). MRI appearances of an ectopic pituitary adenoma: case report and review of the literature. Neuroradiology 35: 546-548.
2397. Slootweg PJ (1987). Carcinoma arising from reduced enamel epithelium. J Oral Pathol 16: 479-482.
2398. Slootweg PJ (1989). Comparison of giant cell granuloma of the jaw and non-ossifying fibroma. J Oral Pathol Med 18: 128-132.
2399. Slootweg PJ (1991). Bone and cementum as stromal features in Pindborg tumor. J Oral Pathol Med 20: 93-95.
2400. Slootweg PJ (1992). Cementoblastoma and osteoblastoma: a comparison of histologic features. J Oral Pathol Med 21: 385-389.
2401. Slootweg PJ (1996). Maxillofacial fibro-osseous lesions: classification and differential diagnosis. Semin Diagn Pathol 13: 104-112.
2402. Slootweg PJ (2002). Malignant odontogenic tumors: an overview. Mund Kiefer Gesichtschir 6: 295-302.
2403. Slootweg PJ, Hordijk GJ, Schade Y, van Es RJ, Koole R (2002). Treatment failure and margin status in head and neck cancer. A critical view on the potential value of molecular pathology. Oral Oncol 38: 500-503.
2404. Slootweg PJ, Lubsen H (1991). Rhabdomyoblasts in olfactory neuroblastoma. Histopathology 19: 182-184.
2405. Slootweg PJ, Muller H (1984). Malignant ameloblastoma or ameloblastic carcinoma. Oral Surg Oral Med Oral Pathol 57: 168-176.
2406. Slootweg PJ, Panders AK, Koopmans R, Nikkels PG (1994). Juvenile ossifying fibroma. An analysis of 33 cases with emphasis on histopathological aspects. J Oral Pathol Med 23: 385-388.
2407. Slootweg PJ, Roholl PJ, Muller H, Lubsen H (1989). Spindle-cell carcinoma of the oral cavity and larynx. Immunohistochemical aspects. J Craniomaxillofac Surg 17: 234-236.
2408. Slootweg PJ, Wittkampf AR (1986). Myxoma of the jaws. An analysis of 15 cases. J Maxillofac Surg 14: 46-52.
2409. Smets G, Warson F, Dehou MF, Storme G, Sacre R, Van Belle S, Somers G, Gepts W, Kloppel G (1990). Metastasizing neuroendocrine carcinoma of the larynx with calcitonin and somatostatin secretion and CEA production, resembling medullary thyroid carcinoma. Virchows Arch A Pathol Anat Histopathol 416: 539-543.
2410. Smith BC, Ellis GL, Meis-Kindblom JM, Williams SB (1995). Ectomesenchymal chondromyxoid tumor of the anterior tongue. Nineteen cases of a new clinicopathologic entity. Am J Surg Pathol 19: 519-530.
2411. Smith EM, Pignatari SS, Gray SD, Haugen TH, Turek LP (1993). Human papillomavirus infection in papillomas and nondiseased respiratory sites of patients with recurrent respiratory papillomatosis using the polymerase chain reaction. Arch Otolaryngol Head Neck Surg 119: 554-557.
2412. Smith EM, Summersgill KF, Allen J, Hoffman HT, McCulloch T, Turek LP, Haugen TH (2000). Human papillomavirus and risk of laryngeal cancer. Ann Otol Rhinol Laryngol 109: 1069-1076.
2413. Smith O, Youngs R, Snell D, Van Nostrand P (1988). Paraganglioma of the larynx. J Otolaryngol 17: 293-301.
2414. Smith PG, Marrogi AJ, Delfino JJ (1990). Multifocal central giant cell lesions of the maxillofacial skeleton: a case report. J Oral Maxillofac Surg 48: 300-305.
2415. Smullen S, Willcox T, Wetmore R, Zackai E (1994). Otologic manifestations of neurofibromatosis. Laryngoscope 104: 663-665.
2416. Snyder ML, Paulino AF (1999). Hybrid carcinoma of the salivary gland: salivary duct adenocarcinoma adenoid cystic carcinoma. Histopathology 35: 380-383.
2417. Snyder RN, Perzin KH (1972). Papillomatosis of nasal cavity and paranasal sinuses (inverted papilloma, squamous papilloma). A clinicopathologic study. Cancer 30: 668-690.
2418. Sobin LH, Wittekind C (2002). TNM: Classification of Malignant Tumours. 6th ed. John Wiley & Sons: New York.
2419. Soga J, Ferlito A, Rinaldo A (2004). Endocrinocarcinomas (carcinoids and their variants) of the larynx: a comparative consideration with those of other sites. Oral Oncol 40: 668-672.
2420. Soga J, Osaka M, Yakuwa Y (2002). Laryngeal endocrinomas (carcinoids and relevant neoplasms): analysis of 278 reported cases. J Exp Clin Cancer Res 21: 5-13.
2421. Soini Y, Kamel D, Nuorva K, Lane DP, Vahakangas K, Paakko P (1992). Low p53 protein expression in salivary gland tumours compared with lung carcinomas. Virchows Arch A Pathol Anat Histopathol 421: 415-420.
2422. Solomon D, Smith RR, Kashima HK, Leventhal BG (1985). Malignant transformation in non-irradiated recurrent respiratory papillomatosis. Laryngoscope 95: 900-904.
2423. Som PM, Brann EA (2003). Tumor and Tumor-like Conditions. In: Head and Neck Imaging, Som PM, Curtin HD, eds.,

Mosby: St. Louis, Mo. pp. 261-373.
2424. Som PM, Shugar JM, Cohen BA, Biller HF (1981). The nonspecificity of the antral bowing sign in maxillary sinus pathology. J Comput Assist Tomogr 5: 350-352.
2425. Som PM, Silvers AR, Catalano PJ, Brandwein M, Khorsandi AS (1997). Adenosquamous carcinoma of the facial bones, skull base, and calvaria: CT and MR manifestations. AJNR Am J Neuroradiol 18: 173-175.
2426. Sonobe H, Taguchi K, Motoi M, Ogawa K, Matsumura M, Ohsaki K (1980). Malignant fibrous histiocytoma of the maxillary sinus. Acta Pathol Jpn 30: 79-89.
2427. Sorensen M, Baunsgaard P, Frederiksen P, Haahr PA (1986). Multifocal adenomatous oncocytic hyperplasia of the parotid gland (unusual clear cell variant in two female siblings.). Pathol Res Pract 181: 254-259.
2428. Sorensen PH, Wu JK, Berean KW, Lim JF, Donn W, Frierson HF, Reynolds CP, Lopez-Terrada D, Triche TJ (1996). Olfactory neuroblastoma is a peripheral primitive neuroectodermal tumor related to Ewing sarcoma. Proc Natl Acad Sci U S A 93: 1038-1043.
2429. Soysal V, Yigitbasi OG, Kontas O, Kahya HA, Guney E (2001). Inflammatory myofibroblastic tumor of the nasal cavity: a case report and review of the literature. Int J Pediatr Otorhinolaryngol 61: 161-165.
2430. Spafford MF, Koch WM, Reed AL, Califano JA, Xu LH, Eisenberger CF, Yip L, Leong PL, Wu L, Liu SX, Jeronimo C, Westra WH, Sidransky D (2001). Detection of head and neck squamous cell carcinoma among exfoliated oral mucosal cells by microsatellite analysis. Clin Cancer Res 7: 607-612.
2431. Spagnolo DV, Papadimitriou JM, Archer M (1984). Postirradiation malignant fibrous histiocytoma arising in juvenile nasopharyngeal angiofibroma and producing alpha-1-antitrypsin. Histopathology 8: 339-352.
2432. Spayne JA, Warde P, O'Sullivan B, Payne D, Liu FF, Waldron J, Gullane PJ, Cummings BJ (2001). Carcinoma-in-situ of the glottic larynx: results of treatment with radiation therapy. Int J Radiat Oncol Biol Phys 49: 1235-1238.
2433. Spector GJ, Ogura JH (1974). Malignant fibrous histiocytoma of the maxilla. A report of an unusual lesion. Arch Otolaryngol 99: 385-387.
2434. Spector JG, Sessions DG, Emami B, Simpson J, Haughey B, Harvey J, Fredrickson JM (1995). Squamous cell carcinoma of the pyriform sinus: a nonrandomized comparison of therapeutic modalities and long-term results. Laryngoscope 105: 397-406.
2435. Spector JG, Sessions DG, Haughey BH, Chao KS, Simpson J, El Mofty S, Perez CA (2001). Delayed regional metastases, distant metastases, and second primary malignancies in squamous cell carcinomas of the larynx and hypopharynx. Laryngoscope 111: 1079-1087.
2436. Speicher MR, Howe C, Crotty P, du Manoir S, Costa J, Ward DC (1995). Comparative genomic hybridization detects novel deletions and amplifications in head and neck squamous cell carcinomas. Cancer Res 55: 1010-1013.
2437. Sperry K (1994). Lethal asphyxiating juvenile laryngeal papillomatosis. A case report with human papillomavirus in situ hybridization analysis. Am J Forensic Med Pathol 15: 146-150.
2438. Spiro JD, Soo KC, Spiro RH (1995). Nonsquamous cell malignant neoplasms of the nasal cavities and paranasal sinuses. Head Neck 17: 114-118.
2439. Spiro RH (1986). Salivary neoplasms: overview of a 35-year experience with 2,807 patients. Head Neck Surg 8: 177-184.
2440. Spiro RH (1995). Changing trends in the management of salivary tumors. Semin Surg Oncol 11: 240-245.
2441. Spiro RH (1997). Distant metastasis in adenoid cystic carcinoma of salivary origin. Am J Surg 174: 495-498.
2442. Spiro RH, Huvos AG (1992). Stage means more than grade in adenoid cystic carcinoma. Am J Surg 164: 623-628.
2443. Spiro RH, Huvos AG, Berk R, Strong EW (1978). Mucoepidermoid carcinoma of salivary gland origin. A clinicopathologic study of 367 cases. Am J Surg 136: 461-468.
2444. Spiro RH, Huvos AG, Strong EW (1974). Adenoid cystic carcinoma of salivary origin. A clinicopathologic study of 242 cases. Am J Surg 128: 512-520.
2445. Spiro RH, Huvos AG, Strong EW (1978). Acinic cell carcinoma of salivary origin. A clinicopathologic study of 67 cases. Cancer 41: 924-935.
2446. Spiro RH, Huvos AG, Strong EW (1979). Adenoid cystic carcinoma: factors influencing survival. Am J Surg 138: 579-583.
2447. Spiro RH, Huvos AG, Strong EW (1982). Adenocarcinoma of salivary origin. Clinicopathologic study of 204 patients. Am J Surg 144: 423-431.
2448. Spiro RH, Koss LG, Hajdu SI, Strong EW (1973). Tumors of minor salivary origin. A clinicopathologic study of 492 cases. Cancer 31: 117-129.
2449. Spiro RH, Thaler HT, Hicks WF, Kher UA, Huvos AH, Strong EW (1991). The importance of clinical staging of minor salivary gland carcinoma. Am J Surg 162: 330-336.
2450. Spitz MR, Hoque A, Trizna Z, Schantz SP, Amos CI, King TM, Bondy ML, Hong WK, Hsu TC (1994). Mutagen sensitivity as a risk factor for second malignant tumors following malignancies of the upper aerodigestive tract. J Natl Cancer Inst 86: 1681-1684.
2451. Spitz MR, Sider JG, Newell GR (1990). Salivary gland cancer and risk of subsequent skin cancer. Head Neck 12: 254-256.
2452. Spitz MR, Sider JG, Newell GR, Batsakis JG (1988). Incidence of salivary gland cancer in the United States relative to ultraviolet radiation exposure. Head Neck Surg 10: 305-308.
2453. Spruck CHI, Tsai YC, Huang DP, Yang AS, Rideout WMI, Gonzalez-Zulueta M, Choi P, Lo KW, Yu MC, Jones PA (1992). Absence of p53 gene mutations in primary nasopharyngeal carcinomas. Cancer Res 52: 4787-4790.
2454. Squires JE, Mills SE, Cooper PH, Innes DJJr, McLean WC (1981). Acinic cell carcinoma: its occurrence in the laryngotracheal junction after thyroid radiation. Arch Pathol Lab Med 105: 266-268.
2455. Stadlmann S, Fend F, Moser P, Obrist P, Greil R, Dirnhofer S (2001). Epstein-Barr virus-associated extranodal NK/T-cell lymphoma, nasal type of the hypopharynx, in a renal allograft recipient: case report and review of literature. Hum Pathol 32: 1264-1268.
2456. Stafford ND, Frootko NJ (1986). Verrucous carcinoma in the external auditory canal. Am J Otol 7: 443-445.
2457. Staley CJ, Ujiki GT, Yokoo H (1971). "Pseudocarcinoma" of the larynx. Independent metastasis of carcinomatous and sarcomatous elements. Arch Otolaryngol 94: 458-465.
2458. Stallmach I, Zenklusen P, Komminoth P, Schmid S, Perren A, Roos M, Jianming Z, Heitz PU, Pfaltz M (2002). Loss of heterozygosity at chromosome 6q23-25 correlates with clinical and histologic parameters in salivary gland adenoid cystic carcinoma. Virchows Arch 440: 77-84.
2459. Stanley RJ, Weiland LH, Olsen KD, Pearson BW (1988). Dedifferentiated acinic cell (acinous) carcinoma of the parotid gland. Otolaryngol Head Neck Surg 98: 155-161.
2460. Stavropoulos F, Katz J (2002). Central giant cell granulomas: a systematic review of the radiographic characteristics with the addition of 20 new cases. Dentomaxillofac Radiol 31: 213-217.
2461. Steinberg BM, Meade R, Kalinowski S, Abramson AL (1990). Abnormal differentiation of human papillomavirus-induced laryngeal papillomas. Arch Otolaryngol Head Neck Surg 116: 1167-1171.
2462. Steiner W (1993). Results of curative laser microsurgery of laryngeal carcinomas. Am J Otolaryngol 14: 116-121.
2463. Stene T, Koppang HS (1981). Intraoral adenocarcinomas. J Oral Pathol 10: 216-225.
2464. Stenman G, Sandros J, Mark J, Nordkvist A (1989). High p21RAS expression levels correlate with chromosome 8 rearrangements in benign human mixed salivary gland tumors. Genes Chromosomes Cancer 1: 59-66.
2465. Stenman G, Sandros J, Nordkvist A, Mark J, Sahlin P (1991). Expression of the ERBB2 protein in benign and malignant salivary gland tumors. Genes Chromosomes Cancer 3: 128-135.
2466. Stephen J, Batsakis JG, Luna MA, von der Heyden U, Byers RM (1986). True malignant mixed tumors (carcinosarcoma) of salivary glands. Oral Surg Oral Med Oral Pathol 61: 597-602.
2467. Stephenson CF, Bridge JA, Sandberg AA (1992). Cytogenetic and pathologic aspects of Ewing's sarcoma and neuroectodermal tumors. Hum Pathol 23: 1270-1277.
2468. Sterman BM, Kraus DH, Sebek BA, Tucker HM (1990). Primary squamous cell carcinoma of the parotid gland. Laryngoscope 100: 146-148.
2469. Stern Y, Braslavsky D, Segal K, Shpitzer T, Abraham A (1991). Intravascular papillary endothelial hyperplasia in the maxillary sinus. A benign lesion that may be mistaken for angiosarcoma. Arch Otolaryngol Head Neck Surg 117: 1182-1184.
2470. Stern Y, Heffelfinger SC, Walner DL, Cotton RT (2000). Expression of Ki-67, tumor suppressor proteins, growth factor, and growth factor receptor in juvenile respiratory papillomatosis: Ki-67 and p53 as predictors of aggressive disease. Otolaryngol Head Neck Surg 122: 378-386.
2471. Stern Y, Hurtubise PE, Cotton RT (1998). Significance of DNA ploidy and cell proliferation in juvenile respiratory papillomatosis. Ann Otol Rhinol Laryngol 107: 815-819.
2472. Stevenson AJ (1994). CJBFMM. CD 99 (p30/32-MIC2) Neuroectodermal/Ewing Sarcoma antigen as an immunohistochemical marker. Review of more than 600 tumours and the literature experience. Appl Immunohistochem Mol Morphol 231-240.
2473. Stevenson AR, Austin BW (1990). A case of ameloblastoma presenting as an exophytic gingival lesion. J Periodontol 61: 378-381.
2474. Stewart CJ, MacKenzie K, McGarry GW, Mowat A (2000). Fine-needle aspiration cytology of salivary gland: a review of 341 cases. Diagn Cytopathol 22: 139-146.
2475. Stillwagon GB, Smith RR, Highstein C, Lee DJ (1985). Adenoid cystic carcinoma of the supraglottic larynx: report of a case and review of the literature. Am J Otolaryngol 6: 309-314.
2476. Stinchi C, Piraccini BM, Pileri S, Lorenzi S, Casavecchia P, Fanti PA, Tosti A (1998). Multiple nodular lesions of the chin and oral mucosa in a patient with Sjogren's syndrome. Eur J Dermatol 8: 350-352.
2477. Stoeckli SJ, Pfaltz M, Steinert H, Schmid S (2002). Histopathological features of occult metastasis detected by sentinel lymph node biopsy in oral and oropharyngeal squamous cell carcinoma. Laryngoscope 112: 111-115.
2478. Stoelinga PJ (2001). Long-term follow-up on keratocysts treated according to a defined protocol. Int J Oral Maxillofac Surg 30: 14-25.
2479. Stolovitzky JP, Waldron CA, McConnel FM (1994). Giant cell lesions of the maxilla and paranasal sinuses. Head Neck 16: 143-148.
2480. Stone DM, Berktold RE, Ranganathan C, Wiet RJ (1987). Inverted papilloma of the middle ear and mastoid. Otolaryngol Head Neck Surg 97: 416-418.
2481. Stone HE, Lipa M, Bell RD (1975). Primary adenocarcinoma of the middle ear. Arch Otolaryngol 101: 702-705.
2482. Struthers PJ, Shear M (1984). Aneurysmal bone cyst of the jaws. (I). Clinicopathological features. Int J Oral Surg 13: 85-91.
2483. Struthers PJ, Shear M (1984). Aneurysmal bone cyst of the jaws. (II). Pathogenesis. Int J Oral Surg 13: 92-100.
2484. Sturm W, Menze B, Krause J, Thriene B (1994). Use of asbestos, health risks and induced occupational diseases in the former East Germany. Toxicol Lett 72: 317-324.
2485. Su L, Weathers DR, Waldron CA (1997). Distinguishing features of focal cemento-osseous dysplasia and cemento-ossifying fibromas. II. A clinical and radiologic spectrum of 316 cases. Oral Surg Oral Med Oral Pathol Oral Radiol Endod 84: 540-549.
2486. Su LD, Atayde-Perez A, Sheldon S, Fletcher JA, Weiss SW (1998). Inflammatory myofibroblastic tumor: cytogenetic evidence supporting clonal origin. Mod Pathol 11: 364-368.
2487. Su W, Ko A, O'Connell T, Applebaum H (2000). Treatment of pseudotumors with nonsteroidal antiinflammatory drugs. J Pediatr Surg 35: 1635-1637.
2488. Suarez PA, Adler-Storthz K, Luna MA, El Naggar AK, Abdul-Karim FW, Batsakis JG (2000). Papillary squamous cell carcinomas of the upper aerodigestive tract: a clinicopathologic and molecular study. Head Neck 22: 360-368.
2489. Suarez PA, Batsakis JG, El Naggar AK (1996). Don't confuse dental soft tissues with odontogenic tumors. Ann Otol Rhinol Laryngol 105: 490-494.
2490. Sudbo J, Bryne M, Johannessen

AC, Kildal W, Danielsen HE, Reith A (2001). Comparison of histological grading and large-scale genomic status (DNA ploidy) as prognostic tools in oral dysplasia. J Pathol 194: 303-310.
2491. Sudbo J, Kildal W, Johannessen AC, Koppang HS, Sudbo A, Danielsen HE, Risberg B, Reith A (2002). Gross genomic aberrations in precancers: clinical implications of a long-term follow-up study in oral erythroplakias. J Clin Oncol 20: 456-462.
2492. Sudbo J, Kildal W, Risberg B, Koppang HS, Danielsen HE, Reith A (2001). DNA content as a prognostic marker in patients with oral leukoplakia. N Engl J Med 344: 1270-1278.
2493. Sudbo J, Ried T, Bryne M, Kildal W, Danielsen H, Reith A (2001). Abnormal DNA content predicts the occurrence of carcinomas in non-dysplastic oral white patches. Oral Oncol 37: 558-565.
2494. Sudhoff H, Bujia J, Fisseler-Eckhoff A, Holly A, Schulz-Flake C, Hildmann H (1995). Expression of a cell-cycle-associated nuclear antigen (MIB 1) in cholesteatoma and auditory meatal skin. Laryngoscope 105: 1227-1231.
2495. Sudhoff H, Bujia J, Holly A, Kim C, Fisseler-Eckhoff A (1994). Functional characterization of middle ear mucosa residues in cholesteatoma samples. Am J Otol 15: 217-221.
2496. Sudhoff H, Fisseler-Eckhoff A, Stark T, Borkowski G, Luckhaupt H, Cooper J, Michaels L (1997). Argyrophilic nucleolar organizer regions in auditory meatal skin and middle ear cholesteatoma. Clin Otolaryngol 22: 545-548.
2497. Sugano H, Sakamoto G, Sawaki S, Hirayama T (1978). Histopathological types of nasopharyngeal carcinoma in a low-risk area: Japan. IARC Sci Publ 27-39.
2498. Sugimoto T, Wakizono S, Uemura T, Tsuneyoshi M, Enjoji M (1993). Malignant oncocytoma of the parotid gland: a case report with an immunohistochemical and ultrastructural study. J Laryngol Otol 107: 69-74.
2499. Sulica RL, Wenig BM, Debo RF, Sessions RB (1999). Schneiderian papillomas of the pharynx. Ann Otol Rhinol Laryngol 108: 392-397.
2500. Sulzner SE, Amdur RJ, Weider DJ (1998). Extramedullary plasmacytoma of the head and neck. Am J Otolaryngol 19: 203-208.
2501. Sumida T, Hamakawa H, Otsuka K, Tanioka H (2001). Leiomyosarcoma of the maxillary sinus with cervical lymph node metastasis. J Oral Maxillofac Surg 59: 568-571.
2502. Summerlin DJ, Tomich CE (1994). Focal cemento-osseous dysplasia: a clinicopathologic study of 221 cases. Oral Surg Oral Med Oral Pathol 78: 611-620.
2503. Sun EC, Curtis R, Melbye M, Goedert JJ (1999). Salivary gland cancer in the United States. Cancer Epidemiol Biomarkers Prev 8: 1095-1100.
2504. Sun Y, Hegamyer G, Colburn NH (1993). Nasopharyngeal carcinoma shows no detectable retinoblastoma susceptibility gene alterations. Oncogene 8: 791-795.
2505. Sunaba K, Shibuya H, Okada N, Amagasa T, Enomoto S, Kishimoto S (2000). Radiotherapy for primary localized (stage I and II) non-Hodgkin's lymphoma of the oral cavity. Int J Radiat Oncol Biol Phys 47: 179-183.
2506. Sunami K, Yamane H, Konishi K, Iguchi H, Takayama M, Nakai Y, Wakasa K, Nakagawa T, Shibata S (1999). Epithelial-myoepithelial carcinoma: An unusual tumor of the paranasal sinus. ORL J Otorhinolaryngol Relat Spec 61: 113-116.
2507. Suoglu Y, Erdamar B, Katircioglu OS, Karatay MC, Sunay T (2002). Extracapsular spread in ipsilateral neck and contralateral neck metastases in laryngeal cancer. Ann Otol Rhinol Laryngol 111: 447-454.
2508. Supance JS, Quenelle DJ, Crissman J (1980). Endolaryngeal neurofibromas. Otolaryngol Head Neck Surg 88: 74-78.
2509. Suster S, Rosai J (1991). Multilocular thymic cyst: an acquired reactive process. Study of 18 cases. Am J Surg Pathol 15: 388-398.
2510. Suzuki H, Fujioka Y (1998). Deletion of the p16 gene and microsatellite instability in carcinoma arising in pleomorphic adenoma of the parotid gland. Diagn Mol Pathol 7: 224-231.
2511. Swain RE, Sessions DG, Ogura JH (1974). Fibrosarcoma of the head and neck: a clinical analysis of forty cases. Ann Otol Rhinol Laryngol 83: 439-444.
2512. Swanson GM, Belle SH (1982). Cancer morbidity among woodworkers in the U.S. automotive industry. J Occup Med 24: 315-319.
2513. Swanson GM, Burns PB (1995). Cancer incidence among women in the workplace: a study of the association between occupation and industry and 11 cancer sites. J Occup Environ Med 37: 282-287.
2514. Swanson GM, Burns PB (1997). Cancers of the salivary gland: workplace risks among women and men. Ann Epidemiol 7: 369-374.
2515. Sykes AJ, Logue JP, Slevin NJ, Gupta NK (1995). An analysis of radiotherapy in the management of 104 patients with parotid carcinoma. Clin Oncol (R Coll Radiol) 7: 16-20.
2516. Syrjanen K, Happonen RP, Syrjanen S, Calonius B (1984). Human papilloma virus (HPV) antigens and local immunologic reactivity in oral squamous cell tumors and hyperplasias. Scand J Dent Res 92: 358-370.
2517. Syrjanen K, Syrjanen S (2000). Papillomavirus Infections in Human Pathology. John Wiley & Sons: Chichester.
2518. Syrjanen S, Puranen M (2000). Human papillomavirus infections in children: the potential role of maternal transmission. Crit Rev Oral Biol Med 11: 259-274.
2519. Szanto PA, Luna MA, Tortoledo ME, White RA (1984). Histologic grading of adenoid cystic carcinoma of the salivary glands. Cancer 54: 1062-1069.
2520. Sze WM, Lee AW, Yau TK, Yeung RW, Lau KY, Leung SK, Hung AW, Lee MC, Chan K (2003). Prognostic significance of primary tumor volume of nasopharyngeal carcinoma on local control. J HK Coll Radiol 6: 119.
2521. Szymas J, Wolf G, Kowalczyk D, Nowak S, Petersen I (1997). Olfactory neuroblastoma: detection of genomic imbalances by comparative genomic hybridization. Acta Neurochir (Wien) 139: 839-844.
2522. Taconis WK (1988). Osteosarcoma in fibrous dysplasia. Skeletal Radiol 17: 163-170.
2523. Taddesse-Heath L, Feldman JI, Fahle GA, Fischer SH, Sorbara L, Raffeld M, Jaffe ES (2003). Florid CD4+, CD56+ T-Cell Infiltrate Associated with Herpes Simplex Infection Simulating Nasal NK-/T-Cell Lymphoma. Mod Pathol 16: 166-172.
2524. Taddesse-Heath L, Pittaluga S, Sorbara L, Bussey M, Raffeld M, Jaffe ES (2003). Marginal zone B-cell lymphoma in children and young adults. Am J Surg Pathol 27: 522-531.
2525. Taguchi Y, Tanaka K, Miyakita Y, Sekino H, Fujimoto M (2000). Recurrent craniopharyngioma with nasopharyngeal extension. Pediatr Neurosurg 32: 140-144.
2526. Tajima Y, Kuroda-Kawasaki M, Ohno J, Yi J, Kusama K, Tanaka H, Fukunaga S, Shimada J, Yamamoto Y (2001). Peripheral ameloblastoma with potentially malignant features: report of a case with special regard to its keratin profile. J Oral Pathol Med 30: 494-498.
2527. Tajima Y, Ohno J, Utsumi N (1986). The dentinogenic ghost cell tumor. J Oral Pathol 15: 359-362.
2528. Takagi M, Ishikawa G, Mori W (1974). Primary malignant melanoma of the oral cavity in Japan. With special reference to mucosal melanosis. Cancer 34: 358-370.
2529. Takahashi H, Fujita S, Okabe H, Tsuda N, Tezuka F (1992). Distribution of tissue markers in acinic cell carcinomas of salivary gland. Pathol Res Pract 188: 692-700.
2530. Takahashi H, Fujita S, Okabe H, Tsuda N, Tezuka F (1993). Immunophenotypic analysis of extranodal non-Hodgkin's lymphomas in the oral cavity. Pathol Res Pract 189: 300-311.
2531. Takahashi H, Kawazoe K, Fujita S, Okabe H, Hideshima K, Tsuda N, Tezuka F (1996). Expression of bcl-2 oncogene product in primary non-Hodgkin's malignant lymphoma of the oral cavity. Pathol Res Pract 192: 44-53.
2532. Takahashi H, Tsuda N, Tezuka F, Okabe H (1989). Primary extranodal non-Hodgkin's lymphoma of the oral region. J Oral Pathol Med 18: 84-91.
2533. Takahashi N, Miura I, Chubachi A, Miura AB, Nakamura S (2001). A clinicopathological study of 20 patients with T/natural killer (NK)-cell lymphoma-associated hemophagocytic syndrome with special reference to nasal and nasal-type NK/T-cell lymphoma. Int J Hematol 74: 303-308.
2534. Takakuwa T, Dong Z, Nakatsuka S, Kojya S, Harabuchi Y, Yang WI, Nagata S, Aozasa K (2002). Frequent mutations of Fas gene in nasal NK/T cell lymphoma. Oncogene 21: 4702-4705.
2535. Takata T, Ito H, Ogawa I, Miyauchi M, Ijuhin N, Nikai H (1991). Spindle cell squamous carcinoma of the oral region. An immunohistochemical and ultrastructural study on the histogenesis and differential diagnosis with a clinicopathological analysis of six cases. Virchows Arch A Pathol Anat Histopathol 419: 177-182.
2536. Takata T, Lu Y, Ogawa I, Zhao M, Zhou ZY, Mock D, Nikai H (1998). Proliferative activity of calcifying odontogenic cysts as evaluated by proliferating cell nuclear antigen labeling index. Pathol Int 48: 877-881.
2537. Takata T, Miyauchi M, Ogawa I, Kudo Y, Takekoshi T, Zhao M, Sato S, Nikai H, Komiyama K (2000). Immunoexpression of transforming growth factor beta in desmoplastic ameloblastoma. Virchows Arch 436: 319-323.
2538. Takata T, Ogawa I, Miyauchi M, Ijuhin N, Nikai H, Fujita M (1993). Non-calcifying Pindborg tumor with Langerhans cells. J Oral Pathol Med 22: 378-383.
2538A. Takata T, Zhao M , Nikai H, Uchida T, WangT (2000). Ghost cells in calcifying odontogenic cyst express enamel-related proteins. Histochem J 32, 223-229.
2539. Takeda Y (1999). Ameloblastic fibroma and related lesions: current pathologic concept. Oral Oncol 35: 535-540.
2540. Takeda Y, Kuroda M, Suzuki A (1990). Ameloblastic odontosarcoma (ameloblastic fibro-odontosarcoma) in the mandible. Acta Pathol Jpn 40: 832-837.
2541. Takeda Y, Sasou S, Obata K (1998). Pleomorphic adenoma of the minor salivary gland with pseudoepitheliomatous hyperplasia of the overlying oral mucosa: report of two cases. Pathol Int 48: 389-395.
2542. Takeda Y, Satoh M, Nakamura S, Matsumoto D (2000). Congenital leiomyomatous epulis: a case report with immunohistochemical study. Pathol Int 50: 999-1002.
2543. Takeichi N, Hirose F, Yamamoto H (1976). Salivary gland tumors in atomic bomb survivors, Hiroshima, Japan. I. Epidemiologic observations. Cancer 38: 2462-2468.
2544. Takeichi N, Hirose F, Yamamoto H, Ezaki H, Fujikura T (1983). Salivary gland tumors in atomic bomb survivors, hiroshima, japan. II. Pathologic study and supplementary epidemiologic observations. Cancer 52: 377-385.
2545. Takes RP, Baatenburg de Jong RJ, van Blommestein R, Hermans J, van Krieken HH, Cornelisse CJ (2002). DNA ploidy status as a prognostic marker and predictor of lymph node metastasis in laryngeal carcinoma. Ann Otol Rhinol Laryngol 111: 1015-1020.
2546. Takes RP, Baatenburg de Jong RJ, Wijffels K, Schuuring E, Litvinov SV, Hermans J, van Krieken JH (2001). Expression of genetic markers in lymph node metastases compared with their primary tumours in head and neck cancer. J Pathol 194: 298-302.
2547. Takimoto T, Tanaka S, Ishikawa S, Umeda R (1988). Infectious mononucleosis in the nasopharynx with a histological picture of malignant lymphoma. Arch Otorhinolaryngol 245: 348-350.
2548. Talamini R, Vaccarella S, Barbone F, Tavani A, La Vecchia C, Herrero R, Munoz N, Franceschi S (2000). Oral hygiene, dentition, sexual habits and risk of oral cancer. Br J Cancer 83: 1238-1242.
2549. Tamada A, Makimoto K, Yamabe H, Imai J, Hinuma Y, Oyagi A, Araki T (1984). Titers of Epstein-Barr virus-related antibodies in nasopharyngeal carcinoma in Japan. Cancer 53: 430-440.
2550. Tamborini E, Agus V, Perrone F, Papini D, Romano R, Pasini B, Gronchi A, Colecchia M, Rosai J, Pierotti MA, Pilotti S (2002). Lack of SYT-SSX fusion transcripts in malignant peripheral nerve sheath tumors on RT-PCR analysis of 34 archival cases. Lab Invest 82: 609-618.
2551. Tambouret RH, Yantiss RK, Kirby R, Eichhorn JH (1999). Mucinous adenocarcinoma of the parotid gland. Report of a case with fine needle aspiration findings and histologic correlation. Acta Cytol 43: 842-846.
2552. Tami TA, Ferlito A, Rinaldo A, Lee KC, Singh B (1999). Laryngeal pathology in the acquired immunodeficiency syndrome: diagnostic and therapeutic dilemmas. Ann Otol Rhinol Laryngol 108: 214-220.
2553. Tanaka H, Westesson PL, Wilbur DC (1998). Leiomyosarcoma of the maxillary sinus: CT and MRI findings. Br J Radiol 71: 221-224.
2554. Tanaka J, Yoshida K, Suzuki M,

Sakata Y (1992). Hodgkin's disease of the maxillary gingiva. A case report. Int J Oral Maxillofac Surg 21: 45-46.

2555. Tanaka N, Odajima T, Mimura M, Ogi K, Dehari H, Kimijima Y, Kohama G (2001). Expression of Rb, pRb2/p130, p53, and p16 proteins in malignant melanoma of oral mucosa. Oral Oncol 37: 308-314.

2556. Tang JY, Wang CK, Su YC, Yang SF, Huang MY, Huang CJ (2003). MRI appearance of giant cell tumor of the lateral skull base: a case report. Clin Imaging 27: 27-30.

2557. Tankere F, Vitte E, Martin-Duverneuil N, Soudant J (2002). Cerebellopontine angle lipomas: report of four cases and review of the literature. Neurosurgery 50: 626-631.

2558. Tapper D, Lack EE (1983). Teratomas in infancy and childhood. A 54-year experience at the Children's Hospital Medical Center. Ann Surg 198: 398-410.

2559. Tarhan NC, Yologlu Z, Tutar NU, Coskun M, Agildere AM, Arikan U (2000). Chondromyxoid fibroma of the temporal bone: CT and MRI findings. Eur Radiol 10: 1678-1680.

2560. Tatagiba M, Samii M, Dankoweit-Timpe E, Aguiar PH, Osterwald L, Babu R, Ostertag H (1995). Esthesioneuroblastomas with intracranial extension. Proliferative potential and management. Arq Neuropsiquiatr 53: 577-586.

2561. Tate DJ, Adler JRJr, Chang SD, Marquez S, Eulau SM, Fee WE, Pinto H, Goffinet DR (1999). Stereotactic radiosurgical boost following radiotherapy in primary nasopharyngeal carcinoma: impact on local control. Int J Radiat Oncol Biol Phys 45: 915-921.

2562. Tatemoto Y, Ohno A, Osaki T (1996). Low malignant intraductal carcinoma on the hard palate: a variant of salivary duct carcinoma? Eur J Cancer B Oral Oncol 32B: 275-277.

2563. Tavani A, Gallus S, La Vecchia C, Talamini R, Barbone F, Herrero R, Franceschi S (2001). Diet and risk of oral and pharyngeal cancer. An Italian case-control study. Eur J Cancer Prev 10: 191-195.

2564. Tavani A, Negri E, Franceschi S, Barbone F, La Vecchia C (1994). Attributable risk for laryngeal cancer in northern Italy. Cancer Epidemiol Biomarkers Prev 3: 121-125.

2565. Taxy JB (1977). Juvenile nasopharyngeal angiofibroma: an ultrastructural study. Cancer 39: 1044-1054.

2566. Taxy JB (1997). Squamous carcinoma of the nasal vestibule: an analysis of five cases and literature review. Am J Clin Pathol 107: 698-703.

2567. Taxy JB, Hidvegi DF (1977). Olfactory neuroblastoma: an ultrastructural study. Cancer 39: 131-138.

2568. Taxy JB, Hidvegi DF, Battifora H (1985). Nasopharyngeal carcinoma: antikeratin immunohistochemistry and electron microscopy. Am J Clin Pathol 83: 320-325.

2569. Tay AB (1999). A 5-year survey of oral biopsies in an oral surgical unit in Singapore: 1993-1997. Ann Acad Med Singapore 28: 665-671.

2570. Taylor GP (1988). Congenital epithelial tumor of the parotid-sialoblastoma. Pediatr Pathol 8: 447-452.

2571. Tazawa K, Kurihara Y, Kamoshida S, Tsukada K, Tsutsumi Y (1999). Localization of prostate-specific antigen-like immunoreactivity in human salivary gland and salivary gland tumors. Pathol Int 49: 500-505.

2572. Tehranzadeh J, Fung Y, Donohue M,

Anavim A, Pribram HW (1998). Computed tomography of Paget disease of the skull versus fibrous dysplasia. Skeletal Radiol 27: 664-672.

2573. Teo P, Tai TH, Choy D (1989). Nasopharyngeal carcinoma with dermatomyositis. Int J Radiat Oncol Biol Phys 16: 471-474.

2574. Teo P, Yu P, Lee WY, Leung SF, Kwan WH, Yu KH, Choi P, Johnson PJ (1996). Significant prognosticators after primary radiotherapy in 903 nondisseminated nasopharyngeal carcinoma evaluated by computer tomography. Int J Radiat Oncol Biol Phys 36: 291-304.

2575. Teo PM, Kwan WH, Lee WY, Leung SF, Johnson PJ (1996). Prognosticators determining survival subsequent to distant metastasis from nasopharyngeal carcinoma. Cancer 77: 2423-2431.

2576. Teo PM, Leung SF, Fowler J, Leung TW, Tung Y, SK O, Lee WY, Zee B (2000). Improved local control for early T-stage nasopharyngeal carcinoma—a tale of two hospitals. Radiother Oncol 57: 155-166.

2577. Teoh TB (1957). Epidermoid carcinoma of the nasopharynx among Chinese: a study of 31 necropsies. J Pathol Bacteriol 73: 451-465.

2578. Terasaka S, Medary MB, Whiting DM, Fukushima T, Espejo EJ, Nathan G (1998). Prolonged survival in a patient with sinonasal teratocarcinosarcoma with cranial extension. Case report. J Neurosurg 88: 753-756.

2579. Terry RM, Lewis FA, Robertson S, Blythe D, Wells M (1989). Juvenile and adult laryngeal papillomata: classification by in-situ hybridization for human papillomavirus. Clin Otolaryngol 14: 135-139.

2580. Thackray AC, Lucas RB (1974). Tumors of major salivary glands. Armed Forces Institute of Pathology: Washington, DC.

2581. Tham KT, Leung PC, Saw D, Gwi E (1981). Kimura's disease with salivary gland involvement. Br J Surg 68: 495-497.

2582. Tharp ME, Shidnia H (1995). Radiotherapy in the treatment of verrucous carcinoma of the head and neck. Laryngoscope 105: 391-396.

2583. Theaker JM (1988). Extramammary Paget's disease of the oral mucosa with in situ carcinoma of minor salivary gland ducts. Am J Surg Pathol 12: 890-895.

2584. Theilgaard SA, Buchwald C, Ingeholm P, Kornum LS, Eriksen JG, Sand HH (2003). Esthesioneuroblastoma: a Danish demographic study of 40 patients registered between 1978 and 2000. Acta Otolaryngol 123: 433-439.

2585. Therkildsen MH, Christensen N, Andersen LJ, Larsen S, Katholm M (1992). Malignant Warthin's tumour: a case study. Histopathology 21: 167-171.

2586. Thirlwall AS, Bailey CM, Ramsay AD, Wyatt M (1999). Laryngeal paraganglioma in a five-year-old child—the youngest case ever recorded. J Laryngol Otol 113: 62-64.

2587. Thomas DM, Wilkins MJ, Witana JS, Cook T, Jefferis AF, Walsh-Waring GP (1995). Giant cell reparative granuloma of the cricoid cartilage. J Laryngol Otol 109: 1120-1123.

2588. Thomas GR, Regalado JJ, McClinton M (2002). A rare case of mucoepidermoid carcinoma of the nasal cavity. Ear Nose Throat J 81: 519-522.

2589. Thomas JA, Cotter F, Hanby AM (1993). Epstein-Barr virus-related oral T-cell lymphoma associated with human

immunodeficiency virus immunosuppression. Blood 3350-3356.

2590. Thomas KM, Hutt MS, Borgstein J (1980). Salivary gland tumors in Malawi. Cancer 46: 2328-2334.

2591. Thomas RL (1979). Non-epithelial tumours of the larynx. J Laryngol Otol 93: 1131-1141.

2592. Thomas WH, Coppola ED (1965). Distant metastases from mixed tumors of hte salivary glands. Am J Surg 109: 724-730.

2593. Thome R, Thome DC, de la Cortina RA (2001). Long-term follow-up of cartilaginous tumors of the larynx. Otolaryngol Head Neck Surg 124: 634-640.

2594. Thompson IO, Phillips VM, Ferreira R, Housego TG (1990). Odontoameloblastoma: a case report. Br J Oral Maxillofac Surg 28: 347-349.

2595. Thompson IO, van Rensburg LJ, Phillips VM (1996). Desmoplastic ameloblastoma: correlative histopathology, radiology and CT-MR imaging. J Oral Pathol Med 25: 405-410.

2596. Thompson L, Chang B, Barsky SH (1996). Monoclonal origins of malignant mixed tumors (carcinosarcomas). Evidence for a divergent histogenesis. Am J Surg Pathol 20: 277-285.

2597. Thompson LD, Bouffard JP, Sandberg GD, Mena H (2003). Primary ear and temporal bone meningiomas: a clinicopathologic study of 36 cases with a review of the literature. Mod Pathol 16: 236-245.

2598. Thompson LD, Gannon FH (2002). Chondrosarcoma of the larynx: a clinicopathologic study of 111 cases with a review of the literature. Am J Surg Pathol 26: 836-851.

2599. Thompson LD, Gyure KA (2000). Extracranial sinonasal tract meningiomas: a clinicopathologic study of 30 cases with a review of the literature. Am J Surg Pathol 24: 640-650.

2600. Thompson LD, Miettinen M, Wenig BM (2003). Sinonasal-type hemangiopericytoma: a clinicopathologic and immunophenotypic analysis of 104 cases showing perivascular myoid differentiation. Am J Surg Pathol 27: 737-749.

2601. Thompson LD, Wenig BM, Ellis GL (1996). Oncocytomas of the submandibular gland. A series of 22 cases and a review of the literature. Cancer 78: 2281-2287.

2602. Thompson LD, Wenig BM, Heffner DK, Gnepp DR (1999). Exophytic and papillary squamous cell carcinomas of the larynx: A clinicopathologic series of 104 cases. Otolaryngol Head Neck Surg 120: 718-724.

2603. Thompson LD, Wieneke JA, Miettinen M (2003). Sinonasal tract and nasopharyngeal melanomas: a clinicopathologic study of 115 cases with a proposed staging system. Am J Surg Pathol 27: 594-611.

2604. Thompson LD, Wieneke JA, Miettinen M, Heffner DK (2002). Spindle cell (sarcomatoid) carcinomas of the larynx: a clinicopathologic study of 187 cases. Am J Surg Pathol 26: 153-170.

2605. Thorp MA, Langman G, Sellars SL (1999). Angiocentric T-cell lymphoma: an extensive lesion involving the posterior tongue, hypopharynx and supraglottis. J Laryngol Otol 113: 263-265.

2606. Tien HF, Su IJ, Tang JL, Liu MC, Lee FY, Chen YC, Chuang SM (1997). Clonal chromosomal abnormalities as direct evidence for clonality in nasal T/natural killer cell lymphomas. Br J Haematol 97: 621-625.

2607. Timon CI, Dardick I, Panzarella T,

Thomas J, Ellis G, Gullane P (1995). Clinicopathological predictors of recurrence for acinic cell carcinoma. Clin Otolaryngol 20: 396-401.

2608. Tiziani V, Reichenberger E, Buzzo CL, Niazi S, Fukai N, Stiller M, Peters H, Salzano FM, Raposo do Amaral CM, Olsen BR (1999). The gene for cherubism maps to chromosome 4p16. Am J Hum Genet 65: 158-166.

2609. To EW, Tsang WM, Pang PC, Cheng JH, Tse GM, Tsang WS (2001). A case of parotid mucoepidermoid carcinoma complicated by fatal gastrointestinal bleeding. Ear Nose Throat J 80: 671-673.

2610. Toda S, Yonemitsu N, Miyabara S, Sugihara H, Maehara N (1989). Polypoid squamous cell carcinoma of the larynx. An immunohistochemical study for ras p21 and cytokeratin. Pathol Res Pract 185: 860-866.

2611. Toda T, Atari E, Sadi AM, Kiyuna M, Kojya S (1999). Primitive neuroectodermal tumor in sinonasal region. Auris Nasus Larynx 26: 83-90.

2612. Toida M, Balazs M, Mori T, Ishimaru JI, Ichihara H, Fujitsuka H, Hyodo I, Yokoyama K, Tatematsu N, Adany R (2001). Analysis of genetic alterations in salivary gland tumors by comparative genomic hybridization. Cancer Genet Cytogenet 127: 34-37.

2613. Toida M, Hyodo I, Okuda T, Tatematsu N (1990). Adenomatoid odontogenic tumor: report of two cases and survey of 126 cases in Japan. J Oral Maxillofac Surg 48: 404-408.

2614. Tomas Carmona I, Cameselle Teijeiro J, Diz Dios P, Fernandez Feijoo J, Limeres Posse J (2000). Intra-alveolar granulocytic sarcoma developing after tooth extraction. Oral Oncol 36: 491-494.

2615. Tomich CE (1974). Oral focal mucinosis. A clinicopathologic and histochemical study of eight cases. Oral Surg Oral Med Oral Pathol 38: 714-724.

2616. Tomita Y, Ohsawa M, Mishiro Y, Itokazu T, Kojya S, Noda Y, Ikehara O, Aozasa K (1997). Non-Hodgkin's lymphoma of Waldeyer's ring as a manifestation of lymphoproliferative diseases associated with human T-cell leukemia virus type 1 in southwestern Japan. Mod Pathol 10: 933-938.

2617. Tomita Y, Ohsawa M, Mishiro Y, Kubo T, Maeshiro N, Kojya S, Noda Y, Aozasa K (1995). The presence and subtype of Epstein-Barr virus in B and T cell lymphomas of the sino-nasal region from the Osaka and Okinawa districts of Japan. Lab Invest 73: 190-196.

2618. Tong AC, Lam KY (2000). Granulocytic sarcoma presenting as an ulcerative mucogingival lesion: report of a case and review of the literature. J Oral Maxillofac Surg 58: 1055-1058.

2619. Tonin PN, Scrable H, Shimada H, Cavenee WK (1991). Muscle-specific gene expression in rhabdomyosarcomas and stages of human fetal skeletal muscle development. Cancer Res 51: 5100-5106.

2620. Torenbeek R, Hermsen MA, Meijer GA, Baak JP, Meijer CJ (1999). Analysis by comparative genomic hybridization of epithelial and spindle cell components in sarcomatoid carcinoma and carcinosarcoma: histogenetic aspects. J Pathol 189: 338-343.

2621. Tornes K, Bang G, Stromme Koppang H, Pedersen KN (1985). Oral verrucous carcinoma. Int J Oral Surg 14: 485-492.

2622. Torske KR, Benson GS, Warnock G (2001). Dermoid cyst of the maxillary sinus. Ann Diagn Pathol 5: 172-176.
2623. Torske KR, Thompson LD (2002). Adenoma versus carcinoid tumor of the middle ear: a study of 48 cases and review of the literature. Mod Pathol 15: 543-555.
2624. Tortoledo ME, Luna MA, Batsakis JG (1984). Carcinomas ex pleomorphic adenoma and malignant mixed tumors. Histomorphologic indexes. Arch Otolaryngol 110: 172-176.
2625. Tosaka M, Hirato J, Miyagishima T, Saito N, Nakazato Y, Sasaki T (2002). Calcified vestibular schwannoma with unusual histological characteristics - positive immunoreactivity for CD-34 antigen. Acta Neurochir (Wien) 144: 395-399.
2626. Totsuka Y, Fukuda H, Tomita K (1988). Compression therapy for parotid haemangioma in infants. A report of three cases. J Craniomaxillofac Surg 16: 366-370.
2627. Tovi F, Hirsch M, Sacks M, Leiberman A (1990). Ectopic pituitary adenoma of the sphenoid sinus: report of a case and review of the literature. Head Neck 12: 264-268.
2628. Toyosawa S, Ohnishi A, Ito R, Ogawa Y, Kishino M, Yasui Y, Kitamura R, Matsuya T, Ishida T, Ijuhin N (1999). Small cell undifferentiated carcinoma of the submandibular gland: immunohistochemical evidence of myoepithelial, basal and luminal cell features. Pathol Int 49: 887-892.
2629. Trattner A, Hodak E, David M, Sandbank M (1993). The appearance of Kaposi sarcoma during corticosteroid therapy. Cancer 72: 1779-1783.
2630. Travis LW, Sutherland C (1980). Coexisting lentigo of the larynx and melanoma of the oral cavity: report of a case. Otolaryngol Head Neck Surg 88: 218-220.
2631. Traweek ST, Arber DA, Rappaport H, Brynes RK (1993). Extramedullary myeloid cell tumors. An immunohistochemical and morphologic study of 28 cases. Am J Surg Pathol 17: 1011-1019.
2632. Tresserra L, Martinez-Mora J, Boix-Ochoa J (1977). Haemangiomas of the parotid gland in children. J Maxillofac Surg 5: 238-241.
2633. Triantafillidou K, Lazaridis N, Zaramboukas T (2002). Epithelioid angiosarcoma of the maxillary sinus and the maxilla: a case report and review of the literature. Oral Surg Oral Med Oral Pathol Oral Radiol Endod 94: 333-337.
2634. Trojanowski JQ, Lee V, Pillsbury N, Lee S (1982). Neuronal origin of human esthesioneuroblastoma demonstrated with anti-neurofilament monoclonal antibodies. N Engl J Med 307: 159-161.
2635. Trott MS, Gewirtz A, Lavertu P, Wood BG, Sebek BA (1994). Sinonasal leiomyomas. Otolaryngol Head Neck Surg 111: 660-664.
2636. Tsai CC, Chen CL, Hsu HC (1996). Expression of Epstein-Barr virus in carcinomas of major salivary glands: a strong association with lymphoepithelioma-like carcinoma. Hum Pathol 27: 258-262.
2637. Tsai MH, Pai HH, Yen PT, Huang TS (1997). Unusual localization of Castleman's disease: report of the first case in the nasopharynx. Ear Nose Throat J 76: 731-5, 739.
2638. Tsai ST, Jin YT, Mann RB, Ambinder RF (1998). Epstein-Barr virus detection in nasopharyngeal tissues of patients with suspected nasopharyngeal carcinoma. Cancer 82: 1449-1453.
2639. Tsang WM, Tong AC, Lam KY, Tideman H (2000). Nasal T/NK cell lymphoma: report of 3 cases involving the palate. J Oral Maxillofac Surg 58: 1323-1327.
2640. Tsang YW, Ngan KC, Chan JK (1991). Primary mucoid adenocarcinoma of the larynx. J Laryngol Otol 105: 315-317.
2641. Tsang YW, Tung Y, Chan JK (1991). Polymorphous low grade adenocarcinoma of the palate in a child. J Laryngol Otol 105: 309-311.
2642. Tsao SW, Liu Y, Wang X, Yuen PW, Leung SY, Yuen ST, Pan J, Nicholls JM, Cheung AL, Wong YC (2003). The association of E-cadherin expression and the methylation status of the E-cadherin gene in nasopharyngeal carcinoma cells. Eur J Cancer 39: 524-531.
2643. Tse GM, Chan KF, Ahuja AT, King AD, Pang PC, To EW (2001). Fibromatosis of the head and neck region. Otolaryngol Head Neck Surg 125: 516-519.
2644. Tsokos M (1994). The diagnosis and classification of childhood rhabdomyosarcoma. Semin Diagn Pathol 11: 26-38.
2645. Tucker KM, Heget HS (1976). The incidence of inflammatory papillary hyperplasia. J Am Dent Assoc 93: 610-613.
2646. Turc-Carel C, Aurias A, Mugneret F, Lizard S, Sidaner I, Volk C, Thiery JP, Olschwang S, Philip I, Berger MP, Philip T, Lenoir GM, Mazabraud A (1988). Chromosomes in Ewing's sarcoma. I. An evaluation of 85 cases of remarkable consistency of t(11;22)(q24;q12). Cancer Genet Cytogenet 32: 229-238.
2647. Tuyns AJ, Esteve J, Raymond L, Berrino F, Benhamou E, Blanchet F, Boffetta P, Crosignani P, del Moral A, Lehmann W, Merletti F, Pequignot G, Riboli E, Sancho-Garnier H, Terracini B, Zubiri A, Zubiri L (1988). Cancer of the larynx/hypopharynx, tobacco and alcohol: IARC international case-control study in Turin and Varese (Italy), Zaragoza and Navarra (Spain), Geneva (Switzerland) and Calvados (France). Int J Cancer 41: 483-491.
2648. Uchino A, Kato A, Yonemitsu N, Hirctsu T, Kudo S (1996). Giant cell reparative granuloma of the cranial vault. AJNR Am J Neuroradiol 17: 1791-1793.
2649. Ueda A, Kage T, Chino T, Komatsu F, Kakajima S, Kawakami T (1998). A case report of peripheral ameloblastoma with unusual invasion. Oral Med Pathol 3: 93-96.
2650. Ueki Y, Tiziani V, Santanna C, Fukai N, Maulik C, Garfinkle J, Ninomiya C, doAmaral C, Peters H, Habal M, Rhee-Morris L, Doss JB, Kreiborg S, Olsen BR, Reichenberger E (2001). Mutations in the gene encoding c-Abl-binding protein SH3BP2 cause cherubism. Nat Genet 28: 125-126.
2651. Ueta E, Yoneda K, Ohno A, Osaki T (1996). Intraosseous carcinoma arising from mandibular ameloblastoma with progressive invasion and pulmonary metastasis. Int J Oral Maxillofac Surg 25: 370-372.
2652. Umeda M, Komatsubara H, Shibuya Y, Yokoo S, Komori T (2002). Premalignant melanocytic dysplasia and malignant melanoma of the oral mucosa. Oral Oncol 38: 714-722.
2653. Umeda M, Yokoo S, Take Y, Omori A, Nakanishi K, Shimada K (1992). Lymph node metastasis in squamous cell carcinoma of the oral cavity: correlation between histologic features and the prevalence of metastasis. Head Neck 14: 263-272.
2654. Ungkanont K, Byers RM, Weber RS, Callender DL, Wolf PF, Goepfert H (1996). Juvenile nasopharyngeal angiofibroma: an update of therapeutic management. Head Neck 18: 60-66.
2655. Unni KK (1996). Dahlin's Bone Tumors: General Aspects and Data on 11,087 Cases. 5th ed. Lippincott Williams & Wilkins: Philadelphia.
2656. Uppal HS, Harrison P (2001). Extramedullary plasmacytoma of the larynx presenting with upper airway obstruction in a patient with long-standing IgD myeloma. J Laryngol Otol 115: 745-746.
2657. Urano M, Abe M, Horibe Y, Kuroda M, Mizoguchi Y, Sakurai K, Naito K (2002). Sclerosing mucoepidermoid carcinoma with eosinophilia of the salivary glands. Pathol Res Pract 198: 305-310.
2658. Uri AK, Wetmore RF, Iozzo RV (1986). Glycogen-rich clear cell carcinoma in the tongue. A cytochemical and ultrastructural study. Cancer 57: 1803-1809.
2659. Urquhart AC, Johnson JT, Myers EN, Schechter GL (1994). Glomus vagale: paraganglioma of the vagus nerve. Laryngoscope 104: 440-445.
2660. Urso C, Ninu MB, Franchi A, Paglierani M, Bondi R (1993). Intestinal-type adenocarcinoma of the sinonasal tract: a clinicopathologic study of 18 cases. Tumori 79: 205-210.
2661. Uzcudun AE, Bravo Fernandez P, Sanchez JJ, Garcia Grande A, Rabanal Retolaza I, Gonzalez Baron M, Gavilan Bouzas J (2001). Clinical features of pharyngeal cancer: a retrospective study of 258 consecutive patients. J Laryngol Otol 115: 112-118.
2662. Valentino J, Brame CB, Studtmann KE, Manaligod JM (2002). Primary tracheal papillomatosis presenting as reactive airway disease. Otolaryngol Head Neck Surg 126: 79-80.
2663. van Damme PA, Mooren RE (1994). Differentiation of multiple giant cell lesions, Noonan-like syndrome, and (occult) hyperparathyroidism. Case report and review of the literature. Int J Oral Maxillofac Surg 23: 32-36.
2664. van der Meij EH, Schepman KP, van der Waal I (2002). Chapter 5: The possible premalignant character of oral lichen planus and oral lichenoid lesions; a prospective study. In: The possible premalignant character of oral lichen planus and oral lichenoid lesions. A clinicopathological study., The possible premalignant character of oral lichen planus and oral lichenoid lesions. A clinicopathological study., Thesis Vrije Universiteit Amsterdam: Amsterdam, The Netherlands .
2665. van der Mey AG, Maaswinkel-Mooy PD, Cornelisse CJ, Schmidt PH, van de Kamp JJ (1989). Genomic imprinting in hereditary glomus tumours: evidence for new genetic theory. Lancet 2: 1291-1294.
2666. van der Mey AG, van Seters AP, van Krieken JH, Vielvoye J, van Dulken H, Hulshof JH (1989). Large pituitary adenomas with extension into the nasopharynx. Report of three cases with a review of the literature. Ann Otol Rhinol Laryngol 98: 618-624.
2667. van der Riet P, Nawroz H, Hruban RH, Corio R, Tokino K, Koch W, Sidransky D (1994). Frequent loss of chromosome 9p21-22 early in head and neck cancer progression. Cancer Res 54: 1156-1158.
2668. van der Velden LA, Schaafsma HE, Manni JJ, Ruiter DJ, Ramaekers CS, Kuijpers W (1997). Cytokeratin and vimentin expression in normal epithelium and squamous cell carcinomas of the larynx. Eur Arch Otorhinolaryngol 254: 376-383.
2669. van der Wal JE, Davids JJ, van der Waal I (1993). Extraparotid Warthin's tumours—report of 10 cases. Br J Oral Maxillofac Surg 31: 43-44.
2670. van der Wal JE, Snow GB, Karim AB, van der Waal I (1989). Intraoral adenoid cystic carcinoma: the role of postoperative radiotherapy in local control. Head Neck 11: 497-499.
2671. van Gorp J, Weiping L, Jacobse K, Liu YH, Li FY, De Weger RA, Li G (1994). Epstein-Barr virus in nasal T-cell lymphomas (polymorphic reticulosis/midline malignant reticulosis) in western China. J Pathol 173: 81-87.
2672. van Hasselt CA, Ng HK (1991). Papillary adenocarcinoma of the nasopharynx. J Laryngol Otol 105: 853-854.
2673. van Heerden WF, Raubenheimer EJ, Swart TJ, Boy SC (2003). Intraoral salivary duct carcinoma: a report of 5 cases. J Oral Maxillofac Surg 61: 126-131.
2674. van Krieken JH (1993). Prostate marker immunoreactivity in salivary gland neoplasms. A rare pitfall in immunohistochemistry. Am J Surg Pathol 17: 410-414.
2675. van Laer CG, Helliwell TR, Atkinson MW, Stell PM (1989). Osteosarcoma of the larynx. Ann Otol Rhinol Laryngol 98: 971-974.
2676. van Oijen MG, Slootweg PJ (2000). Oral field cancerization: carcinogen-induced independent events or micrometastatic deposits? Cancer Epidemiol Biomarkers Prev 9: 249-256.
2677. van Rees BP, Rouse RW, de Wit MJ, van Noesel CJ, Tytgat GN, van Lanschot JJ, Offerhaus GJ (2002). Molecular evidence for the same clonal origin of both components of an adenosquamous Barrett carcinoma. Gastroenterology 122: 784-788.
2678. van Schothorst EM, Beekman M, Torremans P, Kuipers-Dijkshoorn NJ, Wessels HW, Bardoel AF, van der Mey AG, van der Vijver MJ, van Ommen GJ, Devilee P, Cornelisse CJ (1998). Paragangliomas of the head and neck region show complete loss of heterozygosity at 11q22-q23 in chief cells and the flow-sorted DNA aneuploid fraction. Hum Pathol 29: 1045-1049.
2679. van Vroonhoven TJ, Peutz WH, Tjan TG (1982). Presurgical devascularization of a laryngeal paraganglioma. Arch Otolaryngol 108: 600-602.
2680. Vargas H, Sudilovsky D, Kaplan MJ, Regezi J, Weidner N (1997). Mixed tumor, polymorphous low-grade adenocarcinoma and adenoid cystic carcinoma of the salivary gland: Pathogenic implications and differential diagnosis by Ki-67 (MIB1), BCL2, and S-100 immunohistochemistry. Appl Immunohist 5: 8-16.
2681. Vargas PA, Gerhard R, Araujo Filho V, de Castro IV (2002). Salivary gland tumors in a Brazilian population: a retrospective study of 124 cases. Rev Hosp Clin Fac Med Sao Paulo 57: 271-276.
2682. Vartanian RK (1996). Olfactory neuroblastoma: an immunohistochemical, ultrastructural, and flow cytometric study. Cancer 77: 1957-1959.
2683. Varvares MA, Cheney ML, Goodman ML, Ceisler E, Montgomery WW (1992). Chondroblastoma of the temporal bone. Case report and literature review. Ann Otol Rhinol Laryngol 101: 763-769.
2684. Vasef MA, Ferlito A, Weiss LM (1997). Nasopharyngeal carcinoma, with emphasis on its relationship to Epstein-Barr virus. Ann Otol Rhinol Laryngol 106: 348-356.

2685. Vawter GF, Tefft M (1966). Congenital tumors of the parotid gland. Arch Pathol 82: 242-245.

2686. Vayego SA, De Conti OJ, Varella-Garcia M (1996). Complex cytogenetic rearrangement in a case of unicameral bone cyst. Cancer Genet Cytogenet 86: 46-49.

2687. Vencio EF, Reeve CM, Unni KK, Nascimento AG (1998). Mesenchymal chondrosarcoma of the jaw bones: clinico-pathologic study of 19 cases. Cancer 82: 2350-2355.

2688. Veness MJ, Morgan G, Collins AP, Walker DM (2001). Calcifying epithelial odontogenic (Pindborg) tumor with malignant transformation and metastatic spread. Head Neck 23: 692-696.

2689. Venkatachalam MA, Greally JG (1969). Fine structure of glomus tumor: similarity of glomus cells to smooth muscle. Cancer 23: 1176-1184.

2690. Verhaagen J, Oestreicher AB, Gispen WH, Margolis FL (1989). The expression of the growth associated protein B50/GAP43 in the olfactory system of neonatal and adult rats. J Neurosci 9: 683-691.

2691. Vetters JM, Toner PG (1970). Chemodectoma of larynx. J Pathol 101: 259-265.

2692. Vicenzi G (1981). Familial incidence in two cases of aneurysmal bone cyst. Ital J Orthop Traumatol 7: 251-253.

2693. Vikram B, Strong EW, Manolatos S, Mishra UB (1984). Improved survival in carcinoma of the nasopharynx. Head Neck Surg 7: 123-128.

2694. Vikram HR, Petito A, Bower BF, Goldberg MH (2000). Parathyroid carcinoma diagnosed on the basis of a giant cell lesion of the maxilla. J Oral Maxillofac Surg 58: 567-569.

2695. Vincenzi A, Rossi G, Monzani D, Longo L, Rivasi F (2002). Atypical (bizarre) leiomyoma of the nasal cavity with prominent myxoid change. J Clin Pathol 55: 872-875.

2696. Voigtlander V, Boonen H (1990). [Squamous cell carcinoma of the lower lip in discoid lupus erythematosus associated with hereditary deficiency of complement 2]. Z Hautkr 65: 836-837.

2697. Vollrath M, Altmannsberger M, Weber K, Osborn M (1986). Chemically induced tumors of rat olfactory epithelium: a model for human esthesioneuroepithelioma. J Natl Cancer Inst 76: 1205-1216.

2698. von Biberstein SE, Spiro JD, Mancoll W (1999). Acinic cell carcinoma of the nasal cavity. Otolaryngol Head Neck Surg 120: 759-762.

2699. Voytek TM, Ro JY, Edeiken J, Ayala AG (1995). Fibrous dysplasia and cemento-ossifying fibroma. A histologic spectrum. Am J Surg Pathol 19: 775-781.

2700. Voz ML, Agten NS, Van de Ven WJ, Kas K (2000). PLAG1, the main translocation target in pleomorphic adenoma of the salivary glands, is a positive regulator of IGF-II. Cancer Res 60: 106-113.

2701. Voz ML, Astrom AK, Kas K, Mark J, Stenman G, Van de Ven WJ (1998). The recurrent translocation t(5;8)(p13;q12) in pleomorphic adenomas results in upregulation of PLAG1 gene expression under control of the LIFR promoter. Oncogene 16: 1409-1416.

2702. Wada S, Yue L, Furuta I, Takazakura T (2002). Leiomyosarcoma in the maxilla: a case report. Int J Oral Maxillofac Surg 31: 219-221.

2703. Wada T, Morita N, Sakamoto T, Nakamine H (2000). Basal cell adenocarcinoma of the minor salivary gland: a case report. J Oral Maxillofac Surg 58: 811-814.

2704. Wade HW, Plotnick H (1985). Xeroderma pigmentosum and squamous cell carcinoma of the tongue. Identification of two Black patients as members of complementation group. J Am Acad Dermatol 12: 515-521.

2705. Wade PMJr, Smith RE, Johns ME (1984). Response of esthesioneuroblastoma to chemotherapy. Report of five cases and review of the literature. Cancer 53: 1036-1041.

2706. Wadhwa AK, Gallivan H, O'Hara BJ, Rao VM, Lowry LD (2000). Leiomyosarcoma of the larynx: diagnosis aided by advances in immunohistochemical staining. Ear Nose Throat J 79: 42-46.

2707. Waghray M, Parhar RS, Taibah K, al Sedairy S (1992). Rearrangements of chromosome arm 3q in poorly differentiated nasopharyngeal carcinoma. Genes Chromosomes Cancer 4: 326-330.

2708. Wahlberg P, Anderson H, Biorklund A, Moller T, Perfekt R (2002). Carcinoma of the parotid and submandibular glands—a study of survival in 2465 patients. Oral Oncol 38: 706-713.

2709. Wain SL, Kier R, Vollmer RT, Bossen EH (1986). Basaloid-squamous carcinoma of the tongue, hypopharynx, and larynx: report of 10 cases. Hum Pathol 17: 1158-1166.

2710. Waldron CA (1993). Fibro-osseous lesions of the jaws. J Oral Maxillofac Surg 51: 828-835.

2711. Waldron CA, el Mofty SK, Gnepp DR (1988). Tumors of the intraoral minor salivary glands: a demographic and histologic study of 426 cases. Oral Surg Oral Med Oral Pathol 66: 323-333.

2712. Waldron CA, Small IA, Silverman H (1985). Clear cell ameloblastoma—an odontogenic carcinoma. J Oral Maxillofac Surg 43: 707-717.

2713. Walker GJ, Hayward NK (2002). Pathways to melanoma development: lessons from the mouse. J Invest Dermatol 119: 783-792.

2714. Wan SK, Chan JK, Lau WH, Yip TT (1995). Basaloid-squamous carcinoma of the nasopharynx. An Epstein-Barr virus-associated neoplasm compared with morphologically identical tumors occurring in other sites. Cancer 76: 1689-1693.

2715. Wanebo JE, Malik JM, VandenBerg SR, Wanebo HJ, Driesen N, Persing JA (1993). Malignant peripheral nerve sheath tumors. A clinicopathologic study of 28 cases. Cancer 71: 1247-1253.

2716. Wang B, Brandwein M, Gordon R, Robinson R, Urken M, Zarbo RJ (2002). Primary salivary clear cell tumors—a diagnostic approach: a clinicopathologic and immunohistochemical study of 20 patients with clear cell carcinoma, clear cell myoepithelial carcinoma, and epithelial-myoepithelial carcinoma. Arch Pathol Lab Med 126: 676-685.

2717. Wang CC (1999). Cancers of the head and neck. In: Clinical Radiation Oncology: indications, techniques, and results, Wang CC, ed., 2nd ed. Wiley-Liss: New York, pp. 153-159.

2718. Wang CC, See LC, Hong JH, Tang SG (1996). Nasopharyngeal adenoid cystic carcinoma: five new cases and a literature review. J Otolaryngol 25: 399-403.

2719. Wang DG, Barros D'Sa AA, Johnston CF, Buchanan KD (1996). Oncogene expression in carotid body tumors. Cancer 77: 2581-2587.

2720. Wang DG, Johnston CF, Anderson N, Sloan JM, Buchanan KD (1995). Overexpression of the tumour suppressor gene p53 is not implicated in neuroendocrine tumour carcinogenesis. J Pathol 175: 397-401.

2721. Wang DG, Johnston CF, Barros D'Sa AA, Buchanan KD (1997). Expression of apoptosis-suppressing gene bcl-2 in human carotid body tumours. J Pathol 183: 218-221.

2722. Wang NS, Seemayer TA, Ahmed MN, Knaack J (1976). Giant cell carcinoma of the lung. A light and electron microscopic study. Hum Pathol 7: 3-16.

2723. Ward BE, Fechner RE, Mills SE (1990). Carcinoma arising in oncocytic Schneiderian papilloma. Am J Surg Pathol 14: 364-369.

2724. Ward PH, Hanson DG (1988). Reflux as an etiological factor of carcinoma of the laryngopharynx. Laryngoscope 98: 1195-1199.

2725. Warner BA, Santen RJ, Page RB (1982). Growth of hormone and prolactin secretion by a tumor of the pharyngeal pituitary. Ann Intern Med 96: 65-66.

2726. Wasef M, Irish JC, Mancer K, Dardick I, Pynn BR, Gullane P (2000). Basal cell adenocarcinoma: a rare malignancy of the salivary glands. J Otolaryngol 29: 102-109.

2727. Wassef M, Kanavaros P, Polivka M, Nemeth J, Monteil JP, Frachet B, Tran Ba Huy P (1989). Middle ear adenoma. A tumor displaying mucinous and neuroendocrine differentiation. Am J Surg Pathol 13: 838-847.

2728. Watanabe K, Ogura G, Suzuki T (2003). Intra-epithelial neuroendocrine carcinoma of the nasal cavity. Pathol Int 53: 396-400.

2729. Watanabe K, Saito A, Suzuki M, Yamanobe S, Suzuki T (2001). True hemangiopericytoma of the nasal cavity. Arch Pathol Lab Med 125: 686-690.

2730. Watanabe N, Yoshida K, Shigemi H, Kurono Y, Mogi G (1999). Temporal bone chondroblastoma. Otolaryngol Head Neck Surg 121: 327-330.

2731. Watzka MA (1963). Uber die Paraganglien in der Plica ventricularis des menschlichen Kelkopfes. Dtsch Med Forsh 1: 19-20.

2732. Webb AJ, Eveson JW (2001). Pleomorphic adenomas of the major salivary glands: a study of the capsular form in relation to surgical management. Clin Otolaryngol 26: 134-142.

2733. Webb AJ, Eveson JW (2002). Parotid Warthin's tumour Bristol Royal Infirmary (1985-1995): a study of histopathology in 33 cases. Oral Oncol 38: 163-171.

2734. Weber A, Langhanki L, Schutz A, Gerstner A, Bootz F, Wittekind C, Tannapfel A (2002). Expression profiles of p53, p63, and p73 in benign salivary gland tumors. Virchows Arch 441: 428-436.

2735. Weiland LH (1978). The histopathological spectrum of nasopharyngeal carcinoma. IARC Sci Publ 41-50.

2736. Weilbaecher TG, Sarma DP (1984). Plasma cell granuloma of the tonsil. J Surg Oncol 27: 228-231.

2737. Weiner JS, Sherris D, Kasperbauer J, Lewis J, Li H, Persing D (1999). Relationship of human papillomavirus to Schneiderian papillomas. Laryngoscope 109: 21-26.

2738. Weinstein GS, Laccourreye O (1994). Supracricoid laryngectomy with cricohyoidepiglottopexy. Otolaryngol Head Neck Surg 111: 684-685.

2739. Weisman RA, Osguthorpe JD (1988). Pseudotumor of the head and neck masquerading as neoplasia. Laryngoscope 98: 610-614.

2740. Weiss LM, Gaffey MJ, Chen YY, Frierson HFJr (1992). Frequency of Epstein-Barr viral DNA in "Western" sinonasal and Waldeyer's ring non-Hodgkin's lymphomas. Am J Surg Pathol 16: 156-162.

2741. Weiss LM, Movahed LA, Butler AE, Swanson SA, Frierson HFJr, Cooper PH, Colby TV, Mills SE (1989). Analysis of lymphoepithelioma and lymphoepithelioma-like carcinomas for Epstein-Barr viral genomes by in situ hybridization. Am J Surg Pathol 13: 625-631.

2742. Weiss MD, deFries HO, Taxy JB, Braine H (1983). Primary small cell carcinoma of the paranasal sinuses. Arch Otolaryngol 109: 341-343.

2743. Weiss MD, Kashima HK (1983). Tracheal involvement in laryngeal papillomatosis. Laryngoscope 93: 45-48.

2744. Weiss SW (1994). Histological Typing of Soft Tissue Tumours. 2nd ed. Springer Verlag: Berlin, Heidelberg.

2745. Weiss SW, Goldblum JR (2001). Enzinger and Weiss's Soft Tissue Tumors. 4th ed. Mosby: St. Louis.

2746. Weissman JL, Myers JN, Kapadia SB (1993). Extramedullary plasmacytoma of the larynx. Am J Otolaryngol 14: 128-131.

2747. Welch TB, Barker BF, Williams C (1986). Peroxidase-antiperoxidase evaluation of human oral squamous cell papillomas. Oral Surg Oral Med Oral Pathol 61: 603-606.

2748. Welkoborsky HJ, Xiao Y, Mann WJ, Amedee RG, Dienes HP, Volk B (1995). Studies for estimating the biologic behavior and prognosis of paragangliomas of the head and neck. Skull Base Surg 5: 149-156.

2749. Wellman M, Kerr PD, Battistuzzi S, Cristante L (2002). Paranasal sinus terato-carcinosarcoma with intradural extension. J Otolaryngol 31: 173-176.

2750. Wells GC, Whimster IW (1969). Subcutaneous angiolymphoid hyperplasia with eosinophilia. Br J Dermatol 81: 1-14.

2751. Wells M, Michaels L (1984). Malignant otitis-externa - a form of otitis-media with complications. Clin Otolaryngol 9: 131.

2752. Wenig B, Heffess C, Adair C, Thompson L, Heffner D (1995). Ectopic pituitary adenomas (EPA): a clinocopathologic study of 15 cases. Mod Pathol 8: 56A.

2753. Wenig BL, Sciubba JJ, Cohen A, Abramson AL (1985). Nasal septal hemangioma. Otolaryngol Head Neck Surg 93: 436-441.

2754. Wenig BM (1993). Malignant melanoma. In: Neoplasms of the Larynx, Ferlito A, ed., Churchill-Livingstone: Edinburgh, pp. 207-230.

2755. Wenig BM (1995). Laryngeal mucosal malignant melanoma. A clinicopathologic, immunohistochemical, and ultrastructural study of four patients and a review of the literature. Cancer 75: 1568-1577.

2756. Wenig BM (1995). Lipomas of the larynx and hypopharynx: a review of the literature with the addition of three new cases. J Laryngol Otol 109: 353-357.

2757. Wenig BM (1996). Schneiderian-type mucosal papillomas of the middle ear and mastoid. Ann Otol Rhinol Laryngol 105: 226-233.

2758. Wenig BM (2000). Tumors of the upper respiratory tract, PartA: Nasal cavity, paranasal sinuses and nasopharynx. In: Diagnostic Histopathology of Tumors, Fletcher CDM, ed., Churchill Livingstone: London .

2759. Wenig BM (2002). Squamous cell carcinoma of the upper aerodigestive tract: precursors and problematic variants. Mod Pathol 15: 229-254.

2760. Wenig BM, Abbondanzo SL, Childers EL, Kapadia SB, Heffner DR (1993). Extranodal sinus histiocytosis with massive lymphadenopathy (Rosai-Dorfman disease) of the head and neck. Hum Pathol 24: 483-492.

2761. Wenig BM, Devaney K, Bisceglia M (1995). Inflammatory myofibroblastic tumor of the larynx. A clinicopathologic study of eight cases simulating a malignant spindle cell neoplasm. Cancer 76: 2217-2229.

2762. Wenig BM, Gnepp DR (1989). The spectrum of neuroendocrine carcinomas of the larynx. Semin Diagn Pathol 6: 329-350.

2763. Wenig BM, Harpaz N, DelBridge C (1989). Polymorphous low-grade adenocarcinoma of seromucous glands of the nasopharynx. A report of a case and a discussion of the morphologic and immunohistochemical features. Am J Clin Pathol 92: 104-109.

2764. Wenig BM, Heffner DK (1990). Contact ulcers of the larynx. A reacquaintance with the pathology of an often underdiagnosed entity. Arch Pathol Lab Med 114: 825-828.

2765. Wenig BM, Heffner DK (1995). Liposarcomas of the larynx and hypopharynx: a clinicopathologic study of eight new cases and a review of the literature. Laryngoscope 105: 747-756.

2766. Wenig BM, Heffner DK (1995). Respiratory epithelial adenomatoid hamartomas of the sinonasal tract and nasopharynx: a clinicopathologic study of 31 cases. Ann Otol Rhinol Laryngol 104: 639-645.

2767. Wenig BM, Heffner DK (1996). Endolymphatic Sac Tumours: Fact or Fiction ? Adv Anat Pathol 378-387.

2768. Wenig BM, Hitchcock CL, Ellis GL, Gnepp DR (1992). Metastasizing mixed tumor of salivary glands. A clinicopathologic and flow cytometric analysis. Am J Surg Pathol 16: 845-858.

2769. Wenig BM, Hyams VJ, Heffner DK (1988). Moderately differentiated neuroendocrine carcinoma of the larynx. A clinicopathologic study of 54 cases. Cancer 62: 2658-2676.

2770. Wenig BM, Hyams VJ, Heffner DK (1988). Nasopharyngeal papillary adenocarcinoma. A clinicopathologic study of a low-grade carcinoma. Am J Surg Pathol 12: 946-953.

2771. Wenig BM, Vinh TN, Smirniotopoulos JG, Fowler CB, Houston GD, Heffner DK (1995). Aggressive psammomatoid ossifying fibromas of the sinonasal region: a clinicopathologic study of a distinct group of fibro-osseous lesions. Cancer 76: 1155-1165.

2772. Wenig BM, Weiss SW, Gnepp DR (1990). Laryngeal and hypopharyngeal liposarcoma. A clinicopathologic study of 10 cases with a comparison to soft-tissue ounterparts. Am J Surg Pathol 14: 134-141.

2773. Wenzel C, Dieckmann K, Fiebiger W, Mannhalter C, Chott A, Raderer M (2001). CD5 expression in a lymphoma of the mucosa-associated lymphoid tissue (MALT)-type as a marker for early dissemination and aggressive clinical behaviour. Leuk Lymphoma 42: 823-829.

2774. Westerbeek HA, Mooi WJ, Hilgers FJ, Baris G, Begg AC, Balm AJ (1993). Ploidy status and the response of T1 glottic carcinoma to radiotherapy. Clin Otolaryngol 18: 98-101.

2775. Westerman DE, Urbanetti JS, Rudders RA, Fanburg BL (1980). Metastatic endotracheal tumor from ovarian carcinoma. Chest 77: 798-800.

2776. Westerveld GJ, van Diest PJ, van Nieuwkerk EB (2001). Neuroendocrine carcinoma of the sphenoid sinus: a case report. Rhinology 39: 52-54.

2777. Westra WH, Sidransky D (1998). Phenotypic and genotypic disparity in premalignant lesions: of calm water and crocodiles. J Natl Cancer Inst 90: 1500-1501.

2778. Wetli CV, Pardo V, Millard M, Gerston K (1972). Tumors of ceruminous glands. Cancer 29: 1169-1178.

2779. Wetmore RF, Tronzo RD, Lane RJ, Lowry LD (1981). Nonfunctional paraganglioma of the larynx: clinical and pathological considerations. Cancer 48: 2717-2723.

2780. Wettan HL, Patella PA, Freedman PD (2001). Peripheral ameloblastoma: review of the literature and report of recurrence as severe dysplasia. J Oral Maxillofac Surg 59: 811-815.

2781. Wharam MD, Beltangady MS, Heyn RM, Lawrence W, Raney RBJr, Ruymann FB, Soule EH, Tefft M, Maurer HM (1987). Pediatric orofacial and laryngopharyngeal rhabdomyosarcoma. An Intergroup Rhabdomyosarcoma Study report. Arch Otolaryngol Head Neck Surg 113: 1225-1227.

2782. Whitaker SB, Waldron CA (1993). Central giant cell lesions of the jaws. A clinical, radiologic, and histopathologic study. Oral Surg Oral Med Oral Pathol 75: 199-208.

2783. White RR, Arm RN, Randall P (1978). A large Warthin's tumor of the parotid. Case report. Plast Reconstr Surg 61: 452-454.

Whittaker JS, Turner EP (1976). Papillary tumours of the minor salivary glands. J Clin Pathol 29: 795-805.

2784 A. Wick MR, Swanson PE, Scheithauer BW, Manivel JC (1987). Malignant peripheral nerve sheath tumor. An immunohistochemical study of 62 cases. Am J Clin Pathol 87: 425-433.

2785. Wieneke JA, Gannon FH, Heffner DK, Thompson LD (2001). Giant cell tumor of the larynx: a clinicopathologic series of eight cases and a review of the literature. Mod Pathol 14: 1209-1215.

2786. Wieneke JA, Thompson LD, Wenig BM (1999). Basaloid squamous cell carcinoma of the sinonasal tract. Cancer 85: 841-854.

2787. Wiernik G, Millard PR, Haybittle JL (1991). The predictive value of histological classification into degrees of differentiation of squamous cell carcinoma of the larynx and hypopharynx compared with the survival of patients. Histopathology 19: 411-417.

2788. Wiest T, Schwarz E, Enders C, Flechtenmacher C, Bosch FX (2002). Involvement of intact HPV16 E6/E7 gene expression in head and neck cancers with unaltered p53 status and perturbed pRb cell cycle control. Oncogene 21: 1510-1517.

2789. Wilhelmsson B, Hellquist H, Olofsson J, Klintenberg C (1985). Nasal cuboidal metaplasia with dysplasia. Precursor to adenocarcinoma in wood-dust-exposed workers? Acta Otolaryngol 99: 641-648.

2790. Williams HB (1975). Hemangiomas of the parotid gland in children. Plast Reconstr Surg 56: 29-34.

2791. Williams HK, Williams DM (1997). Oral granular cell tumours: a histological and immunocytochemical study. J Oral Pathol Med 26: 164-169.

2792. Williams RR, Horm JW (1977). Association of cancer sites with tobacco and alcohol consumption and socioeconomic status of patients: interview study from the Third National Cancer Survey. J Natl Cancer Inst 58: 525-547.

2793. Williams SB, Ellis GL, Auclair PL (1993). Immunohistochemical analysis of basal cell adenocarcinoma. Oral Surg Oral Med Oral Pathol 75: 64-69.

2794. Williams SB, Foss RD, Ellis GL (1992). Inflammatory pseudotumors of the major salivary glands. Clinicopathologic and immunohistochemical analysis of six cases. Am J Surg Pathol 16: 896-902.

2795. Williamson IG, Ramsden RT (1988). Angiosarcoma of maxillary antrum—association with vinyl chloride exposure. J Laryngol Otol 102: 464-467.

2796. Willman CL, Busque L, Griffith BB, Favara BE, McClain KL, Duncan MH, Gilliland DG (1994). Langerhans'-cell histiocytosis (histiocytosis X)—a clonal proliferative disease. N Engl J Med 331: 154-160.

2797. Winnepenninckx V, Debiec-Rychter M, Jorissen M, Bogaerts S, Sciot R (2001). Aneurysmal bone cyst of the nose with 17p13 involvement. Virchows Arch 439: 636-639.

2798. Winzenburg SM, Niehans GA, George E, Daly K, Adams GL (1998). Basaloid squamous carcinoma: a clinical comparison of two histologic types with poorly differentiated squamous cell carcinoma. Otolaryngol Head Neck Surg 119: 471-475.

2799. Wiseman SM, Popat SR, Rigual NR, Hicks WLJr, Orner JB, Wein RO, McGary CT, Loree TR (2002). Adenoid cystic carcinoma of the paranasal sinuses or nasal cavity: a 40-year review of 35 cases. Ear Nose Throat J 81: 510-517.

2800. Witkin GB, Rosai J (1991). Solitary fibrous tumor of the upper respiratory tract. A report of six cases. Am J Surg Pathol 15: 842-848.

2801. Wittekind C, Henson DE, Hutter RVP, Sobin LH (2001). TNM Supplement: A commentary on uniform use. 2nd ed. Wiley & Sons: New York.

2802. Wojno KJ, McCarthy EF (1994). Fibro-osseous lesions of the face and skull with aneurysmal bone cyst formation. Skeletal Radiol 23: 15-18.

2803. Wolden SL, Zelefsky MJ, Kraus DH, Rosenzweig KE, Chong LM, Shaha AR, Zhang H, Harrison LB, Shah JP, Pfister DG (2001). Accelerated concomitant boost radiotherapy and chemotherapy for advanced nasopharyngeal carcinoma. J Clin Oncol 19: 1105-1110.

2804. Wolf BA, Gluckman JL, Wirman JA (1985). Benign dermal cylindroma of the external auditory canal: a clinicopathological report. Am J Otolaryngol 6: 35-38.

2805. Wolf GT, Fisher SG, Truelson JM, Beals TF (1994). DNA content and regional metastases in patients with advanced laryngeal squamous carcinoma. Department of Veterans Affairs Laryngeal Study Group. Laryngoscope 104: 479-483.

2806. Wolfe JTI, Scheithauer BW, Dahlin DC (1983). Giant-cell tumor of the sphenoid bone. Review of 10 cases. J Neurosurg 59: 322-327.

2807. Wolfe SG, Lai SY, Bigelow DC (2002). Bilateral squamous cell carcinoma of the external auditory canals. Laryngoscope 112: 1003-1005.

2808. Wollner N, Mandell L, Filippa D, Exelby P, McGowan N, Lieberman P (1990). Primary nasal-paranasal oropharyngeal lymphoma in the pediatric age group. Cancer 65: 1438-1444.

2809. Wolvius EB, van der Valk P, van der Wal JE, van Diest PJ, Huijgens PC, van der Waal I, Snow GB (1994). Primary extranodal non-Hodgkin lymphoma of the oral cavity. An analysis of 34 cases. Eur J Cancer B Oral Oncol 30B: 121-125.

2810. Wong KF, Chan JK, Cheung MM, So JC (2001). Bone marrow involvement by nasal NK cell lymphoma at diagnosis is uncommon. Am J Clin Pathol 115: 266-270.

2811. Wong KF, Chan JK, Kwong YL (1997). Identification of del(6)(q21q25) as a recurring chromosomal abnormality in putative NK cell lymphoma/leukaemia. Br J Haematol 98: 922-926.

2812. Wong KF, So CC, Wong N, Siu LL, Kwong YL, Chan JK (2001). Sinonasal angiosarcoma with marrow involvement at presentation mimicking malignant lymphoma: cytogenetic analysis using multiple techniques. Cancer Genet Cytogenet 129: 64-68.

2813. Wong N, Hui AB, Fan B, Lo KW, Pang E, Leung SF, Huang DP, Johnson PJ (2003). Molecular cytogenetic characterization of nasopharyngeal carcinoma cell lines and xenografts by comparative genomic hybridization and spectral karyotyping. Cancer Genet Cytogenet 140: 124-132.

2814. Wood RM, Markle TL, Barker BF, Hiatt WR (1988). Ameloblastic fibrosarcoma. Oral Surg Oral Med Oral Pathol 66: 74-77.

2815. Woodhead P, Lloyd GA (1988). Olfactory neuroblastoma: imaging by magnetic resonance, CT and conventional techniques. Clin Otolaryngol 13: 387-394.

2816. Woodruff JM, Senie RT (1991). Atypical carcinoid tumor of the larynx. A critical review of the literature. ORL J Otorhinolaryngol Relat Spec 53: 194-209.

2817. Woolgar JA (1997). Detailed topography of cervical lymph-note metastases from oral squamous cell carcinoma. Int J Oral Maxillofac Surg 26: 3-9.

2818. Woolgar JA (1999). T2 carcinoma of the tongue: the histopathologist's perspective. Br J Oral Maxillofac Surg 37: 187-193.

2819. Woolgar JA, Rogers SN, Lowe D, Brown JS, Vaughan ED (2003). Cervical lymph node metastasis in oral cancer: the importance of even microscopic extracapsular spread. Oral Oncol 39: 130-137.

2820. Woolgar JA, Scott J (1995). Prediction of cervical lymph node metastasis in squamous cell carcinoma of the tongue/floor of mouth. Head Neck 17: 463-472.

2821. World Cancer Research Fund (WCRF) (1997). Lung. In: Food, Nutrition and the Prevention of Cancer: A Global Perspective (Part II, Cancers, nutrition and food), Food, Nutrition and the Prevention of Cancer: A Global Perspective (Part II, Cancers, nutrition and food), American Institute for Cancer research: Washington, D.C. pp. 130-147.

2822. Worley NK, Daroca PJJr (1997). Lymphoepithelial carcinoma of the minor salivary gland. Arch Otolaryngol Head

Neck Surg 123: 638-640.
2823. Wotherspoon AC, Finn TM, Isaacson PG (1995). Trisomy 3 in low-grade B-cell lymphomas of mucosa-associated lymphoid tissue. Blood 85: 2000-2004.
2824. Wotherspoon AC, Pan LX, Diss TC, Isaacson PG (1992). Cytogenetic study of B-cell lymphoma of mucosa-associated lymphoid tissue. Cancer Genet Cytogenet 58: 35-38.
2825. Wright BA (1978). Median rhomboid glossitis: not a misnomer. Review of the literature and histologic study of twenty-eight cases. Oral Surg Oral Med Oral Pathol 46: 806-814.
2826. Wright D, McKeever P, Carter R (1997). Childhood non-Hodgkin lymphomas in the United Kingdom: findings from the UK Children's Cancer Study Group. J Clin Pathol 50: 128-134.
2827. Wu SB, Hwang SJ, Chang AS, Hsieh T, Hsu MM, Hsieh RP, Chen CJ (1989). Human leukocyte antigen (HLA) frequency among patients with nasopharyngeal carcinoma in Taiwan. Anticancer Res 9: 1649-1653.
2828. Wu SJ, Lay JD, Chen CL, Chen JY, Liu MY, Su IJ (1996). Genomic analysis of Epstein-Barr virus in nasal and peripheral T-cell lymphoma: a comparison with nasopharyngeal carcinoma in an endemic area. J Med Virol 50: 314-321.
2829. Wu TT, Barnes L, Bakker A, Swalsky PA, Finkelstein SD (1996). K-ras-2 and p53 genotyping of intestinal-type adenocarcinoma of the nasal cavity and paranasal sinuses. Mod Pathol 9: 199-204.
2830. Wu TT, Swerdlow SH, Locker J, Bahler D, Randhawa P, Yunis EJ, Dickman PS, Nalesnik MA (1996). Recurrent Epstein-Barr virus-associated lesions in organ transplant recipients. Hum Pathol 27: 157-164.
2831. Wulling M, Engels C, Jesse N, Werner M, Delling G, Kaiser E (2001). The nature of giant cell tumor of bone. J Cancer Res Clin Oncol 127: 467-474.
2832. Wyatt-Ashmead J, Bao L, Eilert RE, Gibbs P, Glancy G, McGavran L (2001). Primary aneurysmal bone cysts: 16q22 and/or 17p13 chromosome abnormalities. Pediatr Dev Pathol 4: 418-419.
2833. Wynder EL, Covey LS, Mabuchi K, Mushinski M (1976). Environmental factors in cancer of the larynx: a second look. Cancer 38: 1591-1601.
2834. Xenellis JE, Linthicum FHJr (2003). On the myth of the glial/schwann junction (Obersteiner-Redlich zone): origin of vestibular nerve schwannomas. Otol Neurotol 24: 1.
2835. Yabut SMJr, Kenan S, Sissons HA, Lewis MM (1988). Malignant transformation of fibrous dysplasia. A case report and review of the literature. Clin Orthop 281-289.
2836. Yaku Y, Kanda T, Yoshihara T, Kaneko T, Nagao K (1983). Undifferentiated carcinoma of the parotid gland. Case report with electron microscopic findings. Virchows Arch A Pathol Anat Histopathol 401: 89-97.
2837. Yamaguchi K, Wu L, Caballero OL, Hibi K, Trink B, Resto V, Cairns P, Okami K, Koch WM, Sidransky D, Jen J (2000). Frequent gain of the p40/p51/p63 gene locus in primary head and neck squamous cell carcinoma. Int J Cancer 86: 684-689.
2838. Yamaguchi M, Kita K, Miwa H, Nishii K, Oka K, Ohno T, Shirakawa S, Fukumoto M (1995). Frequent expression of P-glycoprotein/MDR1 by nasal T-cell lymphoma cells. Cancer 76: 2351-2356.
2839. Yamaguchi T, Dorfman HD (2001). Giant cell reparative granuloma: a comparative clinicopathologic study of lesions in gnathic and extragnathic sites. Int J Surg Pathol 9: 189-200.
2840. Yamaguchi T, Dorfman HD, Eisig S (1999). Cherubism: clinicopathologic features. Skeletal Radiol 28: 350-353.
2841. Yamamoto E, Miyakawa A, Kohama G (1984). Mode of invasion and lymph node metastasis in squamous cell carcinoma of the oral cavity. Head Neck Surg 6: 938-947.
2842. Yamamoto H, Oda Y, Saito T, Sakamoto A, Miyajima K, Tamiya S, Tsuneyoshi M (2003). p53 mutation and MDM2 amplification in inflammatory myofibroblastic tumours. Histopathology 42: 431-439.
2843. Yamamoto Y, Virmani AK, Wistuba II, McIntire D, Vuitch F, Albores-Saavedra J, Gazdar AF (1996). Loss of heterozygosity and microsatellite alterations in p53 and RB genes in adenoid cystic carcinoma of the salivary glands. Hum Pathol 27: 1204-1210.
2844. Yamamoto Y, Wistuba II, Kishimoto Y, Virmani AK, Vuitch F, Albores-Saavedra J, Gazdar AF (1998). DNA analysis at p53 locus in adenoid cystic carcinoma: comparison of molecular study and p53 immunostaining. Pathol Int 48: 273-280.
2845. Yamase HT, Putman HCI (1979). Oncobytic papillary cystadenomatosis of the larynx: a clinicopathologic entity. Cancer 44: 2306-2311.
2846. Yang WT, Kwan WH, Li CK, Metreweli C (1997). Imaging of pediatric head and neck rhabdomyosarcomas with emphasis on magnetic resonance imaging and a review of the literature. Pediatr Hematol Oncol 14: 243-257.
2847. Yankauer S (1924). Angiosarcoma of the larynx removed by indirect laryngoscopy. Laryngoscope 34: 488-493.
2848. Yavuzer R, Ataoglu O, Sari A (2001). Multiple congenital epulis of the alveolar ridge and tongue. Ann Plast Surg 47: 199-202.
2849. Ye YL, Zhou MH, Lu XY, Dai YR, Wu WX (1992). Nasopharyngeal and nasal malignant lymphoma: a clinicopathological study of 54 cases. Histopathology 20: 511-516.
2850. Yellin SA, Weiss MH, Kraus DH, Papadopoulos EB (1995). Tonsil lymphoma presenting as tonsillitis after bone marrow transplantation. Otolaryngol Head Neck Surg 112: 544-548.
2851. Yeoh GP, Bale PM, de Silva M (1989). Nasal cerebral heterotopia: the so-called nasal glioma or sequestered encephalocele and its variants. Pediatr Pathol 9: 531-549.
2852. Yeung WM, Zong YS, Chiu CT, Chan KH, Sham JS, Choy DT, Ng MH (1993). Epstein-Barr virus carriage by nasopharyngeal carcinoma in situ. Int J Cancer 53: 746-750.
2853. Yilmaz T, Hosal AS, Gedikoglu G, Onerci M, Gursel B (1998). Prognostic significance of vascular and perineural invasion in cancer of the larynx. Am J Otolaryngol 19: 83-88.
2854. Yip TT, Lau WH, Chan JK, Ngan RK, Poon YF, Lung CW, Lo TY, Ho JH (1998). Prognostic significance of DNA flow cytometric analysis in patients with nasopharyngeal carcinoma. Cancer 83: 2284-2292.
2855. Yip TT, Ngan RK, Lau WH, Poon YF, Joab I, Cochet C, Cheng AK (1994). A possible prognostic role of immunoglobulin-G antibody against recombinant Epstein-Barr virus BZLF-1 transactivator protein ZEBRA in patients with nasopharyngeal carcinoma. Cancer 74: 2414-2424.
2856. Yoo GH, Eisele DW, Askin FB, Driben JS, Johns ME (1994). Warthin's tumor: a 40-year experience at The Johns Hopkins Hospital. Laryngoscope 104: 799-803.
2857. Yoo GH, Xu HJ, Brennan JA, Westra W, Hruban RH, Koch W, Benedict WF, Sidransky D (1994). Infrequent inactivation of the retinoblastoma gene despite frequent loss of chromosome 13q in head and neck squamous cell carcinoma. Cancer Res 54: 4603-4606.
2858. Yoo J, Robinson RA (2000). H-ras gene mutations in salivary gland mucoepidermoid carcinomas. Cancer 88: 518-523.
2859. Yoo J, Robinson RA (2000). ras gene mutations in salivary gland tumors. Arch Pathol Lab Med 124: 836-839.
2860. Yoshihara T, Shino A, Shino M, Ishii T (1995). Acinic cell tumour of the maxillary sinus: an unusual case initially diagnosed as parotid cancer. Rhinology 33: 177-179.
2861. Yoshikawa DK, Kollar EJ (1981). Recombination experiments on the odontogenic roles of mouse dental papilla and dental sac tissues in ocular grafts. Arch Oral Biol 26: 303-307.
2862. Yoshimura Y, Tawara K, Yoshigi J, Nagaoka S (1995). Concomitant salivary duct carcinoma of a minor buccal salivary gland and papillary cystadenoma lymphomatosum of a cervical lymph node: report of a case and review of the literature. J Oral Maxillofac Surg 53: 448-453.
2863. Yoshino T, Nakamura S, Suzumiya J, Niitsu N, Ohshima K, Tsuchiyama J, Shinagawa K, Tanimoto M, Sadahira Y, Harada M, Kikuchi M, Akagi T (2002). Expression of cutaneous lymphocyte antigen is associated with a poor outcome of nasal-type natural killer-cell lymphoma. Br J Haematol 118: 482-487.
2864. Young SK, Markowitz NR, Sullivan S, Seale TW, Hirschi R (1989). Familial gigantiform cementoma: classification and presentation of a large pedigree. Oral Surg Oral Med Oral Pathol 68: 740-747.
2865. Yousem SA, Shaw H, Cieply K (2001). Involvement of 2p23 in pulmonary inflammatory pseudotumors. Hum Pathol 32: 428-433.
2866. Yu GY, Liu XB, Li ZL, Peng X (1998). Smoking and the development of Warthin's tumour of the parotid gland. Br J Oral Maxillofac Surg 36: 183-185.
2867. Yu GY, Ubmuller J, Donath K (1998). Membranous basal cell adenoma of the salivary gland: a clinicopathologic study of 12 cases. Acta Otolaryngol 118: 588-593.
2868. Yu MC, Garabrant DH, Huang TB, Henderson BE (1990). Occupational and other non-dietary risk factors for nasopharyngeal carcinoma in Guangzhou, China. Int J Cancer 45: 1033-1039.
2869. Yu MC, Ho JH, Lai SH, Henderson BE (1986). Cantonese-style salted fish as a cause of nasopharyngeal carcinoma: report of a case-control study in Hong Kong. Cancer Res 46: 956-961.
2870. Yu MC, Huang TB, Henderson BE (1989). Diet and nasopharyngeal carcinoma: a case-control study in Guangzhou, China. Int J Cancer 43: 1077-1082.
2871. Yu MC, Nichols PW, Zou XN, Estes J, Henderson BE (1989). Induction of malignant nasal cavity tumours in Wistar rats fed Chinese salted fish. Br J Cancer 60: 198-201.
2872. Yu MC, Yuan JM (2002). Epidemiology of nasopharyngeal carcinoma. Semin Cancer Biol 12: 421-429.
2873. Yu RC, Chu C, Buluwela L, Chu AC (1994). Clonal proliferation of Langerhans cells in Langerhans cell histiocytosis. Lancet 343: 767-768.
2874. Yuan BW (1988). [Correlation between nasopharyngeal carcinoma and HLA in Sichuan]. Zhonghua Zhong Liu Za Zhi 10: 263-266.
2875. Yuan JM, Wang XL, Xiang YB, Gao YT, Ross RK, Yu MC (2000). Preserved foods in relation to risk of nasopharyngeal carcinoma in Shanghai, China. Int J Cancer 85: 358-363.
2876. Zaatari GS, Santoianni RA (1986). Adenoid squamous cell carcinoma of the nasopharynx and neck region. Arch Pathol Lab Med 110: 542-546.
2877. Zachariades N (1989). Neoplasms metastatic to the mouth, jaws and surrounding tissues. J Craniomaxillofac Surg 17: 283-290.
2878. Zak FG, Lawson W (1972). Glomic (paraganglionic) tissue in the larynx and capsule of the thyroid gland. Mt Sinai J Med 39: 82-90.
2879. Zak FG, Lawson W (1982). The Paraganglionic Chemoreceptor System: Physiology, Pathology and Clinical Medicine. Springer Verlag: New York.
2880. Zarate-Osorno A, Jaffe ES, Medeiros LJ (1992). Metastatic nasopharyngeal carcinoma initially presenting as cervical lymphadenopathy. A report of two cases that resembled Hodgkin's disease. Arch Pathol Lab Med 116: 862-865.
2881. Zarbo RJ (2002). Salivary gland neoplasia: a review for the practicing pathologist. Mod Pathol 15: 298-323.
2882. Zarbo RJ, Crissman JD, Venkat H, Weiss MA (1986). Spindle-cell carcinoma of the upper aerodigestive tract mucosa. An immunohistologic and ultrastructural study of 18 biphasic tumors and comparison with seven monophasic spindle-cell tumors. Am J Surg Pathol 10: 741-753.
2883. Zarbo RJ, Prasad AR, Regezi JA, Gown AM, Savera AT (2000). Salivary gland basal cell and canalicular adenomas: immunohistochemical demonstration of myoepithelial cell participation and morphogenetic considerations. Arch Pathol Lab Med 124: 401-405.
2884. Zarco C, Lahuerta-Palacios JJ, Borrego L, Toscano R, Gil R, Iglesias L (1993). Centroblastic transformation of chronic lymphocytic leukaemia with primary skin involvement—cutaneous presentation of Richter's syndrome. Clin Exp Dermatol 18: 263-267.
2885. Zatonski W, Becher H, Lissowska J, Wahrendorf J (1991). Tobacco, alcohol, and diet in the etiology of laryngeal cancer: a population-based case-control study. Cancer Causes Control 2: 3-10.
2886. Zbaeren P, Lehmann W, Widgren S (1991). Acinic cell carcinoma of minor salivary gland origin. J Laryngol Otol 105: 782-785.
2887. Zbaren P, Schar C, Hotz MA, Loosli H (2001). Value of fine-needle aspiration cytology of parotid gland masses. Laryngoscope 111: 1989-1992.
2888. Zeitoun IM, Dhanrajani PJ, Mosadomi HA (1996). Adenomatoid odontogenic tumor arising in a calcifying odontogenic cyst. J Oral Maxillofac Surg 54: 634-637.
2889. Zellers RA, Bicket WJ, Parker MG (1992). Posttraumatic spindle cell nodule of the buccal mucosa. Report of a case. Oral

Surg Oral Med Oral Pathol 74: 212-215.

2890. Zeng YX, Jia WH (2002). Familial nasopharyngeal carcinoma. Semin Cancer Biol 12: 443-450.

2891. Zerris VA, Annino D, Heilman CB (2002). Nasofrontal dermoid sinus cyst: report of two cases. Neurosurgery 51: 811-814.

2892. Zhang C, Cohen JM, Cangiarella JF, Waisman J, McKenna BJ, Chhieng DC (2000). Fine-needle aspiration of secondary neoplasms involving the salivary glands. A report of 36 cases. Am J Clin Pathol 113: 21-28.

2893. Zhang F, Zhang J (1999). Clinical hereditary characteristics in nasopharyngeal carcinoma through Ye-Liang's family cluster. Chin Med J (Engl) 112: 185-187.

2894. Zhang JX, Chen HL, Zong YS, Chan KH, Nicholls J, Middeldorp JM, Sham JS, Griffin BE, Ng MH (1998). Epstein-Barr virus expression within keratinizing nasopharyngeal carcinoma. J Med Virol 55: 227-233.

2895. Zhang JZ (1986). [Correlation between nasopharyngeal carcinoma (NPC) and HLA in Hunan Province]. Zhonghua Zhong Liu Za Zhi 8: 170-172.

2896. Zhang L, Michelsen C, Cheng X, Zeng T, Priddy R, Rosin MP (1997). Molecular analysis of oral lichen planus. A premalignant lesion? Am J Pathol 151: 323-327.

2897. Zhang Y, Wang S, Song Y, Han J, Chai Y, Chen Y (2003). Timing of odontogenic neural crest cell migration and tooth-forming capability in mice. Dev Dyn 226: 713-718.

2898. Zhao M, Takata T, Ogawa I, Yada T, Kimata K, Nikai H (1999). Immunohistochemical evaluation of the small and large proteoglycans in pleomorphic adenoma of salivary glands. J Oral Pathol Med 28: 37-42.

2899. Zhao Y, Collins BT, Ramos RR (2003). Ciliated epithelial cells in Warthin's tumor on fine-needle aspiration. Diagn Cytopathol 28: 71.

2900. Zheng JW, Song XY, Nie XG (1997). The accuracy of clinical examination versus frozen section in the diagnosis of parotid masses. J Oral Maxillofac Surg 55: 29-31.

2901. Zheng W, Blot WJ, Shu XO, Gao YT, Ji BT, Ziegler RG, Fraumeni JFJr (1992). Diet and other risk factors for laryngeal cancer in Shanghai, China. Am J Epidemiol 136: 178-191.

2902. Zheng W, Shu XO, Ji BT, Gao YT (1996). Diet and other risk factors for cancer of the salivary glands:a population-based case-control study. Int J Cancer 67: 194-198.

Zheng X, Yan L, Nilsson B, Eklund G, Drettner B (1994). Epstein-Barr virus infection, salted fish and nasopharyngeal carcinoma. A case-control study in southern China. Acta Oncol 33: 867-872.

2903 A. Zhong PQ, Zhi FX, Li R, Xue JL, Shu GY (1998). Long-term results of intratumorous bleomycin-A5 injection for head and neck lymphangioma. Oral Surg Oral Med Oral Pathol Oral Radiol Endod 86: 139-144.

2904. Zhu K, Levine RS, Brann EA, Hall HI, Caplan LS, Gnepp DR (2002). Case-control study evaluating the homogeneity and heterogeneity of risk factors between sinonasal and nasopharyngeal cancers. Int J Cancer 99: 119-123.

2905. Zhu Q, Tipoe GL, White FH (1999). Proliferative activity as detected by immunostaining with Ki-67 and proliferat-ing cell nuclear antigen in benign and malignant epithelial lesions of the human parotid gland. Anal Quant Cytol Histol 21: 336-342.

2906. Zidar N, Gale N, Cor A, Kambic V (1996). Expression of Ki-67 antigen and proliferative cell nuclear antigen in benign and malignant epithelial lesions of the larynx. J Laryngol Otol 110: 440-445.

2907. Zidar N, Gale N, Kambic V, Fischinger J (2001). Expression of tenascin and fibronectin in benign epithelial hyperplastic lesions and squamous carcinoma of the larynx. Anticancer Res 21: 451-454.

2908. Znaor A, Brennan P, Gajalakshmi V, Mathew A, Shanta V, Varghese C, Boffetta P (2003). Independent and combined effects of tobacco smoking, chewing and alcohol drinking on the risk of oral, pharyngeal and esophageal cancers in Indian men. Int J Cancer 105: 681-686.

2909. Zohar Y, Shem-Tov Y, Gal R (1988). Salivary duct carcinoma in major and minor salivary glands. A clinicopathological analysis of four cases. J Craniomaxillofac Surg 16: 320-323.

2910. Zong Y, Liu K, Zhong B, Chen G, Wu W (2001). Epstein-Barr virus infection of sinonasal lymphoepithelial carcinoma in Guangzhou. Chin Med J (Engl) 114: 132-136.

2911. Zong YS, Li QX (1986). Histopathology of paracancerous nasopharyngeal carcinoma in situ. Chin Med J (Engl) 99: 763-771.

2912. Zong YS, Zhang CQ, Zhang F, Ruan JB, Chen MY, Feng KT, Yu ZF (1993). Infiltrating lymphocytes and accessory cells in nasopharyngeal carcinoma. Jpn J Cancer Res 84: 900-905.

2913. Zou XN, Lu SH, Liu B (1994). Volatile N-nitrosamines and their precursors in Chinese salted fish—a possible etiological factor for NPC in china. Int J Cancer 59: 155-158.

2914. Zukerberg LR, Rosenberg AE, Randolph G, Pilch BZ, Goodman ML (1991). Solitary fibrous tumor of the nasal cavity and paranasal sinuses. Am J Surg Pathol 15: 126-130.

2915. Zulman J, Jaffe R, Talal N (1978). Evidence that the malignant lymphoma of Sjogren's syndrome is a monoclonal B-cell neoplasm. N Engl J Med 299: 1215-1220.

2916. Zunt SL, Tomich CE (1989). Oral condyloma acuminatum. J Dermatol Surg Oncol 15: 591-594.

2917. zur Hausen H, de Villiers EM (1994). Human papillomaviruses. Annu Rev Microbiol 48: 427-447.

2918. Zur KB, Brandwein M, Wang B, Som P, Gordon R, Urken ML (2002). Primary description of a new entity, renal cell-like carcinoma of the nasal cavity: van Meegeren in the house of Vermeer. Arch Otolaryngol Head Neck Surg 128: 441-447.

Subject index

A

ABC *See* Aneurysmal bone cyst

Abrikossoff tumour 154

Acantholytic squamous cell carcinoma **129**, **175**

Acinic cell carcinoma 24, 98, 134, 190, 214, **216**, 232-234, 259, 265, 266, 303

Acinic cell tumour 216

Acinous cell carcinoma 216

Ackerman tumour 122

Acoustic neurinoma 351

Acoustic neuroma 351

Acoustic schwannoma 351

Acquired cholesteatoma 342, 343

Acromegaly 100

ACTH 26, 100

Acquired cholesteatoma of the middle ear **342**

Actinic keratosis 334

Acute myeloid leukaemia 63, 203, 204

Adenocarcinoma, not otherwise specified **238**

Adenoid cystic carcinoma 16, 24, 98, 124, 125, 129, **134**, 190, 191, 214, 215, **221-223**, 230, 231, 253, 255-267, 297, 331-333

Adenoid cystic carcinoma, sarcomatoid transformation 222

Adenoid cystic-like carcinoma 124

Adenoid squamous cell carcinoma 15, 17, 129

Adenolymphoma 263

Adenolymphoma in laryngocele 146

Adenoma of ceruminous glands **331**

Adenoma of the middle ear **345**

Adenoma, canalicular type 267

Adenomatoid odontogenic tumour 297, 302, **304**

Adenomatosis of minor salivary glands 267

Adenomatous pharyngeal pituitary 100

Adenomyoepithelioma 225

Adenosquamous carcinoma 15, 17, 24, 77, 125, 129, **130**, 131, **175**, 220

Adult papillomatosis 144

Adult rhabdomyomas 152

AFO *See* Ameloblastic fibro-odontoma

Aggressive epithelial ghost cell odontogenic tumour 293

Aggressive fibromatosis 43

Aggressive papillary middle ear tumour **346**, 355

Aggressive papillary tumour 346

Aggressive papillary tumour of temporal bone 346

ALK 151

Alveolar rhabdomyosarcoma 38-40

Alveolar soft parts sarcoma 153, 275

Ameloblastic carcinoma – primary type **287**

Ameloblastic carcinoma – secondary type (dedifferentiated), intraosseous **288**

Ameloblastic carcinoma – secondary type (dedifferentiated), peripheral **288**

Ameloblastic dentinosarcoma 294

Ameloblastic fibrodentinoma **308**

Ameloblastic fibrodentinosarcoma **294**

Ameloblastic fibroma 294, **308**, 309

Ameloblastic fibro-odontoma **309**

Ameloblastic fibro-odontosarcoma **294**

Ameloblastic fibrosarcoma **294**, 308

Ameloblastic odontoma 312

Ameloblastic odontosarcoma 294

Ameloblastic sarcoma 294

Ameloblastoma **56**, 296, 298

Ameloblastoma – desmoplastic type **298**

Ameloblastoma of mucosal origin 298

Ameloblastoma of the gingiva 298

Ameloblastoma, desmoplastic type 298

Ameloblastoma, extraosseous / peripheral type **298**

Ameloblastoma, solid / multicystic type **296**

Ameloblastoma, unicystic type **299**

Anaplastic carcinoma 19, 85, 133, 247, 365

Anaplastic large cell lymphoma 36, 58, 74, 199, 202

Anaplastic lymphoma kinase *See* ALK

Aneurysmal bone cyst 54, 56, 57, 320, **326**, 336

Angiocentric immunoproliferative lesion 58

Angiofibroma 47, 102

Angioleiomyoma 46, 152

Angiolymphoid hyperplasia 339

Angiolymphoid hyperplasia with eosinophilia 41, 47, **338**

Angiomyoma 46, 275

Angiosarcoma **40**, 47, 74, 129, **148**, 275

Angiosarcoma-like squamous cell carcinoma 129

Anosmia 29, 35, 48, 67, 102

Antoni A areas 48, 351

Antoni B areas 48

AOT *See* Adenomatoid odontogenic tumour

Atypical carcinoid 26, 69, 135, **137**

Aural polyp 335

B

Bacillary angiomatosis 47

Basal cell adenocarcinoma 25, 191, 214, **229**

Basal cell adenoma 192, 222, 229, 253, **261**, 267, 269

Basal cell carcinoma 153, 229, 298

Basal/parabasal cell hyperplasia 140, 177

Basaloid adenocarcinoma 253

Basaloid carcinoma 124

Basaloid salivary carcinoma 229

Basaloid squamous cell carcinoma 15, 16, 84, 85, 94, **124**, 139, **175**